Teaching Today's Health

Teaching Today's Health

Fifth Edition

David J. Anspaugh
University of Memphis

Gene Ezell
University of Tennessee—Chattanooga

Allyn and Bacon
Boston • London • Toronto • Sydney • Tokyo • Singapore

Vice-President, Editor-in-Chief, Social Sciences: Sean W. Wakely
Publisher: Joseph E. Burns
Editorial Assistant: Sara Sherlock
Production Administrator: Joe Sweeney
Editorial-Production Service: Thomas E. Dorsaneo
Composition Buyer: Linda Cox
Manufacturing Buyer: Megan Cochran
Text Designer and Composition: Andrea Miles-Thoma/Menagerie Design & Publishing
Cover Administrator: Linda Knowles

Copyright © 1998, 1995 by Allyn & Bacon
A Viacom Company
160 Gould Street
Needham Heights, MA 02194-2310

Internet: www.abacon.com
America Online: Keyword: College Online

Library of Congress Cataloging-in-Publication Data
Anspaugh, David J.
    Teaching today's health/David J. Anspaugh, Gene Ezell. — 5th ed.
        p.   cm.
    Includes bibliographical references and index.
    ISBN 0-205-27413-7
    1. Health education (Elementary) — United States.   I. Ezell, Gene.
    II. Title.
LB1588.U6A83   1998
372.3'7044'0973—dc21   97-22719
                                                                         CIP

Printed in the United States of America
10 9 8 7 6 5 4 3 2 1 RRDV 01 00 99 98 97

To Dad, Susan, our children, and to Conner—the special one who touches all our lives

To my Mom, Hilda Ezell Tate. Thanks for all your love throughout the years, and for believing in me

To our students over all the years with whom it has been our privilege to serve. We hope that in some small way we have been the wind beneath their wings

Photo Credits:

Contents

The fifth edition of *Teaching Today's Health* seeks to present the background, content, and strategies necessary for optimal teaching of health education in the middle and elementary schools. Health education must originate with a solid knowledge base. From this cognitive base, teachers can provide a plethora of opportunities for students to personalize information. It is through the personalizing of basic information that children can begin to develop their critical thinking skills, value wise decision making, and make decisions that will ultimately result in more positive potential for leading a higher quality of life. Through a strong health education program at the elementary and middle school level, students can begin to foster positive health behaviors, accept the responsibility for their behaviors, develop self-confidence, and enhance the self-esteem necessary for living a more healthy, productive lifestyle.

The U.S. Department of Health and Human Services reported in 1989 in *Healthy People - 2000: National Health Promotion and Disease Prevention Objectives* that the nation's health goals were to increase the span of healthy life for Americans, reduce health disparities among Americans, and to achieve access to preventive services for all Americans. Obviously one answer to helping to achieve these goals is the implementation of a comprehensive health education program that includes dissemination of accurate, current information accompanied by ample opportunities for the student to personalize the information so that positive health attitudes will be developed with more positive behaviors resulting. Ingrained in this concept is the development of critical thinking skills. Decisions concerning smoking, drugs, alcohol, exercise, nutrition, safety, and sexual behaviors have potential for both negative and positive consequences. This fifth edition of *Teaching Today's Health* provides a broad range of content and strategies required to assist teachers in the difficult process of health educating our nations children.

Problems persist that are a threat to the nation and its youth. Drugs, teenage pregnancies, sexually transmitted diseases, and HIV are threats to this generation. Conditions that were unknown only a few years ago are currently classified as epidemic. As they try to deal with controversy and are continually bombarded by new and more information in many areas, it is difficult for teachers to remain on the cutting edge of the health field. *Teaching Today's Health* recognizes this need and, therefore, includes the material needed for a solid foundation in teaching middle and elementary health.

Organization

The fifth edition, like its predecessors, has been divided into two parts to aid they teacher in developing the skills and theory required to become a competent health teacher. Chapters 1 - 3 cover the necessity for health education, the role of the teacher, planning effective health education, and strategies for teaching, and implementing effective evaluation. All these topics are covered within the framework of the contemporary theory of wellness and optimal well-being.

Chapters 6 - 25 consist of specific content areas, followed by strategies for making the content come alive for the student. The strategies include value clarification activities, dramatizations, decision stories, experiments and demonstrations, puzzles, games, as well as suggestions for World Wide Web sites, references, and videos for teaching in each of the content areas. The theme developing high level wellness and the importance of establishing lifelong positive practices pervades throughout the text.

It is our sincere desire that a great many middle and elementary children will benefit from the information gathered in this text

Finally, we appreciate the worthwhile comments and suggestions of our reviewers: Joan M. Couch, University of Delaware; Charles F. Denny, University of South Carolina at Sumter; Jean Denney, California State University - Chico; Susan Giarratano, California State University - Long Beach; Onie Grosshans, University of Utah; Bill Hyman, Sam Houston State University; Frank Schabel, Iowa State University; Barbara Wilks, University of Georgia; Clay Williams, Bowling Green State University; David White, East Carolina University; and Elaine Armour Wolo, Tulane University. Our thanks also to Suzy Spivey and Amy Braddock for keeping us on task and providing excellent guidance during the process.

Chapter One

The Need For Health Education

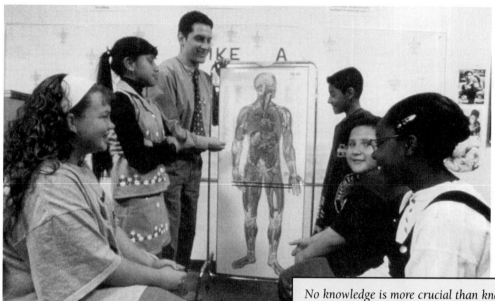

> No knowledge is more crucial than knowledge
> about health . . . . Without it, no other life goal can
> be successfully achieved.
> —*Carnegie Foundation Report on Secondary*
> *Education in America*

Valued Outcomes

After reading this chapter, you should be able to

○ define *health, health promotion,* and *health education*

○ discuss how locus of control and self-efficacy affect health education

○ describe how health education is to be accomplished

○ identify why health education is necessary

○ discuss the significance of the Healthy People 2000 campaign

○ discuss the components of a comprehensive health education program

The Evolution of Health Education

During the latter part of the nineteenth century, epidemics took a drastic toll among the school population of the United States. Children who survived these epidemic diseases often had a diminished capacity to learn as a result of their illnesses. Unsanitary conditions in the schools played a part in the spread of disease.

Alarmed, school physicians instructed teachers to become more involved with the health of their students. At that time, health education was not yet part of the school curriculum. In fact, there was no such thing as health education as we know it. The first efforts in this direction were more crisis oriented than preventive. Teachers were instructed to make daily health inspections of their students and report any suspected cases of serious disease (Haag 1972). In some schools, lunch programs were also instituted; with proper nutrition, students would be less susceptible to illness.

By the turn of the century, these concerns led to the realization of the need for health education. Actual measures were slow in coming, however. In 1924, only four states had certification requirements for health education teachers in the secondary school (Haag 1972).

Formal health education first took the form of instruction in anatomy and physiology. Health was taught purely as a science, and emphasis was placed on retention of facts. As health education evolved, health teachers became more concerned with the attitudinal and behavioral aspects of students' health as well. Today, the emphasis is on a preventive approach, as opposed to the crisis-oriented approach of yesteryear.

Americans are currently in the middle of a health promotion movement. It is virtually impossible to read a magazine, listen to radio, or view television without being bombarded with information on some health-related topic or activity.

Health education has come a long way since its early history. As teachers, the charge today is to motivate students to improve their own health status through positive self-direction. Health education offers students an opportunity for personal growth and enhancement that is not duplicated anywhere else in the school curriculum.

It is interesting to note that, since the 1970s, early-age death rates have declined at a significant rate. This decline reflects a decrease in deaths due to cardiovascular disease. This also coincides with the declining use of tobacco, the reduction in dietary intake of fats and cholesterol, and increased exercise among adults. Society is in a period where lifestyle, more than medicine, can lead to decreases in death ratios.

What Is Health?

Health topics are everywhere we turn. On the television, radio, Internet, and in popular magazines, Americans are continually bombarded with health-related information. What is meant by the term *health*? A definition formulated by the Joint Committee on Health Education Terminology (1991) points to the essence of the concept: The committee stated that **health** "is an integrated method of functioning which is oriented toward maximizing the potential of which the individual is capable.** It requires that the individual maintain a continuum of balance and purposeful direction with the environment where he (sic) is functioning." This concept goes beyond simply not being ill or sick. It implies, as Hoyman suggested in 1975, that health has several dimensions, each having its own continuum. Each continuum ranges from desirable to undesirable, as illustrated in Figure 1.1.

The definition of health has evolved over the years. One very influential individual in its evolution was a physician by the name of Dunn (1991). His definition is almost verbatim the same as the one developed by the Joint Committee on Health Education Terminology (1991). Dunn refers to this conceptualization of health as **wellness**, implying that individuals engage in attitudes and behaviors that enhance quality of life and maximize personal potential. The components of this conceptualization are

1. *Spiritual*—the belief in some force that unites human beings. This force can include nature, science, religion, or a higher power. It includes morals, values, and ethics. Optimal spirituality is the ability to discover, articulate, and act on a (your) basic purpose in life (Chapman 1987).

2. *Social*—the ability to interact successfully with people and one's personal environment. It is the ability to develop and maintain intimacy with others and to have respect/tolerance for those with different opinions and beliefs.

3. *Emotional*—the ability to control stress and to express emotions appropriately and comfortably. It is the ability to recognize and accept feeling, and to not be defeated by setbacks and failures.

4. *Intellectual*—the ability to learn and use information effectively for personal, family, and career development. It means striving for continued growth and learning to deal with new challenges effectively.

5. *Physical*—the ability to carry out daily tasks, develop cardiovascular fitness, muscular fitness, maintain adequate nutrition and proper weight, avoid abusing drugs/alcohol, and not use tobacco products.

The first assumption of the wellness approach to living is that good health is achieved by balancing each of these dimensions. A second assumption is that each individual is ultimately responsible for her or his well-being. That is, we—not the government, physicians, nurses, or some other institution—must accept personal responsibility. Each person must foster attitudes that will improve the quality of life and expand the human potential. To accomplish this, teachers must

Figure 1.1
Levels of Wellness

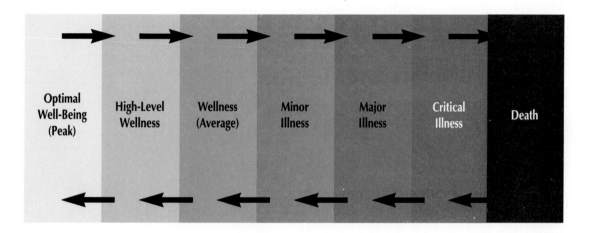

empower their students to see themselves as being *in control* of improving their quality of life. Such students have an internal **locus of control**. (This trait contrasts with external locus of control, in which an individual believes that he or she cannot control many of the factors that contribute to a higher level of wellness.)

Another vital concept in a wellness lifestyle is **self-efficacy**. Self-efficacy is the belief in one's ability to accomplish a specific task or behavior. Self-efficacy is something each student can give him- or herself, if the teacher can provide the support and encouragement necessary to acquire a personal sense of competence.

The sooner children begin the lifelong process of becoming healthy, the greater the possibility they will be successful. Teachers must recognize that children bring to schools many values and behaviors. These values represent both the beneficial and negative aspects of a child's living practices. At the same time, teachers should be aware of the powerful influence they exert on the lives of their students. Nowhere in the entire educational spectrum can a teacher make such an

Health Highlight

What Health Education Is—And Is Not

What Health Education Is Today

Health education is an applied science basic to the general education of all children and youth. Its body of knowledge represents a synthesis of facts, principles, and concepts drawn from biological, behavioral, sociological, and health sciences but interpreted in terms of human needs, human values, and human potential. Acquisition of information is a desired purpose but not the primary goal of instruction.

Rather, growth in critical-thinking ability and problem-solving skills are both the process and the product of instruction. Information can be quickly outdated, but cognitive skills remain an always dependable means of discovering fresh data when they are needed. The ultimate goal of health education is the development of an adult whose lifestyle reflects actions that tend to promote his or her own health as well as that of family and the community.

What Health Education Is Not

Sometimes objects or phenomena of any kind are defined as effectively by explaining what they are not as by describing what they are. Health education is not simply a minor aspect of physical education nor is it hygiene with a new name. It is not a program in physical fitness although physical fitness surely is one of its goals. It is not the inculcation of health habits. It is not watered-down anatomy, physiology, biology or any combination of these sciences. It is not one or two short units specific to certain health concerns and temporarily hosted by another course as a means of satisfying state requirements or local concerns with the health crisis of the month or year. It most certainly is not an assembly lecture program, a rainy day activity, or incidental teaching in response to momentary health problems or concerns.

Source: M. Pollock and M. Hamburg. 1984. Health education: The basic of the basics. Paper presented at Delbert Oberteuffer Centennial Symposium, April, Atlanta, GA.

impression as at the elementary level. Consequently, the teacher who exemplifies a lifestyle conducive to high-level wellness, who exhibits a style of living that is physically, socially, and psychologically healthy, enhances the probability that his or her students will attempt to incorporate those beneficial aspects in their own lives.

What Is Health Education and Health Promotion?

Like **health**, the term **health education** has taken on new meanings over the years. Although there are many ways of defining health education, the Joint Committee on Health Education Terminology (1991, 103) stated that the health education process is the "continuum of learning which enables people, as individual members of social structures, to voluntarily make decisions, modify, and change social conditions in ways which are health enhancing." Green and Kreuter (1991) have defined health education as "any combination of learning experiences designed to facilitate voluntary actions conducive to health."

The term **health promotion** is sometimes used incorrectly in reference to health education. Health promotion is defined by the Joint Committee on Health Education Terminology as "the aggregate of all purposeful activities designed to improve personal and public health through a combination of strategies, including the competent implementation of behavioral change strategies, health education, health protection measures, risk factor detection, health enhancement and health maintenance" (Joint Committee on Health Education Terminology 1991, 102). It can be seen that health promotion is broader in scope than health education, and that health education is an intricate part of health promotion. Health education is one of several different formats that can be used to influence health and quality of life for people.

From the elementary teacher's perspective, health education is the process of developing and providing planned learning experiences in such a way as to supply information, change attitudes, and influence behavior. In other words, health education is helping children develop the concept of wellness (discussed in the previous section). This process should result in children developing a sense of individual responsibility for their health, leading to health enhancement or high-level wellness.

All this is accomplished through the teacher creating and facilitating learning experiences that develop the child's decision-making ability. With good decision-making skills, the child will make better choices, about the personal, family, peer, and societal factors that influence the child's quality of life. An effective school health program must have a direct influence on children's lives and behavior.

Health education is a lifelong process. As people develop awareness of the many components of health and incorporate them into their own lives, they

- assume responsibility for their health and health care and participate in the decision-making process
- respect the benefits of medical technology but are not in awe of medical equipment and tests
- seek information regarding health matters
- try new behaviors and modify others
- are active partners with the physician in the decision-making process
- are skeptical of health fads and trends
- ask questions, seek evidence, and evaluate information
- strive for self-reliance in personal health matters
- voluntarily adopt practices consistent with a healthy lifestyle

Accomplishing Health Education

With the school day already crowded, many elementary teachers wonder how to find time to teach health education. But time must be found. Our nation's children are an invaluable resource. Health education can help ensure that this generation is fit physically, psychologically, and socially to assume the difficult tasks of adulthood. Still, the problem remains: When and how should health education be taught in the classroom? How can it be accomplished?

Health education that is relevant and motivating for the student requires careful planning. The quality of health instruction is reflected in the amount of planning and organization done by the teacher. There are many approaches to teaching health, several of which will be discussed in a later chapter. However, the responsibility rests with each teacher to create and facilitate direct instruction in health and to infuse other health-related topics whenever the opportunity arises.

As previously stated, time must be allotted for direct health instruction during the school day. There is no substitute for this. However, if the time that can be allotted is minimal, health instruction can be incorporated into other parts of the curriculum, such as reading, mathematics, science, geography, art, social studies, and physical education. There are some advantages to integrating a part of health instruction into other subject areas, including opportunities for a significant amount of creativity in learning and teaching. However, the greatest need is for health to receive its just place in the elementary school day.

To accomplish health education, the topic selected must be appropriate to the developmental level of the child. Health must be taught every semester at every grade level from kindergarten through grade six. Only in this way can it become a meaningful part of each child's learning experience. Meaningful health education is education that influences a child's decision-making skills. To do this, health instruction must blend information giving with attitudinal experiences. Brown (1974, 4) describes this balance of information and attitude assessment as *confluent education*, which he defines as "the integration of cognitive learning with affective learning." In short, a child will be better able to make personal decisions concerning health behavior if the teacher has provided cognitive and affective opportunities for growth.

Presenting factual information alone—the cognitive aspect of health education—is not enough. Knowledge of facts *alone* does not lead to changes in behavior. The failure of so many cognitive drug education programs in the past is evidence of this. Knowledge must become personalized if it is to have an effect. This personalization is the affective aspect of health education. Strategies for accomplishing this personalization component will be presented throughout this text.

To accomplish its objectives, health education must be:

1. *Sequential*—taught throughout the educational experience, grades K through 12. The curriculum at each level should be based on what has been learned in previous years and serve as the basis for curricula in future years.

2. *Planned*—instruction should be based on goals, outcome-related objectives, and evaluation criteria. It should be taught within the total curriculum framework, not substituted for by teaching within other subjects such as science.

3. *Comprehensive*—instruction should include all the identified health content areas. More important than the individual subjects, however, is an understanding of how all subjects interrelate with the components of high-level wellness and quality of life.

4. *Taught by qualified health teachers*—individuals who have a concern for the total wellness of their students and who have been trained in the content as well as the strategies of health education. Effective health teaching requires more than the accumulation of knowledge. It requires that students have opportunities to personalize and incorporate positive health habits into their daily lives.

Regular exercise is an important part of total health.

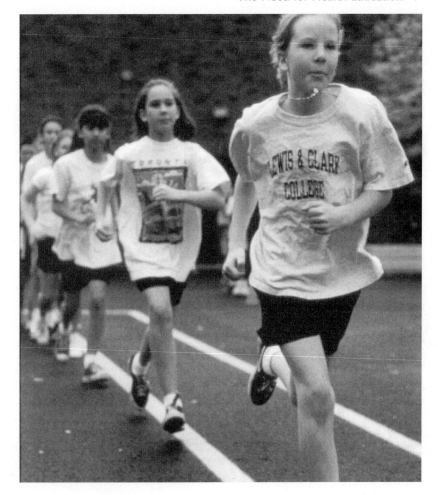

The need for health education continues to grow each year. It is important to remember that in the last twenty years, topics such as drug abuse, smoking, heart disease prevention, teenage pregnancy, adolescent suicide, stress control, incest, child abuse, HIV, and CPR have been added to an already long list of topics that includes nutrition, disease, mental health, sexuality, personal health, environmental health, first aid, and quackery (Purdy and Tritsch 1985).

It would seem that the task of creating health education programs is overwhelming. How does the school help children acquire knowledge, develop awareness and skills, provide personalizing experiences, and reinforce healthful behaviors? Equally important, how does the school interact with the community and the family to maximize the potential for assuming healthful behaviors? These issues were addressed by Kane (1993) when he suggested the relationship shown in Figure 1.2.

The wheel illustrates the student as the center of the focus in the classroom, school, home (family), and community efforts to promote high-quality health. The spokes represent the ingredients that enable the student to assimilate healthful behaviors through support from the school, community, and home. The concept of the wheel recognizes that the family and community play important roles in children's learning and provide opportunities to practice and reinforce health lifestyles. The school must recognize the importance of working within the community and with the family in attaining the healthy development of each child.

Figure 1.2

The Wheel of Comprehensive Health Education

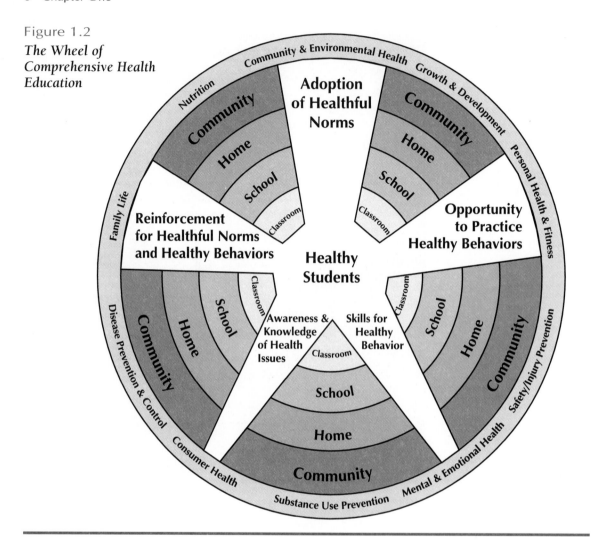

Why Health Education?

Perhaps the best argument for teaching health education is that health behaviors are the most important determinant of health status. Since health-related behaviors are both learned and changeable, there is no better time to start formal health education than in the elementary school years, when the child is more flexible and more apt to accept positive health behaviors. In addition, many of the negative aspects of a lifetime of abuse could be avoided. This avoidance becomes increasingly important with mounting evidence that most health problems are due to smoking, poor nutrition, being overweight, lack of exercise, stress, abuse of drugs and alcohol, and unsafe personal behavior (O'Rourke 1985).

Unfortunately, health education still suffers from a lack of importance in the school curriculum and a lack of adequately trained teachers. If we wish to help prevent many of the conditions that are now the leading causes of death (accidents, cardiovascular disease, cancer, and so on), then we must emphasize prevention in our educational efforts.

The following list outlines some of the problems our society faces. The problems noted help to underscore the need for effective health education.

○ For children and youths aged one to twenty-four years, unintentional injuries are the leading cause of death, accounting for almost half of the total deaths. Motor vehicle accidents were the leading cause of unintentional deaths, followed by drowning, fires, and burns (*Accident facts* 1994).

○ From 1988 to 1991, the firearm death rate for persons fifteen to twenty-four years of age increased 40 percent (*Accident facts* 1994).

○ Almost two-thirds of youths had had at least one drink of alcohol in their lifetime, one-third had used some type of illegal drug in their lifetime, 27 percent had tried marijuana, and 5.9 percent had tried cocaine. Over one-fourth of eighth graders reported they had used alcohol within the past two weeks, and 13.5 percent indicated that they had been involved in binge drinking (Adams and others, 1995).

○ Marijuana is used by 19 percent of tenth graders. Most widely used drugs by eighth graders were the inhalants, alcohol, and tobacco (USD, HHS, 1990).

○ In 1992 48 percent of adolescent males and 29 percent of adolescent females reported physical fighting, while almost 15 percent of teens reported having carried a weapon at least one day during the past month. It is estimated that 1 million teenagers are victims of crime each year. In the 5–14 age group, homicide was the cause of death for 519 children (Adams and others, 1995).

○ Six out of ten (60.9 percent) never-married youth aged 14–21 years have had sexual intercourse, ranging from 31.6 percent for youth fourteen to fifteen years of age to 78.9 percent for youth eighteen to twenty-one years old (Adams and others, 1995).

○ In 1993 there were 4,645 cases of AIDS in children under thirteen years of age and 2,501 deaths (Division of STD Prevention, 1996).

○ Seventy-five percent of all sexually transmitted diseases are found in the fifteen- to twenty-four-year age group (Adams and others, 1995).

○ It is estimated that 1 out of 100 girls between the ages of twelve and eighteen years of age suffers from anorexia nervosa. Researchers estimate that 4 percent of adolescent and college women suffer from bulimia (Wardlaw, Insel, and Seyler 1994).

○ In the past 20 years, the incidence of obesity among teenagers has increased 39 percent (Wardlaw, Insel, and Seyler 1994).

○ One million teenage girls become pregnant each year. This represents 12 percent of all females ages fifteen to nineteen years of age (117 per 1,000) (Alan Guttmacher Institute, 1994).

○ Over 19 percent of U.S. children ages three to seventeen years, or nearly 10.2 million children, have had a developmental delay, learning disability, or an emotional or behavioral problem. Boys were more likely than girls to have one or more of these disorders—23 percent versus 16 percent (*Health of our nation's children* 1994).

○ Children in low-income families are more likely to be in poor health, lose more school days due to chronic health problems, have been hospitalized, and remain in the hospital longer than high-income children (*Health of our nation's children* 1994).

○ Statistics indicate that about one million children in America are abused and neglected. Between 100,000 and 200,000 are physically abused, 60,000 to 100,000 are sexually abused, and the remainder are neglected (*The answer is at school* 1993).

○ The leading causes of death among Americans—heart disease, hypertension, and cancer—are related to lifestyle factors that our children must learn to assume responsibility for controlling. These factors include lack of exercise, use of tobacco products, diet, weight, and stress.

Not every area of concern in a comprehensive health education program has been touched on here. But it is hoped that the pressing need for health education has been established. The scope of health education is a broad one. Personal, family, and community problems must be effectively addressed if we are to live personally and socially satisfying lives. The beginning for effective health education is in the elementary school.

Today parents, administrators, and students no longer perceive health education as a peripheral or secondary activity. More than 90 percent of administrators believe that it is at least as useful as other subjects in the curriculum. Parents and students alike believe that the same amount, or even more time, should be devoted to teaching health education relative to other subjects taught in the curriculum (Seffrin 1994). The window of opportunity is there for providing comprehensive health education. As teachers, parents, and as a society, we must begin to effectively

Health Highlight

Every Day in America
(most recent available data as of September 24, 1996)

1 mother dies in childbirth	466 babies are born to mothers who received late or no prenatal care
3 people under 25 die from HIV	788 babies are born at low birthweight
6 children and youths commit suicide	1,420 babies are born to mothers younger than 20
14 children and youths are murdered	2,444 babies are born to mothers who are not high school graduates
16 children and youths are killed by firearms	2,556 babies are born into poverty
37 children and youths die from accidents	3,086 public school students are corporally punished
92 babies die	3,356 high school students drop out
144 babies are born at very low birthweight	3,533 babies are born to unmarried mothers
326 children are arrested for alcohol offenses	5,500 high school graduates do not go on to college
342 children are arrested for violent crimes	6,042 children are arrested
359 children are arrested for drug offenses	10,829 babies are born
	13,076 public school students are suspended every school day

Source: Children's Defense Fund, © 1995. Washington, DC.

deal with the challenges facing children and youth today. The previous page shows some facts (see the Health Highlight "Every Day in America") and statistics that help emphasize the continuing need for health education.

Many educators share this philosophy. They know that a comprehensive health education program can provide both immediate and long-term benefits for the children of our country. In terms of monetary costs, Americans spend an average of $1,100 per person per year on health care. In 1988, this represented 11.1 percent of the gross national product for the United States. In 1992 the United States spent 14 percent of the GNP on health (Consumers Union of the United States, 1992). In 1985, $1.6 billion was spent to aid teenage mothers through various government programs ("Why School Health" 1985, 3).

More tragic is the loss in human potential. Today, the diseases that are killing Americans are the chronic diseases such as cancer, heart disease, and HIV. Many of these unnecessary deaths could be prevented by helping people alter their lifestyles through improved eating habits, regular exercise, eliminating smoking, and practicing safer sex. Decreasing the incidence of these diseases will be achieved not through additional medical care or greater medical expenditures but through educating people to live healthful lives and, thereby, prevent disease. As a nation, our resources must be invested in helping people take control of their lives.

Health Objectives for the Year 2000

The U.S. Department of Health and Human Services through the Public Health Service issued a statement in the fall of 1990 listing the national health objectives for the year 2000. _Healthy People 2000: National Health Promotion and Disease Prevention Objectives_ listed the opportunities for improving the quality of life for the citizens of the United States. The purpose of these objectives is to commit the nation to the attainment of three broad goals. These goals are (1) increase the span of healthy life for Americans, (2) reduce health disparities among Americans, and (3) achieve access to preventive services for all Americans (_Healthy People 2000_ 1990, 6).

The objectives to accomplish these goals by the year 2000 are organized into twenty-two priority areas. The first twenty-one of these areas are grouped into three broad categories consisting of health promotion, health protection, and preventive services. The _Health Promotion Strategies_

Figure 1.3

Leading Causes of Death for Children Aged One Through Fourteen

Injuries	Pneumonia/Influenza
Cancer	Suicide
Congenital Anomalies	Meningitis
Homicide	Chronic Lung Disease
Heart Disease	HIV Infection

Source: National Center for Health Statistics, 1992. _Statistical bulletin_ 73(1)2–9.

are related to individual lifestyle—personal choices made in a social context that can have a powerful influence over the quality of life (see Table 1.1 for an overview of the areas of concern). The priorities under this heading include physical activity and fitness, nutrition, tobacco, alcohol and drugs, family planning, mental health and mental disorders, violent and abusive behavior, and education. *Health Protection Strategies* are related to environmental or regulatory measures that confer protection on U.S. citizens. The areas of concern include unintentional injuries, occupational safety and health, environmental health, food and drug safety, and oral health. The preventive services include counseling, screening, immunization, or chemoprophylactic intervention for individuals in clinical settings. Some of the areas included are heart disease and stroke, cancer, HIV infections, and sexually transmitted diseases.

Many of the objectives listed under each of these headings are directly related to a comprehensive school health instructional plan. Some of the objectives that apply directly to or have implications for health education have been extrapolated by the American School Health Association. The areas identified include (1) school health education, (2) healthy school food services, (3) physical education, (4) a healthy school environment, (5) school health services, (6) counseling and school psychology, (7) integrated school and community health promotions efforts, and (8) schoolsite health promotions for faculty and staff. Selected examples of the objectives that have implications for elementary health education are found in the following sections. The entire list can be found in the *Journal of School Health*, 61(7): 298–328.

School Health Education

1. Increase to at least 75 percent the proportion of the nation's schools that provide nutrition education from preschool through twelfth grade, preferably as part of quality school health education (baseline data available in 1991).

Table 1.1
Healthy People 2000
Priority Areas

Health Promotion
1. Physical Activity and Fitness
2. Nutrition
3. Tobacco
4. Alcohol and Other Drugs
5. Family Planning
6. Mental Health and Mental Disorders
7. Violent and Abusive Behavior
8. Educational and Community-Based Programs

Health Protection
9. Unintentional Injuries
10. Occupational Safety and Health
11. Environmental Health
12. Food and Drug Safety
13. Oral Health

Preventive Services
14. Maternal and Infant Health
15. Heart Disease and Stroke
16. Cancer
17. Diabetes and Chronic Disabling Conditions
18. HIV Infection
19. Sexually Transmitted Diseases
20. Immunization and Infectious Diseases
21. Clinical Preventive Services

Surveillance and Data Systems
22. Surveillance and Data Systems

Age-Related Objectives
Children
Adolescents and Young Adults
Adults
Older Adults

Health Highlight

Adolescents' Health Knowledge, Attitudes, and Behaviors

The need for a comprehensive health education program in the elementary school can be seen when viewing a survey recently taken. The survey was titled the "National Adolescent Student Health Survey (NASHS)." Published in 1988, the research was the first survey in more than twenty years to determine the knowledge, attitudes, and behavior of the nation's youth. "NASHS" questioned over 11,000 eighth and tenth graders on eight topics: AIDS, injury prevention, violence, suicide, alcohol, drug and tobacco use, sexually transmitted disease, consumer health, and nutrition. Some of the highlights of the survey are listed for each content area.

AIDS

○ 94 percent of the students surveyed know there is an increased risk of AIDS from having intercourse with someone who has the AIDS virus.

○ 91 percent know there is an increased risk of AIDS by sharing drug needles.

○ 82 percent know there is an increased risk of AIDS by having more than one sex partner.

○ 86 percent know that condoms are an effective way to reduce the risk of being infected with the AIDS virus.

○ 91 percent agree that people their age should use condoms if they have sex.

○ 71 percent mistakenly believe that blood transfusions are a common way to get AIDS today.

○ 47 percent mistakenly believe that there is an increased risk of AIDS when donating blood.

○ 51 percent are either unsure or mistakenly believe that washing after sex reduces one's chances of being infected with the AIDS virus.

○ 94 percent of the girls and 76 percent of the boys believe it is acceptable to say no to having sex.

Sexually Transmitted Diseases

○ 44 percent of students do not know or are unsure that a discharge of pus from the sex organs is an early sign of an STD.

○ 33 percent of students do not know that a sore on the sex organs is an early sign of an STD.

○ 55 percent of students do not know that taking birth control pills is ineffective in avoiding STDs.

Violence

○ 34 percent of students report that someone threatened to hurt them, 4 percent report having been robbed in school, and 13 percent report having been attacked while at school or on a school bus during the past year.

○ 33 percent of the students report that someone threatened to hurt them, 15 percent report having been robbed, and 16 percent report having been attacked while outside of school during the past year.

○ Nearly one in five girls report that during the past year someone tried to force them to have sex when they did not want to.

○ 23 percent of boys report having carried a knife to school at least once in the past year. 7 percent of the boys report carrying a knife to school on a daily basis.

○ 3 percent of boys report having carried a handgun to school at least once during

| Health Highlight–cont'd |

the past year. 1 percent of the boys report carrying a handgun on a daily basis.

○ 67 percent did not know that alcohol is involved in half of all murders.

Suicide

○ 42 percent of girls and 25 percent of boys report that they had "seriously thought" about committing suicide at some time in their lives.

○ 34 percent of girls and 15 percent of boys report that they often feel sad and hopeless.

Tobacco, Drug, and Alcohol Use

○ 51 percent of 8th grade students report having tried cigarettes.

○ 12 percent of boys report having chewed tobacco or used snuff during the past month.

○ 77 percent of 8th grade students and 53 percent of 10th grade students report having tried an alcoholic beverage.

○ 34 percent of 8th grade students and 53 percent of 10th grade students report having had an alcoholic beverage during the past month.

○ 26 percent of 8th grade students and 38 percent of 10th grade students report having had five or more drinks on one occasion during the past two weeks.

○ 15 percent of 8th grade students and 35 percent of 10th grade students report having tried marijuana.

○ 6 percent of 8th grade students and 15 percent of 10th grade students report having used marijuana during the past month.

○ 5 percent of 8th grade students and 9 percent of 10th grade students report having tried cocaine.

○ 2 percent of 8th grade students and 3 percent of 10th grade students report having used cocaine during the past month.

Nutrition

○ 51 percent of students who diet report that they fast to control their weight.

○ 39 percent of students eat fried foods four or more times a week.

○ On average, students report eating three snacks a day. More than half of these snacks (59 percent) are foods high in fat and/or sugar.

○ 73 percent of the students knew that eating foods high in saturated fats may be related to heart problems.

○ 48 percent of girls and 33 percent of boys report having eaten breakfast on two or fewer days during the past week.

Consumer Education

○ 57 percent of the students given a cereal box label were unable to determine which cereal ingredient was present in the largest amount.

○ 58 percent of students did not know the meaning of the date stamped on dairy products.

Source: National Adolescent Student Survey (NASHS), 1988. *Health education* 19(4):408. Reprinted by permission.

2. Increase the proportion of high school seniors who perceive social disapproval associated with the heavy use of alcohol, occasional use of marijuana, and experimentation with cocaine.

3. Increase the proportion of high school seniors who associate *risk* of physical or psychological harm with the heavy use of alcohol, regular use of marijuana, and experimentation with cocaine, as follows:

    Heavy use of alcohol—70 percent
    Occasional use of marijuana—85 percent
    Trying cocaine once or twice—95 percent

4. Provide to children in all school districts and private schools primary and secondary school educational programs on alcohol and other drugs, preferably as part of quality school health education.

5. Increase to at least 85 percent the proportion of people aged ten through eighteen who have discussed human sexuality, including values surrounding sexuality, with their parents and/or have received information through another parentally endorsed source, such as youth, school, or religious programs (baseline: 66 percent of people aged thirteen through eighteen have discussed sexuality with their parents; reported in 1986).

6. Increase to at least 50 percent the proportion of elementary and secondary schools that teach nonviolent conflict resolution skills, preferably as a part of quality school health education (baseline data available in 1991).

7. Increase to at least 75 percent the proportion of the nation's elementary and secondary schools that provide planned and sequential, kindergarten through twelfth-grade, quality school health education (baseline data available in 1991).

8. Provide academic instruction on injury prevention and control, preferably as part of quality school health education, in at least 50 percent of public school systems (grades K through 12) (baseline data available in 1991).

9. Increase to at least 95 percent the proportion of schools that have age-appropriate HIV education curricula for students in fourth through twelfth grade, preferably as part of quality school health education (baseline: 66 percent of school districts required HIV education, but only 5 percent required HIV education in each year for seventh through twelfth grade in 1989).

10. Include instruction in sexually transmitted disease transmission prevention in the curricula of all middle and secondary schools, preferably as part of quality school health education (baseline: 95 percent of schools reported offering at least one class on sexually transmitted diseases as part of their standard curricula in 1988).

Healthy School Food Services

1. Increase to at least 90 percent the proportion of school lunch and breakfast services and child care food services with menus that are consistent with the nutrition principles in the *Dietary Guidelines for Americans* (baseline data available in 1993).

School Physical Education

1. Increase to at least 50 percent the proportion of children and adolescents in first through twelfth grade who participate in daily school physical education (baseline: 36 percent in 1984–86).

Healthy School Environment

1. Establish tobacco-free environments and include tobacco use prevention in the curricula of all elementary, middle, and secondary schools, preferably as part of quality school health education (baseline: 17 percent of school districts totally banned smoking on school premises or at school functions in 1988; antismoking education was provided by 78 percent of school districts at the high school level, 81 percent at the middle school level, and 75 percent at the elementary school level in 1988).

Health Highlight

Healthy People 2000

Healthy People 2000: National Health Promotion and Disease Prevention Objectives, released in September 1990, offers a vision for the new century, characterized by significant reductions in preventable death and disability, enhanced quality of life, and greatly reduced disparities in the health status of populations within our society.

Healthy People 2000 does not reflect the policies or opinions of any one individual or any one organization, including the federal government. It is the product of a national effort involving professionals and citizens, private organizations, and public agencies from every part of the country. It is deliberately comprehensive in addressing health promotion and disease prevention opportunities to allow local communities and states to choose from among its recommendations to address their own highest priority needs. Schools offer the most systematic and efficient means available to improve the health of youth and enable young people to avoid

health risks. They provide an avenue for reaching more than 46 million students each year, as well as more than five million instructional and noninstructional staff. The American Public Health Association noted that the school, as a social structure, provides an educational setting in which the total health of the child during the impressionable years is a priority concern. No other community setting even approximates the magnitude of the kindergarten through grade twelve school education enterprise; thus, it seems that the school should be regarded as a focal point to which health planning for all other community settings should relate.

Planned and sequential quality school health education programs help young people at each appropriate grade to develop increasingly complex knowledge and skills they will need to avoid important health risks, and to maintain their own health, the health of the families for which they will become responsible, and the health of communities in which they will reside.

Source: Healthy people 2000: National health promotion and disease prevention objectives. (Conference ed.). 1990. Washington, DC: U.S. Department of Health and Human Services.

School Health Services

1. Increase to at least 90 percent the proportion of all children entering school programs for the first time who have received an oral health screening, referral, and follow-up for necessary diagnostic, preventive, and treatment services (baseline: 66 percent of children aged five visited a dentist during the previous year in 1986).

2. Increase immunization levels as follows:

   Basic immunization series among children under age two: at least 90 percent (baseline: 70–80 percent estimated in 1989).

   Basic immunization series among children in licensed child care facilities and kindergarten through postsecondary education institutions: at least 95 percent (baseline: For licensed child care, 94 percent; for children entering school for the 1987–88 school year, 97 percent; and for postsecondary institutions, baseline data available in 1992).

   Elementary school children are at a point in development where they are acquiring habits that will remain with them throughout life. It is far easier to acquire desirable patterns of living early rather than to change ingrained habits later in life. The part played by health education holds great potential if early in life a sense of values coupled with knowledge and appropriate decision-making skills are developed.

The Comprehensive School Health Program

A total school health program is needed if the school is to function as an effective institution for promoting high-level wellness. A comprehensive school health program includes eight components: (1) a healthful school environment, (2) school health instruction, (3) school health services,(4) school physical education, (5) school nutrition and food services, (6) school-based counseling, (7) schoolsite health promotion, and (8) school, family, and community health promotion partnerships (see Figure 1.4). Each component involves planning, administration, and evaluation. Adequate planning for all eight components ensures their comprehensiveness. Effective leadership coordinates the components and ensures proper staffing, budgeting, policy fulfillment, and evaluation.

A Healthful School Environment. This aspect of the school health program includes the physical and psychological environment in which students and faculty exist. Issues addressed include the emotional and social environment of the classroom, the development of self-worth and self-esteem, and the fostering of positive relationships for students and school personnel. In addition, safety hazards on the school grounds and within the buildings are of concern. This includes chemical agents, temperature, humidity, noise, lighting, and radiation found within the building and classroom environment.

Few teachers are fortunate enough to be able to work in ideal situations. However, it is desirable to do all that is possible to enhance the teaching environment. The classroom should be physically adequate, pleasant, attractive, and comfortable for the children. When the classroom setting is bright, lively, and dynamic, morale is improved.

Teachers should require a quality environment in which to work. This is important not only for the teaching/learning process but also for teacher and student morale. Whenever possible, teachers should volunteer as consultants in planning and maintaining the school site and surroundings. Fostering a cooperative relationship with the custodial staff, lunchroom staff, and

Figure 1.4
*The Comprehensive
School Health
Program*

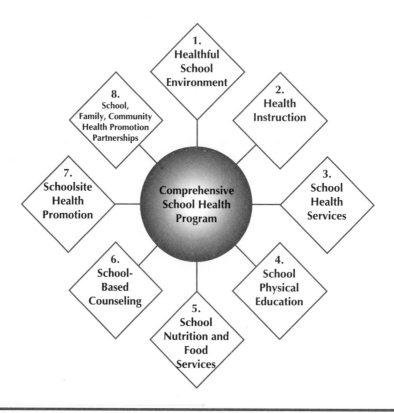

administrators in charge of the various aspects of the environment is beneficial. Working with the custodians by keeping the classroom sanitary and by diplomatically suggesting improvements can enhance the environment significantly.

The psychological setting is just as important as the physical one, and the teacher is responsible for establishing the emotional tone within the classroom. The overall atmosphere should be one of acceptance, one in which the teacher knows the children well and is sensitive to their individual needs. The classroom should be nonthreatening. Stress is reduced when there is a relaxed approach to instruction, one in which there is less emphasis on competition that pits child against child. Students should feel free to express their feelings honestly without fear of ridicule or rebuke. They should also feel free to fail occasionally without punishment. A teacher can promote the children's well-being by being kind but fair in promoting teacher–pupil relationships, setting reasonable goals for each student, praising positive behavior, challenging children within their capabilities, and tolerating occasional frustration. Allowing the students to assist in planning health learning opportunities is also very important. If they are involved in planning, they will become more interested in the subject matter. When children are interested, discipline is less likely to become a problem.

Although emphasis in this section has been on the classroom environment, there are other considerations that are part of the healthy school environment. An issue of particular importance is the safety of students when transported on school buses. Guidelines are needed for daily bus rides, as well as for special occasions, such as field trips or extracurricular events. Safety in the classroom, the cafeteria, the gymnasium, and within the general school physical plant is an important aspect of a healthy school environment.

School Health Instruction. The second area of the school health program is health instruction, in which information is presented to students in a way that fosters desirable health knowledge, attitudes, and practices. Strategies, information, and methods concerning this aspect of a comprehensive school health program are described later in the text.

School Health Services. These programs seek to promote the children's health through screening, intervention, and remediation of various health conditions. The school nurse most often coordinates and provides the services of this component. Screenings for visual or auditory problems and scoliosis, as well as first-aid procedures, illness protocol, and services for the handicapped are part of health services. Professionals who make up the school health services team include the school physician, dentist, social worker, speech pathologist, and the nurse.

School Physical Education. A comprehensive physical education program is one that offers a daily program of activities. These programs should be based on developing cardiovascular fitness, strength, flexibility, and agility. A sound program can help reduce stress and promote social development.

School Nutrition and Food Services. This component involves training the food preparation personnel and developing nutritionally sound food programs for the school. Part of this component is helping children to select nutritionally balanced meals and ensuring that food served in the school cafeteria is nutritional, attractive, and palatable.

School-Based Counseling. This aspect of the comprehensive health program seeks to meet the needs of children by providing services such as assertiveness, problem solving and self-esteem training. Services also are provided by school psychologists for children who experience learning difficulties and behavioral problems.

Schoolsite Health Promotion. Programs for faculty and staff can provide benefits by reducing health care costs, improving morale, and increasing productivity of the faculty and staff. Health promotion programs are a natural for the school, because facilities and personnel for conducting programs are already in place. Health educators, physical educators, nurses, counselors, and nutritionists are available to aid in program development.

School, Family, and Community Health Promotion Partnerships. An effective strategy for promoting the health of school-age students is the development of collaborative efforts between the community agencies and the school. These coalitions can coordinate and advocate for improving the various aspects of the comprehensive school health program.

Teachers should consider themselves as part of a team whose main mission is to provide optimal conditions to enhance the wellness of each student. Each member of the health team has a particular role to play. Like a chain, the health team is only as strong as its weakest link. Everyone involved with the health of students, including the students themselves, must take that personal responsibility seriously. Each member must work cooperatively with other members in order to reach the ultimate goal of total high-level health.

School-Based Health Centers—The School Nurse

School-based health centers (SBHCs) are a fairly recent innovation in the health care of children. The concept is for students to receive primary and preventive care in the school setting and thus to increase quality care. Currently there are more than 600 SBHCs nationally, with some of these facilities serving as primary care providers while others are preventive in function (*Making the Grade* 1995). A U.S. Government Accounting Office (GAO) report in 1994 indicated that SBHCs do improve students' access to quality care. These facilities help overcome financial barriers, lack of health insurance, and transportation difficulties associated with students receiving appropriate health care (U.S. General Accounting Office 1994). Many problems are associated with establishing SBHCs in the school setting. Most current facilities have links with health maintenance organizations (HMOs). Problems with reimbursement, permission to treat, nature of services, and financing are just some of the obstacles to establishing effective SBHCs (Hacker 1996). Yet despite the many problems, the school-based health center approach to student health care may gain much greater acceptance in the future.

Even if such facilities are not available on a broad scale, schools should have access to a school nurse. Unfortunately, many school districts have been forced to cut back or underdevelop the role of the school nurse by assigning one nurse responsibility for several schools. This does not allow nurses sufficient time in a given school to completely develop the school health service. Even worse, in some communities school health services are performed by parents, school secretaries, or some other untrained person.

The services provided by school nurses are extremely important to the children's welfare. Most frequently, they provide direct care to sick or injured children. Important functions are information gathering through assessment of the children, recordkeeping, and routine assessments. These assessments should help provide for appropriate follow-up care and some type of interpretation to the parent.

Nurses are excellent resources. They should be included on any health education curriculum planning committee and should be involved in planning the education of special populations. Nurses have become increasingly involved in planning the educational program of handicapped children. Nurses can assist these children in becoming self-sufficient in the classroom and help alleviate the fears and concerns of the teachers. Finally, the nurse should see that emergency procedures for injuries, accidents, and sickness are developed, because there are obvious legal concerns when undertaking aid in any of these situations. The nurse can help ensure proper care will occur by helping to develop guidelines and workshops for teachers, aids, and office personnel in emergency procedures.

▤ *Summary*

○ Health is defined as an integrated method of functioning that is oriented toward maximizing the potential of which the individual is capable.

○ Wellness implies that individuals engage in attitudes and behaviors that enhance quality of life and maximize personal potential.

○ Wellness consists of five components: spiritual, social, emotional, intellectual, and physical.

○ To achieve wellness, students must feel they can control their lives (locus of control) and believe in their ability to accomplish a specific task or behavior (self-efficacy).

○ Health promotion is the aggregate of all purposeful activities designed to improve personal and public health through a combination of strategies, including the competent implementation of behavioral change strategies, health education, health protection measures, risk factor detection, health enhancement, and health maintenance.

○ Health education is the process of developing and providing planned experiences to supply information, change attitudes, and influence behavior.

○ To accomplish its goals, health education must be sequential, planned, comprehensive, and taught by qualified health teachers.

○ Factual information does not ensure behavioral change.

○ Opportunities must be provided for personalizing information learned so that attitudes can be formulated as precursor to behavior.

○ Problems that indicate the need for comprehensive health education include child and adolescent accident rates, HIV, smoking, poor nutrition, STDs, drug and alcohol use, suicide, and chronic diseases.

○ An effective school health program has eight components and includes healthful school environment, school health instruction, school health services, school physical education, school nutrition and food services, school-based counseling, school site health promotion, and school, family and community health promotion partnerships.

○ A school-based health center can be an important component of an effective school health program.

Discussion Questions

1. Why is health a difficult concept to define?
2. What is meant by the term *wellness*?
3. What is the difference between health promotion and health education?
4. How would you justify the need for health education in our schools?
5. Why is prevention the best approach to affecting the quality of health in the United States?
6. Why is self-responsibility so important to develop in health education?
7. Discuss why the Healthy People 2000 objectives are vital to health education.
8. Why is a comprehensive school health program important?
9. Discuss the various components of a school health education program.
10. How can the classroom teacher aid in the development of a healthy school environment?

References

Accident facts. 1994. Chicago: National Safety Council.

Adams, P. F., Schofenborn, C. A., Moss, A. J., Warren, C. W., and Kann, L. 1995. *Health risk behaviors among our nation's youth: United States, 1992.* National Center for Health Statistics. Vital Health Statistics, 109–120. Hyattsville, MD.

Alan Guttmacher Institute. 1994. *Teenage reproductive health in the U.S: Facts in brief.* New York: Alan Guttmacher Institute.

Allensworth, D. D., and L. J. Kolbe. 1987. The comprehensive school health program: Exploring an expanded concept. *Journal of school health* 57(10):409–412.

American School Health Association. 1983. *A healthy child: The key to the basics.* Kent, OH: ASHA.

American School Health Association. 1983. *Selected school health support statements.* Kent, OH: ASHA.

The answer is at school—bringing health care to our students. 1993. Washington, DC: The School-Based Adolescent Health Care Program.

Brown, G. I. 1974. *Human teaching for human learning: An introduction to confluent education.* New York: Viking Press.

Carlyon, W. H., and D. E. Cook. 1981. Science instruction and health instruction. *BSCS journal* 4:1.

Chapman, L.E. 1987. Developing a useful perspective on spiritual health:love, joy, peace and fulfillment. *American journal of health promotion* 2(22):12–17.

Children's Defense Fund. 1997. *The health of American children yearbook.* Washington, DC: The Fund.

Consumers Union of United States, Inc. 1992. Wasted health care dollars. *Consumer reports.* 435–448.

Creswell, W. H., Jr., and I. M. Newman. 1989. *School health practice.* St. Louis: Times Mirror/Mosby College Publishing.

Division of STD Prevention, U. S. Department of Health and Human Services, Public Health Service. 1996. *Sexually transmitted disease surveillance, 1995.* Atlanta: Centers for Disease Control and Prevention, September 1996.

Dunn, H. L. 1991. *High level wellness.* Arlington, VA: Beatty.

Educational Research Service.1983. Local school district budget items by type of community. *Spectrum: Journal of school research and information* 1(3):16.

Feld, Jon. 1988. Sports survey tracking the trends in club-related sports. *Club industry* 4(12):20–25.

Green, L. W. 1990. *Community health.* St. Louis: Times Mirror/Mosby College Publishing.

Green, L. W., and M. W. Kreuter. 1991. *Health education planning: An educational and environmental approach.* Palo Alto: Mayfield.

Haag, J.H. 1972. *School health program.* 3d ed. Philadelphia: Lea and Febiger.

Hacker, K. 1996. Integrating school-based health center into managed care in Massachusetts. *Journal of school health,* 66(9):317-321.

Healthy people 2000—National health promotion and disease prevention objectives (Conference ed.) 1990. Washington, DC: U.S. Department of Health and Human Services.

Healthy people 2000—National health promotion and disease prevention objectives. 1991. *Journal of school health* 61(7):298–328.

Hoyman, H.S. 1975. Rethinking an ecologic-system model of man's health, disease, aging, death. *Journal of school health* 45:9.

Joint Committee on Health Education Terminology. 1991. Report of the 1990 joint committee on health education terminology. *Journal of health education* 22:97–108.

Kane, W. M. 1993. *Step by step to comprehensive school health.* Santa Cruz: ETR Associates.

Kreuter, M. W. 1984. Health promotion: The public health role in the community of free exchange. Paper presented at the 4th annual colloquium in health promotion, 21 March, Columbia University, New York. 5.

Making the Grade. 1995. *Medicaid managed care and school-based health center: Proceeding of a meeting with policy makers and providers.* Washington, DC: Robert Wood Johnson Foundation.

McKenzie, J. F., and Smeltzer, J. L., 1997. *Planning, implementing, and evaluating health promotion programs.* Boston: Allyn and Bacon.

National Adolescent Student Health Survey (NASHS).1988. *Health education* 19(4):4–8.

National Center for Educational Statistics (NCES).1984. *The condition of education.* NCES Pub. No. 84–401, Washington, DC: U.S. Government Printing Office.

Objectives that can be attained directly by schools, arranged under the eight components of multidimensional school health program. 1991. *Journal of school health* 61(7):298–311.

O'Rourke, T. W. 1985. Why school health education? The economical point of view. Paper presented at the Delbert Oberteuffer Centennial Symposium, 21 April, 1985, Atlanta, GA. Cosponsored by Association for the Advancement of Health Education and the Office of Disease Prevention and Health Promotion. 25–28.

Planned Parenthood of America (PPA). 1981. *Teenage pregnancy: The problem that hasn't gone away.* New York: Planned Parenthood of America.

Purdy, C., and L. Tritsch. 1985. Why health education? The practical point of view. Paper presented at the Delbert Oberteuffer Centennial Symposium, 21 April, 1985, Atlanta, GA. Cosponsored by Association for the Advancement of Health Education and the Office of Disease Prevention and Health Promotion. 25–28.

Seffrin, J. R. 1994. America's interest in comprehensive school health education. *Journal of school health* 64(10): 397–399.

U.S. Bureau of the Census. 1992. *Statistical abstract of the United States: 1992.* Washington, DC: U.S. Government Printing Office.

U.S. Department of Health, Education, and Welfare. 1979. *Sexually transmitted disease fact sheet.* Atlanta: Public Health Science, Centers for Disease Control.

U.S. Department of Health and Human Services. 1986. *Data for the 1990 objectives, estimates from the national health interview survey of health promotion and disease prevention: United States, 1985.* Washington, DC: U.S.Government Printing Office.

U.S. Department of Health and Human Services (USDHHS). 1990. *Teenagers and drug abuse.* NIDA Capsules, 1990. Washington, DC.

U.S. General Accounting Office. 1994. Report to the chairman, committee on government operations, U.S. House of Representatives: Health care reform school-based health centers can promote access to care. Washington, DC: U.S. General Accounting Office.

Wardlaw, G. M., Insel, P. M., and Seyler, M. F. 1994. *Contemporary nutrition—issues and insights.* St. Louis: Mosby-YearBook.

Chapter Two
The Role of the Teacher in Health Instruction

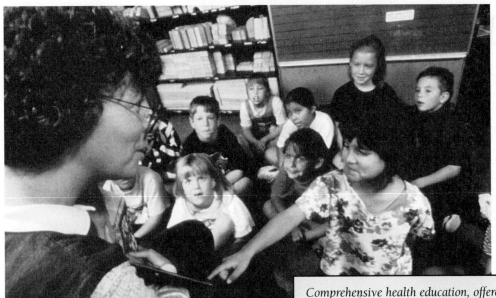

> *Comprehensive health education, offered early and reinforced throughout a student's school career, is fundamental to promoting healthy behaviors*
> —Marx and Northrop, 1995

Valued Outcomes

After reading this chapter, you should be able to

○ discuss the academic and personal qualifications of an effective health educator

○ describe how a teacher of health has an opportunity to be a significant and positive role model in students' lives

○ explain the barriers that make health instruction more difficult to teach than other subjects in the curriculum

○ discuss the minimum competencies needed by a health educator

○ describe the legal liability associated with teaching

○ discuss how the educator can work with other members of the school staff to enhance the wellness of each student

○ describe the qualities of a teacher needed to ensure the proper education of students with special needs

The Challenge of Health Education

"Initiatives have taken place over the past 25 years to enhance the profession and the practice of health education" (Schima and Ames 1996). Health education has become a focal point during the last few years as our nation has worked toward reaching specific health goals (such as the Healthy People 2000 objectives for the nation, discussed in Chapter 1) for the citizens of our country. The emphasis on health education has, in turn, led to an increased awareness of the need for effective health educators.

To be effective, an educator must concentrate not only on academic preparation, but also on personal qualifications. Personal qualifications of an educator are important because of the significance of and emphasis on the teacher's behavior and attitudes.

Teaching health is unlike teaching any other topic in the curriculum. For example, in other classes the teacher may get immediate feedback from the students regarding the learning of a concept. However, in health education the teacher may never know if a student actually applies a health concept in his or her life, because the opportunity to apply that concept may not surface until several years later. Furthermore, the methodology used in health education is unlike other subject areas in that it demands an open, accepting environment in the classroom during instruction.

A philosophy that should govern every teacher is the following: "Every teacher is a health teacher"; that is, every teacher in the school is a health teacher, regardless of what discipline he or she is actually teaching. This implies that, regardless of the subject matter you happen to be teaching, you are making an impact on your students through your behavior. Health education may be the only subject matter in which the teacher must embody the content. You can teach as much by what you do as what you say in the classroom. In other words, you as a teacher are on display before your students, and you have the opportunity to portray a positive health image through your behavior. For example, if the students observe you eating a good diet in the lunchroom, they will see that health, at least that aspect, is important to you; therefore, they are more likely to adopt the same value. You should emphasize positive health behavior in your own life as well as teach students to make wise decisions about their own health.

Elementary school children are very impressionable, and you can teach skills and influence behavior positively through your own behavior and attitudes. You have an excellent opportunity to become a good health role model by practicing safe and healthy habits.

You must emphasize to students that they cannot become healthy passively. Involving them in active learning opportunities, in which they are allowed to clarify their values and taught how to make wise decisions, will personalize their health education. Your students will then be better able to make their own responsible choices for healthful behavior.

Barriers to Successful Health Teaching

Planning and implementing school health education that is comprehensive often demands perseverance, commitment by an individual, and sometimes a fair amount of good luck. Health educators face shrinking budgets and competing priorities and must be aware of and responsive to cultural diversity and value differences. Almost every school that decides to implement a new health education program will face challenges (Marx and Northrop 1995).

For example, elementary education majors in most colleges receive very little instruction in health content and in methodology that specifically relates to health instruction. Because the elementary teacher must teach many subjects, most college programs emphasize methods and materials instead of specific subject areas. This puts the elementary teacher at a distinct disadvantage because teaching health requires a different methodology from other subjects. Teaching content alone is not sufficient in health education. Students may be able to pass a paper-and-pencil test on health knowledge, but this does not ensure that the student will put that knowledge into practice. This phenomenon, known as "cognitive dissonance," concerns the discrepancy between personal health knowledge and general health behavior. For example, there is a common knowledge regarding protective factors related to wearing safety belts in cars, yet a significant number of Americans do not wear them regularly.

Therefore, health instruction requires an active involvement of the student in the learning process; that is, you must give the student opportunities to experience situations (even though they may be simulated) in which they focus their values and make decisions regarding health behavior. Again, this teaching process is no guarantee that every student will make a healthy decision in each case, but it will more effectively help the student learn the concept being taught as well as apply the concept to his or her lifestyle. Health instruction further demands the inclusion of teaching methodologies that enable the student to consider a healthy behavior valuable enough to incorporate into his or her lifestyle. To overcome these specific barriers, take as many courses as you can that emphasize health content and health instruction. For a more detailed discussion of value-based instruction, see Chapter 4, "Strategies for Implementing Health Instruction."

Effective health instruction is hindered by the tremendous wealth of health information. Health education is by its nature interdisciplinary, in that it borrows not only from educational theory but also from many social sciences, such as psychology and sociology, as well as from physical science, biology, and even religion. It is difficult enough for a health education specialist to stay current in health, much less the elementary teacher, who must master several other subject areas. This barrier is compounded by the fact that health information is changing constantly—the results of new studies related to health information appear virtually every day. The teacher has an obligation to follow these new developments. One way to do this is to attend educational seminars and workshops.

Further, some health information is conflicting; two studies on the same health topic might reach different conclusions. Some physicians consider megadoses of vitamin C to be the answer to preventing colds; other physicians disagree. Such disagreements between authorities cause a dilemma for the conscientious teacher who wishes to present *all* the information. Also, the conflicting information can be confusing for the student who is trying to make a wise, informed decision.

Another problem surfaces when teachers must deal with information that is inconclusive. For example, much information about AIDS has not yet been discovered. Normally teachers think it is imperative to know everything in order to command the respect of students, but this is impossible in situations where even the authorities have not discovered all the answers.

Another barrier to effective health instruction is that so many issues in health education are controversial. Teachers who handle controversial issues risk offending students and/or parents. Even in some subjects that would not appear controversial, such as nutrition, you might offend some groups, say vegetarians, if you teach that servings of meat are recommended for a balanced diet. Further, controversial topics tend to polarize students. The more controversial the topic, the more emotional the students become about the issue. When this occurs, there is a greater likelihood of dissension and ill feeling among the students. Such dissension can disrupt the optimal teaching/learning environment that is necessary in health instruction.

Many times, as an instructor, you will be battling against students' negative image of health and health education. Health educators are sometimes viewed as "warriors against pleasure," which means that students thinks of health educators as those who tell them to quit doing what they like to do, such as eat desserts, and to do what they don't like to do, such as exercise. This may translate into negative feelings that the teacher must overcome, especially when the student perceives that the teacher's ideas conflict with those of parents or the peer group. Also, some students come into the health education classroom with preconceived notions, habits, and misconceptions about health information. This misinformation might have come from the home, media, older siblings, or peers. Teachers should be very knowledgeable of their students' backgrounds and subcultural perspectives. This understanding is critical in understanding a student's behavior and knowing what will motivate a student.

This makes the job of the educator doubly difficult because not only must she or he provide the correct information, but she or he may be spending much of the time in the classroom dispelling many myths that the students bring with them.

Finally, some administrators place a low priority on health education by allowing other activities to substitute for health instruction, or by not placing health education in the curriculum at all. One way to overcome this problem is to help other teachers integrate health education with the other main subjects in the curriculum. There are many ways to integrate health into content and activities at the elementary level. For example, figuring one's heart rate can be integrated into mathematics. For language arts, the students can read a story about a health topic. The students can do many experiments in health class that are related to science.

Professional Preparation

Health education is not a new profession. "Health education has evolved from a wide assortment of roots over the past 170 years. Some of these roots can be recognized as responses by professional and voluntary organizations to the many health problems confronting a [society]. Other responses come from families and citizen groups demanding protection for the health and well-being of communities" (Schima and Ames 1996).

Although standards for professional training of health educators have been set in the past, school health education has been criticized as being ineffective. This is largely the result of poorly prepared teachers.

Ideally, a preschool or elementary school health teacher should be a specialist, but this is not feasible when so many subjects must be taught. Therefore, the elementary teacher is forced to teach subjects such as health with less professional preparation than their secondary colleagues. Many states still allow teachers with dual certification in health and physical education to teach health at the secondary level, and those with a general elementary certification to teach health at the elementary level.

There are several reasons for recommending that a teacher of health be a specialist. Health is different from other subjects in that the content comes from a variety of sources and is not limited to one distinct discipline. Also, the behavioral outcomes desired of the student in a health class differ remarkably from other subjects. Because these outcomes are not easily measured, a health teacher should have specific training in making empirical observations that indicate whether the desired outcomes are being acquired.

Even when a teacher is dually prepared—say, in health and physical education—the health portion is typically slightly in favor of the physical education portion. The reduced number of courses in this dual major hinders effective teacher preparation.

A course dealing with the personal health of the individual is also desirable. In this course, prospective teachers learn more about their own personal behavior. Further, a basic course in first aid and emergency is very helpful.

The National Task Force on the Preparation and Practice of Health Educators, composed of professionals from several national organizations with an interest in health education, has been working since 1978 to develop a framework of minimum competencies that should be required of health educators. These competencies are included in the document *A Framework for the Development of Competency-based Curricula for Entry-Level Health Educators* (later revised and retitled *A Competency-Based Curriculum Framework for the Professional Preparation of Entry-Level Health Educator*—National Task Force 1988) and are intended to guide certifying institutions in the professional preparation of students intending to teach health. This curriculum was developed with a generic health educator in mind, that is, an individual who might be teaching health in a variety of settings, including the school classroom. Eventually, NCATE accreditation of teacher credential programs in health will require the use of the guidelines specified in this framework.

As an outgrowth of the work of this task force, the National Commission for Health Education Credentialing (NCHEC) was formed to oversee the professional credentialing process for health educators. Certification is granted through a process of both meeting basic academic eligibility requirements and receiving a passing score on the certified health education specialist national examination. The certification exam itself consists of questions developed around responsibilities of health educators. These responsibilities are discussed more thoroughly in the following Health Highlight.

Health Highlight

Responsibilities of the Health Educator

Area 1. Assess individual and community needs for health education. The emphasis in this competency is placed on the identification of factors that are most likely responsible for unfavorable health behaviors within a particular group such as peer pressure, and cultural or religious factors.

Area 2. Plan effective health education programs. The health educator needs to be able to develop a detailed plan for the most effective use of educational resources.

Area 3. Implement health education programs. Once an educational plan has been completed, the health educator needs to be able to present and describe the program to groups such as local school boards who would approve the plan. Then, assuming approval, the health educator needs to be able to assist teachers in translating the program into classroom learning experiences.

Area 4. Evaluate the effectiveness of health education programs' competency. The health educator needs to be able to demonstrate the effectiveness of the health educa-

tion program that has been planned and implemented.

Area 5. Coordinate the provision of health education services. Many health education programs involve many people and are often based within larger organizations. Both of these characteristics require the health educator in various settings to assist and encourage personnel in carrying out the educational aspects of a health education program.

Area 6. Act as a resource person in health education. The health educator should be able to collect and organize general information to meet routine requests, and should become aware of community resources for referring more complex requests.

Area 7. Communicate health and health education needs, concerns, and resources. Health educators should be able to communicate many different types of messages involving different types of media. Bear in mind that these messages will need to be communicated to a wide variety of individuals and groups.

Source: Kerry J. Redican and Elyzabeth J. Holford. 1996. The certified health education specialist and malpractice." *Journal of health education* 27(4): 257-260.

As discussed earlier, a teacher's preparation does not end upon receipt of a diploma and teaching certificate. You can continue to educate yourself by taking graduate courses, either in specific content areas or in advanced teaching methods, joining local, state, regional, and national health education professional organizations and attending professional health conferences. Staying current also requires reading up-to-date textbooks, journals, and other health education publications. Finally, in-service workshops that deal with health-related topics are extremely valuable.

To continue professional development beyond undergraduate training, many school health educators join one of the following professional associations:

○ American Association for Health Education (AAHE), 1900 Association Drive, Reston, VA 22091-1599. This organization is housed currently under the umbrella of the American Alliance for Health, Physical Education, Recreation and Dance. This organization began as a professional organization for the health and physical education teacher. Its current emphases includes the health professional in several types of work environments, such as K–12 school, university, hospital, business and industry, and community.

○ American School Health Association (ASHA), 7263 State Route 43, P.O. Box 708, Kent, OH 44240. This professional organization emphasizes all areas of school health, including services and environment as well as education. Therefore, its membership includes health educators as well as school nurses, physicians, dentists, and dental hygienists.

In addition to the previous two professional organizations, which primarily attract school health educators, there are other health organizations in which a variety of health professionals may enhance their professional development:

○ American College Health Association (ACHA), 1300 Picard Drive, Suite 2000, Rockville, MD 20850. This organization primarily focuses on providing health services for college students, but also provides an emphasis in health education of college students.

○ American Public Health Association (APHA), 1015 15th Street, NW, Washington, DC 20015. This organization includes health professionals in the public sector, such as public health administrators, public health services, and community sanitation and environmental control; however, it includes sections both in public health education and in school health.

○ Society for Public Health Education (SPHE), 1100 Connecticut Avenue, Suite 430, Washington, DC. Although formerly restricted to professionals with graduate degrees in public health, this organization has now opened its membership to include health educators from a variety of settings.

Personal Qualities of the Health Teacher

There are many influences on a child, such as the media and peer pressure, that may be detrimental. Teachers should be a positive role model, because educators are an important factor in students' health behavior development. Students desire positive role models who are honest, sincere, energetic, knowledgeable, and caring.

The following is a list of characteristics and actions that will help you become a quality health educator:

1. *Stay motivated.* Examples start with the teacher. If you hope to motivate your students to work hard, your own efforts should reflect your commitment to hard work. Motivation for teachers includes "finding ways to get students to do things they might not want to do on their own." Also, this means finding ways to get students to do more than "know" health—to get them to put into *action* what they know. It is necessary to consider motivating techniques to discover

A teacher's task is to motivate students to want to learn.

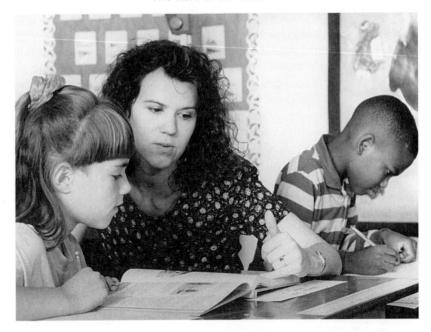

new ways to persuade youngsters to act in healthy ways. If the students are motivated about the subject, we can teach them the skills they'll need to make healthy decisions, and to act in healthy ways. No small part of our task as teachers has become to motivate them beyond apathy. The problem lies in fostering the kind of attitude that includes sacrifice and discipline—among the students and yourselves.

There is probably no phase of teaching health that is more grossly misunderstood by teachers than the area of motivation. Teachers tend to be highly motivated individuals, and they sometimes have trouble understanding or dealing with students who do not share equally their enthusiasm and love for education or health behaviors.

Realize that you can motivate dedicated students, and students who believe in you and your program. You cannot motivate students who feel no sense of responsibility or commitment to you or your program. Your task then, is obvious, to motivate your students to want to learn, and to want to be healthy. Students will more likely be motivated when they know you care enough about them to work as hard as you can to try to improve their skills.

In too many cases, we as health educators accept as truth the contention that students don't care about acting in healthy ways. Many young people are simply waiting for someone to guide them and care about them, and those are the students we have to find and motivate. If we accept as true that none of them will accept the challenge of excelling in an age of mediocrity, we're doing them a grave disservice—we're prejudging them toward the same mediocrity we want them to avoid. Not all young people are selfish and apathetic—many have not had the opportunity to challenge themselves to a higher purpose beyond mediocrity.

Teachers should understand that there are no shortcuts to success—no magic techniques known only to a few select teachers that will ensure effective teaching. The best teachers are, always have been, and always will be, those teachers who have worked hardest to motivate their students. Motivation is as important a part of any teacher's teaching as any part of their lesson plan. One cannot overstate or overestimate the effect of motivation (or lack of motivation) on the level of intensity of a student's performance.

2. *Be organized.* Students—especially young students—want and need the kind of guidance, leadership, and professionalism that is evidenced in teachers' efforts to organize their classes. Practice organization and attention to detail convey to your students in terms more vivid than you could ever express in words your concern for your program.

   Good organization is a habit. It's a copout to attempt to excuse away poor organization and administration in your program by saying "I'm just not an organized person."

3. *Be consistent in your relations with your students.* This doesn't mean that you have to treat all students alike. Students are not alike, and you should not treat them as if they are. Their motivations as well as their personalities vary widely. Some students thrive on praise and compliments, while others react as if a compliment were a signal that it's all right to quit working in class. Be alert to know the differences in your students, and learn what motivates them best.

   Students have the right to fair and equitable treatment, attention, and discipline. Treat all of them with dignity and respect.

4. *Avoid forming hasty (or permanent) negative opinions of students.* This sometimes happens when we pay attention to the teacher's lounge gossip about students that we are going to have in class. When we prejudge, the student never has a chance. Once we label a student, they tend to live up (or down) to that level of expectation.

5. *Never be too busy to listen to your students. Communication is a two-way street.* A Greek proverb says, "Whatever kind of word thou speakest, the like shalt thou hear."

   Students are expecting—or demanding through various forms of behavior—that teachers be concerned about them as human beings as well as students. When a student has a problem, the teacher should be willing to talk with him or her about it, and give the student a chance to talk it out. Sometimes all a youngster needs is an adult to give him a loving pat on the back that says, "I care," and to listen when the youngster needs someone to talk to. Genuine communication does not always require words; it grows out of a mutual sense of concern for others.

6. *Show love, care, and concern to your students.* Teachers may view their teaching as just a job, but students need guidance and a sense of belonging that grows out of a teacher's personal and professional behavior toward his or her students.

   Many teachers prefer not to become involved in the personal lives of their students. Increasingly, however, teachers are being required to deal with problems in students' personal lives that affect their in-class performances—and this is as it should be.

7. *Be a success yourself.* Success, like inventions, is 1 percent inspiration and 99 percent perspiration. Successful people invest in themselves. They go to seminars, read a lot, and consult with others. They are natural and eager learners. This doesn't mean they must go back to school, but they believe there's something to be learned from every encounter they have with other people and their ideas. They make sure there are lots of those encounters. Successful people believe they're in control of their lives (internal locus of control) and their fates. They know that effort means more than luck ("Luck is the loser's way of explaining the winner's victory"). Good luck comes from hard work. A surprising number of golden opportunities seem to open up for those people who work hardest at putting themselves on a successful path.

   Successful people help others succeed. Successful people extend themselves to others, but not with the thought of immediate return. Successful people aren't jealous or resentful of other people's success. Successful people are encouraged, not discouraged by the good things that happen to people around them. Successful people have self-confidence. They believe they can overcome obstacles.

8. *Be positive.* A key ingredient of success is the ability to eliminate from your own environment things that tend to put you in a negative or unresourceful state, while installing positive ones in

yourself and in others. Positive thinking and unswerving dedication to making a dream a reality will provide the incentive to carry through whatever hard times and negativism on the part of others that lies in your path. A teacher can't quit during the hard, frustrating times—you don't want your students to give up, so neither should you. You can and will learn more from the hard times than from those when things came easily. Change your vocabulary. Instead of "Why don't they do something about it?" make it "I know what I'm going to do." Expect, anticipate and welcome change. Change is normal and inevitable. With every change there is the unfamiliar and the unexpected. Risk it!

Use positive self-talk on a daily basis. Don't dwell on small ailments (positive thoughts can heal illnesses—negative thoughts bring on psychosomatic ills). Think highest and most uplifting thoughts. This is especially true regarding your students.

9. *Seek role models.* Benefit from others—If you think about why you are the way you are, chances are it has a lot to do with trying to be like someone you admired. Teachers usually have a teacher in their past that inspired them—therefore, they became teachers.

We never stop needing role models. Even superstars study them, copy them, compete with them, and try to surpass them. Goad yourself to meet new challenges, set new goals, then top your previous behavior.

10. *Set goals.* Another key to success is knowing what you want. People's abilities to fully tap their resources are directly affected by their goals. Before you can operate efficiently, you must develop specific goals. Outline your goals clearly. Concrete goals are easily understood by you and by students. Goals don't have to be elaborate. Set goals and develop a plan to achieve those goals.

11. *Work hard.* The road to success is never easy. To be a success, you have to work. This is not popular advice. Work and achievement are irrevocably linked.

12. *Stay mentally fresh.* No matter how well you are doing what you are doing, you can do it better by exposing yourself to interests and ideas outside your immediate, day-to-day activities. These ideas will spark your imagination and give you ideas you can use in your own work.

One excellent way to stay mentally fresh and get physically healthy at the same time, is to exercise. This is productive time away from work, time spent away from problems.

The Teacher as Part of the Health Team

Legal Responsibilities of the Teacher

One major concern of today's teacher is liability, because we live in a litigious society. Negligence can be charged when children are under your care and supervision, such as in the classroom, on the playground, and entering or departing buses. You are considered *in loco parentis* (or "in the place of parents") when a child is under your supervision. Your primary responsibility is to act responsibly to prevent injury to students. You should be well aware of first-aid and emergency procedures in order to care for a student in your charge, so as not to aggravate an existing injury or illness. You should follow your school system's procedure for filing a report for each accident. Each school should provide in-service preparation of faculty for preventing and handling accidents, and should have an active safety program. (Safety procedures and accident reports are discussed further in Chapter 18, "Intentional and Unintentional Injuries.")

Health Highlight

The Third Phi Delta Kappa Poll of Teachers' Attitudes toward the Public Schools

○ Teachers give their local public schools higher grades than the nation's schools.

○ Teachers says the biggest problem they face in their classrooms is lack of support from parents. Teachers' second biggest problem is funding for public education.

○ Less than half of all teachers say they would encourage the brightest student they know to become a teacher.

○ Practically all teachers agree that it is important for the nation's schools to prepare students to be responsible citizens.

○ Teachers agree that teachers are more committed to improving education than are state and local officials.

○ Teachers say discipline is the main reason teachers leave the profession. The second reason is low salaries.

Source: Carol A. Langdon. 1996. The third Phi Delta Kappa poll of teachers' attitudes toward the public schools. *Phi Delta Kappan* 78(3), 225-227.

Working with Students

One of the teacher's responsibilities is counseling students in health-related matters. Counseling should be straightforward, and free of moral judgment, preaching, or scare tactics. In the role of counselor, you must develop good listening skills and communication skills. Sometimes it is difficult to get to the heart of the problem; these skills will help you offer sound advice. Also, you need to show genuine empathy toward a student's problem.

No matter how concerned you are about a student's problem, you must recognize the limitations of your ability to help. If you cannot provide effective counseling, or if you realize that more help is necessary than you can give, refer the student to another teacher or an administrator. The student may also require additional guidance beyond the initial crisis counseling you can supply. Make sure you are familiar with available services in the school or community so you can refer the student to the most appropriate one. Most teachers are not professionally trained in counseling, nor are they expected to replace those who are. A teacher's personal attributes are as important as his or her knowledge of the subject.

Working with Parents

Always notify a student's parents when an illness or serious deviation from normal health occurs. School policy should be followed when parents are notified. Some schools require teachers to contact parents through the administrative offices. A good policy is to ensure that a member of the school administration is present at any parent–teacher conference. The third party can clear up any confusion in communication and can serve as an arbitrator in case of misunderstanding. Explain to the parents the significance of the child's health condition, and encourage them to obtain needed care for the child. If a parent asks for guidance in seeking care, refer the person to the proper agency or individual. Be sure to take an active role in following up any case reported to parents.

Health educators can involve parents in the health education of their children by sending information home in a newsletter and designing activities in which the parents help the children.

Working with Other Teachers and the School Administration

A major responsibility of the health teacher is to keep the other teachers and the administrators informed of health matters related to the community and students. This information will help the other faculty members and the administration to understand the students, and will also help them recognize the need for health education in the school.

The educator can represent the school on health-related committees of teacher–parent and community organizations. You can help other faculty and administrators be aware of the environmental conditions in the school that might be unhealthy to the students, staff, and faculty. You should also attempt to become involved in textbook selection committees. Look for sound, up-to-date content, but beware of textbooks that propagate stereotypes.

A primary duty of the health educator is to plan the health education curriculum and make recommendations to the administration regarding the health education program within the school. You can help interpret and implement any state requirement for the health curriculum. Also make suggestions concerning the health service program and health environment.

The teacher must also work closely with the school administration when notifying parents about a child's health, referring parents to appropriate health resources, and following up on student cases. Principals often request that the teacher be included in health-related referrals. The teacher should keep the administration informed about a child's progress in school after the child returns from an illness.

Working with the School or Clinic Nurse

Because you daily observe each child in your class, you can help the school nurse understand the health behavior of students. You can also assist the nurse in various aspects of the screening program—by preliminary screening in the classroom, by preparing students for screening tests to reduce their anxiety, and by referring students who are in particular need of screening. Teacher and nurse can cooperate in in-service workshops for the other faculty members. Finally, teachers who are properly trained can complement the school's emergency care program by offering their services when needed.

Working with Outside Agencies

One of your objectives should be to promote health education and awareness in the community. You can help volunteer organizations educate the community in health matters. Many of these agencies, such as the Heart Association and American Dental Association, have health curricula and need help to implement their programs in the schools. Through this cooperation, you can learn about other health professionals in your community and can acquaint yourself with the services offered to students by these agencies.

You should also become involved with the local public health department and cooperate with department staff members in providing services to the students and community.

Health educators can keep other professionals informed of health matters.

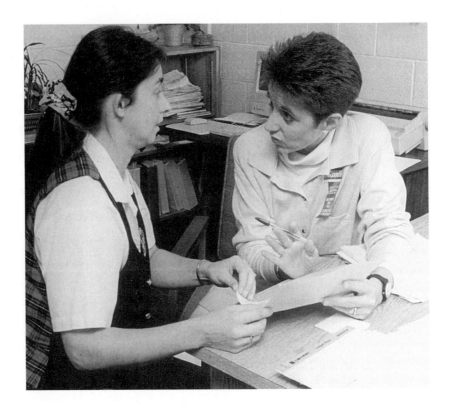

Finally, in this time of budget cuts and termination of health programs, you are strongly urged to become active in lobbying for health services and programs. Work with local teacher groups to educate legislators about health matters.

The Teacher's Responsibility in Education of the Disabled

Teacher Qualities. Teachers may have varying skills for accommodating individual differences when teaching specific content. Teacher attitudes toward acceptance of students with disabilities in their class and their ability to accommodate students with disabilities are important. Research shows that the majority of teachers believe that they are not equipped to deal with youngsters with special conditions. Further, studies indicate that teachers harbor generally negative attitudes toward students with disabilities whose ability levels and needs differ from those of most students. It is therefore extremely important that the teacher become knowledgeable about students with disabilities. A close working relationship should be established with the special education teacher, who has been trained and will be able to answer questions about most disabling conditions. The special education teacher should act as a consultant when specific information about a student is required.

As a teacher, help each child to understand and appreciate that he or she is unique and each of the other students in the class is unique. Emphasize what students *can* do rather than what they cannot do, and provide ways to let each student display his or her talents to the group. These positive actions will both help each student adjust to the regular classroom, and encourage students to accept each other.

▤ *Summary*

○ Health education has evolved from a diverse background over the past 170 years.

○ The nation's emphasis on health education has, in turn, led to a need for effective educators.

○ An effective educator must concentrate on academic preparation and personal qualifications.

○ Teaching health is different from other disciplines in the curriculum.

○ Each teacher must be aware that he or she is modeling health behavior to students through his or her lifestyle.

○ There are several barriers to successfully implementing health education.

○ Teachers can overcome these hindrances by keeping their knowledge of health current, by learning how to present controversial information in the classroom, and by helping administrators see how health education can be integrated with other required subjects.

○ Educators who model good health behavior have a positive impact on their students.

○ Several specific characteristics and actions will help a teacher become a quality educator.

○ Teamwork with parents, the school nurse, the school physician, administrators, community organizations, and students is the key to a successful school health program.

○ As part of the team, the teacher

is aware of his or her legal responsibilities

observes each student for any deviation from normal health

reports to the proper authority within the school

is available to refer the student and parent to the appropriate community resource or to counsel the student and/or parent concerning the child's health.

○ Teaching students with special needs is a challenge for all educators, including health educators.

Discussion Questions

1. Describe the challenges in the role of the elementary health teacher.
2. How does health education differ from other subject area instruction?
3. Discuss the interdisciplinary nature of health as a barrier to implementing good health instruction.
4. Describe the role of the National Commission for Health Education Credentialing in promoting the health education profession.
5. Why is it crucial for any teacher to be a positive role model in health behavior to the students?
6. List the characteristics and actions that will help you become a quality educator.
7. Discuss the ways in which a teacher can work with other teachers to improve the comprehensive school health program.
8. Why should an administrator be present at any parent–teacher conference?
9. Describe the teacher qualities needed to work effectively with handicapped students.
10. Discuss how a teacher can involve parents in their child's health education.

References

Allensworth, Diane, Cynthia Symons, and R. Scott Olds. 1995. *Healthy students 2000: An agenda for continuous improvement in America's schools.* Kent, OH: American School Health Association.

Langdon, Carol A. 1996. The third Phi Delta Kappa poll of teachers' attitudes toward the public schools. *Phi Delta Kappan,* 78(3): 225-227.

Marx, Eva, and Daphne Northrop. 1995. *Educating for health: A guide to implementing a comprehensive approach to school health education.* Newton, MA: Education Development Center.

National Task Force on the Preparation and Practice of Health Educators. 1988. *A Framework for the Development of Competency-based Curricula for Entry-Level Health Educators.* New York: National Task Force on the Preparation and Practice of Health Educators.

Redican, Kerry J., and Elyzabeth J. Holford. 1996. The certified health education specialist and malpractice. *Journal of health education,* 27(4): 257-260.

Schima, Marilyn, and Evelyn E. Ames. 1996. The health education profession in the twenty-first century: Setting the stage. *Journal of health education:* 27(6): 358.

Chapter Three

Planning for Health Instruction

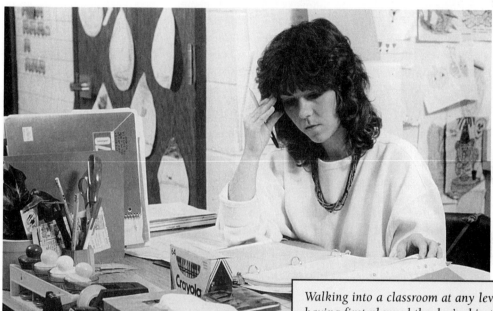

> Walking into a classroom at any level without having first planned the day's objectives is like beginning an automobile trip with an empty gas tank.
>
> —Donald A. Read and Walter H. Greene

Valued Outcomes

After reading this chapter, you should be able to

○ list the content areas of health education

○ describe the scope and sequence of health education

○ discuss the factors that influence what is taught in elementary health education

○ identify the variety of curricular approaches used in school health education

○ design an effective lesson plan

○ compare the various classifications of objectives

○ write instructional objectives

○ discuss how to plan and teach controversial health education topics

Content Areas in the Elementary School ———

Teaching health education, like teaching any subject, requires careful planning. Teachers must know what to teach, when to teach it, and how to teach it so that the content is internalized, or personalized, by the students. First graders are vastly different from eighth graders. Health instruction at each grade level must be tailored to the maturational, intellectual, and interest levels of the students.

Virtually every state department of education has a health education curriculum that can be used as a guide for planning. It should be read carefully, for in it can be found a recommended list of topics to be presented at each grade level.

Teachers must recognize the complexity of life and attempt to incorporate the dimensions of wellness (physical, social, intellectual, emotional, spiritual) into health instruction.

The general public often visualizes elementary health instruction merely in terms of rules for brushing teeth and riding bicycles safely. It is, of course, far more. Various health education authorities cite from ten to twenty different content areas, depending on how the areas are grouped or separated. Most health educators agree on the content areas for elementary health instruction shown in Figure 3.1.

The ultimate reason for all health education is to increase in each student the **health literacy** or "the capacity of the individual to obtain, interpret, and understand basic health information and services and the competence to use such information and services in ways which are health enhancing" (AAHE, 1995, 75).

Content areas and topics also change in emphasis to reflect current knowledge and health concerns.

Grade Placement for Health Education Topics

Once basic content areas have been charted, it must be determined how much emphasis will be placed on each area at each grade level. Emphasis should be based on the developmental level,

Figure 3.1
Content Areas
of Health Education

- ○ Mental/emotional health
- ○ Body systems and the senses
- ○ Nutrition
- ○ Family life
- ○ Alcohol, drugs, and tobacco (substance use and abuse)

- ○ Safety and first aid
- ○ Personal health
- ○ Consumer health
- ○ Diseases: chronic and communicable
- ○ Environmental health

health needs, and interests of the students. A planned cycle of presentation of content areas ensures that necessary topics will be included and will receive appropriate emphasis at each grade level.

A cycle plan helps eliminate useless repetition and ensures that topics are covered to the depth necessary for a particular grade. A cycle plan also prepares children for the subject matter awaiting them in their remaining educational experiences.

Developing Scope and Sequence

Content areas must not only be identified, they must also be ordered and organized. That is, the scope and sequence of the health education curriculum must be determined. **Scope** refers to the depth or difficulty of the material—the "what" to teach. **Sequence** refers to the order in which the material is to be covered—the "when" to teach it. Here again the state department of education health guide or the local guide can be of great use. Such guides usually spell out the scope and sequence of health education for each grade level. They may also indicate what competencies a child should possess after completing the course of study.

Planned health instruction should attempt to ensure that each previous learning experience provides the basis for new learning. Topics should build on one another and not be presented as discrete bits of information. Concepts within each lesson should relate to each other, lessons within a unit should relate to each other, and units within the course should relate to each other. In this way, students will see health education as a whole rather than as seemingly unrelated fragments.

Scope also refers to the arrangement of the curriculum from kindergarten through senior high school. As such, it serves as a reminder that everything done in the classroom should be built on what has been previously accomplished so that initial learning becomes the basis for subsequent learning.

The National Health Education Standards can be found in the Health Highlight on pages 41-47. These standards should serve as the foundation for curriculum development and instruction in health education. Not shown in this excerpt, but contained in the original document are the performance indicators for the National Health Education Standards. These standards are a framework for health educators in the United States. The goal is to create an instructional program that will enable students to experience comprehensive health education, which in turn will enable them to become/remain healthy and to achieve academic success (AAHE, 1995, p. 1).

Determining What to Teach

Although state health education guidelines are helpful in determining the scope and sequence of the health curriculum, they should not be the sole planning aid. In developing the curriculum, other factors, such as the social mores of the community, student interest, and student health needs, must be considered. Curriculum needs may vary according to community, state, or region.

Social Mores

The curriculum that is developed must be acceptable to the community in which it is located. Ascertaining the social mores of the community demands careful judgment. Teachers have an advantage if they are well acquainted with the community, perhaps through long-term residence.

Even then, however, it may be difficult to assess feelings within the community about how best to teach certain health topics, such as substance abuse or family life education. Controversial topics should be discussed with administrators before any course of instruction is implemented.

Another community influence on curriculum development comes from special interest groups, which may be national, state, or local. Their charge is to promote or protect their own philosophy or special interests. Most of these groups are sincere about bringing beneficial services to the children in a community, but such groups can also have a detrimental influence on curriculum development. For example, groups that form to stop family life education can be formidable opponents to the development of a comprehensive health education program. Regardless of content area, it is wise to be familiar with local and state guides and recommendations for teaching health education.

Student Interest

Children are more interested in certain health topics than in others, depending on their age. For example, younger children are apt to be more interested in the parts and functions of their bodies than are older children. Also, because primary age children are more self-centered, they are less concerned about social topics than are upper elementary age children.

Questionnaires, checklists, and direct questioning can all aid in determining student interest in the classroom. In fact, there is no substitute for interacting directly with a class to gauge interest in various topics. Familiarity with professional literature on the subject is equally important. There are basic health interests common to all students, regardless of locality or socioeconomic class.

Later in elementary school, children's abstract reasoning becomes better developed, and students are capable of dealing with more than immediate life situations. Then, increasingly abstract health concepts, such as pollution or aging, can be taught. Reasoning and insight into causal relationships also develop.

Learning activities help children internalize the content and form concepts. The teacher must select the activities that are best suited to each class.

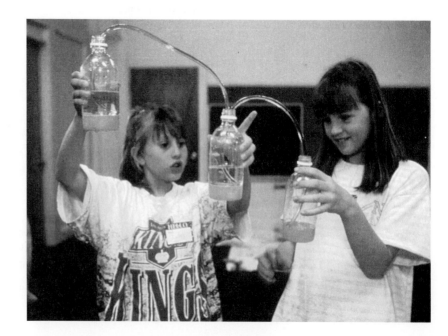

Health Highlight

The National Health Education Standards
Health Education Standard 1:

Students will comprehend concepts related to health promotion and disease prevention.

Rationale

Basic to health education is a foundation of knowledge about the interrelationship of behavior and health, interactions within the human body, and the prevention of diseases and other health problems. Experiencing physical, mental, emotional, and social changes as one grows and develops, provides a self-contained "learning laboratory." Comprehension of health promotion strategies and disease prevention concepts enables students to become health-literate, self-directed learners, which establishes a foundation for leading healthy and productive lives.

Performance Indicators

As a result of health instruction in grades K–4, students will

1. describe relationships between personal health behaviors and individual well being.
2. identify indicators of mental, emotional, social, and physical health during childhood.
3. describe the basic structure and functions of the human body systems.
4. describe how the family influences personal health.
5. describe how physical, social, and emotional environments influence personal health.
6. identify common health problems of children.
7. identify health problems that should be detected and treated early.
8. explain how childhood injuries and illnesses can be prevented or treated.

As a result of health instruction in grades 5–8, students will

1. explain the relationship between positive health behaviors and the prevention of injury, illness, disease, and premature death.
2. describe the interrelationship of mental, emotional, social, and physical health during adolescence.
3. explain how health is influenced by the interaction of body systems.
4. describe how family and peers influence the health of adolescents.
5. analyze how environment and personal health are interrelated.
6. describe ways to reduce risks related to adolescent health problems.
7. explain how appropriate health care can prevent premature death and disability.
8. describe how lifestyle, pathogens, family history, and other risk factors are related to the cause or prevention of disease and other health problems.

Health Highlight

The National Health Education Standards
Health Education Standard 2:

Students will demonstrate the ability to access valid health information and health-promoting products and services.

Rationale

Accessing valid health information and health-promoting products and services is important in the prevention, early detection, and treatment of most health problems. Critical thinking involves the ability to identify valid health information and to analyze, select, and access health-promoting services and products. Applying skills of information analysis, organization, comparison, synthesis, and evaluation to health issues provides a foundation for individuals to move toward becoming health-literate and responsible, productive citizens.

Performance Indicators

As a result of health instruction in grades K–4, students will

1. identify characteristics of valid health information and health-promoting products and services.

2. demonstrate the ability to locate resources from home, school and community that provide valid health information.

3. explain how media influences the selection of health information, products, and services.

4. demonstrate the ability to locate school and community health helpers.

As a result of health instruction in grades 5–8, students will

1. analyze the validity of health information, products, and services.

2. demonstrate the ability to utilize resources from home, school, and community that provide valid health information.

3. analyze how media influences the selection of health information and products.

4. demonstrate the ability to locate health products and services.

5. compare the costs and validity of health products.

6. describe situations requiring professional health services.

Health Needs

All children, regardless of community, have certain basic health needs. These include the need for love and nurturing, sound nutrition, intellectual stimulation, proper dental care, and safety. However, specific health needs vary from community to community, and the curriculum that you plan should take into account these special needs. For example, inner-city children may need to receive emphasized instruction about the dangers of lead poisoning, as many inner-city dwellings still contain lead-based paint. Similarly, the safety instruction provided will vary, depending on whether the community is a rural or an urban one.

Health Highlight

The National Health Education Standards
Health Education Standard 3:

Students will demonstrate the ability to practice health-enhancing behaviors and reduce health risks.

Rationale

Research confirms that many diseases and injuries can be prevented by reducing harmful and risk-taking behaviors. More importantly, recognizing and practicing health-enhancing behaviors can contribute to a positive quality of life. Strategies used to maintain and improve positive health behaviors will utilize knowledge and skills that help students become critical thinkers and problem solvers. By accepting responsibility for personal health, students will have a foundation for living a healthy, productive life.

Performance Indicators

As a result of health instruction in grades K–4, students will

1. identify responsible health behaviors.
2. identify personal health needs.
3. compare behaviors that are safe to those that are risky or harmful.
4. demonstrate strategies to improve or maintain personal health.
5. develop injury prevention and management strategies for personal health.
6. demonstrate ways to avoid and reduce threatening situations.
7. apply skills to manage stress.

As a result of health instruction in grades 5–8, students will

1. explain the importance of assuming responsibility for personal health behaviors.
2. analyze a personal health assessment to determine health strengths and risks.
3. distinguish between safe and risky or harmful behaviors in relationships.
4. demonstrate strategies to improve or maintain personal and family health.
5. develop injury prevention and management strategies for personal and family health.
6. demonstrate ways to avoid and reduce threatening situations.
7. demonstrate strategies to manage stress.

Textbooks and Courses of Study

Most elementary health textbooks contain detailed suggestions for developing curricula. The teacher's editions of these texts provide outlines and units for teaching health and identify major concepts to be taught at a given grade level. Like state health guidelines, however, textbooks cannot provide a course of study tailored to a specific community and a specific classroom. Because textbooks are developed for use nationally, they may lack sufficient depth of coverage on topics of particular relevance to a given setting.

Health Highlight

The National Health Education Standards
Health Education Standard 4:

Students will analyze the influence of culture, media, technology, and other factors on health.

Rationale

Health is influenced by a variety of factors that coexist within society. These include the cultural context as well as media and technology. A critical thinker and problem solver is able to analyze, evaluate, and interpret the influence of these factors on health. The health-literate, responsible, and productive citizen draws on the contributions of culture, media, technology, and other factors to strengthen individual, family, and community health.

Performance Indicators

As a result of health instruction in grades K–4, students will

1. describe how culture influences personal health behaviors.

2. explain how media influences thoughts, feelings, and health behaviors.

3. describe ways technology can influence personal health.

4. explain how information from school and family influences health.

As a result of health instruction in grades 5–8, students will

1. describe the influence of cultural beliefs on health behaviors and the use of health services.

2. analyze how messages from media and other sources influence health behaviors.

3. analyze the influence of technology on personal and family health.

4. analyze how information from peers influences health.

To supplement the textbook you use, you will probably wish to obtain pamphlets, filmstrips, CD-ROMs, and other learning aids from government or private health-related agencies such as the U.S. Department of Agriculture or the National Safety Council. Most health-related agencies will make classroom materials available free of charge or at a nominal cost. Be sure, however, to screen all materials before classroom use to determine their appropriateness, currentness, and possible biases.

Barriers to Quality Health Education

Providing a quality, comprehensive health education experience for students is not an easy task. Because health education is in constant change, it is imperative to understand that there are potential and real obstacles to achieving quality health education. Some of the barriers, identified by the Gallup Organization (1994) are

Health Highlight

The National Health Education Standards
Health Education Standard 5:

Students will demonstrate the ability to use interpersonal communication skills to enhance health.

Rationale

Personal, family, and community health are enhanced through effective communication. A responsible individual will use verbal and nonverbal skills in developing and maintaining healthy personal relationships. Ability to organize and to convey information, beliefs, opinions, and feelings are skills that strengthen interactions and can reduce or avoid conflict. When communicating, individuals who are health literate demonstrate care, consideration, and respect of self and others.

Performance Indicators

As a result of health instruction in grades K–4, students will

1. distinguish between verbal and nonverbal communication.

2. describe characteristics needed to be a responsible friend and family member.

3. demonstrate healthy ways to express needs, wants, and feelings.

4. demonstrate ways to communicate care, consideration, and respect of self and others.

5. demonstrate attentive listening skills to build and maintain healthy relationships.

6. demonstrate refusal skills to enhance health.

7. differentiate between negative and positive behaviors used in conflict situations.

8. demonstrate nonviolent strategies to resolve conflicts.

As a result of health instruction in grades 5–8, students will

1. demonstrate effective verbal and nonverbal communication skills to enhance health.

2. describe how the behavior of family and peers affects interpersonal communication.

3. demonstrate healthy ways to express needs, wants, and feelings.

4. demonstrate ways to communicate care, consideration, and respect of self and others.

5. demonstrate communication skills to build and maintain healthy relationships.

6. demonstrate refusal and negotiation skills to enhance health.

7. analyze the possible causes of conflict among youth in schools and communities.

8. demonstrate strategies to manage conflict in healthy ways.

Health Highlight

The National Health Education Standards
Health Education Standard 6:

Students will demonstrate the ability to use goal-setting and decision-making skills to enhance health.

Rationale

Decision making and goal setting are essential lifelong skills needed in order to implement and sustain health-enhancing behaviors. These skills make it possible for individuals to transfer health knowledge into healthy lifestyles. When applied to health issues, decision-making, and goal-setting skills will enable individuals to collaborate with others to improve the quality of life in their families, schools and communities.

Performance Indicators

As a result of health instruction in grades K–4, students will

1. demonstrate the ability to apply a decision-making process to health issues and problems.

2. explain when to ask for assistance in making health-related decisions and setting health goals.

3. predict outcomes of positive health decisions.

4. set a personal health goal and track progress toward its achievement.

As a result of health instruction in grades 5–8, students will

1. demonstrate the ability to apply a decision-making process to health issues and problems individually and collaboratively.

2. analyze how health-related decisions are influenced by individuals, family, and community values.

3. predict how decisions regarding health behaviors have consequences for self and others.

4. apply strategies and skills needed to attain personal health goals.

5. describe how personal health goals are influenced by changing information, abilities, priorities, and responsibilities.

6. develop a plan that addresses personal strengths, needs, and health risks.

○ lack of appreciation for the relationship between health status and success in academic and work performance

○ low levels of commitment by school board members and administrators

○ inadequately prepared teachers

○ insufficient funding for resources and staff development

Health Highlight

The National Health Education Standards
Health Education Standard 7:

Students will demonstrate the ability to advocate for personal, family, and community health.

Rationale

Quality of life is dependent on an environment that protects and promotes the health of individuals, families, and communities. Responsible citizens, who are health literate, are characterized by advocating and communicating for positive health in their communities. A variety of health advocacy skills are critical to these activities.

Performance Indicators

As a result of health instruction in grades K–4, students will

1. describe a variety of methods to convey accurate health information and ideas.

2. express information and opinions about health issues.

3. identify community agencies that advocate for healthy individuals, families, and communities.

4. demonstrate the ability to influence and support others in making positive health choices.

As a result of health instruction in grades 5–8, students will

1. analyze various communication methods to accurately express health information and ideas.

2. express information and opinions about health issues.

3. identify barriers to effective communication of information, ideas, feelings, and opinions about health issues.

4. demonstrate the ability to influence and support others in making positive health choices.

5. demonstrate the ability to work cooperatively when advocating for healthy individuals, families, and schools.

○ lack of parent and community involvement and support

○ overcrowded curricula with little or no time for health education

○ impersonalized school environment

○ unconnected and seemingly irrelevant health instruction

○ lack of recognition of the contribution made by health education to the achievement of the academic goals of schools

○ failure to adequately document student performance in achievement of health literacy

○ failure to make connections between health instruction and other disciplines and to the world outside of school

Health literacy is the ability of the student to obtain, interpret, and understand basic health information and services and the competence to use information and services in ways that are health enhancing (AAHE, 1995, 75).

Teaching for Values

Values give direction to life and determine behavior. Members of our society share many of the same values. However, each community, family, and individual has a more specific set of values. Values are closely linked with personal feelings and must be carefully considered when planning health instruction. Failure to do so can result both in the blocking of effective learning and opposition from parents and community organizations. Values are learned through a variety of experiences and interactions with the environment. The family, peer group, school, church, and media all influence personal value formation. In other words, value formation is a continual process. Yet many parents become concerned when formal teaching about values takes place in the schools. There is concern that values contrary to the parents' values will be inculcated. Any recommendation or point of emphasis by a teacher can be construed as the imposition of values. Conversely, to take no stand at all can imply an anything-goes attitude.

Therefore, in planning health instruction, it must be made clear how values will be a part of the teaching. A teacher's job is not to impose his or her values; it is to help children develop their own values by making wise decisions about health-related matters. Children will form values with or without their teacher's assistance, but their teacher can help them make positive decisions that will lead to high-level wellness by providing factual knowledge about health and by allowing children to clarify their own feelings.

Attitudes and behavior are intertwined. If a balance between knowledge and attitudes toward health education is to be achieved, student feelings must be addressed in teaching. In other words, the study of health must be personalized if it is to have an impact. By providing opportunities for children to identify feelings and personalize health information, teachers can help them understand how information, attitudes, and behavior affect quality of life. In doing so, children become better equipped to deal with peer pressure, communicate more effectively, and develop sound decision-making skills.

Each person must weigh the importance or value of a decision against perceived rewards and costs involved. To brush one's teeth regularly, to smoke, to have regular physical examinations, and to experiment with drugs are all examples of decisions that affect health. Decisions must be made by the individual; consequently, teachers must make a planned effort to help children think through the possible consequences of health-related decisions.

Curriculum Approaches

Beginning teachers will probably find many helpful resources they can use to plan a course of health education for the class. As noted, these resources include the state health education guidelines, commercial health education textbook series, and materials from government and private health-related agencies.

School Health Education Study (SHES)

SHES is mentioned because it holds historical significance and serves as a reference for several curriculum projects. Although dated, it still reflects an excellent conceptualization of health education.

SHES is a comprehensive kindergarten through twelfth grade health education curriculum that was developed in the 1960s. The project developers visualized health as having physical, mental, and social dimensions, as shown in Figure 3.2. In this conceptual model, health is seen as "dynamic interaction and interdependence among the individual's physical well-being, his mental and emotional reactions, and the social complex in which he exists" (School Health Education Study 1967).

This interaction and interdependence are reflected in the key concepts shown in the model: growing and developing, interacting, and decision making. Growing and developing are defined as a dynamic life process by which the individual is in some ways like all individuals, in some ways like some individuals, and in some ways like no other individual. Interacting is an ongoing process in which the individual is affected by and in turn affects certain biological, social, psychological, economic, and physical forces in the environment. Decision making is a uniquely human process of consciously opting to take or not to take an action or of choosing one alternative rather than another.

The scope of the SHES curriculum is embodied in the ten concept statements shown in Figure 3.2 as Cl, C2, and so on. These statements are as follows:

1. Growth and development influence and are influenced by the structure and functioning of the individual.

2. Growing and developing follow a predictable sequence, yet are unique for each individual.

3. Protection and promotion of health is an individual, community, and international responsibility.

4. The potential for hazards and accidents exists, whatever the environment.

5. There are reciprocal relationships involving humankind, disease, and environment.

6. The family serves to perpetuate humankind and to fulfill certain health needs.

7. Personal health practices are affected by a complexity of forces, often conflicting.

8. Utilization of health information, products, and services is guided by values and perceptions.

9. Use of substances that modify mood and behavior arises from a variety of motivations.

10. Food selection and eating patterns are determined by physical, social, mental, economic, and cultural factors (School Health Education Study 1967, 21–23).

Subconcepts of these ten conceptual areas serve as guides in the selection and ordering of subject matter, as well as in the development of appropriate instructional or behavioral objectives. Each subconcept is viewed through physical, mental, and social dimensions. For each of the concepts, long-range goals are stated in terms of behavioral objectives. These goals represent desired student outcomes for the total sequential curriculum.

The SHES curriculum marked an important breakthrough in comprehensive kindergarten through twelfth grade health education. The emphasis is on the conceptualization of concepts rather than facts, because facts become dated and require constant revision.

The National Diffusion Network (NDN)

There are many approaches to health education at the national, state, and local level. There are so many that it is difficult for teachers to determine what is an excellent, good, or (sometimes) a poor program. State and local districts often have their own plans for curriculum, but teachers who are asked to review or select a new program may find it a difficult task based on the overwhelming number of plans available.

Figure 3.2
Conceptual Model of the SHES Curriculum

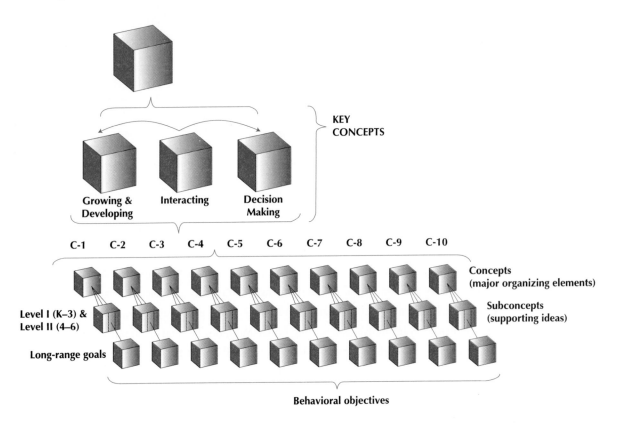

One of the best ways to approach the task is by becoming familiar with the **National Diffusion Network (NDN).** This federally funded program is designed to improve educational opportunities and achievement for all levels of education. NDN's philosophy is to identify exemplary programs from their development sites and transfer them to other educational settings. NDN provides educational institutions with a wide array of offerings from which to select those that best meet their respective philosophies, needs, and resources. Limited funds are also available to help create awareness of outstanding programs, help with adoption decisions, and provide in-service training and follow-up assistance. Some funds are also available for the purchase of teaching aids.

To be classified as an "exemplary program," a program must be reviewed by the Program Effectiveness Panel (PEP), which represents the U.S. Department of Education. Approval by PEP means that the panel has examined objective evidence of effectiveness submitted by the developers of the program. The panel must be convinced that the program has met its stated objectives at the developmental site. In addition, the developers must prove that the program will meet the educational needs of others in similar locations (NDN 1995, 9). Approved programs are eligible for NDN funds or from other federal funding programs.

To help public and private schools identify NDN programs, the U.S. Department of Education supports facilitators' projects in every state, the District of Columbia, and several territories throughout the world. These facilitators help schools determine their problems, determine their needs, and select NDN programs appropriate for their situation. The facilitators can aid in providing training and follow-up and in either monitoring or evaluating the program(s) selected by the schools. Limited funds also are available to support travel to demonstration sites.

Health Programs Approved by NDN

Although programs are certified and recertified for NDN exemplary program status, the 1995 edition of *Education Programs That Work* lists the following elementary health programs: (1) Healthy for Life (HFL), (2) Know Your Body (KYB) School Health Promotion Program, (3) Social Decision Making and Problem Solving, (4) Project Choice, (5) Growing Healthy, (6) Me-Me Drug and Alcohol Prevention Education Program, and (6) Ombudsman. All descriptions of the programs are those provided by NDN in the 1995 edition of *Education Programs That Work,* pages 9-2 to 9-11.

Healthy for Life (HFL). A program designed to help students in grades 6-8 to manage situations that are high risk. The program seeks to improve health behaviors in nutrition, tobacco, alcohol, marijuana use, and sexuality.

Description Healthy for Life (HFL) is a comprehensive program composed of four components: (1) **curriculum** that is cumulative, sequenced, and focused on health promotion lessons, activities, and teaching strategies; (2) **peer leadership** to employ students to teach through their words and actions; (3) **family** to facilitate communication between the adolescent and one significant family member or other adult; and (4) **community** to enlist community people actively working to reinforce the behavioral messages of the curriculum and launch an attack on the pervasive double messages about the target behaviors that most communities transmit. Games, role plays, videos, cooperative learning activities, and hands-on demonstrations keep students engaged and participating. Homework, which involves students "interviewing" parents, encourages the sharing of family values and rules. Fifty-eight lessons in sequence everyday for four weeks, first to one cohort of sixth graders and then to the same cohort as seventh and eighth graders. In this version, topics are addressed when they are most salient in the adolescent's life, and students build on their skills and experiences in previous grades. The intensive version delivers the lessons in one sequential, twelve-week block to an entire cohort of seventh graders.

Know Your Body (KYB) School Health Promotion Program. A multicomponent comprehensive school health promotion program for students in grades K–6 with the goal of empowering students with the skills they need to make their own positive health choices.

Audience Approved by PEP for students in grades K–6.

Description The Know Your Body (KYB) School Health Promotion Program consists of five basic components: (1) skills-based health education curriculum, (2) teacher/coordinator training, (3) biomedical screening, (4) extracurricular activities, and (5) program evaluation.

The curriculum and the teacher/coordinator training are considered the "core" components of the program, while the others are considered optional components or "enhancements." Although implementation of the full KYB program is recommended, the program may be effectively implemented without the additional components. The American Health Foundation will assist schools to customize a program that best suits their needs, goals, philosophies, and capacities.

KYB curriculum materials include age-appropriate teacher's guides (grades K–6), student master sheets (grades K–3); student activity books (grades 4–6); a class Big Book (grade 1); and puppet sets (grades K–3). A comprehensive user's guide (*Coordinator's Guide*) is also available, which provides detailed instructions for implementing all of KYB's program components.

The program stresses individual responsibility for health and provides the basis for making health-promoting and disease-preventing decisions. Behavioral goals are geared toward outcomes that children of this age can realistically affect, such as breakfast and snack choices, and asking adults not to smoke in their presence.

It is recommended that the KYB program be taught a minimum of 40 minutes per week. Most teachers are able to use the program much more often because of its interdisciplinary approach.

The KYB program addresses the National Goals for Education in several ways. Through its substance use prevention, healthy relationship, and skill modules, the program can help reduce drug use and violence (Goal 7). As part of the KYB training, program coordinators learn how to improve their school food service programs as well as how to achieve a smoke-free campus, thereby creating an "environment conducive to learning."

Me-Me Drug & Alcohol Prevention Education Program. A school-based, multidisciplinary, year-long prevention program that helps improve children's self-esteem, their ability to solve problems and make responsible decisions, and increases their knowledge about the dangers of all drugs, in grades 1–6.

Description The Me-Me Drug & Alcohol Prevention Education Program was developed to improve low self-esteem and other conditions found to be evident in most young people and adults who abuse drugs and alcohol. The program places great emphasis on enhancing the self-esteem of children during their formulative years when most of their learning and identifying who they are takes place. Children learn to make responsible decisions by learning how to predict the consequences of their choices and to recognize and resist negative peer influences. They receive the most up-to-date information about the dangers of all drugs including prescription, over-the-counter medicines, and alcohol. The Me-Me Program meets the National Goals for Education that pertain to (1) student achievement and citizenship; and (2) safe, disciplined, drug-free schools. All classroom teachers (K–6) are responsible for implementing the program and coordinating their teaching styles with the program's goals. Activities are incorporated into all areas of the curriculum as well as noncurriculum areas. An entirely new curriculum has been written and expanded to include other areas of concern. A parent component has been added that includes areas not previously explored in other programs. All teachers must attend a six-hour training conducted at their site. Program expenses include manuals for each teacher costing $48 per set ($18 for kindergarten teachers), travel, lodging, and meal expenses for the trainer. Everything used in the program is found in the manuals. Technical assistance is available. General information about the program is available at no cost, and program staff are available to conduct awareness sessions.

Ombudsman. A school-based drug education/primary prevention program. Grades 5-6.

Description Ombudsman is a structured course designed to reduce certain psychological and attitudinal states closely related to drug use. Through experiential activities, *Ombudsman* teaches healthy living skills and emphasizes information about drugs.

The course has three major phases. The first phase focuses on self-awareness and includes a series of exercises permitting students to gain a wider understanding and appreciation of their values as autonomous individuals.

The second phase teaches group skills and provides students with an opportunity to develop communication, decision-making, and problem-solving techniques that can be applied in the immediate class situation as well as in other important group contexts such as with family and peers.

The third phase is in many ways the most important: The class uses the insights and skills gained during the first two phases to plan and carry out the program within the community or school. During this phase, students have an opportunity to experience the excitement and satisfaction of reaching out to others in a creative and constructive way. The program is designed for thirty 50-minute implementation sessions.

Growing Healthy®. Comprehensive health education program (designed to foster student competencies to make decisions enhancing their health and lives. Grades K–6.

Description Growing Healthy includes a planned sequential curriculum, a variety of teaching methods, a teacher training program, and strategies for eliciting community support for school health education. Through group and individual activities, children learn about themselves by learning about their bodies. There is one 8-12-week unit for grades K through 6. Each grade studies a separate unit specifically designed for that age group. The units include an introduction of the five senses, feelings, caring for health, wellness, and general health habits; the senses of taste, touch, and smell and their roles in communicating health information; the emotions and communication methods with regard to sight and hearing; the skeletal and muscular systems; the digestive system; the respiratory system; the circulatory system; and the nervous system. Throughout all grades, health information about safety, nutrition, environment, drugs and alcohol, hygiene, fitness, mental health, disease prevention, consumer health, wellness and lifestyle is explored and reinforced. Access to a variety of stimulating learning resources, including audiovisuals, models, community health workers, and reading materials, is abundantly provided. The curriculum is designed to integrate with the lives and personality development of children by providing situations in which they may assume responsibility, research ideas, share knowledge, discuss values, make decisions, and create activities to illustrate their comprehension and internalization of concepts, attitudes, and feelings. The curriculum has been developed to enhance other school subjects such as reading, writing, arithmetic, physical education, science, and the creative arts. Twenty-four separate studies have been completed including a ten-year longitudinal study. These studies indicate that Growing Healthy was effective in increasing health-related knowledge and providing positive health-related attitudes. Growing Healthy requires a school team comprised of two classroom teachers, the principal, and one or more curriculum support persons to receive training in the grade level being adopted.

CASPAR Alcohol and Drug Education Series. Curriculum to improve attitudes and cognitive knowledge related to alcohol and alcoholism. Grades 7-12.

Description The CASPAR Alcohol and Drug Education Series has modules for elementary grades K–3 and 3–6, intermediate grades 7–8, and high school grades 9–12. Each unit is designed for seven to ten 45-minute teaching periods, with flexibility for expansion or contraction. Factual information, personal and societal attitudes about alcohol, and decision-making and refusal skills are covered during the first six or seven periods, with alcoholism covered only during the last one to three periods, when children who are experiencing family problems will be more ready to accept this information. The curricula emphasizes high student involvement through participatory activities such as debates, role plays, polls, drawings, and small-group discussions. Activities focus on real-life issues and situations, and convey repeated and consistent messages about safe behavior and responsible decision making. Evaluation evidence from a number of sites indicates that proper implementation facilitates referrals, increases knowledge, and affects attitudes, and that these changes remain for at least a year. Published evidence also suggests that repeated exposure may decrease rates of problem drinking.

CASPAR has revised its curricula to include drug education units at all grade levels to be used in conjunction with its alcohol units. The drug lessons include participatory activities, age-appropriate information, and emphasize a nonuse message.

Project CHOICE.   A cancer prevention program for students grades K–12. Grades K–12.

Description   Project CHOICE is a cancer prevention and risk-reduction curriculum for students in grades K–12. The program lessons are taught during a two-week time period at each grade level. The Project CHOICE curriculum consists of comprehensive, sequential units that promote three primary learning goals: (1) Students will learn cancer information and components of cancer risk, (2) students will learn a rational process of information evaluation and decision making, and (3) students will assume the locus of responsibility for behaviors leading to cancer risk reduction and wellness.

The curriculum kits include original filmstrips, experiments, decision-making scenarios, group work, classroom reports, debates and discussions. The overall program emphasis is on positive health promotion, personal responsibility for health, the role of health professionals, and an understanding of risk and risk reduction concept. The lesson themes attempt to replace a fear of cancer with a positive and active approach to maintaining health. At different grade levels the units deal with seven broad areas of cancer risk: host factors; drugs, including alcohol and tobacco; occupational hazards; stress; environmental factors, including radiation exposure; nutrition; and sun exposure.

Not all cancers can or will be eliminated by cancer risk reduction practices; therefore, students are taught to understand and recognize cancer warning signs, methods of early detection, appropriate treatment, and unproven methods of cancer treatment. By developing their own personal cancer risk reduction plans, students enhance their awareness of their own responsibility for their health. Teachers are provided with complete lesson plans, student learning objectives, a *Cancer Resource Guide* with information that corresponds to lesson content, and all teaching materials.

Social Decision Making and Problem Solving.   This program teaches all children to "think clearly" when under stress. The program is curriculum-based and occurs in three developmental phases. The readiness phase targets self-control, group participation, and social awareness skills. The instructional phase teaches an eight-step social decision-making strategy to students. The application phase teaches children to use these skills in real-life interpersonal and academic situations.

Audience   Approved by PEP for teachers, administrators, guidance, child study team staff, and parents of children in grades K–6, both in regular and special education programs.

Description   Social Decision Making and Problem Solving works by training educators and parents to equip children with skills in self-control and group participation, the use of an eight-step social decision-making strategy, and the practical know-how regarding the use of these skills in real life and academic areas.

The program is curriculum based and occurs in three developmental phases. The readiness phase targets self-control, group participation and social awareness skills. The instructional phase teaches an eight-step social decision-making strategy to students. The application phase provides practice to help children apply these skills in real-life interpersonal and academic situations.

The primary objective is to teach children a set of heuristic social decision-making thinking steps. Lessons are taught to the children on a regular basis by their classroom teacher. Extensive guided practice and role playing are used, as is skill modeling and the use of hypothetical social problem situations. Facilitative questioning and dialogue stimulates the integration of the techniques. And cooperative group projects and writing assignments further advance that process.

The Social Decision Making program targets the National Goals for Education, which address substance abuse and violence, the rights and responsibilities of citizenship, productive employment, and the critical thinking skills inherent in all aspects of academic and social learning.

Commercial Programs

Health Activities Project (HAP). HAP is under development at the University of California, Berkeley (Lawrence Hall of Science 1987). Currently it consists of sixty-four student-centered activities grouped into thirteen modules for use in grades 4 through 8. Each module represents from six to eight weeks of classroom activity. Titles of the modules are as follows:

1. Breathing Fitness
2. Sight and Sound
3. Heart Fitness
4. Action/Reaction
5. Balance in Movement
6. Skin Temperature
7. Flexibility and Strength
8. Personal Health Decisions
9. Growth Trends
10. Consumer Health Decisions
11. Nutrition and Dental Health
12. Your Heart in Action
13. Environmental Health and Safety

HAP modules are packed in a kit, and each kit contains materials for twenty-seven students (Figure 3.3). Each module includes a teacher's guide that states the purpose of the activity, describes the activity itself, gives procedures for setting up, provides an introduction to the activity, and suggests evaluation and follow-up procedures. One advantage of the HAP materials is that they are reusable and can thus be shifted from class to class. Each module comes with the necessary apparatus, games, wall charts, and other materials.

HAP is not an all-inclusive curriculum, but it is an excellent student-centered project that provides a wide range of low-cost activities. Additionally, the student-centered approach allows children to learn concepts that will better enable them to control their own health behavior.

Health Skills for Life. Health Skills for Life is a relatively new approach to health education. The emphasis is on skill acquisition rather than knowledge acquisition. Ten major health content areas consisting of 118 units are used in a comprehensive kindergarten through twelfth grade curriculum. The ten content areas are titled

1. Health Services and Consumer Health (6 units)
2. Fitness (2 units)
3. Dental Health (4 units)
4. Environmental Health (4 units)
5. Disease Prevention (9 units)
6. Growth and Development (12 units)
7. Nutrition (12 units)
8. Substance Use and Abuse (9 units)
9. Safety and First Aid (27 units)
10. Mental Health, Family Life, and Human Sexuality (33 units)

Each unit is independent of the other units in the curriculum. Any teaching aids needed for the program can be found locally. Units are bound in three-ring binders to facilitate revisions to the various units. Evaluation plans and tests for pretesting and posttesting, as well as skill tests, are included. An administrative guide is also included. A section of each unit includes the sequence for teaching, goals, performance indicators, estimated teaching time, content, student handouts, preparations needed, and information on integrating the unit with other subjects. The developers of the curriculum offer training to school districts that purchase the materials. The entire program was certified by the Oregon State Department of Education in 1982. The program is offered, either in parts or in its entirety, in more than thirty states.

Figure 3.3
The HAP Modules

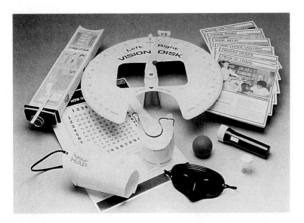 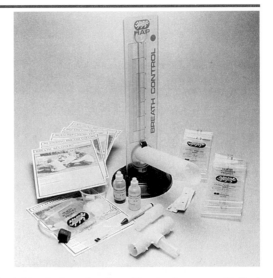

Source: Equipment and materials shown are from the Health Activities Project developed by the Lawrence Hall of Science and published by the Hubbard Scientific Company of Northbrook, IL.

The Best Program. A series of three innovative programs that seek to develop the message that alcohol, drugs, and tobacco are not to be used. The first component focuses on grades 2 through 4 and is titled "Just for Me." This program consists of six 15-minute videotapes for classroom use. Also included is a twenty-minute utilization video for teachers, a comprehensive teacher's guide, and a facilitator's manual to assist teacher educators in providing in-service workshops on using the materials. A peer helper handbook and three videos designed for parents help improve strategies that contribute to prevention. A parent guide as well as a parent workshop leader's guide are included.

"Your Choice . . . Our Chance" is designed for fifth and sixth graders. For these grade levels, there are three 30-minute video programs for the community, which demonstrates how a particular community developed a process for helping prevent/delay young people from using alcohol, drugs, and tobacco. In this component there are 10 fifteen-minute videos and a facilitator's manual for use with the children.

"Project Alert" is for grades 7 and 8. This segment includes thirteen weekly lessons, 10 for grade 7, and three additional lessons for grade 8. Like the other components for the lower grades, videotapes and posters are the basis for the program.

For all three components, the videos are based on "real-life" situations and are geared toward developing good decision-making skills, resisting peer pressure, and engaging in critical thinking activities. The videotapes are multicultural, which allows a wide range of diverse students to relate to the presentations.

Contemporary Health Series. Developed by ETR associates, the Contemporary Health Series was designed as a K–12 comprehensive program. Three components make up the series, including "Actions for Health" (K–6), "Into Adolescence" (middle school), and "Entering Adulthood" (high school). The ten content areas in the program are accompanied by specific objectives, lesson plans, teaching strategies, reference materials, implementation strategies, evaluation procedures, and suggested follow-up activities are found in the instructor guides for each series.

Other Teaching Materials

Agencies such as the American Cancer Society, American Heart Association, March of Dimes, American Red Cross, American Dental Association, and American Dairy Association provide free and inexpensive materials through their local affiliates.

Developing a Health Curriculum

A health curriculum is a comprehensive plan for kindergarten through twelfth grade, designed to encompass pertinent health concerns and provide learning experiences throughout the school years. Such a plan should help promote responsible decisions and practices regarding personal, family, and community health. A comprehensive school health education plan should be prepared for each local school district and then developed for the individual schools within the district. Although a district may elect to use a state-developed or other existing curriculum, in some cases, the decision may be made to develop a new curriculum approach.

The Michigan Model—A State Model

Although there is not an officially mandated national curriculum, several models have been suggested as possibilities. An excellent model that several states have adopted is the Michigan Model for Comprehensive School Health Education. The model was a result of a coalition of eight state agencies that included the Department of Education, Department of Public Health, Department of Social Services, Department of Mental Health, Department of State Police, Office of Substance Abuse Services, Office of Health and Medical Affairs, and Office of Highway Safety Planning. In addition, over 120 voluntary and professional groups agreed to promote comprehensive health education.

Currently 85 percent of Michigan's public schools have implemented the model. The model also is being implemented in 129 of Michigan's private schools. Throughout the United States other public and private school systems have also adopted the program. Over one million students have been reached through implementation of the Michigan Model. The parent/family involvement component of the curriculum has been expanded to include a forty-eight-page magazine that is available to parents, community groups, physcians, and youth-serving groups to inform people concerning the content of school and community resources. In addition, a series of videos are being developed for use by school libraries, parent groups, and local video stores. These videos are designed both to be watched by families and to inform parents on health and parenting topics. Table 3.1 contains the scope and sequence plan for the content areas offered through the Michigan Model. Table 3.2 lists the classroom time required at each grade level.

Teaching Units

A *teaching unit* is an organized method for developing lesson plans for a particular group of students and thus can be tailored to each classroom. The resource unit serves as a guide, whereas the

Table 3.1

Content Areas and
Grade-Level Concerns
of the Michigan Model

Curriculum addresses the following at each grade level(s):

	K	1	2	3	4	5	6	7	8	9	10	11	12
Sexual Behavior						√	√	√	√				
• HIV	√	√	√	√	√	√	√	√	√				
• Other STDs					√	√		√	√				
• Teen Pregnancy							√	√	√				
Tobacco Use													
• Smoking	√	√	√	√	√	√	√	√	√				
• Smokeless			√			√			√				
Substance Abuse	√	√	√	√	√	√	√	√	√				
Injury Prevention	√	√	√	√	√	√	√	√	√				
Suicide Prevention								√	√				
Nutrition	√	√	√	√	√	√	√	√	√				
Physical Activity	√	√	√	√	√	√	√	√	√				

Table 3.2

*Classroom Time
Required at Each
Grade—Michigan Model*

How much classroom time does the curriculum require at each grade level?

	Average Minutes per Session	Number of Sessions per Year
K	30	39
1	30	40
2	30	37
3	40	40
4	40	39
5	40	44
6	40	40
7	50	59
8	50	63

teaching unit is the plan for student learning. Unlike the resource unit, which is prepared by a curriculum committee, the teaching unit is developed by the classroom teacher. It is specific; the resource unit is general. The teacher selects the specific concepts to be studied, as well as the objectives, content, learning strategies, evaluation methods, and references that will be used in class. Given a well-developed resource unit that identifies major concepts, creating a teaching unit is fairly easy. In addition to the resource unit, the state health education guidelines, the teacher's edition of the classroom textbook, and various materials from health-related agencies can all be used to develop the teaching unit.

In preparing a teaching unit, a variety of formats can be used, depending on individual preference. Figure 3.4 illustrates a typical format.

Lesson Planning—Selected Strategies

Once the teaching unit has been developed, plans are made for how to teach the unit. This is done by creating daily lesson plans that provide for a logical progression of the unit from start to finish. Each lesson plan must be based on concepts taught in previous lessons so that learning builds on the established base.

Figure 3.5 shows a typical daily lesson plan for grade 3. Notice that the format of this lesson plan parallels the format used for the teaching unit. A conceptual statement and objectives are stated for that day. The content outline provides a summary of the main topics to be covered. The strategies are the heart of the lesson plan. They should be described in detail and listed in the order in which they are to be used.

As shown in the daily lesson plan example, each strategy should be followed by an evaluation activity. Through this activity, the teacher will be able to judge to some extent how well the students have learned the concept presented. Because the strategy is a performance in nature, it can also be used to determine how well the objectives have been achieved.

Figure 3.4
Typical Unit Format

Grade Level: K-3		Title of Unit: Eating for Good Health		
		Conceptual Statement: Food Selection and eating patterns are determined by social, economic and cultural factors.		
Objectives: student will	Content	Strategies Learning Activities	Evaluation methods	References: A. Student B. Teacher
Identify foods that belong to the four food groups.	Food Groups A. Milk 1. milk 2. cheese 3. ice cream 4. cottage cheese B. Meat 1. pork 2. beef 3. fish 4. eggs C. Fruits and Vegetables 1. citrus fruit 2. green vegetables 3. beets D. Bread and Cereal 1. whole grains 2. bread 3. rice	1. Discuss the four food groups, why they are important and what foods are in each group. 2. Have students play grocery store with empty cartons, cans etc., and place one food from each of the food groups in their sack. 3. By using wrappers from a fast food restaurant, the students pretend that they are at a fast food hamburger restaurant and they choose one food from each of the basic food groups to form a nutritious meal. Follow up with a field trip to a hamburger restaurant.	1. List four foods for each group. 2. From a group of pictures, ask the students to choose a food from each food group to form a nutritious menu for a day.	A. Student Filmstrips "The Fruits and Vegetables" Encyclopedia Britannica Educational Corporation, 1997 "Foods from Grains." Coronet Books Richmond, et al., You and Your Health, II Scott Foresman, 1997 Fodor, et al., Being Healthy Laidlaw Bisc., 1996. Chapter 6, B. Teacher You and Your Health, II Scott Foresman, 1997 Chapter 3. Fodor, et al., Being Healthy Laidlaw Bisc., 1996. Chapter 6,

Following the daily lesson, teachers should also evaluate their own performance, as indicated at the bottom of the daily lesson plan example. How well has the content been presented? How effective were the activities? Were the instructional objectives fulfilled? From such an evaluation, teachers can improve their teaching skills and thus better meet the needs of students.

The Hunter Approach to Lesson Planning

Another approach is the instructional model developed by Madeline Hunter. The design of this model consists of seven components used either in their entirety or in some workable combination, depending on appropriateness for a particular objective. The model begins with a statement of the *long-range objective or goal,* of which a particular lesson is a part, and is written for the teacher as a focus for the intent of the lesson. Next is the *instructional objective,* which specifically tells in behavioral terms the desired learning outcome. An instructional objective is written in the form of "the student will list four characteristics of good mental health" or "the student will correctly demonstrate CPR techniques."

The *set* begins the actual instructional portion of the strategy. The purpose of set is to prepare the student to learn and to describe what is going to be taught. Set should label the learning and involve all the students through some kind of activity. Set should also relate to both previous

Figure 3.5
Daily Lesson Plan

Unit Title: Mental Health - Getting to know me   Date: February 19, 1997
Conceptual Statement: There are healthy and   Time: 10am
          unhealthy ways to express emotions.   Grade: Three
Objectives: The student will identify several   Teacher: Goodman
          emotions and state acceptable ways   Teaching points: Write role
          to express them.   player situations
Teacher Needs: Pictures of people expressing   on index cards.
          emotions, crayons, paper.

Content (progression)	Learning activities	Evaluation for activities

Emotion - the way we feel
  A. Anger   D. Fear
  B. Love   E. Excitement
  C. Sadness
Expressing Emotions
A. Facial expression
  1) Smile   3) Tears
  2) Frown   4) Eyes
B. Talking
  1) Soft voice 4) Fast voice
  2) Loud voice 5) Slow voice
  3) Excited voice
C. Body language
  1) Using arms
  2) Kissing
  3) Clapping
	1. Discuss what feelings are and list on the board. Show pictures of people displaying different emotions. Several pictures that reflect certain emotions.
	
	2. Discuss ways we express emotions. Ask students to give ways that are acceptable/unacceptable means of expressing feelings. Have students role play these ways to express the various emotions.
		1. Give children a crayon and have them draw a face of the emotion requested.
		
		2. Give the children a situation which smacks of expression of a particular emotion. Have them role play an acceptable way to express the emotion.

Teacher evaluation
1. Keep the lesson as taught? yes _ no _   2. What I need to improve _____
3. Next time make sure _____
_____   4. Strengths of lesson _____
_____
_____   _____
                                                  _____

learning and real-life experiences. Instruction is composed of actual teaching of new information, taking time to monitor the students through interaction, and adjusting instruction according to student needs. *Modeling* should occur while labeling the learning. Modeling is composed of the teacher doing an example, the teacher doing one with student help, the students doing one with teacher help, and students doing one alone. It is imperative that interaction with students take place. Supervised practice is also necessary to ensure an accurate and successful introduction to new information. Closure involves students verbally summarizing what they have learned and then doing one more example.

The final component in this strategy is called *options*. At this point, the teacher has the option to reteach the lesson if there seems to be a need, to go on to the next step, or to provide independent practice. Independent practice should be performed without major errors or confusion and may be oral or written. The principles of learning involved in the Hunter approach are motivation, retention, reinforcement, active participation, set, and closure. Figure 3.6 shows a lesson plan based on the Hunter model.

Developing Objectives

The terms *goals, behavioral objectives,* and *instructional objectives* are not synonymous. A *goal* is a statement of instructional intent. Goals give direction and purpose to educational efforts. Goals are long range and may take years to accomplish. They are useful in developing long-term objectives for curriculum and grade-level expectations. *Behavioral objectives* are for more than one lesson and are written for long-term or unit objectives. They do not tell the teacher what or how to teach, but they do provide a framework for selecting appropriate content, learning activities, and evaluation procedures. *Instructional objectives* indicate the learning or behavior to be demonstrated in a particular lesson. An instructional objective, which is specific and short range, is taught within the framework of each health class.

In the current climate of evaluation and school reform, many educational leaders are moving toward what is called **outcome-based education (OBE).** The emphasis is on the learning outcomes the students are expected to exhibit at the end of their twelve-year school experience (McCown, Driscoll, and Roop 1996). Outcome-based education is predicated on the development of state and national standards in education. An example of OBE can be found in the Health Highlight—The National Health Education Standard, which shows the National Health Education Standards. States, districts, and individual schools usually form councils or school improvement teams whose charge is to develop specific plans for the indicators demonstrating improvement.

From these writers' perspective, an excellent way of measuring OBE is through the development of sound instructional objectives. In particular, broad-scope measurable objectives are most helpful in assessing fulfillment of OBE standards. Instructional objectives can help identify potential assessment areas, particularly when viewed within the three areas of framework found in Bloom's Taxonomies of Educational Objectives (Bloom 1956). The three domains are **cognitive** or knowledge; **affective** or **attitudes/values**; and **behavioral**, which focuses on skills or behavior. The problem in using this framework is that the emphasis may be only on the cognitive or knowledge component. However, it is imperative in the teaching of health education to recognize that learning is reflected in other ways than simply in recalling the content of health education. The ability to think, judge, evaluate, and act on the information is more important than simple recall of facts. Nonetheless, instructional objectives can provide a framework for performance-based evaluation, as mentioned in Chapter 5.

Figure 3.6

Lesson on Friendship Utilizing the Hunter Model of Daily Lesson Planning

Long-Range Objective: Understands the importance of various types and patterns of interpersonal relationships to maintenance of good health.

Instructional Objectives: The learner will (TLW) define *friendship* and identify and write five qualities or characteristics of a friend.

Objective	Method	Materials	Evaluation
TLW identify some characteristics of and ways to be a friend: visualize a friend.	**Set:** 1. *Label Learning:* We will be thinking and talking about friends. 2. *Relate to Previous Learning:* In our last health class we talked about communication and relationships in your family. 3. *Involve All Students:* Respond to questions about friends by raising and lowering pencils (questions in teacher's manual). 4. *Relate to Real-life Experiences:* Close your eyes and think about someone who is your friend.	Pencils	*Student correctly identifies characteristics of and ways to be a friend*
TLW write definitions of words.	**Instruction:** 1. Using a transparency, teacher will project vocabulary words. 2. Teacher leads discussion of word meanings, monitors, and checks for understanding as students write definitions.	Transparency Screen Overhead Projector	*Definitions correctly written*
TLW complete worksheet; contribute to class discussion. **TLW** write a list of qualities important to her or him in a friend.	3. Read directions to worksheet, explain, and provide examples. Lead class discussion upon completion Worksheet (monitor as students work). 4. "Use the back of your vocabulary list for this activity. We all have qualities we want our friends to possess. I like for my friends to be nice. What are some qualities you like for your friends to exhibit?" Write suggestions on board. Have each student write own list (monitor and adjust as needed).	Worksheet	*Student produces list and discusses these characteristics*
TLW watch a film about friends and subsequently discuss it.	5. Show film about friends and lead discussion after. Film projector	Film Projector	
TLW list on paper five qualities important in a friend; read her or his answers to a partner.	**Closure:** 1. "Today we have defined a friend and listed many qualities. I want you to complete the following . . ." (display sentence using overhead). 2. Divide class into partners and have each student read her or his answers to the partner.	Attachment III Overhead Projector Transparency	*Student lists and reads answers. Answers are appropriate for discussion.*

Writing Instructional Objectives

To consider important only what can be measured results in the trivialization of instruction. What can be accomplished through well-planned instructional objectives is exposure to all three domains so that students can make decisions that have the potential to enhance the overall quality of health throughout life. Children can be helped to internalize information so that it helps them make decisions that lead to positive health behaviors. The use of instructional objectives is a start in the right direction.

It is useful to think of instructional objectives in terms of having five components. Definitions and examples of these components follow:

1. *Who:* The student or the one who is to exhibit the knowledge, attitude, or behavior as the result of the teaching/learning process.

2. *Behavior expected:* What the student will do to show that learning has taken place.

3. *Learning requirement:* What the student will know, feel, or do when the learning is completed. For example, "the student will label the diagram." It is generally a good idea to keep the verb as action-oriented as possible. However, the preciseness demanded by many educators in the 1970s and 1980s has been replaced by the concept that the objective should be as broad in scope as possible, salient and measurable (Popham 1995). An example of a broad-scope objective might be as follows: "After reading a selected article on the social and physiological effects of alcohol, the student will compose a critical essay on the potential dangers of alcohol use associated with their personal use."

4. *Conditions:* The specific conditions under which the student will be expected to do the activity; for example, on a test, orally, or working in a group.

5. *Standard of performance:* The minimum level of achievement, either quantitative or qualitative, that will be accepted as meeting the requirements for demonstrating successful achievement; for example, 80 percent correct, writing a critical essay, constructing an exhibit, judged acceptable by a group of peers (peer evaluation).

In using instructional objectives, the teacher should strive to develop a reasonable number of manageable, broad, yet measurable objectives that will help in assessing whether students have achieved the desired learning. Attempting to become too precise in stating the objective may limit or obscure other valid indicators of a skill or ability. Instructional objectives should be viewed as starting points; they are not the totality of quality education. An alternate behavior exhibited by the student at the end of instruction may be an equally valid indicator that learning has taken place. With performance-based evaluation (see Chapter 5), the use of many different indicators of learning is now being fully recognized and appreciated.

≣ *Summary*

○ Teachers must recognize the complexity of life and seek to incorporate the dimensions of wellness into the teaching of health education.

○ Content must be organized to ensure comprehensive coverage of grades K through 12.

○ Scope and sequence must be considered when developing curriculum.

○ The National Health Education Standards provide the foundation for curriculum development and instruction.

O Health topics should be based on the needs, interests, and comprehension ability of the students.

O Health literacy is the ability of the student to obtain, interpret, and understand basic health information and services and the competence to use information and services in ways that enhance health.

O Effective health education requires a balance between factual information and the attitude or valuing component.

O Time must be allotted for examining values and for practicing critical thinking skills.

O Many useful curriculum approaches are offered through the National Diffusion Network, commercial organizations, and state departments of education.

O The Michigan Model is an excellent example of a curriculum plan that used a coalition of state and voluntary agencies to develop a comprehensive approach to health education.

O Outcome-based education is the direction in which Health education is moving in the 1990s.

Discussion Questions

1. What determines the nature of the content for a given grade level?
2. What is meant by the "scope and sequence" of health education?
3. Why are the National Health Education Standards important?
4. What are some barriers to quality health education?
5. Describe what is meant by the phrase "teaching for values."
6. What is the National Diffusion Network?
7. Discuss what advantages/disadvantages commercial programs might have over state- or NDN-developed programs.
8. How does your state curriculum model for health education compare with the Michigan Model?
9. What purpose do objectives fulfill in the educational process?
10. What is outcome-based education?

References

Association for the Advancement of Health Education (AAHE). 1995. *National health education standards—achieving health literacy.* Reston, VA: AAHE.

Bloom, B. S. 1956. *Taxonomy of educational objectives, handbook I: Cognitive domain.* New York: McKay.

Bruess, C. E., and J. S. Greenberg. 1981. *Sex education—Theory and practice.* Belmont, CA: Wadsworth.

Byler, R., G. Lewis, and R. Totman 1969. *Teach us what we want to know.* Hartford, CT: Connecticut State Board of Education.

Creswell, W. H., and I. M. Newman. 1992. *School health practice.* St Louis: Mosby.

Fodor, J. T., and G. T. Dalis. 1989. *Health instruction: Theory and application.* 4th ed. Philadelphia: Lea & Febiger.

————. 1992. *Growing healthy—A comprehensive school health education curriculum.* New York: National Center for Health Education.

Gallup Organization. 1994. *Values and opinions of comprehensive school health education in U.S. public schools: Adolescents, parents, and school district administrators.* Atlanta: American Cancer Society.

Harbeck, M. B. 1970. Instructional objectives in the affective domain. *Educational technology* 10 (49):52.

Hunter, M. 1976. *Improved instruction.* El Segundo, CA: TIP Publications.

Kibler, R. J., D. J. Cegala, L. L. Barker, and D. T. Miles. 1974. *Objectives for instruction and evaluation.* Boston: Allyn and Bacon.

Krathwohl, D. R., P. R. Bloom, and B. B. Masia. 1964. *Taxonomy of educational objectives, handbook II: Affective domain.* New York: McKay.

Lawrence Hall of Science.1987. *Health activities project.* Northbrook, IL: Hubbard.

McCown, R., M. Driscoll, and P. G. Roop. 1996. *Educational psychology—A learning-centered approach to classroom practice.* Boston: Allyn and Bacon.

Miller, D. F., and S. K. Telljohann. 1992. *Health education in the elementary school.* Dubuque, IA: W.C. Brown.

(NDN). 1995. *Education programs that work—The catalogue of the National Diffusion Network,* 21st ed. Longmont, CO: Sopris West.

Newman, I. M., and K. A. Farrell. 1991. *Thinking ahead: Preparing for controversy.* Lincoln: Nebraska Department of Education.

Popham, W. J. 1995. *Classroom assessment—What teachers need to know.* Boston: Allyn and Bacon.

Read, D. A., and W. H. Greene. 1989. *Creative teaching in health.* Prospect Heights, IL: Waveland Press.

School Health Education Study. 1967. *Health education: A conceptual approach to curriculum design.* St. Paul, MN: 3M Education Press.

U.S. Bureau of Health Education. 1977. *The school health curriculum project.* Washington, DC: U.S. Government Printing Office.

Zais, R. S. 1986. *Curriculum principles and foundations.* New York: Crowell.

Chapter Four

Strategies for Implementing Health Instruction

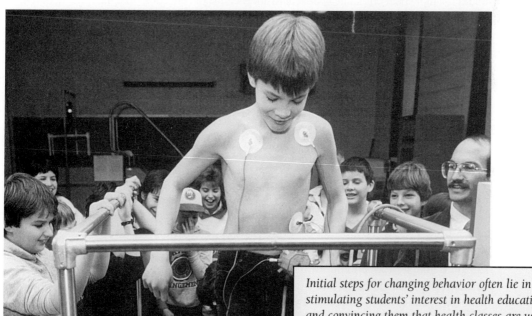

> Initial steps for changing behavior often lie in stimulating students' interest in health education and convincing them that health classes are useful in their daily lives.
>
> —Humphrey Taylor, Louis Genevie, and Xiaoyan Zhao (1988)

Valued Outcomes

After reading this chapter, you should be able to

○ list the factors that affect teaching strategy selection

○ discuss criteria and salient points of using values clarification strategies

○ describe effective use of decision stories in the classroom

○ explain the importance of using verbal strategies to implement health instruction

○ identify the elements necessary to prepare for discussion

○ list action-oriented strategies used in health instruction

○ discuss ways to utilize the computer in the classroom

○ describe the use of media in the classroom

○ identify different strategies to foster health instruction

The Relationship of Strategies to Learning ——————————

Learning strategies are things that make content and objectives come alive. This enlivening involves selecting strategies and techniques that make learning exciting and motivating. Carrying this out is the direct responsibility of teachers, who, having established a working knowledge of the many strategies available in health education, are limited only by their own creativity.

A **strategy** is any activity or experience that teachers use to interpret, illustrate, or facilitate learning. Foder and Dalis (1989) view a strategy as anything used with or on students to accomplish the objectives of the program. For the most effective learning to take place, teachers should seek strategies that are student-centered and provide for group involvement. Additionally, they should use more than one strategy or activity for each major concept so that their instruction more fully encompasses the variety of student abilities and aptitudes.

The teacher must remember that selecting a variety of strategies does not ensure learning. Several other factors influence effective learning and must be considered, such as a relationship with the students that is conducive to learning. Treating students fairly is the first step in facilitating learning and creating a proper classroom atmosphere. Many techniques to help promote creative learning are available. With proper preparation, the strategies listed in Table 4.1 can be useful.

Factors Affecting Strategies

In selecting strategies to provide learning experiences, keep the following criteria in mind:

○ Select strategies that contribute to total learning. Some activities lend themselves to acquiring knowledge, whereas others are better suited to attitude assessment and decision making. Ideally, the strategies selected should help the student develop the ability to reason and assess the information being presented. Any strategy selected should involve the students as participants in the activity.

○ The more complex the concept, the more activities are needed to develop the concept. As a general rule, for each concept, two strategies or activities should be employed. If the material being studied is difficult, more than two strategies or activities should be used. Another reason for using more than one strategy is that students learn in a variety of ways and through different means. Thus, a variety of strategies will help all students to grasp the concept under examination.

○ The strategies selected should begin with the simple and move to the more complex. Once the teacher has prepared the class for the activity through a proper introduction, the students should become part of the learning activity. With simple activities, students should be able to learn by means of group involvement, self-assessment, and class–teacher interaction. As the students become better able to deal with more difficult topics, more complex strategies can be used that require self-discovery or analysis of materials and conclusions.

○ Audiovisual aids should be included whenever possible. These can include models, classroom exhibits, videos, filmstrips, CD-ROMs, and so forth. Audiovisual aids add another dimension to teaching concepts and are excellent for reinforcing learning.

Strategies can be classified into many different categories. Some authorities distinguish between strategies, media, and instructional materials, whereas others group all three into one category. Classification is unimportant as long as you can identify the strengths and weaknesses of each available technique. Your objective should be to select those strategies that are most appropriate and effective with your class and based on the learning styles of the student.

Table 4.1

Instructional Strategies
for Health Education

• Audiocassettes	• Dramatization	• Resource speakers
• Brainstorming	• Exhibits	• Role-playing
• Bulletin boards	• Field trips	• Self-appraisals
• Buzz groups	• Filmstrips	• Slides
• Case studies/committee work	• Magazines	• Specimens/models
• CD-Roms	• Newspapers	• Storytelling
• Charts/maps	• Panel discussion	• Television
• Computers	• Peer helpers	• Transparencies
• Cooperative learning	• Posters	• Values clarification
• Debates	• Puppet shows	• Video tapes
• Demonstrations/experiments	• Radio	• Word searches/crosswords

A Positive Climate for Learning

Regardless of the strategy employed, the teacher must strive to create a classroom environment that is conducive for learning. Students should look forward to class, feel emotionally/intellectually unthreatened, and realize that they will be supported in their learning efforts. There are several things a teacher can do to facilitate a positive learning climate:

○ Identify appropriate instructional goals and discuss them with the student so that the intent is clear concerning what is expected.

○ Insist that work be completed satisfactorily to agreed-on standards.

○ Refuse to accept excuses for poor work.

○ Communicate acceptance of imperfect initial performance when students struggle to achieve new learning.

○ Convey confidence in the student's ability to do well.

○ Display a "can do" attitude that generates student excitement and self-confidence.

○ Avoid comparative evaluations, especially of lower-ability students, that might have them conclude they cannot meet expectations (Evertson, Emmer, Clements, Worsham 1997, 123).

Values Clarification Strategies

To personalize health concepts, students must relate to health instruction from the affective domain. An excellent strategy for achieving this end is through the use of valuing strategies activities. By examining and clarifying values, children can learn positive health behavior. As mentioned earlier, however, the use of values clarification techniques is not without some controversy. Values cannot and should not be avoided when teaching health education, but the teacher must be adequately prepared to do the job right.

Begin by recognizing that values are relative, personal, and often situational. You should not attempt to teach your own personal values or the "correct" values; instead, your goal should be to assist students in assessing and developing their own values so that these values lead to positive health behavior. It is essential that any value judgment made by the students be made through their own cognitive process. According to Hochbaum, Rosenstock, and Kegeles (1960), for a value judgment or health practice to evolve, the following criteria must apply:

1. Students must perceive the issue as being important.

2. Students must believe that they are susceptible to the problem.

3. Students must believe that the problem is serious.

4. The intensity of the threat and resultant anxiety must not be so great as to paralyze the ability to act.

5. There must be an action to take that the individual believes will be effective.

For students to function effectively when using values clarification strategies, they also must be prepared. Greenberg (1989, 43) states that the following are requisites of learner-centered instruction.

1. familiarity with and trust of other program participants (students)

2. friendship with at least one other participant

3. listening skills

4. knowledge of and experience with roles assumed by members and leaders of groups

5. knowledge of and experience with the decision-making process

6. cooperation and participation among all members of the program

7. an understanding and appreciation of both one's own feelings and the feelings of others

8. open communication among disagreeing factions and empathy with those of opposing viewpoints

9. recognition of unfulfilled needs of program participants and means of satisfying those needs

10. appreciation of individual differences and unique potential

When engaging in any values clarification activity, the teacher must allot sufficient time for students to assess their own feelings about the issue under examination. Students must also feel free to assess their values without fear of being ridiculed or forced to pay lip service to the opinions of others, including the teacher. Keep these points in mind:

○ Values clarification activities do not lead to one "correct" solution to a problem; they are open ended. The purpose of these activities is to open the doors to additional assessment.

○ As a teacher, you are a participant in the activities and a role model for the students.

○ Every student has the right to decline from speaking, without having to give a reason for declining. Respect individual feelings and keep the activity nonthreatening.

Many instructional devices are available for incorporating values clarification activities into the health curriculum. The ones you choose should be appropriate for the developmental level of the students. As already discussed, young children are not capable of dealing with highly abstract issues. Further, they do not have the experiential background to deal knowingly with topics far

Health Highlight

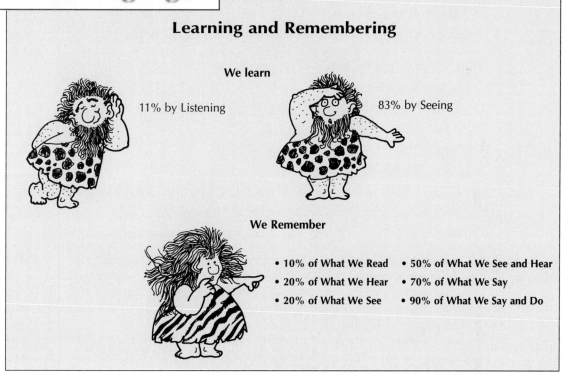

Learning and Remembering

We learn

11% by Listening   83% by Seeing

We Remember

- 10% of What We Read
- 20% of What We Hear
- 20% of What We See

- 50% of What We See and Hear
- 70% of What We Say
- 90% of What We Say and Do

removed from their everyday world. Therefore, it is not realistic to attempt to grapple with such values-related issues as euthanasia or world hunger at the primary level.

Simple Values-Related Strategies

One of the simplest and most appropriate activities for younger students involves what is known as a shield activity, which is excellent for teaching children the ten prerequisites suggested by Greenberg. The major objective of this activity is to assist children in identifying values they have. A typical shield is illustrated in Figure 4.1. Each child is given a prepared form as shown in the figure. The activity consists of filling in each segment of the shield with a values-related response, either in words or with drawings. For younger children, you should read the instructions aloud.

The following steps may be used to help children work through the activity.

1. After students have filled out the shield, ask students to cross out any area of the shield they are unwilling to discuss.

2. Ask the students to move about the room in silence, holding the shield in front of themselves so other students can see them. Remind them that they should not talk.

3. After five to ten minutes, ask each student (teacher may pair them) to select someone standing close by. Tell students to sit together to discuss the shield. The process begins with one student asking the other a question concerning his or her shield. After answering the question, the other

student asks a question. The process continues until all the areas in the shield have been covered. This usually takes five to ten minutes.

4. Ask the students who were paired to introduce one another as each feels his or her partner would want to be introduced.

5. To bring closure, you might ask the children the following questions:

○ How many of you knew the name of your partner?

○ Did you introduce yourself?

○ Did you find some things that you shared with your partner?

○ Did you find some things that were different from your partner?

○ How did you feel about your introduction?

○ What would you change about your introduction?

○ Did you feel you were a good listener when your partner answered your questions?

○ Can you write down one thing you learned about yourself?

○ Can you write down one thing you learned about your partner? the group?

In presenting such an activity, it is essential that you thoroughly introduce, carry out, and summarize the experience. If this is not done, the activity becomes nothing more than a game. Through careful introduction, a psychological set is established so that the activity will be meaningful and the students will understand why they are doing it. By careful summation, you can help students assess their feelings and clarify existing values.

Asking children to complete open-ended statements is another simple values-related activity. This kind of activity is appropriate for children at a slightly higher developmental level. Examples of typical open-ended statements include the following:

○ I think that smoking is _____

○ If my friend did something wrong, I would _____

_____

_____

Decision Stories

Decision stories are open-ended vignettes that describe a values-related dilemma which ask students to suggest a course of action. The stories should reflect real-life circumstances and should be appropriate to the age level of the children. No easy answer should suggest itself in the story, but viable courses of action must be possible for the activity to be meaningful. If only unacceptable or repugnant alternatives seem possible, children will be unable to incorporate positive decision-making skills into their own behavior repertoires. A decision story that children can identify with and relate to can provide an excellent springboard for values discussion. A good decision story not only encourages students to sort out opinions, values, and feelings but also requires students to think about them, test them, and try them out. The real test of the importance of values comes with application.

In preparing decision stories, follow these guidelines:

Figure 4.1
Shield Activity for Identifying and Assessing Values

1. **Name or draw something that you do well.**

2. **Name or draw something that you are trying to get better at.**

3. **Write down a feeling that would be very hard for you to change.**

4. **Write the thing that you are most proud of having done.**

5. **Tell about a happy thing that happened to you.**

6. **Tell about a sad thing that happened to you.**

7. **Tell what you want to do with your life.**

8. **Write three words that best tell about who you are.**

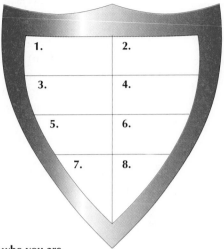

1. The story should be between 50 and 150 words in length. It should include enough detail to establish realism and character, but it should not be so long as to obscure the central issue.

2. Establish a focus on the main issue with relevant supportive facts and events.

3. Do not slant the story so that only one solution or course of action is implied.

4. Provide a descriptive title.

5. End with a focus question that asks each student to suggest a course of action. This question is also the basis for discussion of the issue. (Hamrick, Anspaugh, and Smith 1980, 455)

Following are examples of decision stories.

Pressure

Jim and Paul are fifth graders in the same classroom. In the past few weeks, they have become friends. One day while walking home from school, Jim and Paul meet some of Paul's other friends by the park. Paul's friends are all smoking. They offer Paul a cigarette. He takes it and lights up. Paul's friends also offer Jim a cigarette, but he says no. The boys start to make fun of him and call him a chicken. Even Paul is laughing at his friend.
Focus Question: What should Jim do?

Hot Spot

Mary's fourth-grade class is taking an important arithmetic test. Mary has studied hard for the test. In the seat next to her is her friend Julia. Julia is worried that she will not pass the test. The teacher leaves the room for a minute. While she is gone, Julia asks Mary for some of the test answers. The other students see and hear this. The teacher will be back in the room soon.
Focus Question: What should Mary do?

Students are an excellent source for developing such decision stories. After being exposed to a few models that you have written or located in values clarification materials, students are usually eager to write vignettes of their own. This should be encouraged, as student-developed stories are highly relevant and motivating to the students themselves.

Presenting Decision Stories in Class. Begin by setting the stage for the story to motivate the class for the activity and to focus the inquiry. Discuss the title of the story and ask the children what it suggests to them. Stimulate the students' curiosity and get them involved from the start. For decision stories to be effective, students must be participants and not merely passive listeners.

After a few minutes of this warm-up phase, present the story itself. Most of the stories can be read aloud. However, in some circumstances, it may help to give copies of the stories to the students, so they can consider the details of the presentation.

Have the students offer individual responses to the focus question: What course of action do you think is most appropriate? Encourage thought and reflection on the matter, but do not force any student to respond unwillingly. A good way to get students thinking is to have each write a response on paper. The writing process facilitates thinking through the situation that has been presented. This process could be structured in a manner that requires students to begin by defining the problem. Below the definition, the options or choices can be listed, along with the possible consequences of each action. Consequences can be either positive or negative or a combination of the two. Writing also requires each student to make a commitment based on the information presented. It should be made clear, however, that the written responses need not be shared with the class at this point.

Pooling Ideas.   Next, generate a list of all possible solutions to the decision story dilemma by asking students to share their responses with the class. This should be done on a volunteer basis. The teacher should not provide feedback to the students such as "That's good" or "I'm not sure that is such a good idea." Attempt to remain noncommittal. Respond with such phrases as "Thank you for sharing that idea with us," or by simply paraphrasing their responses. Then collect the responses and compile a list of solutions on the chalkboard without revealing which student offered any particular solution. You should also add possible solutions to the list that the students have overlooked.

Consider all the ideas put forth. Do not be judgmental, and do not reject any solution out of hand. Remember that the teacher's role is to help students clarify their own values, not to impose values on them.

Now divide the class into small groups and have each group discuss the possible solutions to the dilemma. Allow time for each group to reach a consensus on the preferred solution. Encourage the students to offer reasons for their choices.

Discussion and Reappraisal. After each small group has come to some sort of agreement, have them present the results of their discussions to the whole class. Different groups will probably opt for different solutions. Ask individual students why one solution seems better than another. Again, refrain from being judgmental and display neutrality. Instead of commenting, "So you think that Mary should just pretend that she didn't hear Julia," you might say, "How could Mary have responded to Julia?"

Finally, have each student reconsider the decision story in light of the class discussion (Smith, Hamrick, and Anspaugh 1981, 637). Some children will want to change their minds at this point. Others may modify their approach to the problem. Again have each student write down his or her solution to the problem along with reasons why the solution seems best. Have the students reflect on the ramifications of their decisions. Without necessarily requiring verbal responses, ask questions such as the following:

○ Have you ever been in a situation like the one in the story?

○ Did you come to the same solution then?

○ Did you or would you carry out your planned decision?

○ What happened or what do you think would happen if you tried out this decision?

○ How did this decision affect your own values? How were you affected by the decision? How were others affected?

○ Would you always make a similar decision?

Using this structured approach to decision stories will help students develop decision-making skills. It will also assist them in applying rational thought to everyday problems involving values.

Other Verbal and Discussion-Oriented Strategies

Values clarification activities rely to a large extent on discussion, as do many other classroom strategies. Discussion is a useful technique, but it must be structured. Always keep in mind your objective in employing any particular discussion strategy so that you do not lose the focus. Following are several other discussion-oriented strategies that have proven effective in health instruction.

Brainstorming

Like valuing strategies activities, brainstorming can be used to improve decision-making skills by having students generate many possible ideas concerning an issue. Freedom of expression and creativity are also encouraged. This strategy can be employed by all age groups and can foster a higher level of thinking. It is imperative that precise instructions be given about "how" and "what" is to be brainstormed. Possible topics for brainstorming sessions include

○ How can you get students to follow safety rules?

○ How can you encourage students to eat nutritious snacks instead of junk food?

○ How can we make our physical environment more healthful and more pleasant?

In conducting a brainstorming session, it is very important to follow these four rules:

1. The problem to be brainstormed must be well defined.

2. Any and all ideas must be accepted.

3. Criticism of any idea put forth is not allowed.

4. All ideas should be evaluated objectively when the session is over.

Brainstorming can be used effectively in the lower as well as upper elementary grades. The biggest drawback is that in a large class, not all children will get to express their thoughts. Nonetheless, the activity can be quite productive. By encouraging and accepting all opinions, new or novel possible solutions to a problem may be found. Even impractical suggestions can lead to new ways of thinking about an issue.

Follow-up is important. In the follow-up session, ask children to elaborate on their ideas. Present additional information that will be useful in making suggestions more practical or realistic. In doing so, emphasize to the class how the freewheeling brainstorming session led to many approaches to the problem.

Buzz Groups

Akin to brainstorming, buzz groups are an effective strategy for examining a specific problem. Generally, this technique is productive if students are mature enough to use the format. It allows for student participation in an atmosphere conducive to discussion. The buzz group strategy should not be overused, however, because too much small-group work can lessen student enthusiasm.

To use this approach, divide the class into groups of three to five students. Avoid putting friends in the same group or the discussion may tend to stray to issues besides the assigned task. Have each group focus on a specific problem that you have introduced and discussed so that the children will have a knowledge base for their discussion. Each group should choose a chairperson and a recording secretary. The chairperson must keep the discussion on the topic, and the secretary records important points. Walk from group to group to help maintain the focus of each group.

Allow three to fifteen minutes for buzz group discussion. Suitable topics for this strategy include the following:

○ How should an accident victim be handled?

○ How can children get along better with brothers and sisters?

○ What can be done to educate children to the dangers of smoking?

○ What can be done about vandalism?

After the discussion time is over, ask the recording secretary for each group to present the results of that group's discussion. The more controversial the topic, the more likely it will be that many diverse opinions will be aired. In the summary discussion, encourage objective consideration of all approaches put forth.

Case Studies

Case studies are actual events that you can use in class for discussion. The decision story format lends itself well to the case study strategy. Just substitute the actual event for the hypothetical one. Good sources for case study materials are health journals, newspapers, news magazines, and television programs.

Cooperative Learning

An excellent strategy for fostering cohesiveness in the classroom is cooperative learning. This technique involves having students work together to solve an identified problem or to work toward some common goal. Divide the class into small groups and instruct each to arrive at a conclusion on a particular problem or situation. This strategy allows students to work together, and each child can provide input to the conclusions. Above all, one or two students should not be allowed to dominate any group. This problem can be overcome by the teacher listening carefully to the group discussions and refocusing them when needed. It is difficult to assign grades for cooperative learning since contribution to solving the problem or arriving at the solution is not easily determined on an individual basis. Topics such as those suggested for the brainstorming or buzz group activities lend themselves to cooperative learning.

Critical Essays

The teacher asks the students to write their evaluation or judgment concerning an issue, product, or concept. This strategy is an excellent way to help students determine their feelings, how they would react, or their perspective on a situation or issue. Critical essays allow the students to express their own personal learning experiences. Teachers might ask the students to write why they feel a certain way, by what path they arrived at their feelings, or what effect the information, insight, or feeling will have on their behavior. This technique allows information gathered to be personalized in such a fashion that it has potential to develop attitudes and change/reinforce behavior.

Debate

Debate focuses on the merits and problems associated with a proposed solution to an issue. Through the use of this technique, you can ensure that both sides of the issue are presented. Although debate can be used in the lower elementary grades, the strategy is more effective when used with older children, who are more articulate and better able to organize their thoughts for oral presentation. Students must also be able to work individually as well as cooperatively in groups.

Topics suitable for debate include the use of nuclear power or its alternatives, the supposed merits of organic foods versus regular produce, and the use of laboratory animals in medical experiments. Environmental issues are also good debate topics.

Thorough preparation for a debate is essential. Students who volunteer to be part of a debate team should be given ample time to become knowledgeable about the issue they will discuss. The whole class should engage in this preparation so that students not on the debate teams are prepared to deal with the pros and cons of the arguments objectively.

In selecting students for debate teams, be sure that both sides are well balanced in ability. The teacher's role is that of moderator. The moderator should keep both debate teams on the topic and also guard against emotions becoming too extreme during and after the debate.

Committee Work

This technique allows small groups of children to research a topic of interest. Each group member has an opportunity to do in-depth research on the topic. For elementary school children, the work must be closely supervised and structured. It is very important that each member of the group contribute to the project if it is to be successful.

Projects that lend themselves well to committee work include investigating different types of pollution, collecting newspaper and magazine articles on a recent medical discovery or health approach, or researching types of foods used in different cultures as sources of essential nutrients.

Results of the committee work are presented orally. Encourage committee members to use exhibits and audiovisual aids to reinforce their presentations.

This strategy can also be used on an individual basis. In such an instance, each student makes a presentation of the research done.

Lecture, Group, and Panel Discussion

Discussion, in one form or another, is probably the most common technique used in education. Lecture discussion is usually thought of as a lecture delivered by the teacher. However, this strategy should not be limited to one-way communication. Lecture discussion can be from teacher to student, student to teacher, or student to student. The technique should be a means for achieving two-way communication.

For group discussion to be effective, the teacher must develop an atmosphere of freedom in the classroom. Without this atmosphere, students will not state their true feelings. And the discussion must be kept on course. Curtis and Papenfuss (1980, 139) offer the following suggestions for conducting group discussion.

1. Present a discussion topic or legitimize an appropriate student-formulated topic.

2. Establish and maintain an atmosphere of thoughtful communication without injecting teaching value judgments.

3. Make the ground rules for the discussion clear and enforce them.

4. Try to understand what students are attempting to say, but do not badger or cross-examine.

Panel discussion offers an opportunity for three to five students to investigate and report on a particular health topic. This strategy is similar to committee work, but it allows more give-and-take between the participating students. Usually fifteen minutes is sufficient time for a panel discussion. Adjust the time allotted to the attention span and developmental level of the class. When using this strategy, be sure that the students who will be panel members have a precise theme to explore. A prepared outline is also necessary so that the presentation is organized.

All three of these discussion techniques allow for the exchange of information and ideas between students. In this way, children are involved in the teaching–learning process. Discussion techniques also help students develop respect and understanding for the feelings and opinions of others.

To be successful, discussion must be guided. Stone, O'Reilley, and Brown (1980, 281) note six elements that must be addressed when preparing for a discussion.

1. Choose a topic that the students can discuss and have options on, such as "violence."

2. Introduce the topic and motivate the class about it. For example, write the word *violence* on the board and ask the students, "What is this word? Can you give me some examples of violence? Where have you seen violence in your own life? Have you ever been in a fight? Have you ever hit anyone? Have you ever thrown something at someone with the intention of hitting them? All of these are acts of violence."

3. Prepare key questions that generate discussion: for example, "If you have been in a fight or hit someone, do you think it was appropriate or necessary? If someone hits you, should you hit back? If not, what should you do? Is it ever necessary or the best option to hit someone else? When might those times be? If not, what course of action can be followed?"

4. Provide structure to the discussion by keeping it going in a predetermined direction. The focus of this topic for each student is to develop his own concept of the appropriateness or inappropriateness of violence. The emphasis needs to remain on these issues, even if the specifics get diverse.

5. Develop closure on the topic discussed. As an activity, students can write a paragraph describing their personal outlook on violence.

6. Summarize and reinforce the key points. After writing the paragraphs, the class members can review the issues discussed. For example, the teacher can write on the board, "We have decided that violence involves these kinds of activities . . ." and list them, along with "We think violence is appropriate/not appropriate in the following situations . . ."

Resource Speakers

Speakers can enrich many areas of health instruction. Possible resource speakers include doctors, nurses, police and fire department personnel, nutritionists, and health researchers. When contacting a resource speaker, be sure to provide that person with information about your class, including grade and developmental level. In this way, a speaker is less likely to talk down to or over the heads of the children. You should also politely emphasize that the speaker stick to the specific topic to be examined because some speakers are apt to digress to a favorite cause or concern not in keeping with your instructional objectives. Suggest that the speaker use audiovisual aids if appropriate, as this will heighten student interest. Also, ask the speaker to allow time for a question-and-answer session.

Before the speaker addresses the class, be sure that adequate instruction has been provided, so the students are not introduced to the topic cold. Also, provide information about the position and background of the resource speaker. For example, what exactly is a nutritionist? What does a nutritionist do, and for whom does the person work?

Resource speakers can be very instructive, especially if the students are properly prepared and the speaker uses visual aids to keep the students' interest.

Action-Oriented Strategies

A variety of action-oriented or student-centered strategies can be used to enliven health instruction. These range from seatwork activities to field trips. Whenever possible, any strategy selected should help students discover concepts through action-oriented means. Strategies that incorporate at least two of the senses can greatly facilitate learning. Listening is fine, but listening plus seeing, tasting, smelling, touching, feeling, and doing is better.

Dramatizations

Plays and skits, role playing, and puppet shows are all effective dramatization techniques. Each of these strategies is an excellent way of allowing students to express their feelings. Thorough preparation and follow-up are essential, however, lest these activities be seen merely as fun, with the point of the exercise being missed.

Presenting a play involves use of a script and props. You can use a commercial script or have students write their own. A skit is much more informal. Only an outline for the story needs to be prepared, not an actual script. Each character speaks extemporaneously. Props are not required. Nonetheless, plays and skits are both quite time consuming.

Role playing, or sociodrama, is a technique whereby students act out roles identified by you or by them. Each student is given a basic description of the role and the situation. The actual role playing is done with little or no rehearsal. A typical sociodrama should last from one to three minutes. It should then be followed by class discussion. Why did the person react to the situation in the particular way that the role was defined? What solutions suggest themselves from the sociodrama? Are these the only possible alternatives? If time permits, have students switch roles, or allow different students to play the same role.

Puppet shows are great motivators for health behavior and attitude development. They are especially effective in the lower grades. Commercial puppets may be used, or children can make their own. Puppets can be used for plays, skits, or role playing (Timmreck 1978, 140).

Storytelling

As a strategy, storytelling is similar to dramatization. However, the teacher is the active participant, and the children are onlookers.

This is nonetheless an effective strategy for helping students identify positive health habits and for shaping attitudes. Using a flip chart or other visual aid can heighten the impact of storytelling, although no props are needed for many stories.

Flannel, Felt, and Magnetic Boards

Flannel or felt boards are made by stretching a piece of either material over a large board or easel. Objects that will cling to the fabric can be placed on the board. Such boards are quite useful as aids in telling a story or developing a concept, because objects can be added or taken off during the presentation. These boards can also be used by the students in developing their own stories or presentations.

Magnetic boards serve the same purpose as flannel and felt boards. A magnetic board is simply a sheet of metal to which objects can be attached by means of small magnets. Chalk can also be used to write directly on a magnetic board.

Crossword Puzzles

Crossword puzzles are useful seatwork devices for building vocabulary and reinforcing concepts. They can be developed by the teacher, the students, or a computer-generated program. Commercial materials are also available. Crossword puzzles for younger children must be kept relatively simple. This technique is best employed with children in grade 3 and above. Figure 4.2 shows an example of a crossword puzzle concerning milk and milk products

Demonstrations and Experiments

Demonstrations and experiments help make verbal explanations more meaningful to students because they involve other senses, for example sight or touch. In a demonstration, the outcome should always be the same; in an experiment, the predicted outcome may vary. Otherwise, the two terms mean much the same. These techniques are especially good for use with elementary school children. Students are always interested in demonstrations and experiments because these strategies help clarify what they have learned.

When you consider either a demonstration or an experiment, careful planning is essential to make sure that it will actually work. All equipment should be set up ahead of time, and it is wise to have a rehearsal before the class actually views the procedure.

Appropriate areas for demonstrations and experiments include the following:

○ typing blood
○ feeding animals
○ determining the starch content of food
○ brushing and flossing teeth

Introduce the procedure to the class and explain what you plan to do. All students should be able to see the activity. Encourage them to ask questions as you go, and be sure to explain what is happening at each stage. After the activity, reinforce the learning by writing important points on the chalkboard.

Figure 4.2

Nutrition Crossword Puzzle

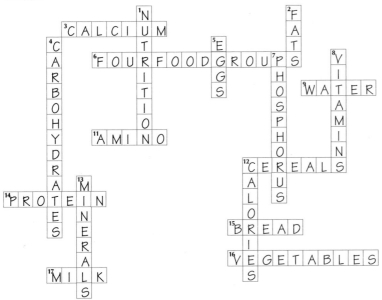

Across

3. A mineral in milk that builds strong bones and teeth.
6. A useful guide for eating daily (three words).
9. Helps regulate body temperature.
11. Parts of protein, called _____ acids.
12. Foods rich in carbohydrates. Oatmeal is an example.
14. A nutrient that builds and repairs body tissue.
15. A food product rich in carbohydrates. Good for making sandwiches.
16. Lettuce and carrots are examples. Can be eaten fresh or cooked.
17. Beverage from cows that is rich in protein.

Down

1. The science of food as it relates to optional health and performance.
2. Food substances that do not dissolve in water.
4. Nutrients found in many foods, especially in the Bread and Cereal Group: a source of energy.
5. Product of chickens that are popular for breakfast. Contain plenty of protein.
7. Helps build strong bones and teeth.
8. A group of nutrients that help other nutrients do their job. Known by letter names.
12. Measure energy provided by food. Dieters count them.
13. Sometimes called the "Structural Framework" of the body.

Source: Developed by the Memphis Nutritional Center, Memphis City Schools.

Exhibits

Exhibits allow students to view, examine, and touch health-related materials. Exhibits are most effective when the children help in the design and construction. Careful planning is essential, as is a central theme. Always ask yourself: What is the point of the proposed exhibit? Your answer will provide a focus for the children, too.

Examples of appropriate exhibits include X-ray plates of broken and healed bones, safety equipment used in different types of sports, dental instruments, and samples of raw foods, such as cereal grains. If the actual objects are unavailable or impractical for classroom display, pictures can be substituted, although they are not as effective.

Everything in an exhibit should be clearly labeled. If sound and motion can be added, student interest will be increased. Use your imagination to make the exhibit as visually appealing and interest provoking as you can.

Field Trips

Field trips can provide rich learning experiences. This strategy must be used sparingly, however, because field trips are time consuming and often expensive. Further, parents and administrators must give their approval for any activity outside the school, and liability must be considered.

A field trip should always be a culminating activity rather than an introductory one. Children should be well prepared for the experience through prior classroom instruction. If the field trip is to be of value, the students must be able to understand what they will be seeing.

Good places for health-related field trips away from the school include the local health department, a dairy farm, a food-processing plant, or a sewage treatment facility. There are also many opportunities for field trips within the school grounds. These are often quite effective as learning experiences for younger children. Although the places themselves are familiar, you can add a new dimension to them by explaining the structure and planning behind the situation. Examples of on-site field trips include visits to the school cafeteria, to a crosswalk area, or to the playground. For instance, at the crosswalk area you can ask children how the crosswalk is planned for safety. Are there school speed limit signs to slow traffic during school hours? Are crosswalk lines painted on the street? Do crossing guards supervise the crossing? These and other questions will help the students see the area in a new light.

Games

Games can stimulate interest while providing a review of concepts learned through other strategies. They are also sometimes a welcome relief from the normal classroom routine. In addition, games especially help younger children understand the importance of following rules and provide useful experience in socialization. Many commercially available games, such as bingo, can be adapted to health-related topics, or you may wish to develop your own games if you have the time.

When using games as part of the health instruction that you provide, be sure that the fun of the activity does not overshadow the health-related content of the game. Also, keep the game from becoming too competitive so that no player feels inferior.

Models and Specimens

Models and specimens allow students to have multisensory experience of health-related topics. The value of models and specimens lies in their degree of accuracy. Many excellent models of body parts are available commercially. These include models of the human eye, heart, lungs, and other organs. Another useful model is Resuscitation Annie/Andy, a functional model used to teach mouth-to-mouth resuscitation.

Specimens can be obtained from biological supply houses. These include tissue samples, animal eyes, and so forth. Commercial slaughterhouses can also supply some of these items. Exercise discretion in the use of specimens. For some children, such exhibits can be too grisly, and models are better employed.

Peer Helpers

Peer helper programs have proven successful in a number of informal settings. Peer helpers are children who have been trained to listen, support, offer assistance, and serve as models in a variety of roles, such as class monitors, tutors, big brothers/sisters, and playground helpers. Peer helpers can serve as excellent conduits between the children and teachers.

The children selected to serve as peer helpers are usually a grade or two ahead of the groups they help. The key to a successful program is the training and supervision peer helpers receive. In the school setting peer helpers can occasionally help to lead discussions or to work one-on-one with other children. They should be trained to help children think about a situation and develop a solution to or attitude about it. Peer helpers have been successful in helping to prevent smoking, drug and alcohol use, and eating disorders.

To be successful, the following ingredients must be present in peer helper programs:

1. *Well-qualified adult leaders:* Leaders must be knowledgeable in all aspects of program development, maintenance, and evaluation. National certifications and training workshops are available to help adults develop the skills for training the children.

2. *Well-established goals:* A needs assessment must be done to determine what the needs are of the school, community, and children. The identified needs should be stated as goals, with the school and community aware of the goals and purposes of the program.

3. *Effective recruitment and selection process:* Some programs will accept everyone who applies for training. Others may find it necessary to screen the students thorough interviews, letters of intent, and input from teachers. The program should represent all the social and ethnic groups in the school community. If a child is not selected he or she should be informed tactfully about the reasons for not having been selected and whenever possible, used in some other aspect of the program.

4. *Training:* Training should be adequate and appropriate. Typical training should include an introduction to the issue or topic based on the students' needs and a skill-building activity designed to help practice, receive coaching, and build on their natural abilities. It is not unusual for the training to require a time framework of twenty-five to thirty hours.

5. *Peer helper involvement:* The ways that peer helpers become involved will depend on the needs of the school. Even if some of the peer helpers have no formal duties, they can act as natural helpers in their own classrooms. The school should have some way to recognize peer helpers.

6. *Supervision:* A most critical element of an effective peer program is supervision. Weekly feedback and contact should be provided. Training should be a continuous process to help provide support and skill development for the peer helpers. The ability of the supervisor(s) to model the use of skills in real-life situations is a crucial ingredient.

7. *Evaluation:* Evaluation should be in terms of the program goals. It should describe how well the program has met its goals and point to possible changes. (Carr 1992, 4)

Self-Appraisals

There are many inventories that children can be given to help them assess their health status or feelings concerning an important issue. These instruments may be teacher developed or commercially prepared. Unfortunately these assessments may not be appropriate for very young children or may provide a false sense of security. There is always the risk that the children will not accurately report their true feelings. For example, a child may state that he does not smoke, realizing that to correctly report that he does would indicate a poor health habit. The strength of such inventories and assessments is that they help make children aware of potentially harmful behaviors and help to provide insight into positive health behaviors.

The Use of Media in Health Instruction

Educational media include everything from videotape to computer-assisted instruction. For the present purposes, the term will be defined as any nonprint vehicle used for instructional intent. Such media include computers, television and videotape, filmstrips, slides, overhead transparencies, and audio tapes.

Computer-Assisted Instruction

The first attempts to employ computers in the classroom were made in the 1960s. A programmed instructional format was generally used—that is, instructional information was provided by the computer in small increments. By responding to questions asked about the material by the computer, the student learned the material and received immediate reinforcement. Programmed instruction, with or without the computer as a vehicle, can be an effective educational tool, but rigid structure and format often lead to student boredom.

The development of microcomputers and CD-ROMs in the last few years has led to an increasing use of computers in the classroom. In fact, many children today come from homes where personal computers are used for a variety of purposes, from preparing business records to playing video games. In the years ahead, we shall no doubt see an increased use of computers in health instruction.

Today there is available to most schools a vast array of information on a global network called the **Internet**. The Internet can be linked to schools through a variety of sources, but one of the most popular is the **World Wide Web (WWW)**. The Web makes extensive use of multimedia, incorporating not only printed matter, but pictures, graphics, animation, and sound. Unfortunately the WWW has become host to much commercial advertising, but it remains a source of increasing health-related information that can be used in school. The computer holds great potential for a variety of activities. Some suggestions for student use in the classroom include:

1. Helping students "handle" large volumes of electronic information stores.
2. Developing skills that help students identify information that is essential and related to the task at hand.
3. Developing information acquisition skills. In this regard the student should be able to analyze information, apply information gathered, and evaluate the information acquired (Rivard 1997, p. 21).

Further benefits of using the computer in health education include active involvement of students and the ability to see knowledge in relational ways to carry out higher-level thinking by selecting and evaluating information, and to delve deeply into subjects and concepts while working either by themselves or in groups. The use of computers provides an excellent tie-in with outcome- or performance-based evaluation. For example, in both performance-based evaluation and in the use of computers the student must prepare, practice, experiment, and evaluate. As a result, students are expected to create a product and demonstrate competence before or among others. In addition, when there are several participants, performance can be interactive, enabling students to learn the impact of their actions through immediate feedback. Finally, outcome-based evaluation is promoted by the ability of peers to provide commentary on how to improve performance (U.S. News & World Report, 1997).

To make better use of computers in the educational setting, the following guidelines should be considered:

1. *Beware of flash.* Software is not enough. Avoid drill or game-oriented programs. Spreadsheet programs are a better choice. They can help teach health, science, or content-related courses.

2. *Use computers only where they make sense.* Use a computer only to help students in a way that would otherwise be difficult.

3. *Train teachers.* Training is the most crucial ingredient of an effective computer program. Technology is wasted without proper training.

4. *Don't expect miracles.* Computers don't always improve test scores, nor do they overcome poor teaching, overcrowded classrooms, or unmotivated students. (Wagner and others 1997, pp. 92–93).

Computer instructional programs tend to follow one of six types. They are

1. *Drill and practice.* In drill and practice, students are presented a series of questions to be answered or problems to be solved. The microcomputer immediately checks the responses and provides feedback to the student. Although drill-and-practice programs are one of the most common educational applications of computers, they can be unnecessarily boring for students, and they tend to promote rote learning. This strategy is most often used to reinforce or review material learned elsewhere.

2. *Tutorial.* The objective of the tutorial is frequently to teach concrete concepts. The microcomputer presents new information to the student, and then it poses a series of questions. Based on the responses provided by the student, the program either presents additional information or reviews the previous lesson. Users of this strategy should ensure that the software does not

Computers can serve as excellent motivational tools for students.

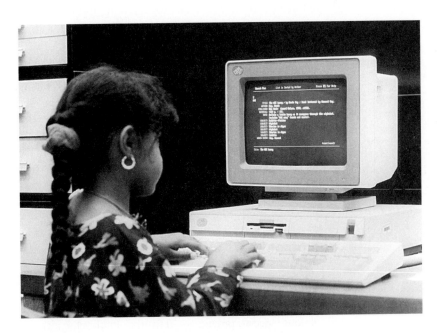

overwhelm the student with screen after screen of text. This repetition can quickly lead to learner fatigue.

3. *Demonstration.* A demonstration program allows students to observe a functioning model or situation. By observation, the student learns how systems work. For example, one commercial program demonstrates the effect of exercise on a graphic representation of a human heart, and another illustrates how nerve impulses travel through the nervous system of the body.

4. *Simulations.* Simulation programs imitate real or imaginary systems based on a modeler's theory of the operation of that system. Students test hypothetical courses of action by manipulating variables and observing the impact of these changes. This process allows the student to formulate realistic projections based on sound theory. Simulations can be used to make defined concepts more understandable. Programs currently available can simulate such things as a nuclear reactor, the human circulatory system, various ecosystems, and a malaria epidemic.

5. *Instructional games.* Games often use one or more of the strategies previously described. Instructional games, unlike arcade games, are designed to meet well-defined instructional objectives. Instructional games have explicit rules and winners, but educational concepts and information must be mastered for the player to become successful. For example, a commercially available game requires a knowledge of human anatomy and physiology to successfully complete a voyage through the human body.

6. *Problem solving.* Many advocates of computer-assisted instruction view the area of problem solving as one of the most powerful for the computer. Research has not indicated that using a computer is a significantly better way to teach problem solving than other strategies because the limited programming environment doesn't automatically guarantee transfer to real life. However, a new kind of problem-solving program has recently been introduced. This strategy is to confront learners with original situations that require the use of already acquired knowledge in new circumstances. Because the computer provides both prompts as needed and immediate response, the computer manages this type of activity well. Make sure that the educational strategy employed by the instructional program is appropriate for the content area and the students' abilities. Most important, consider whether the program being reviewed is superior to other strategies of teaching the same content.

Computers have great potential in the classroom. However, there are potential concerns of which teachers must be aware. Obviously, the high cost of computer hardware and software, as well as the incompatibility of different systems, is a problem. Gold (1991) also expressed concern at the possibility of dehumanizing the health education process. However, with the advent of outcome-based evaluation this seems less of a problem, because teachers must assist in developing objectives for the project and serve as overseer and interact with the student as the work progresses. Finding good software is another formidable task. The abundance of software programs makes finding quality software even more difficult. Because of cost, anything purchased must be used for a long time. Nevertheless, computer instruction is here to stay. The new technology that is coming on line everyday is adding to the potential that computers have in the classroom.

Television, Videotape, and Videodisk

It is probably safe to state that every school in the United States has access to television and videocassette recorders (VCRs). Many fine health-related programs, designed with the elementary school child in mind, are available. These include "Sesame Street," "Mr. Rogers' Neighborhood," and various special programs. Both the Public Broadcasting Service (PBS) and National

Educational Television (NET) regularly provide programs that can be used in health education. The commercial networks also occasionally produce suitable programs.

In addition to scheduled broadcasts, public and commercial agencies also make many programs available on film or videotape. For example, *Straight Up* (1987) was produced by KCET in Los Angeles and is distributed through Educational Enterprises. The series was developed for grades 4 through 6. It is composed of six 15-minute segments on substance abuse prevention and includes ancillary instructional materials, a comprehensive teacher's guide, student materials, and a comic book. The Best Foundation for a Drug-Free Tomorrow distributes three programs through the Agency for Instructional Technology in Bloomington, Indiana. The programs are *Just for Me* (1992), *Your Choice Our Chance* (1989), and *My Best* (1993). *Just for Me* is designed for grades 2, 3, and 4. This series of six fifteen-minute video programs consists of a teacher component, peer component, and home component. *Your Choice Our Chance* consists of ten fifteen-minute videos for students in grades 5 and 6 showing realistic situations involving children their age and the use of tobacco, alcohol, or marijuana. The emphasis is on positive skills for dealing with stress, peer and media pressure, self-esteem, and self-responsibility. A teachers' guide, informational video, and community component are included in the package. The third program, *My Best*, is designed for grades 7 and 8. This series of six videos deals with the same issues covered in the *Your Choice Our Chance* series.

Making your own videotapes for health instruction is also a useful approach although an expensive one because of the equipment involved. If your school has the equipment, however, you should consider using it. Record class plays, skits, and sociodramas. Also, suggest that students produce their own health public service messages or "commercials" for use in conjunction with consumer health discussions.

Choosing Videotapes and Videodisks

Most films used in the classroom are 16 mm, but this type of media is rapidly being replaced with videotape. Standard 16-mm films use a regular 16-mm projector, a piece of equipment to which virtually every school has access. Probably within the next decade, the 16-mm film will be replaced by the video cassette or the newer videodisk technology.

Videodisks are large vinyl disks that represent some of the latest technology being used in the classroom. The problem is that the equipment is quite expensive and the selection of disks is rather limited. The technology is extremely interactive and can be programmed to move quickly from one segment to another. In theory, they are less easy to damage than videotapes and easier to store. Selection should be based on similar criteria as for videotapes or CD-ROMs.

In considering videotape or disk as instructional devices, keep in mind that they should not serve as the sole basis of instruction and that every video must be carefully chosen and previewed. The following questions should be considered when selecting either films or videos for use in the classroom.

○ Is the tape or disk interesting and appropriate to the age and grade level?

○ Does the tape or disk convey the desired facts and concepts, and is it likely to contribute to the formation of positive health attitudes or behavior?

○ Is the tape or disk accurate and up-to-date?

○ Can the tape or disk be correlated with and integrated into the course of study at the particular grade level?

○ Is the language suited to the intended audience?

○ Does it meet reasonable standards of technical excellence in terms of quality, sound, and acting?

○ Is the videotape or disk of appropriate length?

○ Are there commercial overtones that are distasteful and detract from the educational message?

Keep a file of all audiovisuals you preview. An example of a typical file entry is shown in Figure 4.3. Such recordkeeping will help you build an index of especially useful films and will alert you to inappropriate ones.

Filmstrips

Filmstrips are continuous strips of 35-mm pictures. Captions or an accompanying sound track on a cassette provides the narrative. Filmstrips are colorful, relatively inexpensive, easy to use, and easy to store because they take up little space. The same criteria for selecting films should be used with filmstrips.

In addition to commercially prepared filmstrips, kits are available for classroom preparation of original filmstrips. This is an activity that upper elementary school children enjoy and find highly motivating. Titles and topics for original filmstrips might include *Ways of Keeping My Body Healthy, Community Health Helpers,* and *Waste Disposal in the Community.*

Slides

Another fairly inexpensive medium is 35-mm slides. These can be purchased from commercial sources, or you can make them yourself if you have a 35-mm camera and a bit of photographic skill. Like filmstrips, slides are colorful and easy to store. Depending on the kind of projector system you have, one slide tray will hold from 40 to more than 100 two-by-two-inch slides.

If you make your own slides, the subject matter can include class activities and field trips, health fairs, environmental problems in the community, and class projects. An advantage to using slides is that you can delete or add slides to the sequence as you desire. In this way, you can keep your slide collection current.

Overhead Transparencies

Used with an overhead projector, transparencies are extremely popular as teaching tools. A transparency consists of a 10-by-10-inch sheet of transparent acetate, usually mounted in a thin cardboard frame. Prepared transparencies can be purchased, or you can make your own either by using special transparency masters or by simply drawing on the acetate with felt-tipped pens. Both permanent and erasable inks are available.

One unique feature of using a transparency is the ability to show a progression by using a series of overlays. Overlays can be employed to show the position of organs within the body or to add or remove captions for informal quizzes.

Audio Tapes

Selectively used, audio tapes can be valuable teaching tools. They are inexpensive and can be stopped as needed for discussion. Finding useful tapes may take some work on your part, however, because relatively few are available that relate directly to health instruction.

Tape recordings are in some ways more versatile than visuals. You can easily make recordings of radio and television programs, for example, or of interviews with health officials, classroom

Health Highlight

Examples of Software/CD-ROMs for Classroom Use

A.D.A.M. Essentials: School Edition
4000 identification labels in approximately 100 layers. Detailed overviews of 13 anatomical systems with classroom activities and animation summaries for each system. Lists of key terminology and student activity sheet. Includes a teacher's guide.
Grades 5–9
Macintosh and PC

Forest Biomes
Complexity of the forest ecosystem is explored with live action video. Study the balanced network of plant and animal relationships that make up the food chain.
Grades 5–9
Macintosh

Scholastic's The Magic School Bus Explores the Human Body
Students travel aboard a bus into a human body, to learn about the parts of the body and how organs and systems work.
Grades 6–10
Windows 3.1 and above

3-D Body Adventures
CD-ROM in which students use 1950s-style 3-D glasses to fly through organs, examining them from every angle and in cross sections of actual human tissue. Students hear complete descriptions of anatomy and systems. "Emergency Room" players can cure patients based on their symptoms and medical history. This aspect provides a great test of what was learned in using the material.
Grades 2–8
Macintosh and Windows 3.1 and above

Grab a Byte
Consists of three separate programs, including (1) *Restaurant*—students enter their height and weight and choose foods for their meal(s). Nutritional values, calories, vitamins, etc. are provided; (2) *Grab a Grape*—three levels of difficulty on six nutritional areas. Examples are food and sports, and weight management; (3) *Nutrition Sleuth*—clues are provided on nutritional mysteries. Each incorrect response results in another clue. Scores are presented as the game continues.
Grades 6, 7, and 8
Windows 3.1 and above

guest speakers, and so forth. Recording commercials for classroom use can be useful when teaching consumer health.

Selecting Appropriate Media

Which of the many available media should you use for a particular instructional situation? How should you prepare yourself and your students for the medium that you have chosen? These are important questions that you must ask yourself before using television, films, videocassettes, or any other instructional medium. Kinder (1973, 29–30) offers some useful guidelines:

Figure 4.3

A Checklist for Audiovisuals and Instructional Software

Title _____ Date Reviewed

Distributor _____ Rent _____ Cost_____

Loan _____ Purchase_____ Cost_____

Media Type

     ○ Videotape   ○ 35-mm slides   ○ Filmstrip   ○ CD-ROM

     ○ Videodisk   ○ Audio tape   ○ Computer software

     ○ Other

Evaluation Instructions

Below are criteria that can be used to rate audiovisuals, CD-ROMS, and other media. Not all sections are appropriate for all types of media. A four-point scale is provided for evaluating the various media.

       4 = Excellent   3 = Good   2 = Average   1 = Poor

Content/Format

1. Is the production technically accurate? _____
2. Accuracy of content _____
3. Grammar/spelling_____
4. Multicultured_____
5. Viewer appeal _____
6. Exude or elicit biases _____
7. Use of special effects _____
8. Length of production _____
9. Music, background, dress _____
10. Sound quality_____
11. Creative production _____
12. Reference or user's guide_____

Overall Rating

       48–43 = Excellent content/format   36–31 = Average content/format

       42-37 - Good content/format   30 and below = Poor content/format

Appropriate for intended audience(s)? ○ Yes   ○ No

Useful for special projects? ○ Yes   ○ No

Comments _____

_____

_____

_____

Computer Software/CD-ROM

Title _____

Distributor _____ Phone _____ Cost_____

License _____ Costs _____

Compatible with what hardware   ○ Mac   ○ Windows 3.1 or higher   ○ Other

Version_____ Updates available_____

Needs for operation

○ RAM   ○ Memory   ○ Modem   ○ Hard Drive   ○ CD-ROM

Grade level_____ Computer skill level required: ○ Beginner   ○ Intermediate   ○ Advanced

Technical information:

Graphics_____ Help screens_____ Personalize database_____ Pulldown menu_____

Information display_____ Help hotline ( )___ - ____ Assessments available_____

Output of individual student data   Yes_____ No_____   Classroom data output   Yes_____ No_____

Manuals provided   Teacher_____   Student_____   Technical_____

Comments _____

_____

_____

_____

Reviewed by _____ Date _____

Recommended purchase   Yes_____   No_____

1. Choose instructional media that fit specific objectives of the instruction. By listing your objectives first, then selecting materials that best further the attainment of those objectives, you will avoid using materials merely for the sake of using materials.

2. Prepare yourself in advance. Once you have selected the media you will use for your lesson, familiarize yourself with them and consult study guides and manuals. Further, integrate the materials you have chosen into your lesson plan, considering sequence, timing, and proper coordination of all learning materials used.

3. Prepare the class in advance. Student readiness ensures an atmosphere conducive to assimilation. Discuss with the class in advance the materials to be used, by name, type, source, and so forth. Make the students aware of the reasons for using those particular materials. Suggest things to look for and associations to consider. Introduce any new or unusual words, phrases, or symbols. Also, explain any negative features of the material beforehand.

4. Prepare the physical facilities in advance. Although students are a captive audience, they are entitled to the use of all learning materials under optimum conditions. All equipment and media should be ready before the class assembles and should be in good working order. Alternative material should be available in case of breakdown. Schedule student equipment operators, if used, and be sure that you and/or the student operator knows how to operate the equipment easily. Attend to seating arrangements, screen placement, lighting control, sound volume, and similar considerations.

5. Ensure student participation either before, during, or after the presentation. The actual degree of participation will depend on the types of material used, their purpose, and the student's age or grade levels. Audio material does not necessarily eliminate student discussion, for example.

6. Follow up the use of instructional media with related activities and an evaluation of the materials by the class. Help the students solidify associations and conclusions, and encourage them to summarize the content. You might test the students on the lesson or repeat the use of the media presentation if necessary. Follow-up projects might involve individual students, committees, the entire school, or even the community.

7. Evaluate the materials that you have used. Judge how well the materials did the job they were intended to do. Consider whether the students responded positively. Then ask yourself what other materials, if any, might do a better job.

≣ *Summary*

○ A strategy is an activity or experience that the teacher uses to interpret, illustrate, or facilitate learning.

○ Proper selection of strategies helps provide interest, motivation, and reinforcement of learning.

○ Strategies should contribute to total learning, more complex concepts should have several strategies, proceed from the simple to the complex, include audiovisual aids, and be based on the learning styles of the students.

○ Regardless of the strategy, an environment that is conducive for learning must be developed and maintained.

○ Values clarification activities help students to determine their feelings concerning issues and concepts.

○ Verbal and discussion-oriented strategies include brainstorming, buzz groups, case studies, cooperative learning, critical essays, committee work, debates, panel discussion, and resource speakers.

○ Action-oriented strategies include dramatizations, storytelling, flannel, felt, and magnetic boards, crossword puzzles, demonstrations/experiments, exhibits, field trips, games, and model/specimens.

○ Peer helper programs are an excellent strategy for offering other children assistance and serving as role models. Peer helpers must be trained.

○ Instructional media are not strategies in themselves, but do serve as valuable approaches for involving students in the learning process. Examples include computers, television, videotapes, filmstrips, transparencies, and audio recordings.

○ The decision to use any strategy should be based on how effective it will be in facilitating learning.

○ A strategy should be chosen because it offers some teaching advantage, not simply novelty.

Discussion Questions

1. What factors should you keep in mind when selecting strategies for classroom use?

2. Discuss the strengths and weaknesses of values clarification techniques.

3. Describe the process for using decision stories in the classroom, from preparation of the stories to discussion and follow-up activities.

4. Select three types of discussion-oriented strategies, such as brainstorming and debate, and discuss the strengths and weaknesses of each approach.

5. Select three types of action-oriented strategies, such as dramatizations and field trips, and discuss the strengths and weaknesses of each.

6. Why must discussion-oriented strategies be structured for greatest effectiveness?

7. How can the computer be effectively used in the classroom?

8. What are the criteria for selecting media for the classroom?

9. Select three types of media, such as computers and television, and discuss the strengths and weaknesses of each.

References

Agency for Instructional Technology (AIT). 1989. *Your choice. . . our chance: Teacher's guide.* Bloomington, IN: AIT.

Agency for Instructional Technology (AIT). 1992. *Just for me: Teacher's guide.* Bloomington, IN: AIT.

Bullough, R.V. 1988. *Creating instructional materials.* 3d ed. Columbus, OH: Merrill.

Carr, R. 1992. *Peer helper handbook to accompany just for me.* Bloomington, IN: Agency for Instructional Technology.

Curtis, J., and R. Papenfuss. 1980. *Health instruction: A task approach.* Minneapolis: Burgess.

Evertson, C. M., E. T. Emmer, B. S. Clements, and M. E. Worsham. 1997. *Classroom management for elementary teachers.* Boston: Allyn and Bacon.

Foder, G. T., and G. T. Dalis. 1989. *Health Instruction: Theory and application.* 4th ed. Philadelphia: Lea & Febiger.

Gold, R. S. 1991. *Microcomputer application in health education.* Dubuque, IA: Brown.

Gold, R. S., and D. Duncan. 1980. Computers and health education. *Journal of school health* 50:503–505.

Greenberg, J. S. 1989. *Health education—Learner-centered instructional strategies.* Dubuque, IA: Brown.

Hamrick, M., D. Anspaugh, and D. Smith. 1980. Decision making and the behavioral gap. *Journal of school health* 50:455–58.

Hubbard, B. M. 1992. *A teacher's guide for my best.* Bloomington, IN: Agency for Instructional Technology.

Kinder, J. 1973. *Using instructional media.* New York: Van Nostrand.

Petosa, R., and Gillespie, J. 1984. Microcomputers in health education: Characteristics of quality instructional software. *Journal of school health* 54:394–396.

Popham, J. W. 1995. *Classroom assessment—what teachers need to know.* Boston: Allyn and Bacon.

Rivard, J. D. 1997. *Allyn & Bacon quick guide to the Internet for educators.* Boston: Allyn and Bacon.

Sager, R. A. 1987. Microcomputer software—The hard part. *Health education* 18(3): 52–56.

Smith, D., M. Hamrick, and D. Anspaugh. 1981. Decision story strategy: Practical approach for teaching decision making. *Journal of school health* 51(10):637–43.

Stone, D., L. O'Reilley, and J. Brown. 1980. *Elementary school health education.* Dubuque, IA: Brown.

Taylor, H., L. Genevie, and X. Zhao. 1988. *Health: You've got to be taught.* New York: Metropolitan Life Foundation.

Timmreck, T. 1978. Creative health education through puppetry. *Health education* 9(1):40–41.

Wagner, B., S. Gregory, M. Daniel and J. Sapers. 1997. "Where computers do work." *U. S. News & World Report* 121(22):82–93.

Chapter Five
Measurement and Evaluation of Health Education

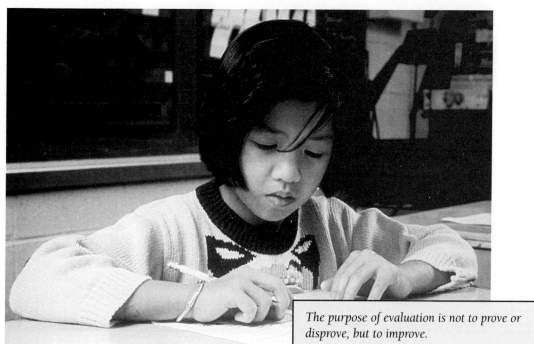

> The purpose of evaluation is not to prove or disprove, but to improve.
>
> —J. Thomas Butler

Valued Outcomes

After reading this chapter, you should be able to

○ explain the difference between measurement and evaluation

○ list the teacher skills needed to be competent in measuring and evaluating student progress

○ discuss the steps necessary for developing a teacher-made test

○ identify alternative methods of assessment

○ discuss the Kentucky model of student evaluation

Measurement and Evaluation

Every instructional effort should be evaluated to determine how successful it has been. Both student learning and teacher effectiveness must be determined. The emphasis in recent years on teacher accountability has made evaluation more important than ever.

Measurement can be defined as the process of obtaining a numerical description of the degree to which an individual possesses a particular characteristic (Gronlund and Linn 1990). Stanley and Hopkins (1990, 3–4) define measurement slightly differently but maintain the same framework of reference when they state that measurement is the construction, administration, and scoring of tests. Measurement generally results in quantitative data in numerical form. The various types of tests, rating scales, attitude scales, checklists, and observation techniques used in the elementary school are all forms of measurement. The resulting raw data, however, must be evaluated before the effectiveness of the instruction can be assessed. Data are not information; they are only the basis for information. They answer the question "How much?"

Evaluation is the process of collecting, analyzing, and interpreting information to determine the extent to which pupils are achieving instructional objectives (Gronlund and Linn 1990). The purpose of evaluation is to arrive at a judgment of value, worth, merit, or effectiveness (Payne 1992). Evaluation can be either objective or subjective. It is a judgment of what the numerical measurement data actually mean. For example, if all the students in a class get a perfect score on a test, has the instruction been successful? Perhaps not. The test might have simply measured what was known before any instruction. Or the test might have been so poorly constructed that the correct answers were obvious whether instruction had been provided or not.

More importantly, evaluation is now seeking to provide more than a score to determine successful learning. Techniques include performance-based evaluation, narrative grading, portfolio evaluation, group projects, individual exhibits, critical thinking essays.

Generally, evaluation has been delineated into three general approaches that are expressed in terms of levels. These are presented in Figure 5.1 and are expressed as (1) process evaluation, (2) impact evaluation, and (3) outcome evaluation (Green and Simons-Morton 1990). For most class-

Figure 5.1
Three Approaches to Evaluation

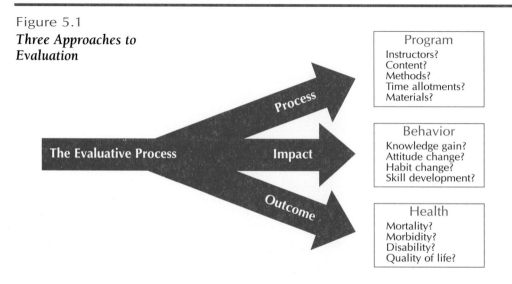

room teachers, the impact level is the one most often addressed. Process and outcome evaluation are important concerns but, because of lack of time, are usually not assessed. For purposes of this text, impact evaluation will receive the major emphasis, because classroom health educators must deal daily with this type of assessment.

Specifically, the purposes of measurement and evaluation are

○ *to assess the effectiveness of the learning activities.* Measurement and evaluation will help determine whether learning activities that have been designed and employed have increased knowledge, helped clarify values or determine attitudes, and promoted decision-making skills. If not, the activities must be revised or replaced.

○ *to motivate the student.* Tests help students recognize how much learning has taken place. Pretests are useful for introducing the scope of a topic and making students aware of the material that will be covered. Posttests then are used to chart actual student progress.

○ *to help develop the scope and sequence of teaching.* Measurement and evaluation can help determine the level of teaching and the order in which it should occur. For example, if the knowledge level of a class is high, a simple review of the factual material may be all that is necessary before moving on to new subject matter. Or, if the factual material is known, the decision may be to work next on developing attitudes toward this knowledge.

Teacher Skills Needed
for Competent Measurement and Evaluation

Becoming competent in measurement and evaluation does not happen overnight. Developing the skills that will be needed occurs in education classes, in educational psychology classes, and during student teaching. As a teacher gains professional experience, these skills will be sharpened. To be competent at measuring and evaluating, the National Council on Measurement in Education (1990) notes that a teacher should be skilled in

1. *choosing assessment methods appropriate for instructional decisions.* Criteria that should be considered include convenience and fairness. A variety of methods should be used, and a teacher should know where to obtain information about them.

2. *developing assessment methods appropriate for instructional decisions.* If high-quality commercial methods are not available, teachers must create them. Methods include classroom tests, oral exams, rating scales, performance assessment, observation schedules, and questionnaires.

3. *administering, scoring, and interpreting the results of both commercially produced and teacher-produced assessment methods.* Knowledge about the common methods of expressing assessments is essential. A large number of quantitative concepts need to be assimilated (for example, descriptive statistical methods, reliability, validity, and so on).

4. *using assessment results in making decisions about individual students, planning instruction, developing curriculum, and school improvement.* Assessments are valueless unless they are applied at both group and individual levels. Planning is a vital part of the education process.

5. *developing pupil-grading procedures that use pupil assessments.* Grades and marks should be data based. Grading, although subjective to a great extent, can be rational, justifiable, and fair. The rules must be the same for everyone.

6. *communicating assessment results to students, parents, other lay audiences, and educators.* Effective communication should include not only the facts but also an indication of the limitations and implications as well. In addition, everyone involved must use terminology in the same way.

7. *recognizing and having knowledge about unethical, illegal, and inappropriate assessment.* Potential dangers of invasion of privacy and discrimination exist, and these—together with legal and professional ethics—should always be in the forefront of a teacher's mind while planning and implementing assessment tasks.

In health education, measurement and evaluation cannot be limited to the cognitive domain but must also be vitally concerned with the formation of attitudes and behavior patterns among students. The emphasis in testing instruments is on quantitative measures, but these measures must also be employed to gain insight into qualitative areas. Selection of an instrument is not simply a matter of locating a test on a specific content. It is important to select the best test available; *best* being defined in terms of most appropriate for specific objectives and for specific students. If a test fails to measure what the teacher wants it to measure, another one needs to be developed.

Tests for assessing knowledge, attitudes, and practices are used to assess the impact of education on children.

Teacher-Made Tests

Teacher-made tests can be tailored to specific purposes and groups of students. This is a primary advantage. On the negative side, teacher-made tests may lack validity and reliability. However, with experience, the tests that teachers develop should become increasingly good indicators of student learning and change.

In constructing tests, each of the following areas must be included:

Validity. Does the test measure what it is supposed to measure? If the desire is to determine changes in student attitudes, for example, a test that asks students for factual information will not fulfill this intent. Validity is a matter of degree, not a characteristic that is absent or present. A test that is currently valid may not necessarily be so in the future. Because tests are designed for a variety of purposes, and because validity can be viewed only in terms of purpose, it is not surprising that there are several types of validity. **Content validity** is defined as the degree to which a test measures an intended content area. **Construct validity** is the degree to which a test measures a hypothetical construct. Intelligence is an example. **Concurrent validity** is the degree to which the scores on a given test are related to the scores on another test. **Predictive validity** is the degree to which a test can predict how well a student will do in a particular situation.

Reliability. Does the test measure accurately and consistently? A test that gives consistent results is said to possess reliability. For example, if a class takes the same test two different days, the scores obtained should be about the same. A reliable test will yield data that are stable, repeatable, and precise (Hastad and Lacy 1989). An intuitive sense of how reliable an instrument is can be gained by comparing test results with classroom observations. Hopkins and Antes (1990, 292) reported that, in general, reliability will be greater for

1. a long test than a short one

2. a test on homogeneous content rather than one on heterogeneous content

3. a set of scores from a group of examinees with a wide ability range rather than from a group that has members much alike

4. a test composed of well-written and appropriate items

5. measures with few scoring errors rather than for measures that vary from test to test or paper to paper because of scoring procedures

6. test scores obtained by proper conditions for testing and students with optimum motivation

Other factors that can affect the reliability of a test include inappropriate test items, the way the test is administered to the students, how the test is scored and interpreted, and the physical condition of the test environment.

Objectivity. Is the test fair to the students? For example, if the readability level is too high, students may be unable to supply correct answers even if they understand the concept being tested. If there is more than one possible correct answer, students should not be penalized for providing reasonable alternatives.

Discrimination. Does the test differentiate among good, average, and poor students?

Comprehensiveness. Is the test long enough to cover the material? Keep in mind that a fifty-item test may be no more comprehensive than a ten-item test if the items tap only certain areas while neglecting others.

Administration and Scoring. Is the test easy to give, use, and score? Keep in mind that the easiest test to administer and score may not be the best test for assessing the area. For example, an essay test, which is more difficult to score, may provide a better assessment of certain concepts than an easier-to-score true/false test.

Developing Tests

Developing good tests is a difficult task. The starting point is to establish a table of specifications. This table serves as the blueprint for the test. The purpose of the table of specifications is to ensure that all the objectives for a unit or lesson are covered on the test. By developing the table, the teacher can ensure that the proper percentage of test items appears in relationship to the emphasis placed on each objective (see Table 5.1).

1. Prepare the table of specifications based on the unit objectives.

2. Draft the test items.

3. Decide on the length of the test.

4. Select and edit the final items.

5. Rate the items in terms of difficulty.

6. Arrange the items in order of difficulty from easiest to most difficult.

7. Prepare the instructions for the test.

8. Prepare the answer key and decide the rules for scoring.

9. Produce the test.

Paper-and-pencil tests are best suited for measuring student progress in the cognitive domain.

The next area of concern is developing the various types of test items. The following represent some of the advantages/disadvantages and rules for development for each type of item.

Several types of test items can be used for assessment purposes. Some teachers may wish to use a variety of types, while others may prefer one or two types. It is wise to employ at least two types of test items because some students don't always do well on a particular type of test item. For example, some students do well on essay tests, while others do better on a multiple choice.

Another important consideration is the order in which the test items appear. Most important, all items should be grouped together. This helps to simplify directions, makes it easier for students to maintain the same psychological set throughout each section, and makes the scoring of the test easier. Test items should proceed from the simpler items to more complex ones. The following order is suggested for sections of test items:

1. *True/false.* Consists of declaratory statements that are either true or false.
   Examples:
   T   A.   Drugs are harmful if they are abused.
   F   B.   A burn on the skin should be bandaged tightly.

2. *Matching.* Answers in one column to be paired with the correct item in another column. A form of multiple-choice test, except that the number of choices is compounded.
   Example:

a	1.	compensation	a.	covering faults by trying to excel in another area.
c	2.	regression	b.	creating make-believe events.
d	3.	rationalization	c.	acting in an immature way.
			d.	making an excuse for a mistake or failure.

3. *Multiple choice.* Requires the student to recognize which of several suggested responses is the best answer. This kind of test provides an opportunity to develop thought-provoking questions. It is considered the best short-answer test format.
   Example:
   c   1.   Which of these nutrients helps repair the body?
           a.   carbohydrates
           b.   fats
           c.   proteins
           d.   vitamins

4. *Short answer questions.* Includes a variety of types of questions ranging from fill-in-the-blank to listing.
   Example:
   A.   List the four chambers of the heart.
                Right atrium
                Left atrium
                Right ventricle
                Left ventricle
   B.   The iris controls the amount of *light* going to the lens.

5. *Essay questions.* Requires the student to organize in a systematic fashion. Allows the teacher to gain insight into the amount of understanding students have developed.
   Example:
   What has been most influential in shaping your perceptions of yourself? Do you feel some of these perceptions are correct?

Regardless of the type of item employed, each item should be evaluated as to that item's effectiveness (Gronlund and Linn 1990, 230). The following questions should be asked concerning each item and the test as a whole.

1. *Is the item format appropriate for the teaming outcome being measured?* The action verb in the statement of each specific learning outcome (*defines, describes, identifies*) indicates which item format is more appropriate.

2. *Does the knowledge, understanding, or thinking skill called forth by the item match the specific teaming outcome and subject matter content being measured?* The response called forth by an item should agree with the purpose for which the item is to be used.

3. *Is the point of the item clear?* Each item should be so clearly worded that all pupils understand the task. Correct responses should be determined solely by whether students possess the knowledge being measured.

4. *Is the item free from excessive verbiage?* Items are generally more effective when the problem is stated concisely. If there are any elements that the pupils may disregard and still respond correctly, they probably should be removed.

5. *Is the item of appropriate difficulty?* The best judgment about item difficulty (unless item analysis data are available) should be based on the nature of the test and the educational background of the pupils.

6. *Does the item have an answer that would be agreed on by experts?* Do not include items that require pupils to endorse someone's unsupported opinion (even if it happens to be yours).

7. *Is the item free from technical errors and irrelevant clues?* An irrelevant clue is any element that leads the nonachiever to the correct answer and thereby prevents the item from functioning as intended.

8. *Is the item free from racial, ethnic, and sexual bias?* A judicious and balanced use of different roles for minorities and males and females should contribute to more effective testing.

Table 5.1

Specifications for Unit on Substance Abuse

Valued Outcome: The learner will . . .	Content	Percentage of items
Define what constitutes substance abuse.	What substance abuse is; what abuse causes; what some symptoms are	15%
List the various substances that can be abused.	Depressants (types); cocaine; marijuana; designer drugs; hallucinogens	35%
Discuss why people use drugs.	Reasons for drug use	15%
List where to get help for substance abuse.	Agencies; organizations; professionals	10%
Develop techniques for avoiding substance abuse.	How to say no to substance abuse	25%

Measuring Health Attitudes

The need to measure attitudes is probably greater in health education than in any other subject area. Attitudes have been defined as "descriptions of how people typically feel about or react to other people, places, things, or ideas" (Kubiszyn and Borich 1990, 156). In other words, an attitude involves feelings, values, and appreciations. An attitude can also be described as a predisposition to actions. Because one of the goals in teaching health is the development of positive health attitudes, it is essential to attempt to assess student attitudes.

This is no easy matter, because attitudes are not within the cognitive domain and are not thus readily tapped by most kinds of tests. Even those that are designed for this purpose often lack validity, as students may respond with answers they think the teacher will favor rather than state their true feelings or predispositions. Thus, it is important to supplement such testing instruments with other means of assessment, such as self-inventories, questionnaires, checklists, observation, informal conferences, small-group discussion, and anecdotal recordkeeping. These strategies produce subjective indications of what the child's attitudes may be. With these limitations in mind, we now examine some of the more common written measures for assessing student attitudes.

Attitude Scales

A scale is a testing instrument that requires the student to choose between alternatives on a continuum. Two polar choices, such as yes/no or agree/disagree, may be offered, or a range of choices may be provided.

Figure 5.2 shows a *forced-choice scale,* one that provides only two options about each statement being considered. This kind of attitude scale is appropriate for use with younger children, who lack the developmental ability to handle more complicated attitude scales.

The major disadvantage of the forced-choice scale test is that students can readily perceive what the "correct" response should be. They will respond accordingly, even if the answer does not reflect their actual attitude toward the issue. This problem can be overcome to a certain degree by establishing an atmosphere in the classroom of warmth, trust, and rapport.

Figure 5.2

***Example of a Forced-
Choice Attitude Scale***

Rating Myself: How I Feel

		Agree	Disagree
1.	My overall physical health is excellent.	_____	_____
2.	I have a positive attitude toward most things.	_____	_____
3.	I have the ability to make my life work.	_____	_____
4.	I relate well to other people.	_____	_____
5.	I have control of my life.	_____	_____

A *Likert scale* is a more sophisticated attitude scale that provides a range of choices about each attitudinal issue. The more choices that are offered, the more discrimination a student must have to complete the scale. Figure 5.3 provides an example of a Likert scale.

Scoring may be done in a variety of ways, depending on how the statements in the scale are phrased. For example, the continuum of responses may be weighted from 1 to 5, with the lowest score for a *strongly disagree* statement and the highest score for a *strongly agree* statement. Thus, if a student checks *strongly agree* to the statement, "Being stoned all the time is no way to live," the score would be a 5. An *undecided* response would rate a 3, and a *strongly disagree* would rate a 1. Note that the scoring rank must be reversed for oppositely worded statements, such as "Experimenting with drugs is not really very risky." In this case, a *strongly disagree* response would score as a 5.

The total numerical score derived from adding the individual response scores offers a measure of how firmly opinions and attitudes are held about the issues examined in the scale. However, this measure, despite its seeming quantitative preciseness, is only a rough indicator of attitude. Bear in mind that the scoring system is arbitrary; that even with five options, students are still making forced choices; and that students may respond with "correct" answers that do not actually reflect their true attitudes. Instruments used for attitude assessment should not be used for purposes of grading, because this will further bias the students' responses.

Observation

As mentioned earlier, the use of attitude scales to assess children's feelings and values has its limitations. The results of such scales are often inconclusive. Scales or other measurement devices,

Figure 5.3

A Likert Scale with a Five-Choice Spread

Feelings about Exercise

	Strongly Agree	Agree	Not Sure	Disagree	Strongly Disagree
1. Exercise is healthy for a person.	____	____	____	____	____
2. I like to run and jump.	____	____	____	____	____
3. I would rather watch TV than engage in exercise.	____	____	____	____	____
4. I feel relaxed after exercising.	____	____	____	____	____
5. Playing sports is fun.	____	____	____	____	____
6. I cannot work on exercise.	____	____	____	____	____
7. Playing sports and games is too much work to program into my daily schedule.	____	____	____	____	____
8. I would rather watch sports than play them.	____	____	____	____	____
9. Exercise helps keep me healthy.	____	____	____	____	____

such as checklists or student surveys, should be augmented with other techniques, including observation and anecdotal recordkeeping.

Observation is an excellent way of assessing behavior. Because observation can be done on an ongoing, daily basis, it can provide important clues as to attitudes and predispositions to actions. A major disadvantage of observation is that it is time consuming. Further, discretion must be exercised so as not to violate student and parent privacy.

In assessing student health attitudes, an attempt to remain neutral in observations should be made. Variations in personal health attitudes and behaviors are not necessarily a cause for concern. Children are still forming their attitudes about health-related issues. They should not be expected to have completely made up their minds about health practices. If they have, there would be far less point to the job of teaching.

Further, attitude formation is a gradual process. Instant changes in behavior patterns are not necessarily going to occur. The teacher's efforts can make a difference. With these thoughts in mind, one method to use in assessing attitudes is the checklist. The checklist allows the observer to note quickly and effectively whether a trait or characteristic is present. Checklists can be useful in evaluating learning activities or some aspects of personal-social interaction. Figure 5.4 is a sample checklist for evaluating student behavior after a unit on respect for others.

As has been noted, measuring attitudes is difficult. Any technique used to measure and evaluate attitudes or health practices should be done carefully and with student input if they are to be part of the grading process. If this is done, students will be more likely to reveal their true feelings or their actual practices. Instead, the evaluation can be used to plan for future instruction and

---

Figure 5.4
*Observation Checklist
for Assessing Respect
for Others*

Name _____   Date of Grade _____

Observation_____

Observer_____

Directions: Listed below are a list of characteristics related to "Respect for Others." For the student listed, check those characteristics that are appropriate.

_____ Respects views and opinions of others

_____ Is sensitive to needs of others

_____ Is sensitive to problems of others

_____ Respects the property of others

_____ Works cooperatively with others

_____ Addresses others in a respectful manner

to help students understand their current level of development. The more aware students become about themselves, the more likely it is that they will use this awareness to make conscious decisions about future behavior.

Traditional Grading Strategies

Grades serve to inform students, parents, teachers, and administrators about the progress and work efficiency of the student. Ideally, grades should not be an end in themselves. Instead, they should act as motivators for students to do their best and as guides to future courses of study. For parents, student grades identify the child's strengths and weaknesses and also help clarify the goals of the school. If parents gain insight through grades as to what the school is attempting to accomplish, they will be in a better position to cooperate with the teacher in enhancing the child's educational process. Administrators can use grades to see how effective the curriculum is and to step in to provide extra help for students who need it by means of special programs, counseling, and so forth.

Each school district has its own approach to grading. Teachers should become familiar with the system used in their district in order to apply the standards objectively and fairly.

The Percentage Method

This grading method is based on 100 percent. It assumes more preciseness than can actually exist and essentially reduces the range of scores from 70 to 100. Any student falling below 70 percent correct responses on a given test fails. Most school districts that employ this method use a scale similar to the following one:

A = 93–100
B = 85–92
C = 78–84
D = 70–77
F = Below 70

The A to F Combination Method

The A to F combination method system of grading is a combination of the percentage method and other descriptors that indicate student performance. With this method, students can be rated in relation to both the group norm and personal development. The A to F combination method better enables students and parents to know whether learning and work are being accomplished at peak capacity. For example, it is possible for students to make a C grade and still have them appreciate that they are working near maximum effort. A typical example of how this method is structured is as follows:

A = excellent work and working at or near capacity; 95–100%
B = good work and working at or near capacity; 85–94%
C = average work or all that should be expected; 77–84%
D = much less than should be expected; 70–76%
F = no noticeable progress; less than 70%

1 = above grade level
2 = at grade level
3 = below grade level

Health Highlight

Guidelines for Effective Grading

1. Describe your grading procedures to pupils at the beginning of instruction.
2. Make clear to pupils that the course grade will be based on achievement only.
3. Explain how other elements (effort, work habits, personal-social characteristics) will be reported.
4. Relate the grading procedures to the intended learning outcomes (instructional objectives).
5. Obtain valid evidence (tests, reports, ratings, and so on) as a basis for assigning grades.

6. Take precautions to prevent cheating on tests, reports, and other types of evaluation.
7. Return and review all test results (and other evaluation data) as soon as possible.
8. Properly weight the various types of achievement included in the grade.
9. Do *not* lower an achievement grade for tardiness, weak effort, or misbehavior.
10. Be fair. Avoid bias and when in doubt (as with a borderline score), review the evidence. If still in doubt, assign the higher grade.

The numbers can be used in conjunction with the letter grades. For example, a child who receives a grade of B-2 is performing near capacity at grade level, whereas a child who receives a grade of B-3 is performing near capacity but below grade level.

Pass/Fail

Some school districts use symbols for giving grades in health education. Most of the symbols are used to indicate a level of achievement. It is very hard for students and parents to interpret what the level of achievement indicates unless there is some information about that level (Mehrens and Lehmann 1984). Some of the symbols used to indicate achievement are O, S, and U for *outstanding, satisfactory,* and *unsatisfactory.* The symbols P and F are also used to indicate *pass* or *fail.* Others may use E, S, N, or U for *excellent, satisfactory, not satisfactory,* and *unsatisfactory.*

Unfortunately, any course using these symbols may be viewed as less important than those courses receiving the traditional A to F grades. Certainly, in the case of health education, this connotation must be avoided, because the knowledge, attitudes, and behaviors developed have the potential to be life enhancing, and, in some cases, life saving.

There are no easy answers in choosing a grading system. The best method is really a combination of systems. Each teacher and school system must weigh the advantages of each type of grading and select the one that best informs students and parents of progress.

Performance-Based Evaluation

In addition to traditional cognitive testing, which generally involves the use of paper-and-pencil tests, teachers must now seek to base their evaluation of students "upon the values, diversity, and ability to make environmentally sound and healthy personal choices" (Read 1997, 148). Most evaluation specialists refer to these types of evaluation as **performance-based evaluation.** Performance-based evaluation is not contingent on what the student recalls but on how they show what they have learned. Several techniques lend to this type of evaluation. Examples include portfolios, exhibitions, group projects, and critical thinking essays. **Portfolios** are defined as a purposeful collection of student work that exhibits effort, progress, and achievement. This effort must include the student's participation in selecting the content, how the material will be assessed, and what will provide evidence of student self-reflection (Woolfolk 1995). **Exhibitions** are considered a performance test or demonstration of learning that is presented before an audience and takes extended time to prepare (Woolfolk 1995). Examples of exhibits might include developing displays, writing skits or plays, or bulletin boards.

Critical thinking essays can be defined as cognitive writing activity that allows the student to analyze or synthesize information in order to make a decision (McCown, Driscoll, and Roop 1996, 382). An excellent way to promote critical thinking in elementary students is to provide the student with what King (1990) referred to as *reciprocal questioning* by having the students work in pairs or small groups to answer questions concerning the health topic. Questions that provide stems such as the following (King):

How would you use . . . to . . . ?
What is a new example of . . . ?
How are . . . and . . . similar?
What are the strengths and weaknesses of . . . ?

To ensure that portfolios will serve as useful tools, the following guidelines should be kept in mind:

1. There must be student involvement in selecting the components that will constitute the portfolio.
2. Students should include information that allows them to self-reflect and self-criticize.
3. Student activities should be reflected in projects, writing, and drawing, and result from the student's learning goals.
4. The portfolio should reflect the growth of the student in progress toward achieving insight and attitude/behavior development. It should reflect the feelings and thinking of the student.
5. Evaluation should be based on each student's established standards, not on comparisons with other students in the class.

Performance-based evaluation is a very important concept in health education, because attitude and ultimately behavior are the culminating factors. Obviously, in both the case of portfolios and exhibitions, group work and critical essays may be an extensive part of the process. Certainly when using this type of evaluation, it is difficult to tell where instruction stops and assessment starts because of the interwoven nature of the two in performance-based evaluation. The goal should be to help the students focus on what they have learned, how they have changed, and what they have achieved as a result of the process. What better way to do this than allow the student to have input on what will constitute learning and evaluation? Perhaps the greatest advantage of performance-based evaluation is that if done properly, children can learn, achieve, and progress in a fashion that does not label or negatively affect their self-esteem.

Peer Evaluation

A trend in the current rethinking of how evaluation should occur is to involve students in the process. One strategy for accomplishing this is through peer evaluation. Peer evaluation occurs when students evaluate each other's work (McCown, Driscoll, and Roop 1996, 457). "If we want people to gain control of important habits of standards and habits of mind, then they have to know . . . how to accurately view those things and to apply criteria to their own work" (Wiggins 1993, 54).

Peer evaluation occurs all the time on an informal basis when students look at one another's work for comparison with their own efforts. For peer evaluation to be effective, students should work together to establish the criteria or standards used for judging their work. By setting the standards for judgment, students have established their own goals, which they expect their work to reflect. Assessment can be done through the use of checklists or questionnaires.

Narrative Grading

Narrative grading has been defined as "serious dialogue between student and teacher about the quality of the work" (Shor 1992). The dialogue should be student generated and should reflect creative options as well as critical thinking. The facts should not be isolated from the student's experience. Effort should be made to help the student personalize the information to ensure positive health-related behavior. The advantage of this type of grading is that once verbalized, ownership of the concept(s) is more likely to occur. This strategy also enables students to assess their feeling on particular topics. The biggest disadvantage is that the process can be very time consuming when working with a large group.

The Kentucky Model

For years health educators have been seeking better ways of assessing student progress. The State of Kentucky may have identified a truly unique method of measuring and evaluating a student's progress. The plan is part of the Kentucky Education Reform package and has been labeled the Kentucky Instructional Results Information System (KIRIS).

Like most states, Kentucky in the past relied on annual achievement tests to measure "what" students knew. The new plan is performance based and seeks to measure not only "what students know" but also "what they can do." The goal is to have students apply what they know in situations they will face throughout their lives.

The actual assessment consists of three parts: (1) multiple-choice test accompanied by short essay questions; (2) performance tasks/situations that require students to either work individually or in groups to solve simulated, real-life problems; and (3) a portfolio that represents each student's best work from the past year. Based on the assessment, each child is placed into one of four performance levels. The identified levels include *novice, apprentice, proficient,* or *distinguished.* No child fails, because the lowest level, novice, recognizes the child as a beginner, not a failure.

Table 5.2 provides a conceptualization of how KIRIS works. The demonstrators are objectives for the elementary and middle school (the high school objectives are not shown). The learning links represent content areas, subjects that would contribute to fulfilling the objectives. Related concepts represent the skill acquisition necessary for meeting the objectives (demonstrators).

The sample teaching/assessment strategies and community resources are ideas to help the teacher develop the teaching strategies to help the student develop competency. The sample instruction and assessment activities are those suggestions specifically for the elementary level. Applications across the curriculum are activities in other learning areas that can be incorporated to help the student develop the valued outcome and objectives.

Table 5.2
*A Conceptualization of
the Kentucky Model*

Valued Outcome: Students will demonstrate positive strategies for achieving and maintaining mental and emotional wellness.

Demonstrators of Valued Outcome:

Elementary

- Practice interpersonal skills that contribute to healthy relationships and self-esteem.
- Recognize the factors that influence self-esteem.
- Demonstrate techniques for stress management.
- Predict consequences of substance abuse and other addictive behaviors.
- Recognize that mental and emotional health problems can be treated.
- Recognize and respect individual differences and take turns.
- Express basic feelings and emotions in a positive way.

Middle School

- Analyze factors that influence self-esteem.
- Practice strategies for achieving stress management.
- Plan strategies for avoiding substance abuse and other addictive behaviors.
- Apply interpersonal relationship skills that contribute to emotional well-being.
- Investigate methods of prevention, intervention, and treatment of mental and emotional disorders.
- Practice expressing self and reacting to others constructively.
- Use strategies to manage stress.

Learning Links

Stress
Substance abuse
Addictive behaviors
Relationships
Mental disorders
Grief
Nutrition
Student service
Organizations
Support groups
Relaxation
Drug therapy
Self-expression
Physical fitness
Counseling
Assertiveness
Arts and crafts

Related Concepts

Self-esteem
Interpersonal relationship skills
Communication
Stress management
Refusal skills
Conflict resolution
Goal setting
Rights and responsibilities
Self-assessment
Time management

Sample Teaching Assessments Strategies

Collaborative: peer tutoring, interviews, brainstorming • **Community-based instruction:** field studies, service learning • **Problem solving:** simulation, role-play, inquiry • **Whole-language approach**

Table 5.2
(*continued*)

Ideas for Incorporating Community Resources

- Invite a representative from a mental health agency to discuss mental and emotional disorders and/or ways to express feelings and emotions constructively.
- Invite a mental health expert to demonstrate the value of humor and other techniques for stress management.
- Tour a substance abuse treatment facility.
- Invite a law enforcement official to discuss the DARE Program and the consequences of a DUI citation.
- Invite a professional counselor to discuss coping with grief.

Sample Instruction and Assessment Activities—Elementary

- Make a class Big Book titled: "It's OK": Describe a situation on one page and on the next page write, "but it's OK to . . . " and identify reactions ("When my ice cream cone gets knocked out of my hand, it's OK . . . to tell Mom/ask for another cone/cry for a minute/expect an apology").
- Graph your positive characteristics and strong points. Develop a plan for self-improvement.
- Identify a situation that causes stress; explore and practice ways to relieve the stress constructively.
- Role-play a "what to do when" game to identify resources of treatment for mental and emotional health problems.
- Create a classroom collage of affirmatives.
- View a television program as a group; analyze ways emotions were expressed, both verbally and nonverbally, and the impact of the expressions on others.

Applications across the Curriculum—Elementary

Language Arts

- Brainstorm ways to deal with stress. Create a bumper sticker.

Science

- Develop and implement a plan to complete a science project. Set realistic short-term goals. Report progress emphasizing positive feelings on task completion.

Social Studies

- Research the elements of physical and emotional health. Produce role-plays to show the correct and incorrect strategies to promote good health.

Arts and Humanities

- Create a visual display to help someone change an unhealthy habit or manage stress. Present your work to a civic group and survey their reactions.

Vocational Studies

- Plan and prepare a comic book that illustrates ways to cope with stress.
- Make a collage using the warning labels from ads for alcohol and tobacco products.
- Mime various emotions (sad, happy, mad, and so on).

Health Highlight

Understanding the Results
of the Kentucky Instructional Results Information System

The table below represents a student's results on KIRIS taken in any given year. Each parent receives a copy of the table. The report does not reflect exactly where a student falls within each category, but each school does receive that information.

Percentage of students statewide achieving at each performance level
Your result is indicated by a √

SUBJECT	Novice	Apprentice	Proficient	Distinguished
Reading	40%	49%√	10%	1%
Mathematics	44%√	45%	9%	2%
Science	30%√	65%	5%	0%
Social Studies	41%	48%	10%√	1%

Interpretation:
Reading: This student was an Apprentice; 49% of the students statewide scored at this level.
Mathematics: This student was Novice; 44% of the students statewide scored at this level.
Science: This student was Novice; 30% of the students statewide scored at this level.
Social Studies: This student was Proficient; 10% of the students statewide scored at this level.

☰ *Summary*

- The purpose of measurement and evaluation is to determine whether instructional objectives have been fulfilled.
- Measurement involves the construction, administration, and scoring of tests.
- Evaluation is the process of interpreting, analyzing, and assessing the data gathered.
- Newer methods used for evaluation include performance-based evaluation, narrative grading, portfolios, group projects, individual exhibits, and critical thinking essays.
- Tests should be valid, reliable, objective, discriminate, comprehensive, and easy to give, use, and score.
- Typical test question types are true/false, matching, multiple choice, short answer, and essay.
- Measuring attitudes is difficult; examples of useful tools include attitude scales, checklists, and critical thinking essays.
- Traditional grading strategies include the percentage method, the A to F combination, and the pass/fail or satisfactory/unsatisfactory method.
- Newer methods include performance-based evaluation, critical thinking essays, peer review, and group projects.
- The state of Kentucky has developed a new model for student assessment that holds a great deal of promise.

Discussion Questions

1. Differentiate between measurement and evaluation.

2. Discuss the purposes of measurement and evaluation, and explain how you can achieve these purposes.

3. Why is a table of specifications necessary when developing a test?

4. Discuss some of the techniques used to assess attitudes in health education. What are the shortcomings of these techniques?

5. What purposes does grading serve in health education?

6. Discuss some of the common methods of grading used in the elementary school. Explain how they have changed in the 1990s.

7. Explain the Kentucky Instruction Results Information System (KIRIS) and the implications of the model for schools throughout the country.

References

Bedworth, A. E., and D. A. Bedworth. 1992. *The profession and practice of health education.* Dubuque, IA: Brown.

Butler, J. Thomas. 1992. *Principles of health education and health promotion.* Englewood, CO: Morton.

Carey, L. M. 1994. *Measuring and evaluating school learning.* Boston: Allyn and Bacon.

Ebel, R. L., and D. A. Frisbie. 1991. *Essentials of educational measurement.* 5th ed. Englewood Cliffs, NJ: Prentice Hall.

Evertson, C. M., E. T. Emmer, B. S. Clements, and M. E. Worshaw. 1997. *Classroom management for elementary teachers.* Boston: Allyn and Bacon.

Green, W. H., and B. G. Simons-Morton. 1990. *Introduction to health education.* Prospect Heights, IL: Waveland Press.

Gronlund, N. E., and R. L. Linn. 1990. *Measurement and evaluation in teaching.* New York: Macmillan.

Hopkins, C. D., and R. L. Antes. 1990. *Classroom measurement and evaluation.* 3rd ed. Itasca, IL: Peacock.

King, A. 1990 Enhancing poor interaction and learning in the classroom through reciprocal questioning. *American educational research journal* 27: 664–687.

Kubiszyn, T., and G. Borich. 1990. *Educational testing and measurement—Classroom application and procedure.* New York: HarperCollins.

McCown, R., M. Driscoll, and P. G. Roop. 1996. *Educational psychology—a learning-centered approach to classroom practice.* 2nd ed. Boston: Allyn and Bacon.

National Council on Measurement in Education (NCME). 1990. *Standards for teacher competence in educational assessment of students.* Washington, DC: NCME.

National Education Association (NEA), National Commission on Teacher Education and Professional Standards. 1955. *The improvement and use of tests by teachers: Implications for teacher education.* Washington, DC: NEA.

Payne, D. A. 1992. *Measuring and evaluating educational outcomes.* New York: Merrill.

Popham, J. W. 1996. *Classroom assessment—What teachers need to know.* Boston: Allyn and Bacon.

Read, D. A. 1997. *Health education—A cognitive-behavioral approach.* Boston: Jones & Bartlett Publishers.

Shor, I. 1992. *Empowering education: Critical teaching for social change.* Chicago: University of Chicago Press.

Stanley, J. C., and K. D. Hopkins. 1990. *Educational and psychological measurement and evaluation.* 7th ed. Englewood Cliffs, NJ: Prentice Hall.

Wiggins, G. P. 1993. *Assessing student performance.* San Francisco: Jossey-Bass.

Woolfolk, A. E. 1995. *Educational psychology.* 6th ed. Boston: Allyn and Bacon.

Chapter Six

Body Systems/
Personal Health

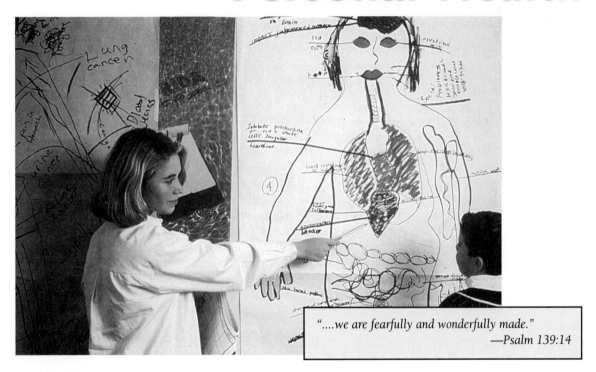

> "....we are fearfully and wonderfully made."
> —Psalm 139:14

Valued Outcomes

After reading this chapter, you should be able to

○ explain the differing roles of the cerebrum and the cerebellum

○ discuss the function of selected components (structures) of the nervous system

○ describe the functions of selected glands and the hormones associated with the endocrine system

○ discuss the role the components of the respiratory system play in the breathing process

○ trace a drop of blood through the circulatory and pulmonary systems

○ describe the major function of the red blood cells

○ explain the function of white blood corpuscles in fighting off infection

○ describe how food travels through the body

○ describe the function of the skeletal system

○ describe how liquid and solid wastes are filtered in the body

○ differentiate between voluntary and involuntary muscles

○ discuss the reasons a person with acne should avoid skin creams with an oil base

○ discuss the hazards of overexposing the skin to the sun

○ describe proper lifting, pushing, and pulling techniques to avoid hurting the lower back muscles

○ describe proper posture while sitting at a desk, walking, bending, and lifting

○ list the possible behavioral indications of vision problems

○ discuss the classroom adjustments a teacher should make for a student with poor vision

○ list the possible behavioral indications of hearing problems

○ discuss the proper health practices to prevent gum disease

○ list the cardiorespiratory benefits of a regular exercise program

A Unique Machine

The human body is an efficient functional organism, a most amazing and well-organized machine. If cared for properly, it will continue to perform well.

At conception, individuals are given the capacity for growth, development, and functioning through genetic factors. However, the environmental factors—especially health-related behaviors—determine the actual growth, development, and functioning.

Health and health enhancement can certainly never be achieved without keeping the body and its systems in good condition. This chapter will provide you with information you can use to help children learn about their bodies and how to care for them. The chapter presents a brief outline and description of several of the major systems of the body and discusses how these systems function. This description is followed by a section on how to care for the body.

The Nervous System

Because all physiological functions, and many psychological ones as well, are controlled in one way or another by the brain, discussion of the nervous system and its structure is a logical and appropriate beginning. The nervous system is composed of two major divisions—the central nervous system and the autonomic nervous system. The central nervous system includes the brain and the spinal cord. The autonomic nervous system includes the peripheral portions of the outlying nerves and nerve pathways not directly connected to the central nervous system.

The Central Nervous System

In conjunction with the sensory systems of the body, such as those responsible for vision and hearing, the central nervous system plays the chief role in altering and guiding individuals through their environments and enabling interaction with the world around them. The central nervous system allows us to perceive, interpret, and react to the various stimuli we come into contact with every day. For example, a message from the ears travels by way of the auditory nerve to the hearing center in the brain, and the brain interprets the message.

The Brain and Spinal Cord

The brain is the "computer center" of the central nervous system. It receives messages from and sends messages to the rest of the body by way of nerves and nerve pathways that originate in the spinal cord and branch to all other organs and tissue. The general structure of the brain and spinal column is shown in Figure 6.1, and a cross section of the spinal cord can be seen in Figure 6.2.

The human brain, weighing about 2 pounds in an adult, is the center for memory, motor activity, and thinking. It contains about 13 billion brain cells. These cells have a greater need for oxygen and are more sensitive to oxygen deprivation than any other cells in the body. The brain is encased and protected by the cranium, or skull. The spinal cord is enclosed and protected by thirty-three bones known as *vertebrae,* which are flexibly joined together to form the spinal column. The cord itself is about three-quarters of an inch in diameter and has thirty-one branching spinal nerves, each of which serves a particular part of the body.

Like the spinal cord, the brain is divided into parts. The major parts are the cerebrum, cerebellum, and brain stem.

The Cerebrum.   The largest part of the human brain, the cerebrum is the center for conscious mental processes. Thought and the ability to learn and reason originate in this part of the brain. In addition, all five of the sensory systems, as well as motor movement and coordination, are controlled by the cerebrum.

The cerebrum is divided into two halves, called *cerebral hemispheres,* in such a way that the left hemisphere controls the right side of the face and body, while the right hemisphere controls the left side of the face and body (see Figure 6.3).

Since each specific area of the cerebrum controls a specific function, brain damage to a portion of the brain may impair one sensory system to varying degrees without harming others. For example, a person's sense of taste, smell, and hearing may be damaged without motor coordination, speech, and vision being adversely affected. Or memory may be diminished without loss of sensation to touch, and so on. The various control centers of the cerebrum are illustrated.

The Cerebellum.   Like the cerebrum, the cerebellum consists of two hemispheres. The cerebellum has two main functions—coordination of muscle groups and maintenance of equilibrium. Damage to the cerebellum may result in jerky or spastic movements. A person may walk with a stagger, as if intoxicated, but memory loss and sensory impairment may not exist, because these functions are mainly controlled by the cerebellum functioning.

As an example of the differing roles of the cerebrum and the cerebellum, a conscious decision to perform a task, such as bicycling, originates in the cerebrum, but the messages sent to the specific muscle groups that perform the task originate in the cerebellum. The directions for accomplishing the task, once it is learned, are then stored in the cerebellum until a conscious order arises from the cerebrum to initiate the task once again.

The Brain Stem.   As the name implies, the brain stem is a tubelike structure located at the base of the brain, and is the center of physiological responses that do not require conscious thought or action in order to be performed. Circulation, respiration, and blood pressure are controlled by the brain stem, as are responses to sensory signals from the internal organs, such as hunger and thirst. In addition, fear, anger, and other emotional reactions are triggered in the brain stem.

In essence, the brain stem acts as a conductor between the spinal column and the cerebrum. The actual connection between the spinal cord and the brain is found at the medulla oblongata, the very bottom of the brain stem.

Figure 6.1
The Brain and Spinal Column

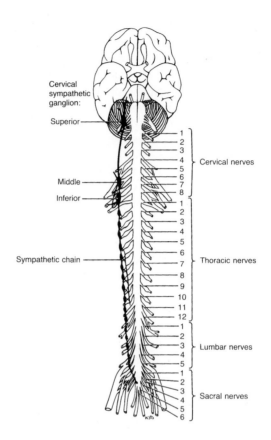

Cervical sympathetic ganglion:

Superior

Middle

Inferior

Sympathetic chain

1
2
3
4
5
6
7
8
} Cervical nerves

1
2
3
4
5
6
7
8
9
10
11
12
} Thoracic nerves

1
2
3
4
5
} Lumbar nerves

1
2
3
4
5
6
} Sacral nerves

Figure 6.2
A Cross-Section of the Spinal Cord

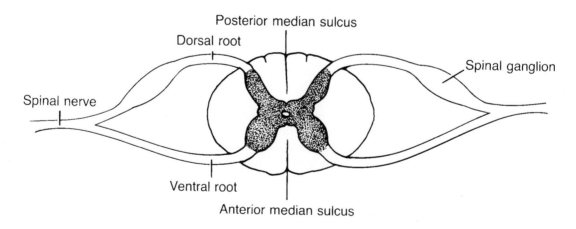

Posterior median sulcus

Dorsal root

Spinal ganglion

Spinal nerve

Ventral root

Anterior median sulcus

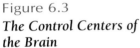
Figure 6.3
*The Control Centers of
the Brain*

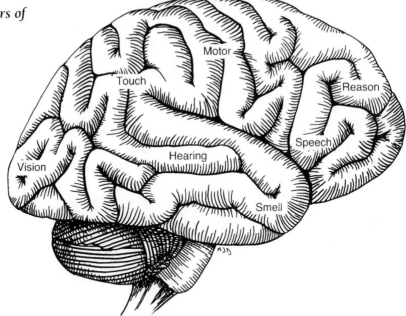

The Autonomic Nervous System

The second major division of the nervous system is the autonomic nervous system. Reflexes, as well as the physiological adaptations the body makes as a whole to its external environment, are largely controlled by skeletal muscles. These functions fall under the jurisdiction of the autonomic nervous system. In addition, the autonomic nervous system helps regulate the internal environments of various vital organs.

The Endocrine System

Closely associated with the nervous system is the endocrine system. This section describes some of the glands associated with the endocrine system.

The endocrine system's role is that of a regulator. Through the production and secretion of chemical substances called *hormones* from thirteen tiny glands dispersed throughout the body, the endocrine system keeps the other body systems and processes in balanced operation. The two "controller" glands of the endocrine system are the hypothalamus and the pituitary. They secrete hormones that in turn signal other endocrine glands to activate. Both the hypothalamus and the pituitary glands are located in the brain, thus establishing the close relationship between the endocrine system and the nervous system.

The Hypothalamus

The hypothalamus is thought to be the conductor and regulator of daily operations of the body. Current research suggests that the hypothalamus is responsible for orchestrating the actions of the pituitary, which in turn triggers other endocrine glands. The hypothalamus lies in the posterior portion of the forebrain. Without signals from this master gland, the pituitary would not activate, resulting in the malfunction of many normal processes.

Apart from directing the pituitary, the hypothalamus also integrates and balances the work of the internal organs governed by the autonomic nervous system by controlling the hormonal secretions of various endocrine glands throughout the body. In addition, the hypothalamus serves as the sleep center, temperature-regulating center, and appetite and hunger center for the body. Other similar centers, not yet clearly identified, are also believed to be regulated by the hypothalamus (Guyton 1992, 450).

The Pituitary.   Once thought to be the master gland, the pituitary is a pea-sized mass lying at the base of the brain. It is composed of three parts that, unlike the hypothalamus, are not seen spatially as separate, distinct bodies but that function as separate, distinct bodies. These are the anterior lobe, the posterior lobe, and the pars intermedia.

Anterior Lobe.   The anterior lobe is the portion of the pituitary most closely associated with the hypothalamus. It is connected to the hypothalamus through a network of specialized vessels and secretes six different hormones. These hormones influence such functions as affecting skin pigmentation, activating the reproductive glands, human growth and development as a whole, and regulating adrenal secretions.

Posterior Lobe.   The posterior lobe of the pituitary, an outgrowth of the brain stem, secretes two hormones that affect the smooth muscles of the body, such as the uterus, muscles involved in circulation, and the constriction of blood vessels.

The Thyroid

The thyroid secretes two hormones that play an important role in bone formation, the production of large amounts of calcium, early childhood development, tissue differentiation during growth and development, and body metabolism. These hormones also affect skin texture, hair production, development of the reproductive organs, bone length, and mental development.

The Adrenals

Set on top of the kidneys, the adrenal glands secrete more than fifty hormones or hormonelike substances. Major hormonal secretions from the medulla include epinephrine and norepinephrine. Epinephrine (adrenaline) is the hormone responsible for the "flight or fight" response people display during times of great danger, anxiety, or stress. Increased production of epinephrine stimulates the heart, dilates the bronchioles, increases the respiratory rate, and increases the rate of metabolism (Marieb and Mallatt 1992, 403–404). Other adrenal hormones regulate normal circulation, and regulate the metabolism of fats, carbohydrates, minerals, and water balance.

The Pancreas

The pancreas, located between the stomach and the small intestine, aids in regulating the blood sugar level through the manufacture of insulin. When food—especially food high in carbohydrate content—is digested, the blood sugar level is elevated. Insulin is then secreted to lower the blood sugar by helping metabolize glucose (sugar). As glucose is used by the body for energy, the secretion of insulin subsides.

If an insufficient amount of insulin is produced, a chronic condition known as *diabetes melli-tus* results. People suffering from this condition must modify their diets by restricting the amount of carbohydrates they ingest daily. In addition, depending on the severity of the insufficiency, some diabetics must take artificial doses of insulin, either orally or by injections, so that a balanced blood sugar level can be maintained. If the blood sugar level of a diabetic remains below normal, insulin shock, characterized by extreme dizziness and weakness, will occur, and death results quickly unless carbohydrates, such as juice or candy, are administered immediately. If the blood sugar level remains above normal, diabetic coma, characterized by a gradual loss of coherence over several days, will occur, and death may result unless insulin is administered.

The Respiratory System

To the elementary school child, many body systems, such as the endocrine system, may appear somewhat abstract, because these systems' functions take place largely unnoticed to a young observer. Nevertheless, all children at an early age can appreciate the important role that breathing plays in their lives. As a result, the respiratory system is more easily grasped at the elementary school level. Components of the respiratory system include the lungs, nose, throat or pharynx, epiglottis, esophagus, trachea, bronchi, alveoli, diaphragm, and rib cage. These components are illustrated in Figure 6.4.

Figure 6.4
The Respiratory System

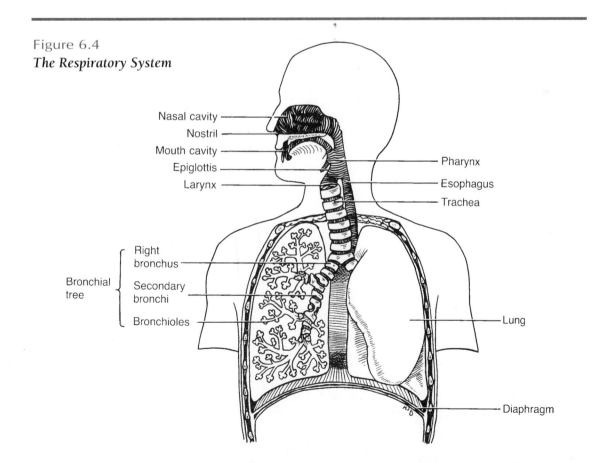

The Nose

The only visible part of the respiratory system is the nose. Through the nose, air is inhaled into and exhaled from the body. In addition, the nose, in which the sense of smell originates, signals olfactory nerves and can thus warn of harmful gases, and it allows drainage of secretions from the sinus cavities within the skull. However, its main function is to filter the air before it passes into the rest of the respiratory tract. The narrow passages of the nasal cavity are lined with fine hairs called *cilia* that sift bacteria and dust and carry these impurities to lymph tissue. Mucous secretions help trap bacteria and dust and also moisten the air being inhaled. The nose helps warm incoming air as well. From the nose, air moves down into the throat, or **pharynx.** The lower portion of the pharynx ends in two tubes, the esophagus and the trachea.

The Esophagus and Epiglottis

Although the esophagus and epiglottis are primarily associated with the digestive system, they also have respiratory functions. The esophagus is the tunnel through which food is transported to the stomach. The epiglottis is a small flap of fibrous cartilage positioned just above the esophagus near the base of the tongue. When food enters the mouth and swallowing begins, the epiglottis covers the entrance to the trachea, the other tubular division of the pharynx, so that food is channeled through the esophagus, preventing choking.

The Trachea, Bronchi, and Alveoli

Inhaled air is conducted from the pharynx to the trachea, a long, narrow pipe often referred to as the *windpipe*. Like the pharynx, the trachea branches into two smaller pipes, called *bronchi*. One bronchus extends toward the right side of the chest cavity into the right lung; the other extends toward the left side of the chest cavity into the left lung. Each bronchus continues to split into smaller and smaller tubules, called *bronchioles,* which penetrate inner lung tissue. The tiny, terminal branches of the bronchioles form enlarged air pockets called *alveolar sacs* that expand into various-sized alveoli. The alveoli are the functional units of lung tissue. Filling with air, they inflate the lungs upon inhalation. Expelling air and carbon dioxide on exhalation, they deflate the lungs (Thibodeau and Patton 1992, 590-591).

The Lungs

The lungs, two fan-shaped structures found on each side of the chest cavity, are gas exchange organs for the entire body. Oxygen, which makes up about 20 percent of the air we breathe, is trapped in the alveoli and transported in the blood via the pulmonary vein back to the heart, where the oxygen-enriched blood is pumped to the rest of the body. Conversely, blood coming from body tissue is rich in waste products, particularly carbon dioxide. Blood from this direction is pumped from the heart into the lung cavity via the pulmonary artery. From the lungs, carbon dioxide is then expelled from the body during exhalation by being forced back out through the respiratory tract and finally released from the nose.

Each lung is enclosed in a protective double membrane known as the *pleura*. Sometimes the pleura, because of infection, become inflamed, causing a painful condition called *pleurisy*. Other infections of the lungs and respiratory passages can result in communicable diseases such as influenza, colds, pneumonia, or tuberculosis. Irritants of the bronchial and lung tissue like pollen, cigarette tar and gases, asbestos, coal dust, or industrial pollutants can also affect or cause a variety of respiratory ailments that vary in degree from bronchitis and allergies to emphysema and lung cancer.

The Diaphragm and Rib Cage

Air is mechanically forced in and out of the lung cavity by means of muscular actions of the diaphragm and the rib cage. The diaphragm, a domelike sheet of muscle, separates the thorax or chest cavity from the abdominal cavity and is attached to the chest wall. Air is inhaled into the lungs when the rib muscles pull the rib cage upward and outward, causing the diaphragm lying below it to contract and flatten. As a result, air is forced into the chest cavity so that the volume of the chest cavity increases and the lungs expand or inflate. Then, as the diaphragm moves upward, relaxing its contraction, and the rib muscles loosen, moving the rib cage downward and inward, the volume of the chest cavity decreases and the lungs deflate (Memmler, Cohen, and Wood 1992, 81). This cyclical action of inhalation and exhalation is what we commonly call breathing. Breathing, or respiration, occurs involuntarily about twelve times a minute for adults and about fifteen times a minute for children. If breathing stops because of injury, death will occur in four to six minutes. Even if breathing is resumed within a few minutes, brain damage may occur due to oxygen deprivation to the brain cells.

The Circulatory System

Life-sustaining oxygen, provided by the respiratory system, is made available to all parts of the body through the circulatory system. The heart pumps oxygen-rich blood to all body tissue. The oxygen is exchanged for carbon dioxide and other waste products of cell functioning. Not only is blood the vehicle for gas exchange, it also aids in stabilizing body temperature, supplying nutrients, furnishing disease-fighting antibodies, transporting hormones, delivering waste products to the kidneys, and regulating the body's acid–base balance. Besides the heart and blood, other components of the circulatory system include the various blood vessels that carry blood from the heart to the body tissue and vice versa. An overall view of the circulatory system is shown in Figure 6.5.

To the elementary child, many body systems may appear somewhat abstract.

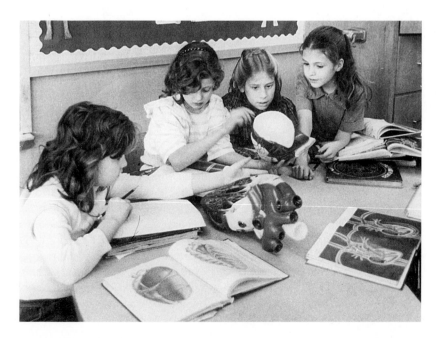

Figure 6.5
The Circulatory System

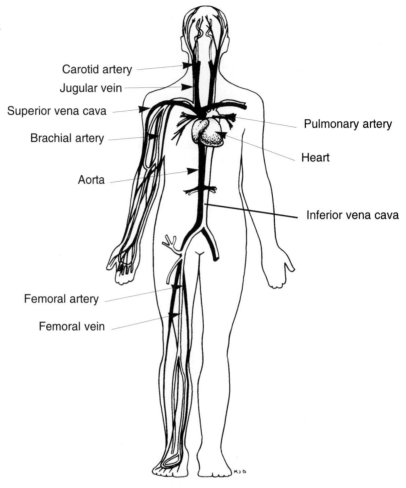

Carotid artery
Jugular vein
Superior vena cava
Brachial artery
Aorta

Pulmonary artery
Heart
Inferior vena cava

Femoral artery
Femoral vein

The Heart

The heart, positioned between the sternum or breastbone and spinal column, is in essence a hollow muscle about the size of a fist. By its rhythmic muscular contractions and relaxations, the heart continuously pumps blood through vessels that circulate the blood from the heart to the rest of the body and then back again. The anatomy of the human heart is illustrated in Figure 6.6.

A wall of muscle also runs through the middle of the heart, separating it into two sides or chambers. The right side of the heart receives incoming blood from the body tissue and channels this blood into the lungs, where it deposits carbon dioxide and picks up oxygen. The left side of the heart receives oxygen-rich blood from the lungs and pumps it to the rest of the body. There is an upper division and a lower division of each chamber. The upper division of each chamber, called the *atrium,* is a thin-walled section that merely receives blood. The lower division of each chamber, called the *ventricle,* is a thick-walled section that exerts a strong contraction or pumping action on the blood. This contraction is associated with heartbeat or pulse.

Figure 6.6
*Flow of Blood Through
the Heart*

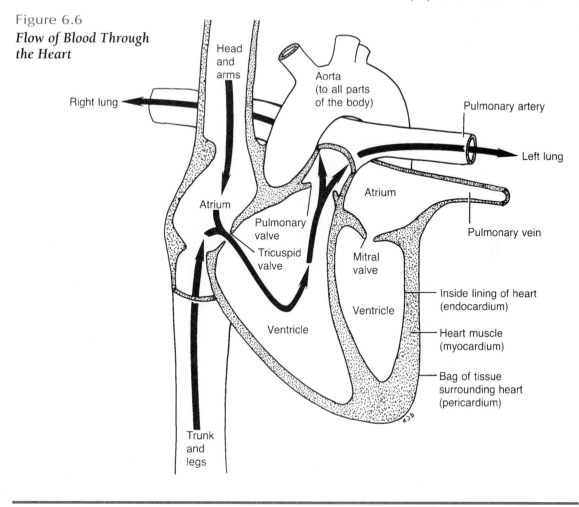

Valves between each atrium and ventricle allow for the flow of blood from the upper section to the lower section. The tricuspid valve, composed of three flaps, is in the right chamber of the heart, and the biscuspid or mitral valve, composed of two flaps, is in the left chamber of the heart. After opening to permit the flow of blood from the atrium to the ventricle, the valves close during the contraction of the ventricles so that blood cannot flow backward into the atrium (Hole 1993, 655). Sometimes a malfunction of the opening and closing mechanism of the valves may occur as a result of a birth defect or illness. When this happens, some backflow can be heard with the use of stethoscope. This condition is called a *heart murmur*. Heart murmurs can vary in their degree of severity.

The Blood

Blood carries oxygen and nutrients to tissue and absorbs tissue waste products, transporting them to the lungs or kidneys. Heat, hormones, and antibodies are also all delivered to cells and tissue by the blood. In addition, the blood provides the body with the proper ratio of buffer systems referred to as *acid balance,* or *pH.*

Blood is made up of two major components—blood corpuscles and plasma. Corpuscles include red blood cells, white blood cells, and blood platelets. Plasma is 90 percent water. The remaining 10 percent is composed of blood proteins, glucose, amino acids, hormones, antibodies, and enzymes, and some waste products.

Red Blood Cells.   Red blood cells, or erythrocytes, are the component that gives blood its color. A main function of these cells is to transport oxygen and carbon dioxide. Oxygen and carbon dioxide combine with hemoglobin, a protein substance that is the most important constituent of red blood cells. Since erythrocytes are the only cells in the human body that do not have a nucleus, they age rapidly, having an average life span of about four months. New red blood cells are constantly being manufactured in bone marrow.

If either an insufficient amount of red blood cells is produced or an insufficient amount of hemoglobin is contained in the red blood cells, anemia results. People suffering from anemia have less physical strength, tire quickly both physically and mentally, have less general body resistance, and are thus more prone to illness. Several specific types of anemia exist, such as sickle cell anemia, a potentially fatal inherited condition found mainly in blacks; pernicious anemia, which arises when the red blood cells that are manufactured are not only insufficient in numbers but mature abnormally and are much larger and more fragile than normal; and nutritional anemia, which occurs when there is an iron deficiency in the diet.

White Blood Corpuscles.   White blood cells, or leukocytes, are specialized blood cells that protect the body by either engulfing foreign substances that enter the bloodstream and tissue or by producing antibodies, specific chemical substances used to fight specific infectious diseases. The white blood cells that engulf foreign substances are called *phagocytes;* the white blood cells that produce antibodies are called *lymphocytes.*

Lymphocytes are a chief component of lymph, a fluid much like blood but lacking erythrocytes, that also helps fight infection. Lymph has its own separate circulation system throughout the body called the *lymphatic system,* which is characterized by specialized clusters of tissue called *lymph nodes* located in specific body regions such as the neck and under the arms.

Blood Platelets.   Blood platelets, or thrombocytes, are tiny oval or spherical cells that are produced in red bone marrow. Thrombocytes are essential for the coagulation of blood. Coagulation is a complex chemical process making use of more than thirty-five compounds. Simply stated, on hemorrhage platelets quickly disintegrate and release or in some way affect the release of many of the chemicals needed for coagulation. In addition, thrombocytes easily clump together to form a sticky lump that entraps white blood cells to form a clot (Guyton 1992, 273-274).

The Blood Vessels

Blood being pumped from the heart to the rest of the body and back again is circulated through a meshlike group of tubes or vessels that can be classified as arteries, or capillaries, or veins. Arteries originate from the heart ventricles and carry oxygenated blood to other parts of the body. The right ventricle gives rise to the pulmonary artery, which transports blood rich in carbon dioxide to the lungs, where it deposits carbon dioxide and receives oxygen. Oxygenated blood is then circulated back to the left atrium via the pulmonary vein, and finally to the left ventricle. The left ventricle gives rise to the main coronary artery, the aorta, which channels blood into smaller and smaller arteries that eventually branch throughout the body into even smaller vessels called *arte-*

rioles. The semilunar valves, positioned at the opening between the pulmonary artery and the aorta, open only into arteries, thus prohibiting backflow of blood into the atria on relaxation of the ventricles (Hole 1993, 655).

The arterioles, the smallest arterial branches, give rise to countless microscopic tubules called *capillaries,* which reach every cell of the body. It is here, at the capillary level, that oxygen and nutrients are delivered and carbon dioxide and other cellular waste products are absorbed. The capillaries merge to form larger vessels called *venuoles,* which in turn unite to form veins. Veins then transport blood rich in carbon dioxide back to the heart through the right atrium, the right ventricle, and into the lungs, where gas exchange takes place and oxygenated blood is ready once again to be pumped from the left chamber of the heart to the rest of the body.

The Digestive/Excretory System

The digestive system, as shown in Figure 6.7, converts the food that we eat into usable substances that can enter the bloodstream and supply the energy needed for fueling all other bodily systems. The excretory system removes nonusable food substances and wastes that are by-products of the body's various chemical processes by eliminating them as feces from the rectum or as urine from the kidneys.

Figure 6.7
The Digestive System

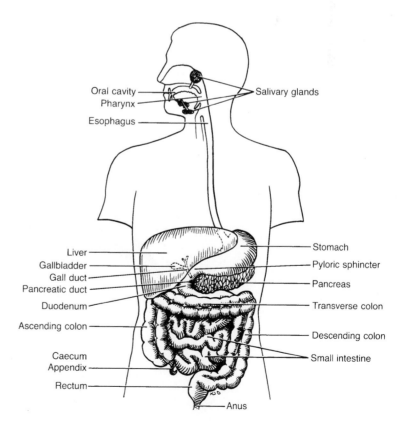

When food is swallowed, it travels from the pharynx to the esophagus and into the stomach, where digestive juices chemically act on it. From the stomach, food is channeled into the upper section of the small intestine and further metabolized by enzymes from the pancreas and liver bile stored in the gallbladder. It then moves through the remaining portions of the small intestine, whose walls absorb the nutrients and pass them into the bloodstream. Food substances not absorbed by the alimentary canal (digestive tract) constitute nondigestible matter, which is funneled into the large intestine, where bacteria decompose it. Additional water in the material is also absorbed. Then the remaining material moves into the rectum, where it is eliminated from the body as feces through the anus.

Toxic or waste substances in the plasma as well as bacteria entering the bloodstream are filtered by the kidneys. Chemical reactions that yield the by-products water, urea, uric acid, and various salts are also filtered by the kidneys, channeled to the bladder, and excreted from the body as urine through the urethra.

The excretory system is illustrated in Figure 6.8.

Figure 6.8
The Excretory System

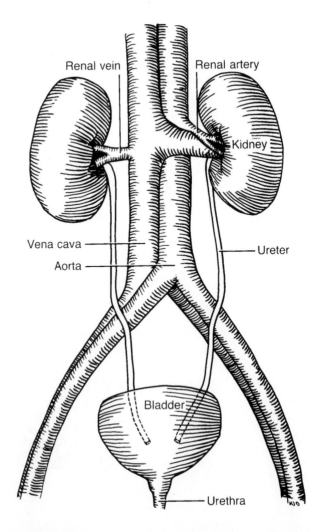

The Stomach

Before entering the stomach, each mouthful of food is mechanically broken into a smaller, moister mass called a *bolus* by the chewing action of the jaw and teeth accompanied by enzymatic secretions from the salivary glands in the mouth. As noted, the epiglottis blocks the trachea during swallowing so that food is automatically channeled from the pharynx to the esophagus, where involuntary peristaltic (wavelike) muscular contractions push it into the stomach.

A special ring of muscle called a *sphincter* joins the esophagus and stomach. The sphincter muscle is signaled by peristalsis of the esophagus to open and allow the passage of food into the stomach. When the sphincter muscle tightens or contracts, it closes the entrance to the stomach. The sphincter generally remains contracted to prevent backflow of stomach contents into the esophagus during digestion (Thibodeau and Patton 1992, 632-634). The stomach is a muscular, saclike organ lying in the upper left portion of the abdominal cavity just below the ribs. It is the only structure in the alimentary canal that can expand. The stomach functions as a storage area for food and as a secretory organ. When completely empty, the stomach cavity is quite small, but when full an adult stomach can hold just in excess of a quart. At the rate of about three per minute, gentle peristaltic waves are triggered a few minutes after food enters the stomach. This churning action mixes the food with gastric secretions such as hydrochloric acid and pepsin until the food becomes a gel-like mixture called *chyme*, which leaves the stomach to enter the small intestine (Memmler, Cohen, and Wood 1992, 209).

The Small Intestine

The most important component of the digestive tract is the small intestine. It is here that the vast majority of food, which leaves the stomach as a soupy mixture, is digested and absorbed. The small intestine is a tightly coiled tube about 22 feet long and is made up of three sections—the duodenum, jejunum, and ileum. The duodenum, the first section, is joined by the stomach and is a much shorter segment (1 foot) than either the jejunum or the ileum (Hole 1993, 531).

The inside of the small intestine contains numerous ridges and folds that are covered by tiny fingerlike projections called *villi*. The chyme is pushed through the small intestine by peristaltic action (Memmler, Cohen, and Wood 1992, 209). As food is being propelled through the upper portion of the small intestine, ducts from the pancreas and gallbladder open into the duodenum to deliver both pancreatic enzymes and liver bile, which aid in breaking down food substances.

In the small intestine, food substances are broken down into their simplest chemical form and are absorbed through the walls of the jejunum and ileum into the bloodstream (Hole 1993, 535). The remaining nonnutritive chyme in the small intestine is then propelled to the cecum, a functionally unimportant projection of the large intestine in the lower right portion of the abdominal cavity, from which the large intestine or colon begins to ascend or move upward. (The appendix lies at the tip of the cecum.)

The Large Intestine

There are three components of the large intestine—the ascending colon, transverse colon, and descending colon—which in essence surround the small intestine and lead into the rectum and anus, also considered parts of the large intestine. One of the main functions of the colon is the reabsorption of water used in the chemical processes of digestion so that it is channeled back into the body. The large intestine is also responsible for secretion of salts, including iron and calcium, that are too high in blood-level concentration. These salts are mixed with the remaining chyme decomposed by bacteria, and converted into feces. Feces are stored in the rectum, in the final portion of the large intestine adjoining the descending colon, until distension triggers rising pressure in the rectum followed by muscular movement. The feces are then expelled from the body through the rectum and its opening, the anus (Marieb and Mallatt 1992, 582).

The Kidneys

While solid waste products are eliminated from the body through the colon, liquid waste products are chiefly excreted as a result of the action of the kidneys in the form of urine. The kidneys, bean-shaped organs about 4 inches long, are located on either side of the lower back region of the spinal column. Microscopic tubules called *nephrons*, collect waste products that have been delivered by the circulatory system and filtered in the kidneys. Waste products are transported to the kidneys in the blood through the renal artery, a major artery leading directly from the aorta to the kidneys. A duct from each kidney called the *ureter* conveys urine to the urinary bladder where it is stored and then excreted through another duct, the urethra, to the outside of the body (Thibodeau and Patton 1992, 705-707).

The Skeletal/Muscular System ─────────────────────

The body and all its organs and systems are given support, protection, and mobility by the skeletal/muscular system. More than 200 bones make up the human skeleton and over 600 muscles attached to these bones allow body movement and act as a protective covering for the trunk or thoracic area. The bones are connected by joints, often containing a lubricating fluid to enhance flexibility. Some joints, such as the hip or shoulder, are extremely movable, allowing a rotation motion. These are called ball-and-socket joints. Other joints, such as the elbow or knee, allow movement in only one direction. These are called *hinge joints*. Many others, like those of the spinal column, provide rather restricted movement. These are called *fixed joints*.

Bones are composed of a porous, inner layer of spongy tissue surrounded by hardened outer compact bone material. The ends of the long bones of the body contain red marrow essential for manufacturing red blood cells. In infancy, bones are elastic, flexible, and soft. Through the maturation process, with the ingestion of minerals like calcium and phosphorous as well as vitamin D, bones become more rigid and also grow thicker and longer.

The skeletal/muscular system gives form and shape to the human body. The most characteristic skeletal feature in humans is the vertebral or spinal column, which gives the support needed for walking upright. Other major human bone structures and their attached muscles of particular importance are the skull, sternum and rib cage, pelvis, bones of the legs and feet, and bones of the arms and hands.

The Spinal Column

Composed of thirty-three bones called *vertebrae*, the spinal column or backbone extends from the base of the head down to the hip region, and allows bending, twisting, and turning motions of the upper body. Because the spinal vertebrae encase the delicate spinal cord that conducts all body messages to the brain, any injury along the spinal column is extremely serious and can lead to paralysis or death.

There are five divisions or groupings of bones in the spinal column. The first seven vertebrae are called the *cervical vertebrae* and comprise the neck. These are followed by twelve other bones

Health Highlight

Black and White Adolescent Females' Perceptions of Ideal Body Size

Perception of body size as it related to actual size may be a critical element of weight regulation for many individuals, including the anorexic, the normal weight, and the obese. In a study of black and white adolescent females, the body size considered ideal by black females was significantly larger than the size selected as ideal by white females. It was found that, although obesity is a risk for health-related problems for black females, they seem more accepting than white females of additional body weight. Black females may evaluate their weight in relation to their heavy peers rather than on a health-based standard. These attitudes, with perceptions of body shape and preferences for certain levels of thinness or fatness, are culturally determined. White females are more influenced by peer group and TV and magazines with regard to their perception of ideal body size, while black females' perceptions are more like their family members' perception. This difference in influencing factors could help to explain the disproportionate rate of obesity between the black and white female population as well as the more frequent occurrence of disordered eating in the white female population. These findings should be used in the development of culturally sensitive intervention activities to help reduce the high rate of obesity in black females and the high rates of disordered eating among white females.

Source: K. Parnell and others. 1996. Black and white adolescent females' perceptions of ideal body size. *Journal of school health,* 66(3), 112–118.

known as the *thoracic vertebrae*, which support the upper trunk region. The five *lumbar vertebrae* extend to the waist and are followed by five fused *sacral vertebrae* in the lower back. The *coccyx*—four relatively small bones—marks the end of the spinal column and is commonly referred to as the *tailbone*. The upper twenty-four bones of the spine, the cervical, thoracic, and lumbar vertebrae, are more flexible structures than the sacral and coccyx vertebrae because they are joined by separate pieces or disks of cartilage that cushion the impact of walking, running, jumping, and similar movements.

The Skull

The human skull, situated above the spinal column, includes the cranium and the bones of the face. The cranium is a group of sixteen large, flat, hard bones that form a domelike structure surrounding and protecting the brain. The bones of the face form protective coverings for the eyes, nasal passages, and the inner face or cheeks. These bones also make up the hinged upper and lower jawbones, the maxilla and the mandible respectively, that give shape to the oral cavity and support the teeth (Memmler, Cohen, and Wood 1992, 55).

The Sternum and Rib Cage

The sternum is a flat, elongated, rigid bone that is very thick because it protects the heart. Attached to both the sternum with cartilage in the front and to the thoracic vertebrae in the back are ten pairs of ribs that form a cagelike structure called the *rib cage*. Two other pairs of ribs are attached to the thoracic vertebrae but are not attached to the sternum, and are thus referred to as *floating ribs*. The rib cage protects the lung cavity.

The Pelvis

The pelvis is formed by connections of the sacral and coccyx vertebrae of the back with the hip-bones in the side and front portions of the body. When joined together, these bones form a large, bowl-like structure. The pelvis helps to protect some of the organs of the reproductive system and the excretory system, as well as to support the upper part of the body. The pelvis, with its ability to rotate, also aids in twisting, turning, and sitting motions.

Bones of the Legs and Feet

Extending from each side of the hip is the upper leg bone or femur. It is the largest bone in the body. The femur is attached to the shin or tibia, the largest bone in the lower leg, at the knee or patella. To the outward side of the tibia lies the fibula, the other lower leg bone. Because the leg bones are porous, they are especially adapted for supporting body weight and providing mobility. Heavier, thicker bones would not be suitable for these functions.

The tibia and fibula are joined to the bones of the feet at the ankles or tarsals. Seven tarsal bones form the posterior part of the foot, the largest being the calcaneus or heel bone (Hole 1993, 221). Extending from the tarsals are the five long bones of the upper foot called the *metatarsals*, which are arched and joined to the fourteen bones of the toes, the phalanges. Because these bones are arched, they provide further support and stability for maintaining the body in an upright position.

Bones of the Arms and Hands

Hinged to the flat, triangular scapula or shoulder blade is the upper arm bone or humerus, which hangs below the collarbone or clavicle. The humerus is attached at the elbow to both the ulna, the longer lower arm bone, and the radius, the shorter inner arm bone. These bones in turn connect with the eight wrist or carpal bones that provide flexibility and rotation for the hands. Attached to the carpals are the five metacarpals that form the palm of the hand. These are then joined to the fourteen phalanges, the bones of the fingers. Because of the multiple joints in the fingers, the hands are ideal for performing clutching and grasping motions.

The Muscles

The 600 muscles responsible for moving the skeletal structures at will are called *voluntary muscles*, because their movements are triggered by conscious thoughts and actions. Many other muscles that act on body systems and internal organs do so without messages from the individual and are therefore referred to as *involuntary muscles*.

The muscles of the body are organized and operate in groups rather than as isolated structures so that a single action, such as lifting the leg, depends on the contraction of certain muscles accompanied by the simultaneous relaxation of others. The most important groups of skeletal muscles are those that move the shoulders, arms, chest, back, and legs.

Although numerous muscles cover the scapula, the major ones are the trapezius in the back of the shoulder blades and the deltoid connected to the front, rounded portion of the shoulder. The triceps on the outer upper arm bone and the biceps on the inner upper arm bone are the chief muscles covering the humerus, while the brachio-radialis of the radius and the aconeus and flexor group of the ulna are the major muscles in the lower arm. The chest is supported by a large muscle group called the *pectorals*, the pectoralis minor covering the sides of the ribs and the pectoralis major covering the chest, while the lattisimus dorsi covers the back and the ribs attached to the thoracic vertebrae. The major muscles of the thigh are commonly called the *hamstring muscles* and include the biceps femoris on the outer thigh and the semimembranesus and the semitendinosis on the inner thigh, all of which flex at the knee and aid in the extension of the hip. The major muscles of the leg include the gastrocnemius or calf muscle and the soleus or ankle muscle (Agur and Lee 1991, 298).

Developing Good Habits Early

It is not enough to know about the structure and function of the human body. The human body must be given daily attention to ensure its continued performance. This attention is the responsibility of the individual. Thus it is essential that personal health habits be learned at an early age. Inattention to personal health practices in childhood has consequences in later life.

This section of the chapter focuses on the areas of personal health that are considered the most crucial for the elementary school child. These areas include personal appearance, care of the senses, dental health, exercise, relaxation, and sleep, and disease control and prevention.

Personal Appearance

A multitude of factors can influence personal appearance, including genetics, socioeconomic status, illness, and so forth. However, in this section of the chapter, only care of the skin, care of the nails, care of the hair, and the importance of posture are discussed. In addition, because of its far-reaching effects on almost all other areas of health, nutrition is presented in a separate chapter.

The Skin

The skin is the largest organ of the body, and is composed of three layers—the outer skin (epidermis), the "true" skin (dermis), and the subcutaneous layer (fat tissue). The outer skin is comprised of sheet upon sheet of scales, overlapping like roof shingles. As the top layer of scales is rubbed off, the next layer below takes its place.

The pigment in the skin is found in the germinative layer of the epidermis. The amount of skin pigment is greater in some people than in others. African Americans have the most amount of pigment, Euro-Americans have the least, and albinos have none. The amount of pigment can vary in one individual from time to time when exposure to ultraviolet rays increases the deposits of pigment in the epidermis. The pigment acts as a screen to protect the delicate structures beneath the epidermis from further action of the ultraviolet rays. Pigment also shows up in the form of freckles when the pigment in the skin is unevenly distributed. Those people with less pigment, or with an uneven distribution of pigment are more susceptible to the damaging effects of ultraviolet radiation.

The bottom layer of the epidermis is connected to the dermis. The dermis contains blood vessels, nerves, muscles, and connective tissue. Also, some glands originate in the dermis and go up through the epidermis to the outer part of the body. The "sweat" gland sends perspiration through the epidermis to the surface of the skin from the purpose of maintaining the proper body temperature. The sebaceous glands secrete sebum, which keeps the skin soft, pliable, and waterproof. Sebum, which is responsible for the oily coating of the skin, passes out to the skin surface along the hairs (through the hair follicles).

The subcutaneous layer of the skin is sometimes called the *hypodermis*. This layer contains adipose tissue, a fatty layer of skin that helps protect the internal structures from injury due to falls and blows. This layer helps retain heat. A person who has an abnormally high body percentage of fat will have difficulty adjusting to warmer temperatures because the layer of fat will retain heat.

Personal appearance is affected by skin cleanliness, general complexion, and any irregularities or infestations. The skin is also highly functional. Its functions include the following:

❍ Protection against foreign matter trying to enter the body

❍ Regulation of body temperature both through delivery of blood (heat) to body surfaces and the secretion of sweat, which produces a cooling effect

❍ Elimination of minute amounts of waste products through perspiration

❍ Absorption of electromagnetic radiation, including ultraviolet, infrared, visible light, and X rays, thus prohibiting passage to underlying structures

❍ Conversion of ultraviolet light to vitamin D

❍ Storage of fat and water in subcutaneous tissue for use as needed

The skin can be damaged in many ways. Common injuries include cuts, abrasions, and burns. Chemical irritants, insect bites, and rashes are also responsible for skin damage.

Skin Conditions

Skin conditions are numerous and vary in degree of severity from sunburn and dandruff to psoriasis and eczema, so only those that are most frequently seen in school-age children will be discussed. These include acne, athlete's foot, boils and carbuncles, impetigo, pediculosis, ringworm, scabies, warts, and sunburn.

Acne. Characterized by blemishes on the face, neck, shoulders, and back, in the form of pimples, whiteheads, and blackheads, acne arises when oil glands become overly active in secretions, thus blocking skin surface ducts. Pimples are small, pus-filled inflammations, whiteheads are oil blockages that lie beneath the skin, and blackheads are hardened, dried plugs of oil at the skin surface.

Acne is generally considered a problem for preteens and teenagers but may affect people in their twenties, thirties, and forties as well. This condition can become a psychological problem as well as physical, especially for teenagers. During the teen and preteen years, the facial appearance is vital because they are beginning to relate to the opposite sex socially. Because they are so concerned about the facial condition and the acne that affects it, teens may start picking at them or try to cover them with makeup. Both these actions make the acne condition worse.

The condition is not contagious. There is no known cure, but a variety of cleansing treatments coupled, if necessary, with the administration of either surface (local) or oral antibiotics can control the condition. Those suffering from acne should be encouraged to keep hands away from the face, because the hands can introduce more oil to the skin, and can increase infection. People with acne should avoid makeup and skin creams with an oil base, as these applications will further block the pores of the skin. Most affected individuals usually "outgrow" the conditions when their oil glands provide a more balanced output.

Ringworm (tinea). The type of fungal infection known as ringworm can affect several parts of the body, such as the scalp and groin area. When the scalp is affected, the hair breaks off at the weakest point, usually just above the surface of the scalp, and patches form on the scalp. The infected areas may be itchy, grayish, and scaly, and are extremely contagious, even through indirect contact. A fungal infection in the groin area, or body ringworm, is characterized by rounded, red patches that are elevated on the skin. These are contagious, and the infection can be spread by clothing and direct contact. Oddly enough, ringworm is more prevalent in young children than in older children and adults, whereas the reverse is true for athlete's foot. Antifungal agents usually stop acute tinea infection, but are unable to completely destroy the fungus. Tinea can be avoided by keeping the skin dry (Thibodeau and Patton 1992, 147).

Impetigo. The highly contagious skin infection impetigo, caused by both streptococcus and staphylococcus bacteria, is characterized by lesions or breaks in the skin usually around the hands and mouth. Initially the lesions appear as wet-looking red sores. The sores then fill with pus and develop a crusted-over appearance (Thibodeau and Patton 1992, 147).

These sores can lead to more serious infections deeper in the system. Since impetigo can be spread quickly through direct and indirect contact—including pencils, papers, books, doorknobs, desk tops, and towels—any afflicted child should be excluded from school and directed to a physician.

Pediculosis. Lice infestation, or pediculosis, arises when head or body lice—extremely small, parasitic insects—attach to hair shafts. They are passed from infested people either through direct contact or contact with an article of clothing or object used by the infested individual. The lice live and lay eggs in seams of clothing and come on to the skin when sucking blood. Lice were formerly responsible for the spread of typhus fever. Also, lice infestation was the major reason for physical inspections of schoolchildren during the earliest years of health education.

Itching results from the blood-sucking action of the lice, and a secondary infection may occur. Application of an appropriate insecticide can destroy the lice. To prevent widespread outbreaks, schoolchildren should be thoroughly inspected for lice.

Sunburn. People with fair or light complexions do not have as much protective pigment in their skin as darker people. Therefore, lighter people should not stay in the sun for extended periods of time because they are more vulnerable to sunburn than others. Overexposure to the sun has been linked with skin cancer. If fair-complexioned people must be in the sun, for a long time during work or exercise, they should cover the exposed areas of the skin with a good sunscreen.

Care of the Skin

Daily personal cleanliness is the best means of caring for the skin. Washing the hands, feet, and face a few times each day with warm water and soap helps remove dirt, bacteria, and oil. Although a daily shower or bath is not necessary, it is a good practice to encourage. Also, emphasize the need to wear proper clothing to suit temperature variations to protect the skin. Different skin types may require different kinds of daily care. For example, people with oily skin may need to clean their faces and wash their hair more often than people with dry skin. Allergic skin reactions to certain soaps, lotions, or creams may result, so that nonallergenic preparations may be necessary. Therefore, be sure to provide instruction concerning general skin care principles as well as information about special needs. In addition, children need to know that a dermatologist is a physician who specializes in care of the skin and skin disorders in the event a problem arises.

The Fingernails and Toenails

Fingernails and toenails are outgrowths of the skin itself that originate from the inner epidermal layers. The nails arise from live roots within these inner layers and die as they grow out from the roots. As a result, fingernails and toenails are hard, horny cells that develop into keratin tissue that can be cut painlessly. Cuticles—softer but nevertheless hardened skin tissue—surround fingernails and toenails and sometimes break or crack because little oil reaches them. Both the nails and cuticles protect the fingers and toes.

Care of the Nails

Nails should be kept long enough to allow them to fulfill their protective function but should be trimmed or cut periodically to avoid both breakage and the collection of bacteria underneath them. When trimming the nails, a straight-across cut rather than a rounded one is recommended so that the fleshy part of the skin is not damaged. If it is damaged, ingrown toenails may result, because the new growth of skin will then overlap the nail, causing the nail itself to dig into inner skin layers.

Nails should be cleaned daily, and the fingers especially should be kept free of dirt and bacteria when eating or handling food. Cuticles should be kept soft and continually pushed away from the nail. If cuticles are not softened or kept pushed back from the nail, rough edges can develop that may tear nearby skin, causing hangnails. Cold cream or oil can keep the cuticle from becoming broken or cracked.

Changes in the normal appearance and growth of nails and cuticles may indicate underlying health problems. For example, nails that become excessively brittle or begin to split may be the result of some form of dietary deficiency or hormonal imbalance (Miller, Telljohann, and Symons 1996, 160). Usually white spots on the fingernails are formed by bubbles of air between the cell layers and have no significance. However, sometimes these spots may be caused by nutritional deficiency.

Some children develop the habit of biting the nails. Children who are easily irritated or restless sometimes develop this habit as an emotional release. Medical attention is suggested if the nail biting persists to the point that the nails and the skin around the nails are constantly damaged.

The Hair

Hair grows on almost all regions of our bodies. Males and females have the same amount of hair in the concentrated areas (such as under the arm and on the scalp), but they differ in the amount of hair on various parts of the body (such as the face). Hair growth, color, and coarseness is determined by heredity and pigment. Those with less pigment usually develop blonde or light brown hair, while those with the most pigment have black hair. Red hair typically has the coarsest texture, while blonde hair is the least coarse.

Like the nails, hair is an outgrowth of the skin itself. It originates from hair follicles in the dermis. The hair root within the follicle is composed of living cells that are nourished by blood vessels. As a result, removal of hair by its roots is painful. However, as is the case with nails, the visible hair shafts themselves are deadened keratin tissue that can be cut painlessly. Hair shafts on the head grow from about 2 to 6 inches before they begin to fall out naturally on being combed or brushed. Except in cases of inherited male pattern baldness, rare illness, or as a result of some forms of chemotherapy, hair that falls out is continually being replaced.

Hair serves a protective role. Hair on the head guards against excessive exposure of the underlying scalp to solar radiation, as does body hair to some degree. Body hair also acts as a skin covering that helps regulate body temperature—a tremendous amount of body heat is lost when the head is uncovered in cold temperatures. In addition, the eyelashes shield the eyes from dust and other irritants.

Care of the Hair

Hair need not be washed or shampooed daily. Sebum, or oil, comes to the surface of the scalp through the hair follicle. Some people secrete more sebum than others, and therefore should wash their hair more often. The hair should not be washed with extremely hot water, as this makes the hair dry and brittle. The hair should be cleaned often and brushed or combed neatly several times a day.

Unnecessary combing, teasing, bleaching, and heat exposure should be avoided. Because dull, brittle-appearing hair, like the nails, may be a signal of underlying health problems, close attention should be paid to changes in its growth patterns and texture.

Hair should be brushed several times a day.

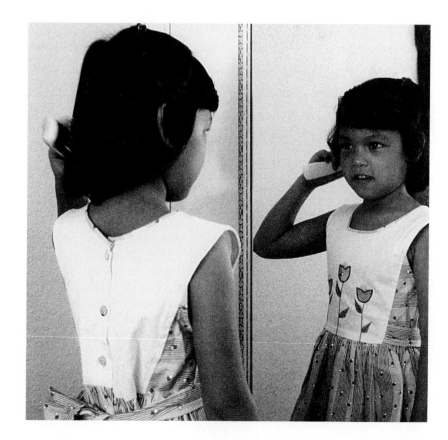

Posture

Posture is more than just standing or sitting straight up. The term *posture* refers to graceful, efficient movement of the body, whether walking, standing, or performing any type of motion. All parts of the body should be used correctly to maintain balance. When a person has poor posture, the muscles, instead of the bones, bear the burden of the off-center weight, and the person becomes fatigued much quicker.

Poor posture may be caused by a number of problems, including weak muscles, chronic fatigue, bone deformities, and careless habits of walking, sitting, and standing. Because students spend so much time during the school day sitting at a desk, it is important to encourage the students to sit properly. Each desk should be at an appropriate height for the individual to allow both feet to touch the floor without straining. The seat of the desk should allow the knees to be higher than the hips to remove stress from the lower back. The back of the chair should encourage the proper spinal curve when the child is seated. The tray of the desk should be slanted sufficiently so the student need not lean forward to write and read.

Posture can be positively influenced through proper nutrition for proper bone growth, exercise to tone the muscles, properly fitting clothing and shoes, well-designed furniture (including desks, chairs, and beds), lifting and carrying objects properly, and proper education.

Poor posture is most often seen in junior high and senior high school students who are self-conscious about height. However, some posture defects are skeletal in nature. For example, scoliosis, or curvature of the spine, may produce posture defects. In addition, sometimes after an illness, injury, or infection, poor muscle tone may cause slouching or slumping. In most instances, however, these types of posture defects can be corrected under the care of an orthopedic surgeon either through surgery, body braces, various exercises, orthotic lifts in the shoes, or a combination of surgery and exercise. Ideally, these defects are discovered very early in life, when correction is much easier.

The Senses

By conveying a myriad of messages to the brain each day, the sensory organs keep us in touch with our physical and emotional environments. Five major senses keep us informed about the world around us. These are vision, hearing, touching, tasting, and smelling.

The Sense of Vision

The ability to see is probably the most important sense of all. Information about images and patterns is recorded in the eyes, the sensory organs for sight, and conveyed to the brain. This information cannot be detected by the eye in the absence of light because light provides the basis for perceiving light and dark gradation, color distinction, and form or shape differentiation.

Proper vision is a key to a child's educational development. Eye problems are frequently found in children who are slow in learning to read. The teacher, more than anyone else, sees students when they are trying to achieve. For this reason, you should observe the students for possible indications of vision problems. Some of the signs of eye trouble in your students are

○ eyes crossed, in or out

○ reddened, itching, or watering eyes

○ frequent sties

Health Highlight

Is School Vision Screening Effective?

Children entering kindergarten in a three-year period were followed retrospectively from kindergarten through twelfth grade to estimate the incidence of abnormal school vision-screening tests and rates of follow-up by community ophthalmologists or optometrists. Over 28 percent of children had at least one abnormal school vision screening test. Abnormal screening with referral increased from 1.2 percent of five-year-olds to 9.1 percent of thirteen-year-olds. Overall, 91 percent of children referred had further evaluation by eye care professionals. However, visits to an eye care professional often were delayed—the median time was 0.8 years for children seeing an ophthalmologist and 1.8 years for children seeing an optometrist. This study suggests that school continue the use of simple visual acuity screening for their students, that consideration should be given to screening children beyond the age of twelve, and developing methods to decrease the amount of time that parents use to respond to referral recommendations.

Source: B. Yawn and others. 1996. "Is School Vision Screening Effective?" *Journal of school health* 66(5): 171-175.

- ○ short attention span
- ○ turning the head to use only one eye
- ○ frowning or placing head close to a book when reading or writing
- ○ sloppy handwriting
- ○ excessive blinking or rubbing of eyes
- ○ losing place while reading
- ○ confusion of similar words
- ○ unusual awkwardness while walking and poor eye–hand coordination
- ○ frequent headaches or dizziness
- ○ blurring of vision
- ○ good performance on oral work, but poor written work

Visual Defects

Problems associated with the eyes and vision are numerous. Visual defects most frequent among schoolchildren include amblyopia, astigmatism, hyperopia, myopia, strabismus, and wall-eye.

Amblyopia. This condition results in dimness of vision without changes in the eye structure. One eye, the "lazy eye," allows the stronger eye to dominate and therefore becomes weakened.

Amblyopia occurs without any known trauma, injury, illness, or physiological impairment necessarily preceding it. Exposure to certain chemical toxins may bring on amblyopia, or a disturbance of the optic nerve may be the cause. Sometimes amblyopia originates with a "blind spot" that grows increasingly larger. Amblyopia can be detected by a thorough eye examination. It is desirable to detect and treat amblyopia at an early age. Remediation includes the use of corrective lenses and vision training to teach the amblyopic eye to function normally. The "lazy eye" is often patched as part of the vision training.

Astigmatism. This condition results from abnormal curvature of the lens and cornea, which inhibits proper focusing. Images appear blurred and, because of strain in attempting to accommodate, discomfort in the form of headaches may result. Astigmatism can be corrected by wearing prescription eyeglasses or hard contact lenses.

Hyperopia. This condition is also called *farsightedness*, because people with hyperopia have no difficulty in seeing objects at a distance. However, because the eyeball is shortened and the image falls behind the retina, the hyperopic individual has trouble focusing on objects close at hand. Severe eye strain and crossing of the eyes may result. Wearing prescription eyeglasses with convex lenses can alleviate this condition (Guyton 1992, 367).

Myopia. Nearsightedness, or myopia, is the opposite of hyperopia. It occurs when images fall in front of the retina because of an elongation of the eyeball. As a result, the myopic individual can focus on objects close at hand but not those farther away. Properly prescribed concave lenses can compensate for eye elongation. Depending on the degree of the condition, nearsighted students may not necessarily show reading difficulty if the task is done at their desks, but they may have difficulty in seeing distant objects, such as a chalkboard, if they are sitting toward the back of the classroom (Guyton 1992, 369).

Strabismus and Wall-Eye. The crossing of the eye inward due to a shortening of the outer muscles surrounding the eye is called *strabismus*. Wall-eye is the opposite of strabismus—with this condition, the eye turns outward instead of inward. Depending on the muscular defect, strabismus may be helped by means of eyeglasses, wearing a patch on the normal eye, surgery, or a combination of procedures. If strabismus is left untreated, visual acuity as well as visual accommodation may be impaired (Hole 1993, 441).

Care of the Eyes

The eyes are among the most sensitive and delicate organs in the body. Because they work together, an injury, infection, or impairment to one eye may result in damage to the other. Therefore, any visual abnormality should be dealt with either by a physician or optometrist.

In your instruction, emphasize individual responsibility for protecting the eyes from harmful chemicals such as dyes, bleaches, cleansing products, insecticides, and cosmetic irritants. Also stress the potential danger of playing with objects that could penetrate or damage the eye, such as air rifles, fireworks, and slingshots. Teach children to keep dirty hands, fingers, and soiled materials away from the eyes and to alert adults to any eye discomfort or visual problem. Students should never self-medicate the eyes with drops, ointments, or creams.

Eye examinations should be given at birth, followed by additional testing around the age of five, during adolescence, and every two years thereafter. More frequent eye examinations may be needed after the age of forty because the aging process usually affects vision. In addition, eye examinations often uncover many underlying health problems such as diabetes, glaucoma, high blood pressure, and systemic infections.

The teacher should make adjustments in the classroom to help remediate some problems of students with poor vision. Have the students sit toward the front of the class so they can see the board more clearly. Some students might need a written handout if they have tremendous difficulty seeing the board.

The Sense of Hearing

The sense of hearing greatly assists communication with others. It also provides information about the environment in the form of sounds, noises, and danger signals. In addition, the ears help an individual maintain a sense of balance and equilibrium.

Hearing Impairments

The inability to hear can arise from a variety of causes, including congenital defects, illness, and injury. The most common hearing disability is classified as conductive. Conductive hearing loss can occur for a variety of reasons and is characterized by some sort of blockage or structural defect in the auditory canal or middle ear that warps or muffles the vibrations. Some conditions of conductive deafness can be corrected, and most are amenable to treatment.

Care of the Ears

The ears should be protected from loud noises, blasts, or other environmental hazards that can cause damage to the eardrum or affect frequency detection. Teach children to recognize the dangers of inserting anything into their ears as well as the importance of informing an adult of any ear discomfort. Children who continually pull on their ears or seem to have trouble with balance and equilibrium should be referred either to an otologist or an otolaryngologist, physicians specializing in care of the ears. Hearing tests should be administered at the preschool level as well as periodically throughout the school years.

Pay close attention to children who seem inattentive or unresponsive; these behaviors may signal hearing impairment rather than intellectual or emotional difficulties. The teacher should watch students for the following indications of hearing problems:

○ chronic nose and throat trouble

○ runny ear

○ complaints of pressure, ringing, or buzzing in the ear

○ frowning when trying to listen

○ leaning forward or turning the head while listening

○ good written work, but poor oral work

The best thing to do for a child with hearing loss is to detect the condition early and get medical attention. In the classroom, the teacher should place the child near the front of the room, look directly at the student, and speak clearly and slowly. Provide the student with a written handout to help the student keep up with any lesson that is presented orally.

The Sense of Touch

Numerous sensory receptor cells in the skin provide the body with the sensations of pain, heat, cold, and touch (pressure). A different type of sensory receptor cell for stimuli causes each of these sensations. Heat receptors obviously trigger sensations very different from those triggered by touch receptors, for example, even though all skin sensory cells send comparable signals through the central nervous system. The difference in sensations occurs because the message from each of the four types of receptor cells is sent by a special nerve ending and is received in a particular region of the brain. That is, heat receptors send electrical impulses through specialized nerve endings to the heat centers in the brain, whereas touch receptors send their messages to the touch centers of the brain. Different areas of the skin vary in their degree of sensitivity, with the fingers being among the most sensitive. The sense of touch arises when unequal pressure occurs between the skin and an object or material in contact with it. This unequal pressure produces a depression in the skin, and thus touch is perceived.

Care of the Sense of Touch

Problems associated with loss of sensation are neurological in nature and are as a result complex and varied. Therefore very little can be done by the individual to affect the sense of touch. However, children should be aware of diminished sensation in any part of the body and should report such an occurrence.

The Senses of Taste and Smell

The senses of taste and smell are closely aligned, because they each enhance and are enhanced by the other. These senses can affect health in many ways—for example, influencing choices of food.

Taste buds are the sensory receptor cells within the visible papillae, or bumps on the tongue. Hairlike projections on the taste buds are stimulated by food entering into the mouth and send impulses to the brain from connecting nerves. The tongue itself contains taste centers, each of which is more sensitive to a particular taste. The tip of the tongue is receptive to food that is sweet, whereas the rear of the tongue keys into bitter-tasting food. Salty foods are more easily tasted on the sides toward the front of the tongue, whereas sour foods are more easily tasted on the sides toward the back. In addition, the tongue differentiates temperature as well as texture of foods, adding greater variety to the sense of taste.

Food is not easily tasted if nasal passages are blocked in some way, as in the case of a head cold. Food in the mouth produces odors in the form of vapors that travel through the nasal passages, where they stimulate receptor cells in the upper nose region. If the passages are blocked, the odors do not reach these cells, and the sense of taste/smell is diminished accordingly. Nerve endings attached to these cells join to form the olfactory nerve (first cranial nerve), the nerve that sends messages concerning smell to the cerebral cortex.

Care of the Senses of Taste and Smell

As with the sense of touch, not much can be done personally to maintain the senses of taste and smell. Impairment because of blockage of the nasal cavity due to colds or infection is temporary and will abate. Impairment due to nerve damage, although rare, cannot be reversed, so loss of taste and smell may be permanent.

Dental Health

Clean, polished-looking teeth and a bright, glowing smile can do much to enhance self-confidence and project a positive image in the minds of others. These emotional benefits are certainly important, but strong, healthy teeth are also essential to overall physical health. Without adequate dental care and upkeep, certain food may not be digested properly or even eaten at all in later life, jaw and facial deformities can result, affecting speech patterns, and personal health in general may suffer. All but a very few schoolchildren experience problems with teeth and gums, such as dental caries and gingivitis (Thibodeau and Patton 1992, 632).

It is imperative that children at an early age learn to follow effective practices that will help ensure the lifelong health of their teeth and oral cavity. They must understand how these habits contribute to good dental health and why teeth are important to preserve and maintain. A tooth has running through its interior core a pulp canal or cavity that serves as the tooth's blood supply. This is surrounded by a bonelike material called *dentin*. Outside the dentin lie roots that fit into sockets of the jawbone. The roots are covered by a material similar to dentin, called *cementum*. The visible portion of the tooth surfacing through the gums is called the *crown* and is covered with a substance called *enamel*.

Dental Problems

By far, the most frequent dental problem among children is dental caries—cavities produced within the teeth due to decay of tooth enamel that, if untreated, may extend into the dentin and pulp canal. Tooth decay leads to the loss of many or all of the permanent teeth. Although false teeth can be fitted, they are generally not as effective, comfortable, or satisfactory as permanent teeth. Tooth decay results from a buildup of plaque, an invisible, sticky film of harmful bacteria whose continual growth in the mouth seems to be enhanced by the presence of foods containing processed sugars. Proper and frequent flossing and brushing of the teeth with a fluoride toothpaste seems to inhibit the buildup of plaque.

Malocclusion. Malocclusion is improper alignment of the upper and lower teeth when the jaw is closed, producing either an overbite or an underbite. Braces fitted by an orthodontist, a dentist who specializes in these problems, can correct malocclusion.

Care of the Teeth

Daily flossing and brushing of the teeth, preferably after each meal but at least once a day, is the best way to maintain good dental health. Flossing should be done first, because it removes plaque from between teeth. Flossing should be done using about 18 inches of floss wound around the middle fingers until only a few inches are left. The ends of the remaining floss section are then grasped between each thumb and forefinger and eased between the gum and tooth so that a scraping motion against the side of the tooth can occur. This procedure should be repeated with each tooth, using a new section of floss each time. Brushing removes plaque from tooth surfaces and is best accomplished by angling the brush against the gumline so that a back-and-forth (side-to-side) motion using gentle strokes can be done on the outside, inside, and biting surfaces of the teeth. A fluoridated toothpaste is recommended.

In addition to daily flossing and brushing, particular attention should be paid to diet. Avoidance of sweets is recommended, and the intake of food high in vitamin D during childhood will help develop strong teeth. Regular dental examinations, preferably twice a year, from childhood through adulthood will also do much to ensure good dental health.

*Exercise can be of value
in a variety of ways.*

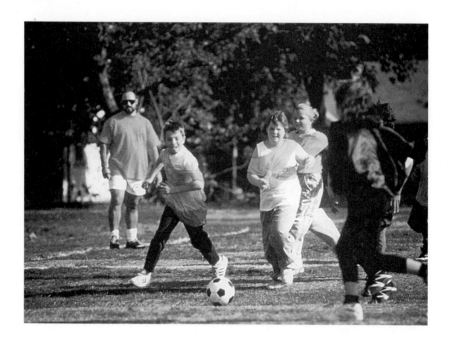

Exercise, Relaxation, and Sleep

Exercise, done according to sound physiological principles in a routine or scheduled regimen, is necessary for maintaining and enhancing personal health. The body also requires relaxation and sleep to renew its energy and strength resources. Body systems that are not allowed to recharge and rejuvenate themselves will ultimately malfunction in ways that can drastically affect the person's general health and well-being. Both short- and long-term personal health can be greatly enhanced by appropriate periods of exercise, relaxation, and sleep.

Exercise

Exercise, when it is an integral component of a person's lifestyle, can be of value in a variety of ways. Fitness not only builds up the strength and resistance to injury of the muscles themselves, it is also beneficial to the entire body. Individuals engaging in planned exercise programs that include not only conditioning or calisthenics, but also extended exercise such as jogging, swimming, or bicycling, show more resistance to chronic ailments, including fatigue, backaches, headaches, anxiety, muscular weakness and atrophy, high blood pressure, and some cardiovascular conditions associated with heart disease.

Cardiorespiratory Fitness. A chief aim of any exercise program should be to develop and improve an individual's aerobic capacity so that intense physical activities can be maintained for longer periods without running short of sufficient oxygen. To do this, exercises that require the heart and lungs to do more work should be stressed, such as running, jogging, and swimming, so that both of these organs become more efficient at delivering oxygen to the cells. Since the heart is a muscular organ, the more strenuously it is taxed with the appropriate type and duration of activity, the larger and stronger its muscle fibers become. Aerobic exercises also improve the muscles of the ribs and diaphragm so that the rib cage is lifted higher, allowing greater expansion of the lungs. Breathing is made easier, and exercise can continue for a longer period of time without adverse effects.

Aerobic exercises that improve cardiorespiratory fitness are not generally lacking in the routine of most elementary school children's lifestyles. However, it is essential that planned, prescribed exercise programs be provided by specialists, such as physical educators and exercise physiologists, to meet individual needs, particularly as the individual grows older.

Skeletal and Muscular Fitness. Although cardiorespiratory fitness should be the foundation for any exercise program because it increases the body's ability to perform strenuous activity, emphasis on muscular strength and skeletal support is also important. Along with aerobic exercises, calisthenics and isotonic exercises (exercise with little or no body movement, such as pushing against a wall) can develop muscular strength and power. Muscle fibers become thicker as a result of regular exercise and therefore stronger. In addition, coordination between muscle groups is improved as well as coordination between muscles and nerves. Static stretching in particular can help produce flexibility of muscles, which enhances skeletal support and fitness.

Relaxation

Relaxation is one of the body's most useful tools in combatting fatigue, either physical, mental, or both. By learning how to relax during the day so that alert and conscious functioning continues, a person can reduce feelings of listlessness, tiredness, apathy, tension, and aches and pains.

Fatigue may be due solely to physical overexertion or to a drain of mental capabilities after engaging in such chores as reading, writing, problem solving, or studying in general. Fatigue can also be produced by adverse environmental conditions, such as improper ventilation or lighting, or by emotional stress.

Relaxation involves the releasing of physical and mental tension through varied and diverse means that can include doing nothing, meditating, watching television, listening to music, taking a hot bath, or relaxing the muscles with a massage. The ways in which an individual chooses to relax should be based on personal interests, environment, or setting, and comfort with the procedure or technique. Regardless of how achieved, relaxation needs to be incorporated into every individual's lifestyle, just as exercise does, so that stress reaction can be minimized and personal health and well-being can be maximized.

Sleep

The body's need for sleep must be met consistently in order to maintain good personal health. Unlike exercise and relaxation, sleep is an involuntary process that does not require a planned or prescribed regimen that must be purposely enacted by the individual. In fact, scientists still cannot fully explain all the mysteries associated with sleep, including its cause and why it is needed.

The amount of sleep needed varies from individual to individual. Most adults need about 8 hours sleep in order to awaken easily and without fatigue. The amount of sleep needed decreases as age increases. Newborn infants spend a majority of their time sleeping, while most older adults sleep less than 8 hours at night but may require short naps during the day. Elementary school children need 8 to 9 hours of sleep a night, and young adults need anywhere from 6 to 8 hours of sleep a night (Hahn and Payne 1997, 86).

▤ Summary

○ Almost every individual begins life with a sound, healthy body, which requires care and maintenance.

○ Knowledge of the body systems and how they interact with one another is important in building and promoting personal health and well-being.

○ Each body system has special roles and functions that directly or indirectly affect all other body systems.

○ The brain and nervous system receive messages from all other parts of the body and act to keep both an internal and external balance.

○ The body's internal balance depends greatly on the release and regulation of hormones from the endocrine system, which strongly influences growth, development, and reproduction.

○ Oxygen, essential to all cells, is channeled into the body by the respiratory system and delivered to all tissues through the actions of the circulatory system.

○ Other chemicals and nutrients are ingested, broken down, and made usable to cells and tissue by the digestive/excretory system so that vital processes can take place.

○ The skeletal/muscular system provides physical shape and structure for the body, assists in protection, and enables movement.

○ Personal health, a most desired and cherished possession, is of concern to everyone.

○ Without good health, the quality of life is diminished considerably and day-to-day existence becomes a burden instead of a joy.

○ To ensure good personal health, each individual must assume responsibility for taking care of his or her own body so that it is kept in good condition.

○ Learning to maintain and enhance one's health and well-being in early childhood through sound health practices is crucial for sustaining high levels of personal health in later life.

○ It is important to teach children the elements of personal health, including

an appreciation for personal appearance

the senses that allow them to relate to their environments

good dental health

○ Children must be taught to exert purposeful, conscious action in incorporating and integrating regular intervals of exercise, relaxation, and sleep into their living patterns.

Discussion Questions

1. What are the two major divisions of the nervous system? Describe and differentiate each.
2. Describe the functions of the cerebrum, cerebellum, and brain stem.
3. What are the overall functions of the endocrine system?
4. Explain why the hypothalamus is considered to be the master gland.
5. Briefly describe the functions of each of these glands: pituitary, pineal, thyroid, parathyroid, thymus, adrenal, and pancreas.

6. Explain how oxygen is transported by means of the respiratory system from the nose, into the lungs, and finally to body tissue. Also explain how the respiratory system expels waste gases.

7. Describe in detail how the blood circulates from the heart to all parts of the body and then back to the heart.

8. Discuss the pumping action of the heart, explaining how the atrium and ventricle in each heart chamber function.

9. Differentiate between red blood cells, white blood corpuscles, and blood platelets.

10. Describe how food moves through the digestive system, from the mouth to the stomach and intestines, and to the rectum.

11. Explain how liquid waste products are filtered and removed from the body by the excretory system.

12. What are the main functions of the skeletal/muscular system?

13. Discuss the importance of the spinal column.

14. Differentiate between voluntary and involuntary muscles.

References

Agur, A. M. R., and M. J. Lee. 1991. *Grant's atlas of anatomy.* 9th ed. Baltimore: Williams & Wilkins.

Guyton, A. C. 1992. *Human physiology and mechanisms of disease,* 5th ed. Philadelphia: Saunders.

Hahn, D. B., and W. A. Payne. 1997. *Focus on health,* 3rd ed. St. Louis: Mosby.

Hole, J. W., Jr. 1993. *Human anatomy & physiology,* 6th ed. Dubuque, IA: Brown.

Marieb, E. N., and J. Mallatt. 1992. *Human anatomy.* Redwood City, CA: Benjamin/Cummings.

Memmler, R. L., B. J. Cohen, and D. L. Wood. 1992. *Structure and function of the human body*, 5th ed. Philadelphia: Lippincott.

Miller, D. F., S. K. Telljohann, and C. W. Symons. 1996. *Health education in the elementary & middle-level school*, 2nd ed. Madison: Brown & Benchmark.

Parnell, K., and others. 1996. Black and white adolescent females' perceptions of ideal body size, *Journal of school health* 66(3): 112–118.

Thibodeau, G. A., and K. T. Patton. 1992. *Anatomy & physiology*, 2nd ed. St. Louis: Mosby.

Yawn, B. and others. 1996. *Journal of school health* 66(5): 171-176.

Chapter Seven
Strategies for Teaching Body Systems/Personal Health

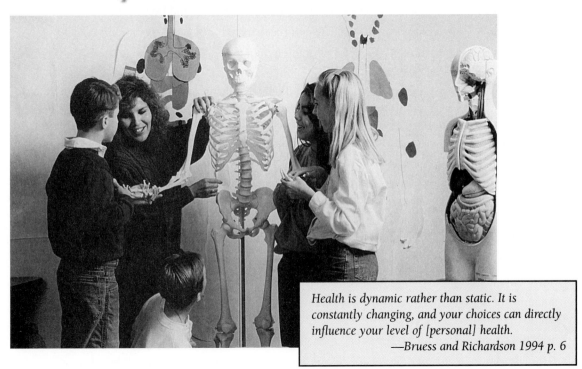

> Health is dynamic rather than static. It is
> constantly changing, and your choices can directly
> influence your level of [personal] health.
> —Bruess and Richardson 1994 p. 6

Valued Outcomes/Body Systems

After doing the activities in this chapter, the student should be able to express and illustrate the following guidelines:

○ The human body is a highly organized and well-developed "machine."

○ The body systems are interdependent and contribute to the healthy functioning of the body as a whole.

○ There is a reciprocal relationship between growth and development.

○ Growth and development as lifelong processes enhanced by responsible behavior.

○ Some growth and development characteristics are common to all living things.

○ Growth and development occur at the level of the cell.

○ Each person is unique in the way he or she grows and develops.

○ Many factors influence physical, mental, and social growth and development.

○ Daily care and maintenance of the human body and an understanding of how its systems operate serve as the foundation for personal health and well-being.

○ The nervous system acts as the body's computer by receiving, interpreting, and sending messages that help direct and guide all other body systems so that the individual can make both internal and external adjustments to the environment.

○ The endocrine system helps maintain balance among all body systems through the secretion from various glands of chemical substances called *hormones* that influence the actions of body organs and structures.

○ The reproductive system becomes activated in puberty and creates and perpetuates human life.

○ The respiratory system provides the pathway and mechanics for oxygen to enter the body.

○ The circulatory system, through the heart's pumping of blood, delivers oxygen and other essential chemicals to all cells and tissue of the body.

○ The digestive/excretory system is responsible for mechanically and chemically breaking down food so that it can be used for all body processes. Substances that cannot be used are eliminated from the body as waste products.

○ The skeletal/muscular system provides the body and its parts with shape, support, protection, and movement.

○ Although body systems operate in standard ways, personal differences in structure and physical functioning affect individual growth and development.

Valued Outcomes/Personal Health

○ Personal health maintenance and enhancement are essential to well-being.

○ Developing of positive health care habits helps maintain the body and promote overall wellness.

○ Attaining of personal health and well-being is an individual responsibility, but can be facilitated by school, community, and social resources.

○ Health care practices promote physical, mental, and social health.

○ Regular visits to health care professionals are important in maintaining personal health.

○ Personal health is influenced by choices made and actions taken based on individual values, attitudes, beliefs, and knowledge.

○ Daily care and upkeep of our personal appearance is an important component of our personal health.

○ Protecting the eyes, ears, teeth, and other body parts is essential to maintaining personal health.

○ Personal appearance is influenced by health habits concerning care of the skin, nails, hair, and posture.

○ Preserving the five major body senses—vision, hearing, touch, taste, and smell—is essential to personal health because the senses keep us in touch with our physical and emotional environments.

○ Adequate dental care may help to prevent jaw and facial deformities, speech abnormalities, and malnourishment in later life, thus safeguarding personal health.

○ Consistent, routinely scheduled, prescribed exercise programs promote personal health and well-being by strengthening cardiorespiratory and muscular fitness.

○ Leisure-time activities promote fitness and contribute to personal health.

○ Relaxation and sleep allow bodily processes and functions to renew their energy sources, thus helping to combat physical and mental fatigue.

Planning Learning Activities

A sound, healthy body is the basis for optimal personal health and well-being. From the instant of birth and throughout life, an individual strives first to meet basic physiological needs. As a result, instruction about the function and care of the human body and its interacting systems is of the utmost importance to children, especially at the elementary school level. Learning opportunities should demonstrate and emphasize health practices that ensure maintenance of body systems so that children develop positive health habits that will enhance their physiological growth and development.

Because children generally enjoy and are interested in participating in physical activity and discovering the unseen "mysteries" of their own body actions, teaching about body systems should be an exhilarating and challenging experience for you. Throughout instruction, children should be made aware of the interrelationships between all body systems and should develop a sense of "ownership" in regard to the body so that personal commitment to its upkeep is fostered.

The Concept of Personal Health

Health education was formerly limited to hygienic practices. Since those days, health education has branched out to include concepts from sociology, psychology, and other disciplines; however, we must not overlook the importance of teaching children about taking care of their bodies. In teaching personal health, emphasize to your students that enhancing well-being is largely an individual responsibility. The concept of personal health is an abstract idea that young children need to be familiarized with, yet many of the practices associated with health maintenance are already familiar to them and can be used as a base for building understanding of the concept. To do this, relate daily health practices to overall well-being. In this way, children will begin to see that discrete practices, such as face washing or tooth brushing, are components of an overall approach to optimum health. That is, a person does not wash simply to clean a part of the body, and tooth brushing and flossing are not simply done to help prevent tooth decay. Rather, these and other personal health practices are parts of an overall maintenance and health enhancement program. To bring this point home, note that personal body cleanliness plays an important role in the prevention of disease, just as proper dental care contributes to overall health.

The strategies described in this chapter are designed not only to teach specific health practices but also to foster good personal health habits. Knowing how to brush one's teeth properly is of little value unless tooth brushing and allied dental care are attended to on a regular basis. For this to occur, children must personalize the information you present and must make decisions to develop good habits. Continually emphasize that personal health is a matter of personal accountability.

Value-Based Activities/Body Systems ───────────

Values Voting

Valued Outcome: The students will be able to clarify values regarding activites related to personal health.

Description of Strategy: The following questions can be posed by the instructor, with the participants voting yes or no on each. Discussion should be allowed to interrupt the voting at any time. How many of you . . .

   . . . use good posture when you sit, stand, walk?
   . . . eat foods that lead to good skeletal development?
   . . . would have a heart transplant if that was needed to lengthen your life?
   . . . get regular physical examinations?
   . . . would smoke if it shortened the length of your life?

Materials Needed: paper and pencil

Processing Question: What health habits most affect your personal health?

Being Good to Me

Valued Outcome: The students will be able to discuss habits they perform to care for the body.

Description of Strategy: Divide students into small groups, and ask each group to list five routine things they do for themselves that they consider beneficial. Compare group listings to see how many listings relate to care of the body. Then write on the board each listing relating to body care, and ask the groups to rank-order them in terms of importance in maintaining body functioning. Follow with general discussion.

Materials Needed: paper and pencil

Processing Question: What are the most important personal health habits necessary to maintain proper body functioning?

Body Drawings

Valued Outcome: The students will be able to draw and label the internal body systems.

Description of Strategy: Provide each student with paper long enough to fit body length. In pairs, have students trace each other's body outlines. Each student then draws and labels the internal body systems. On the reverse side, under each body system heading, have the student list at least two reasons why he or she feels the system is important. Tack the completed body drawings to the wall, interspersing the body parts side of some with the written side of others.

Materials Needed: butcher paper, drawing instruments (crayons)

Processing Question: What is the relative significance of each body system?

Rank-Ordering Health Practices

Valued Outcome: The students will be able to list in order of priority (rank-order) practices that affect each body system.

Description of Strategy: Prepare a handout that lists each body system and three health practices that affect it. Ask students to rank-order the practices according to the positive influence each practice has on that system, "1" being the most positive.

Examples:
> Digestive/Excretory System
>> eating fresh fruits and vegetables
>> eating foods high in fiber
>> limiting sweet snacks
> Skeletal/Muscular System
>> sitting and standing straight
>> getting plenty of exercise
>> relaxing during the day

In the class discussion that follows, indicate that all the practices are important but that some more directly influence specific body systems than others.

Materials Needed: paper and pencil

Processing Question: What practices are significant in affecting the body systems?

Body Systems Position Statement

Valued Outcome: The students will be able to explain the importance of each body system.

Description of Strategy: Divide the class into six groups, each representing a different body system, with the exception of the reproductive system. Have each group be responsible for developing and presenting a five-minute statement that argues for the position that their system "is number 1." After all the positions have been presented, have the students vote to determine a "winner." Follow with a discussion of why students voted the way they did.

Materials Needed: none

Processing Question: Is any one body system really more important than the others, or do we need the functions that each of the body systems provide?

Body Care Collage

Valued Outcome: The students will be able to explain how proper care of the body can influence growth and development.

Description of Strategy: Provide students with poster board, and ask the students to make a collage of people with diverse body types and habits that may influence body functioning. Collages should be made from magazine pictures and newspaper clippings, and should depict the varying health status of the people depicted. Accompanying each collage should be a brief written description that summarizes the student's attitudes and opinions regarding how care of the body can influence growth and development.

Materials Needed: poster board for each student, magazines, newspapers

Processing Question: What are some health habits we can perform that will positively affect our growth and development?

Body Image Sentence Completion

Valued Outcome: The students will be able to complete sentences with their own thoughts about several statements related to body image.

Description of Strategy: Provide students with handouts containing incomplete statements such as the following:

> My body is . . .
> I like my body because . . .
> I take good care of my body by . . .

The bones of my body are . . .
I help my muscles by . . .
When I breathe, I . . .
When I eat, . . .

Materials Needed: pencil

Processing Question: What do you feel are the strengths and weaknesses about your body shape?

Value-Based Activities/Personal Health

Happy Health Activities

Valued Outcome: The students will be able to record personal health activities.

Description of Strategy: Have children record their happy and fun activities related to personal health (such as exercises) with paint or crayons. This activity strengthens the importance of valuing health-related activities.

Materials Needed: marking instruments (such as crayons) and paper

Processing Question: Which personal health activities are important in enhancing one's health?

Sad and Glad

Valued Outcome: The students will be able to discern which personal health behaviors they most enjoy.

Description of Strategy: Mount pictures of various personal health behaviors on large cards. With cards face down, a student chooses one and tells the group that he would be sad or glad if he were participating in this behavior. Older students may describe the activity to the class, emphasizing the sad and/or glad aspects of the behavior, and have the class guess the behavior from the student's description.

Materials Needed: pictures of people involved in health behaviors and large cards on which to post these pictures.

Processing Question: Which personal health behaviors do you most enjoy participating in?

Exercise and Sleep Attitude Scale

Valued Outcome: The students will be able to clarify their attitudes toward exercise, relaxation, and sleep.

Description of Strategy: Present the following forced-choice attitude scale to discover the students' attitudes about the concepts of exercise, relaxation, and sleep:

	AGREE	DISAGREE
1. Exercise makes me feel good.	_____	_____
2. Sleep is important to my health.	_____	_____
3. I take time during the day to do something I enjoy.	_____	_____
4. I sleep eight or nine hours a night.	_____	_____

	AGREE	DISAGREE
5. Exercise can be fun.	_____	_____
6. Taking time during the day to do something enjoyable keeps me healthy.	_____	_____
7. My body can benefit from exercise all my life.	_____	_____
8. I often feel tired when I awake in the morning.	_____	_____

Materials Needed: pencil
Processing Question: How are sleep, relaxation, and exercise beneficial to you?

Personal Health Voting

Valued Outcome: The students will be able to clarify their values regarding personal health habits.
Description of Strategy: Each student will have a card with green on one side and red on the other side. Explain to the students that the green is for "agree" and the red is for "disagree." Remember that there are no right or wrong answers. When the teacher asks the question, the students hold up green cards if they agree with the question (or would answer yes), and hold up red cards if they disagree with the question (or would answer no).

How many of you . . .

. . .would rather go to a birthday party than keep your dentist appointment?
. . .would encourage your brother or sister to clean their teeth?
. . .think it is funny to bump someone at the drinking fountain?
. . .feel that brushing your teeth is necessary to prevent cavities?
. . .feel that eating snacks are harmful to your teeth?
. . .would rather eat a sweet snack than fruit or a raw vegetable?
. . .go to sleep when you are very tired without brushing your teeth?

Materials Needed: pencil
Processing Question: How important are personal health habits to you?

Smiley/Sad Face

Valued Outcome: The students will be able to differentiate between activities they like and those they dislike.
Description of Strategy: An activity similar to voting involves giving the students yellow circle "smiley faces" and blue circle "sad faces." Ask volunteer students to describe to the class an exercise they do for fun and fitness. After the student describes the exercise, have the other students hold up a "smiley face" if they would like to try that exercise, or a "sad face" if they would not. Explain that it is all right to have different preferences for exercises.
Materials Needed: smiley face stickers and sad face stickers for each student
Processing Question: In what activities do you most like to participate?

Dental Health/Self-Confidence

Valued Outcome: The students will be able to differentiate between good and bad dental care.
Description of Strategy: On a piece of paper, have students make two columns—one with the heading "Good Dental Care" and the other with "Bad Dental Care." Under each heading, the students should list different ways that dental care can affect self-confidence. *Example*:

	Good Dental Care	**Bad Dental Care**
Smiles frequently	_____	_____
Covers smile	_____	_____
Positive self-image	_____	_____
Negative self-image	_____	_____
Good first impression	_____	_____
Poor first impression	_____	_____

This activity could be repeated with other personal health behaviors.
Materials Needed: paper and pencil
Processing Question: In what ways can practicing good dental health make you feel better about yourself?

Good Health/Bad Health

Valued Outcome: The students will be able to differentiate healthy from unhealthy behaviors.
Description of Strategy: Divide the class into small groups. Distribute magazines, glue, and scissors. Each group receives a sheet of paper divided in two. One part is headed "Good Health" and the other "Poor Health." Instruct the students to look through the magazines and find pictures that show people involved in healthy and unhealthy behaviors, and then paste the pictures under the appropriate heading. This is a team activity, and the children will have to discuss among themselves which heading would be appropriate for the behaviors.
Materials Needed: magazines, glue, paper, and scissors
Processing Questions: What variables make a behavior healthy or unhealthy?

Before and After

Valued Outcome: The students will be able to explain how personal appearance can be improved.
Description of Strategy: Have students either draw or cut out pictures illustrating facets of personal appearance that need improvement. These are the "before" pictures. Each student describes how he or she believes personal appearance could be improved and then draws an "after" picture to illustrate these opinions and ideas.
Materials Needed: magazines, scissors
Processing Question: What are some ways in which personal appearance can be improved?

What Sleep Means to Me

Valued Outcome: The students will be able to interpret the value of sleep.
Description of Strategy: Have students sketch or paint a picture showing their interpretation of the value of sleep. Have them write a statement about their picture, such as

I smile more when I get enough sleep.

I can run faster when I get my sleep regularly.

I am always tired, but I hate to go to bed.

I get sleepy in school when I stay up too late.

Materials Needed: crayons and paper
Processing Question: How important is sleep to one's personal health?

Self-Portrait

Valued Outcome: The students will be able to describe their strengths in narrative form and pictorially.
Description of Strategy: Provide large pieces of paper and crayons to each student. Ask the students to draw a picture of themselves. (This may best be done at home where a mirror is available and time constraints are removed.) On the reverse side, have students list what they perceive to be their positive attributes. Also have them describe the measures they take to promote personal health.
Materials Needed: large pieces of paper, crayons for each student
Processing Question: What are your positive attributes?

Relaxation Ranking

Valued Outcome: The students will be able to list ways to relax.
Description of Strategy: Prepare a list of ten ways people can relax during the day. Ask each student to rank-order the measures from most effective to least effective. Divide students into small groups, and indicate that each group must come to a consensus ranking. Record each group's ranking on the board and allow for explanations, questions, and summarization.
Materials Needed: chalk, chalkboard
Processing Question: What are the most effective ways to relax?

Personal Health Sentence Completion

Valued Outcome: The students will be able to verbalize their feelings regarding several personal health habits.
Description of Strategy: Have students provide endings to statements such as the following:

I like the way I look because . . .

Sleep is . . .

I take care of my eyes by . . .

If I lost my sense of hearing, . . .

Sitting, standing, and walking straight helps to . . .

Lack of exercise makes me . . .

Materials Needed: pencil
Processing Question: How important do you think it is to take care of your personal health?

Decision Stories/Body Systems

Present decision stories such as the following to the class. Follow the procedure discussed in Chapter 5 for using the stories as a values clarification activity.

Rita's Dilemma

Rita comes from a large, loving family. She has three brothers and four sisters. Her family is poor, but her parents do the best they can. After studying about body systems in class, Rita is aware that it is important to have a physical exam regularly, to make sure that the body is functioning properly. She is now in the fifth grade but hasn't seen a doctor since kindergarten. Rita knows her parents are having a hard time taking care of all the children. There never seems to be enough money to live on. Rita is feeling fine and has only missed one day of school this year, because of a cold.
Focus Question: Should she mention anything to her parents about getting a checkup?

Mary's Father

Mary's father smokes tobacco cigarettes. Mary has just learned how important the heart and lungs are for the proper functioning of the body. How can Mary tell her father about the bad effects on her father's and her own body from his smoking cigarettes?

Decision Stories/Personal Health

Present decision stories such as the following, using the procedures outlined in Chapter 5.

Vision Problems

Kathy is the youngest member in her family. She has two older brothers. Both her parents and her brothers wear eyeglasses. Kathy has felt sorry for them because she thinks that glasses make people look funny and they seem to be such a nuisance. You can't run or play games as easily, because they are always falling off. Kathy has just found out that she is going to have to wear glasses, too, and she is having trouble getting used to the idea.

You are a good friend of Kathy's. You have perfect vision and don't wear eyeglasses. You sense that Kathy is feeling sorry for herself and feeling jealous of your good vision.
Focus Question: What would you say to Kathy?

Teeth and Truth

It's been over a year since Danny has been to the dentist. Danny knows that his mother forgot about his regularly scheduled dental appointment, because he answered the phone when the hygienist called to remind them about the appointment. He didn't tell his mother because he didn't want to go back. But for the last few weeks, one area of Danny's mouth has been feeling funny every time he eats. Danny hates going to the dentist. He is also afraid that he will be punished if he tells his mother what he did.
Focus Questions: What should Danny do? Why?

The Christmas Party

Elizabeth's teacher has asked her to be in charge of the sixth-grade Christmas Party in her room this year. This is really an honor for Elizabeth, and she wants to do everything just right. But Elizabeth cannot eat sugar, and most of the holiday treats are loaded with sugar. Elizabeth thought of maybe having a "Sugarless Christmas Party" with lots of vegetables and dips and other foods without sugar. But Elizabeth is really worried that the other students would turn up their noses at this idea. She certainly doesn't want the party to be a flop.
Focus Question: What do you think she should do?

Enhancing Your Health

Valued Outcome: Students will be able to make decisions that will enhance their health.
Description of Strategy: Read the following situation to the students, and have them write their answers down. Ask the students to share their answers on a volunteer basis and discuss the answers given as a class. Emphasize to the students that the time to rest is when the signs of illness first appear, because this might enable the body to eliminate the illness before it really takes hold.

When Roger woke up one morning, his throat felt scratchy. His nose was a little sniffly, too. He did not seem to have much energy. But his class at school was going on an exciting field trip that day. Roger really wanted to go on the trip.
Materials Needed: pencil and paper
Processing Questions: What should Roger do? Why?

Source: HBJ Health. 1983. Teacher's edition, Level 5, Orlando, FL: Harcourt Brace Jovanovich, p. 186.

Dramatization/Body Systems————————————————————

Have students dramatize different body systems as if they actually were the body system in question. Use your creativity in outlining these activities. The following examples may be helpful:

Dramatizing the Circulatory System

Valued Outcome: The students will be able to describe the function of the circulation system.
Description of Strategy: The students will dramatize how the heart and blood work together. Several students will be required for this activity. Three students will represent the blood, four for valves, two for ventricles, two for atriums, two for the vena cavae, one for the aorta, and one each for the pulmonary artery and pulmonary vein. Have the students stand in the proper position of a heart. Have the "blood" follow the proper path of blood through the heart's structure.
Materials Needed: none
Processing Questions: What role does the circulatory system play in helping our body function?

Digestion Dramatization

Valued Outcome: Students will learn the names of the organs of the digestive system and what they do.

Description of Strategy: Write the following words, each on a separate piece of cardboard: *mouth, esophagus* (make three of these signs), *stomach, small intestine* (make four of these), and *large intestine*. Punch two holes near the top of each card, and thread a piece of string through the holes. The children will hang these signs around their necks. Select three or four children to be the food. Have them wear the brightly colored beaded necklaces to represent the nutrients of the food. The other children playing digestive organs will be wearing their respective signs and standing in the order that matches the path the food takes. Select one child to be the mouth. He or she will wear the "mouth" sign. Instruct this child to pour imaginary saliva (give the student the empty pitcher) on the food and to mash the food down. Then the student will push the food into the esophagus. Have the children playing the role of food squat down. The students acting as the esophagus will push the food down the line to the stomach. The stomach student will add more fluids (provide a pitcher) and mash the food even smaller. Have the food students crawl. The children playing the small intestine will suck out fluids (give them straws) and take the food's nutrients. Have the food students pass the necklaces to the small intestine students. The small intestine players will push the waste to the large intestine, who will push the waste out of the body. Be sure everyone has a chance to be in the digestion line, to be the food, and to be an observer. Help the class move through the process at first, then let them do it by themselves. Ask the observers to tell you what is happening at each step. This will help them understand the digestive system and how it works.

Materials Needed: marker, 10 pieces of cardboard (8" x 3"), hole punchers, string, empty pitchers, brightly colored beaded necklaces, drinking straws

Processing Questions:

1. What is the purpose of the digestive system?

2. What are the organs involved in the digestive process?

3. How do these organs work together?

Source: K. L. Siepak. 1995. *Body systems and organs,* Step-by-Step Science Series, Grades K-3. Greensboro, NC: Carson-Dellosa, p. 31.

The Nervous System

Valued Outcome: The students will be able to describe the function of the nervous system.

Description of Strategy: Tell students that they are going to act like the parts of the nervous system that send and receive information or signals. Form the class into a circle, with each student standing arm's length apart. Have the students cup their hands in front of them to form a pouch or "mailbox." Drop a message in one student's pouch and have that student pass the message along to the student to his or her right, and so on. Explain that the students are acting as the nerve pathways. Stop the message by tapping a student on the head. This student represents the brain. The student then reads the message, which gives a command such as to touch your toes or stand on one leg. Everyone follows the directions. Send additional messages, indicating that the class is functioning like the nerve pathways and brain of the nervous system.

Materials Needed: bits of paper for the nerve messages

Processing Question: What role does the nervous system play in helping our bodies function?

Inside-Out

Valued Outcome: The students will be able to illustrate, through creative writing, the functions of different body systems.

Description of Strategy: Divide the students into groups of five and ask each group to write a fantasy play about a girl or boy who is able to travel through a human body, meeting different body systems along the way. You should serve as a resource, but avoid giving too much direction, thus stifling creativity. Have the students perform their plays, with one acting as the traveler, while the others represent body systems or specific organs.

Materials Needed: paper, pencils

Processing Question: How are the body systems positioned in the body?

Dramatization/Personal Health

Tanning Booths

Valued Outcome: The students will be able to explain the hazards of tanning booths.

Description of Strategy: Instruct the students to work in small groups, and write a script about tanning booths. One group could role-play a conversation between a potential customer and a tanning parlor attendant about the safety precautions practiced by the salon. Another group could enact a situation where a customer fails to follow proper precautions in the tanning booth. A third group could role-play a person who seeks counsel from a dermatologist after several visits to the tanning booth.

Materials Needed: none

Processing Questions:

1. What are the dangers to the skin and other body systems from exposure to tanning booths?

2. What are the proper precautions to follow when using tanning booths?

Wearing Braces

Valued Outcome: The students will be able to verbalize the benefits of wearing dental braces.

Description of Strategy: Have a student role-play the part of a parent who is trying to convince his or her child (another student) of the benefits of wearing dental braces. Another dramatization regarding braces could involve one student role-playing a child who wears braces to school for the first time and another student reacting to the braces with ridicule.

Materials Needed: none

Processing Questions:

1. What are the benefits of wearing braces?

2. How can a person be prepared to handle ridicule from friends when he or she is wearing braces?

Health Teams

Valued Outcome: Students will demonstrate an understanding of teamwork and apply it to careers in health.
Description of Strategy: Explain that the task is to develop a "health team." Ask students what the goal might be for their personal health team. Have each student portray a role, and report on the responsibilities of that health professional.
Materials Needed: a blank team roster
Processing Questions:

1. Who are health professionals who can contribute to a health team?

2. What are their roles?

Source: L. Meeks & P. Heit. 1996. *Totally awesome health,* Sixth grade manual. Blacklick, OH: Meeks Heit, pp. 107–108.

Cover Your Mouth When You Cough

Valued Outcome: The students will be able to explain the personal health consequences when one does not cover the mouth when one coughs.
Description of Strategy: Have students role-play a situation where one child with a contagious cough sits in the desk behind (or next to) a "well" student. This situation could be enacted with two different scenarios. In the first, the "sick" student does not cover his or her mouth, and the "well" student reacts. In the second situation, the "sick" student always covers the mouth, and is questioned by the "well" student. The "sick" student then responds with the appropriate answer.
Materials Needed: facial tissues
Processing Questions:

1. How are respiratory diseases spread?

2. What can we do personally to prevent the spread of airborne diseases?

Discussion and Report Techniques/Body Systems————————

Body Systems True/False

Valued Outcome: Students will take a true/false test to indicate their level of knowledge concerning the skin.
Desciption of Strategy: Provide copy of the following test, leaving the answers blank. Have students take the test, then follow this activity with a discussion of the correct answers to the test, noting that caring for your skin is an important part of personal health.

	True	False
1. The largest organ in the body is the skin.	____	____
2. The most effective over-the-counter (OTC) treatment for acne is to use products that contain benzoyl peroxide.	____	____

	True	False
3. Medicated soaps are a great treatment for acne because the medication seeps into the pores.	_____	_____
4. Acne occurs when skin pores become clogged with dead skin cells and dirt.	_____	_____
5. Products containing lanolin are best to use if you have acne.	_____	_____
6. Acne is caused by eating fatty foods and chocolate.	_____	_____
7. Antibacterial soaps are excellent in treating acne.	_____	_____
8. If you have acne, it is best to use water-based cosmetics or no cosmetics at all.	_____	_____
9. The most active sebaceous (oil-producing) glands are located in the scalp.	_____	_____
10. Look for products containing sulfur, resorcinol, or salicylic acid to treat the more severe cases of acne.	_____	_____

Materials Needed: a copy of the true/false activity

Source: Adapted from P. R. Toner. 1993. *Consumer health and safety activities.* Just for the Health of It. Health Curriculum Activities Library. West Nyack, NY: The Center for Applied Research in Education, p. 108.

Apple Stories

Valued Outcome: Students will work as a group to write and illustrate a story about what happens when someone eats an apple.
Description of Strategy: Have the students write the story for a first grader. It should include a title, main character, descriptions of at least four parts of the digestive system, and illustrations. A couple days later, choose two members of each group to read and show their story to the class.
Materials Needed: drawing and construction paper; scissors; markers or crayons
Processing Questions:

1. What are the parts of the digestive system?
2. What happens in each part?
3. Where does digestion begin and end?

Source: National Center for Health Education (NCHE). 1996. *Growing healthy,* teaching manual, Grade 5. New York: NCHE, p. 20

Taking Care of the Covering System

Valued Outcome: Students will learn the importance of hair and skin care.
Description of Strategy: Explain that it is important that we take good care of our covering system so our skin can keep germs out of our bodies and keep our organs inside us. Ask the chil-

dren to help list ways they can care for their covering system. The list should include good hygiene habits such as washing the body and hair regularly, washing hands before eating or other times they need it, and wearing clean clothes. The hair needs to be brushed or combed to keep it from becoming matted and making the scalp sore. The list should also include ways to protect the skin. A few suggestions are to wear protective gear such as elbow, wrist, and knee pads when skating, helmets when skating or biking, and shoes when walking where our feet would be cut. Explain that another way to care for our skin is to cleanse and cover any cuts. This will help our skin heal more rapidly. When a scab forms, it is important to leave it in place so the skin under it can heal.

Materials Needed: none
Processing Questions:

1. What is the skin's purpose?

2. Why is it important to take good care of our covering system?

3. How can first aid play a part in caring for our skin?

Source: K. L. Siepak. 1995. *Body systems and organs,* Step-by-Step Science Series, Grades K–3. Greensboro, NC: Carson-Dellosa, p. 10.

Which Organ Am I?

Valued Outcome: The students will be able to identify the different organs of the body.
Description of Strategy: Make large cards with names of organs printed on each. Distribute cards to several students and have them stand in front of class, wearing or holding his or her card. Have the students each tell what the job of his or her organ is in the body. This activity could be made for just one system—naming parts of one system.
Materials Needed: large cards
Processing Question: What are the specific jobs of each body organ?

Body Systems Matching

Valued Outcome: Students will match each body system to its function.
Description of Strategy: Have students write the correct numbers of the body systems by the body system definitions on the right. Tell them to use each number once, and look for key words to help them.

1. skeletal system	4. urinary system	7. digestive system
2. muscular system	5. respiratory system	8. endocrine system
3. circulatory system	6. nervous system	9. reproductive system

_____ separates **liquid waste** from the blood and removes it from the body.

_____ is made up of glands that make hormones that help us **grow** and **reproduce.**

_____ makes **egg** cells in women and **sperm** cells in men.

_____ breaks **food** down into small pieces that can move into the bloodstream.

_____ carries food and oxygen to all parts of the body through the **bloodstream.**

_____ **supports** and **protects** the body.

_____ is made of **nerves** that carry messages throughout the body.

_____ works with the bones to **move** the body.

_____ contains the **lungs** that bring oxygen into the body and take carbon dioxide out of the body.

Materials Needed: a worksheet with the preceding activity
Processing Questions:

1. What are the nine body systems? Their functions?
2. How do the body systems work together to keep the body going?

Source: National Center for Health Education (NCHE). 1996. *Growing healthy*, teaching manual, Grade 5. New York: NCHE, p. 10

Skeleton Word List

Valued Outcome: Students will demonstrate an understanding of the skeletal system.
Description of Strategy: Students will use the provided word list to complete the paragraph about the skeleton.

heart   femur   muscles   lungs   skull   vertebrae   cartilage   ribs

The human skeleton is made of more than 200 bones. The _____ is at the top of the skeleton and protects the soft brain. The main support of the skeleton is the backbone. It is made up of smaller bones called _____. Each vertebra is cushioned by _____ , a pad of soft material. Twenty-four curved _____ are attached to the backbone. These form the chest cavity that protects the _____ and _____. The body is able to move because the _____ are attached to the bones.

Materials Needed: a worksheet with the preceding activity.
Processing Questions:

1. What would happen if there were no cartilage between your vertebrae?
2. Why is the femur the largest bone in the body?
3. Why do you think the skull completely covers the brain?

Source: National Center for Health Education (NCHE). 1996. *Growing healthy*, teaching manual, Grade 5. New York: NCHE, p. 18.

Handicapped Does Not Mean Unhealthy

Valued Outcome: Students will learn that "handicapped" does not mean "unhealthy."
Description of Strategy: Invite a disabled person to the class to share the things he or she does to stay well. Ask him or her to explain the aspects of his or her life that are actually quite "normal". Follow this with a question-and-answer period. Encourage the students to share stories of people in their lives who are handicapped.
Materials Needed: none
Processing Questions:

1. Do people who are handicapped feel any differently from those who are not?

2. What are some things I can do to better understand different types of handicaps?

Source: Adapted from Agency for Instructional Technology (AIT). 1985. *A teacher's guide to well, well, well with Slim Goodbody*, Bloomington, IN: AIT, p. 6.

Review of the Senses

Valued Outcome: Students will review the five senses and describe what each sense does. Students will recognize that the senses are interdependent.

Description of Strategy: Name some things that people enjoy doing (or name some things that you enjoy)—for example, listening to music, eating strawberries, petting kittens, smelling flowers, or watching the snow fall. Or show the class pictures that illustrate the senses. Have students recall each of the five senses and how each is used. Then have them identify which sense is used in each enjoyable activity or picture. Use the examples to explain how the senses work together.

As a review activity, have the class make a display about the senses. Divide the class into five groups. Assign each group to make a collage representing one of the senses. They should cut out magazine pictures or draw pictures about the sense. Then each group should paste their pictures on a large sheet of construction paper. Add captions to the completed collages, and display them in the classroom. Have members of each group explain their pictures. Each group may also explain how we take care of senses (eye checkups, hearing tests, and so on).

Materials Needed: optional: one picture to illustrate each of the senses; For collages, magazines and/or drawing materials, five large sheets of construction paper (one for each sense), and glue

Processing Questions:

1. What senses are involved when we eat strawberries (touch, taste, smell, sight)?

2. Can you name something we do or eat that requires all five senses?

Source: G. Ezell. 1992. *Healthy living 2: Healthy and growing*. Grand Rapids, MI: Christian Schools International, p. 99.

Nervous System Demonstration

Valued Outcome: The students will research a division of the nervous system and will demonstrate what they have learned for the other students.

Description of Strategy: The students will discuss their prior knowledge of the nervous system. Then the teacher will tell them that the nervous system coordinates and regulates all the body's other systems. It allows the body to adjust to changes that occur within itself and its surroundings. It has three main divisions—the central nervous system, the peripheral nervous system, and the autonomic nervous system. The teacher will divide the students into three groups. Each group will be assigned a division. As a group, the students will research and prepare a report about the system. They will also prepare some visuals to use in explaining the purpose of their division. The students will then as a group discuss what they have learned with the rest of the class. They will show their visuals and demonstrate if needed. Then, after all the groups have made their presentations, the class as a whole will discuss what the students have learned about the three systems. If desired, the teacher can add information during the discussion.

Materials Needed: paper, pencils, encyclopedias, science books, poster board, markers, construction paper, scissors, glue

Source: N. Christen and D. Peppk. 1994. *Body systems*, Science Mini-Unit. Grand Rapids, MI: Instructional Fair, p. 3.

Effects of Smoking on the Lungs

Valued Outcome: Students will discuss the negative effects of smoking cigarettes, especially the effects smoking has on the lungs.

Description of Strategy: Discuss with the students the effects of cigarette smoke on human lungs. Have students find statistics of smoking related to the human body. Show the students pictures of a human lung affected by cigarette smoke and one without any effects. Have the students divide into small groups and make a list of positive and negative effects of smoking. Then the students will discuss and compare their lists with the rest of the class.

Materials Needed: paper, pencil, resource material and statistics on smoking, pictures comparing lungs

Processing Questions:

1. What is the job of our lungs?
2. What are the effects of smoking cigarettes?
3. What do statistics show is the proper thing to do regarding smoking?

Introducing Body Systems

Valued Outcome: Students will recognize that the body has various systems.

Description of Strategy: Discuss with the students that each person is living and growing— although each individual has his or her own growth rate and pattern. Explain that our bodies have several intricate body systems. Define *system* as "a set or parts or things that form a whole," and give examples such as a stereo system, school system, solar system, or transportation system. In this activity we will be talking about some of the systems that keep our bodies functioning and of which we aren't even aware. Start out by having the students feel a few of their bones—the long bones running along the front of their legs, their ankle and wrist bones, and their cheekbones. Then show the students the handouts of the bone system. Tell the students that this whole bone system is called a *skeleton*. Explain that the skeleton gives the body shape; some bones protect other body parts (give example of the skull protecting the brain). Tell students that the skeleton consists of about 206 bones. Ask students to recall how their bones felt—hard or soft? Explain that bones are hard on the outside, but soft on the inside. Tell students that our bones keep growing. Ask, "How do we know our bones are growing?" Well, the answer is because we become taller. Explain that some bones will continue to grow for almost twenty years; however, a few that are in the inner ear are full size at birth. Explain to students, "We are going to do an activity to make us all aware of our muscles. We are going to practice tension and relaxation of muscles." Have students stand in rows with an arm length of space between each student. Have students curl their toes tightly, and then make all the muscles in each leg hard. Tell them to hold the position. Let it go. Observe to make sure all the students are doing it.

Tell them, "We are going to work the arm muscles next." Tell them to clench their fists tightly so that nails bite into palms. Make sure every muscle in the arm is tightened. After this activity is finished, have students relax their muscles.

Tell them they are now going to work other muscles that they may not normally be aware of using. Tell them to tighten their stomachs so it feels like they are sucking in their stomachs. Hold the position. Let it go. In using the neck muscles, tell the students to tighten their jaw bone as if they have just been scared or eaten a sour lemon. Hold it. Let it go.

Tell the students to relax and sit down. Use this discussion period to explain how we use our muscles and bones every day without even thinking about it as we do it. By using these body systems, we are able to do everyday activities such as stretching, walking, writing, and so on. Without these systems, our bodies would not be able to be active, as we are today.

Materials Needed: Teacher made visuals of muscle and skeleton systems.

Processing Questions:

1. Why is it important to be aware of our muscular system?
2. What happens when we overuse our muscles?
3. Name three muscle areas that we use every day in school.
4. What other muscles do we use?
5. What is the main purpose of our skeletal system?

Source: G. Ezell. 1992. *Healthy living,* Second grade manual. Grand Rapids, MI: Christian Schools International, p. 97.

How Does the Heart Work?

Valued Outcome: Students will understand the concept of circulation: Blood is pumped through tubes (blood vessels) through the body and back to the heart; the heart beats faster when you exercise.

Description of Strategy: On the chalkboard or on chart paper, draw a picture of a train with an engine and at least two cars. Draw tracks under the train, extending in both directions. Ask children to identify the picture and tell about what a train does. Explain that a train's job is to transport. It picks up things at one place, carries them along a route, and delivers them to another place. Write the word *blood* on one train car. Ask the children, "How is the circulatory system like a railroad?" Tell them to imagine that the train is the blood. Encourage children to extend the analogy. The tracks are the blood vessels; the stations along the route are the heart, lungs, and body. The circulatory system carries and delivers blood to all body parts of the body following a particular route, just as the train carries and delivers goods to stations along its route. Display the poster "Your Heart Has Many Parts." Explain that the blood follows a certain route each time it returns to the heart. Point to and name the four chambers of the heart as you describe the route that the blood travels: right atrium, right ventricle, lungs, left atrium, left ventricle, rest of body. Encourage children to say the names with you.

Then give children a handout with a picture of the heart on it. Have them use the poster to help trace the route that the blood travels as it passes through the heart. Ask the children why oxygen is important. Ask them what carries oxygen all around the body. Also, ask the children what happens to the heart if it needs more oxygen. Show the children how to place a stethoscope to listen to their own hearts. Then ask the children to work with a partner to listen to each other's hearts. Have partners take turns using the stethoscope, counting the number of beats in one minute. Have them listen to their own hearts, count, and write the number down for one minute.

Next, have the children jump up and down for one minute. Have them listen to their own hearts, count, and write down the number of heartbeats. Have the children add other categories to their charts at home. Some of the categories can be "after walking or eating."

Materials Needed: large picture of the heart, a picture of the heart for each student, and stethoscopes

Processing Questions:

1. Why is oxygen important?
2. What happened to your heartbeat when you exercised?

3. What happened to your heartbeat when you ate, or after walking?

Source: American Heart Association (AHA). 1996. *Heart power*, second grade level. Dallas, TX: AHA, p. 39.

Muscular System Debate

Valued Outcome: The students will identify the importance of voluntary and involuntary muscles and be able to give examples of each kind of muscle.
Description of Strategy: Divide the class into two groups for a debate. One group will argue that voluntary muscles are the most important to the human body, and the other group will contend the involuntary muscles are most important. Each group should have several minutes to get its arguments ready, and should be able to support its particular muscle group with specific examples of a muscle and its function. After the debate, provide time for a rebuttal from the other group.
Materials Needed: paper and pencils
Processing Question: How does the importance of voluntary muscles compare with involuntary muscles?

Voluntary Health Organization Panel

Valued Outcome: The students will identify organizational purposes and duties of the American Heart Association, the Kidney Foundation, and the American Lung Association.
Description of Strategy: Invite representatives from several voluntary health organizations that deal with a specific organ or body system, such as the Heart Association, Kidney Association, and Lung Association, to address the class. Their presentations should be geared to the age of the students and should include facts about each organization's founding, purpose, and projects. Use a panel discussion format.
Materials Needed: none
Processing Question: How do voluntary health organizations help promote our health?

Respiratory System Demonstration

Valued Outcomes:

1. The students will describe the parts of the respiratory system.

2. The students will be able to explain how air is prepared for the lungs on its way through the respiratory tract.

3. The students will describe the muscular action that results in breathing.

Description of Strategy: The teacher will instruct the students to take two deep breaths, one breathing through the nose and one through the mouth. The teacher will explain that these two air passageways are connected. The students should understand the connection of the air pathways. The teacher will provide the students with a ditto sheet that will show the pathway of the respiratory system. The teacher will have the students trace the pathway of air through the body (nasal passages, trachea, bronchial tubes, air sacs). The students will trace the path on their own bodies starting with their nose and mouth, to the throat, and to the upper chest. Discuss with the students what happens to air as it enters the body. (It's moistened, cleaned, and warmed.) The teacher provides the students with a worksheet on the respiratory system. The teacher has the students fill in names of the parts of the respiratory system and then write a paragraph describing the process of respiration.

Materials Needed: ditto sheet, worksheet
Processing Questions:

1. How is air cleaned?

2. What gas do you breathe in?

3. What gas do you breathe out?

Tracing the Blood Flow

Valued Outcomes:
1. The students will be able to describe the path of blood through the heart and the parts of the heart.

2. The students will be able to describe how to care for the circulatory system.
Description of Strategy: The teacher will instruct the students on the path of blood in the heart. The teacher will provide the students with two worksheets that will help the students understand the pathway of the blood in the heart. The students will trace the pathway with their fingers. The students should be able to say what part of the heart the blood flows through as they trace the pathway. The teacher will provide the students with a worksheet that will have them label the parts of the heart. They will also shade blue the sections of the heart that transport blood carrying carbon dioxide to the lungs. They will also shade red the sections that carry blood with a fresh supply of oxygen from the lungs to the body.
Materials Needed: worksheets, book
Processing Questions:

1. What is the main job of the circulatory system?

2. What are the main parts of the blood?

3. What are the main parts of the circulatory system?

Discussion and Report Techniques/Personal Health

Personal Health Newsletter

Valued Outcome: Students will write a newspaper geared to health in general or to a particular facet of health that is being studied.
Description of Strategy: Every part of a regular newspaper can be written with a health emphasis. Students can create puzzles, poems, stories, drawings, want ads, and so on. These can be transferred to dittos, after your inspection, and reproduced for class members or, money permitting, to the student body and parents. A trip to the library or use of health books and pamphlets can provide a source of information. The real excitement comes when students see their ideas in print—and be sure to let them sign their names to their work. Depending on the age group with which you are working, you may wish to include health advice columns, fashions, sports information, travel, collaged photos (these reproduce very well on a photocopying machine), and even obituaries (deaths due to various poor health practices). Be sure to keep each column geared toward health, fitness, and so on.
Materials Needed: dittos; writing instruments; magazine pictures; scissors

Processing Questions:

1. What health topic is of greatest interest to me?

2. In what way might I be creative in making my contribution to the "Health Newspaper"?

Source: K. Tillman and P. R. Toner. 1990. *How to survive teaching health*. West Nyack, NY: Parker Publishing Company, pp. 35-36.

Presentation by Health Professionals

Valued Outcome: The students will identify the duties of various health professionals.
Description of Strategy: Invite various health professionals, such as dentist, orthodontist, optometrist, ophthalmologist, or audiologist, to address the class and describe their activities and to inform students about sound personal health practices in their field.
Materials Needed: none
Processing Questions: How do health professionals help promote our health?

Sensory Awareness

Valued Outcome: Students will become aware of their senses.
Description of Strategy: Show students magazine pictures related to one of the senses (flower, food, pet, fire, beverage, sand, smoke), and have students decide which sense is involved. In many cases, more than one sense can be named.) Explain that the senses work together.
Materials Needed: magazine pictures depicting each of the five senses
Processing Question: Which body part is associated with each of the five senses?

Source: G. Ezell. 1992. *Healthy living—Kindergarten: God's Healthy Child*. Grand Rapids, MI: Christian Schools International, p. 81.

Accepting Personal Responsibility for Personal Health

Valued Outcome: Students will participate in taking responsibility for their health.
Description of Strategy: Ask the students to do some things to care for themselves without being asked by their parents. Some examples may include: washing your hands before you eat, brushing your teeth on your own, getting to bed by yourself, and so on. Ask the students to pay close attention to their families' reactions and to come to class the next day prepared to share their experiences.
Materials Needed: none
Processing Questions:

1. How does it make me feel to be able to care for myself?

2. How do my parents' reactions make me feel?

Source: Julius B. Richmond, et al. 1990. *Health for life*. Grade 1. Glenview, IL: Scott, Foresman, p. 141.

Building a Family Tree

Valued Outcome: Students will learn of their family histories with regard to health.

Description of Strategy: Have the students construct a family tree that includes their parents, brothers and sisters, aunts and uncles, and grandparents. For each person, write in the names of any chronic or serious diseases that person has had. Explain that some diseases tend to occur often in certain families. Some are due to the families' habits and environment, and some are inherited.

Materials Needed: construction paper; scissors; markers, etc.

Processing Question: How does my family's history contribute to my health and well-being?

Source: Being healthy, teacher's edition. 1990. Orlando, FL: Harcourt Brace Jovanovich.

Time to Brush Your Teeth

Valued Outcome: Students will determine when are good times to brush their teeth.

Description of Strategy: Read the following passage to the students, and follow it with class discussion.

Betsy and her best friend are going out to dinner with their families. After dinner they plan to see a movie. The girls will not have time to go home between dinner and the movie. How should they take care of their teeth? Should they wait until after the movie to brush their teeth? Should they take their toothbrushes and toothpaste to the restaurant with them? What else might they do to keep their teeth safe from cavities?

Materials Needed: If possible, obtain some pictures of people who have taken care of their teeth, and some pictures of people who have not taken care of their teeth. Show to the students to emphasize the importance of taking care of their teeth.

Processing Questions:

1. How often do I currently brush my teeth?

2. What habits do I have that contribute to good care of my teeth?

3. What might I do differently to care for my teeth better?

Source: HBJ health, Level 5. 1983. Orlando, FL: Harcourt Brace Jovanovich, p. 156.

Screening Procedures

Valued Outcome: The students will list and describe a screening procedure used in school systems.

Description of Strategy: Prepare an outline of the various screening procedures that are commonly used in school systems. Include screening measures that may not necessarily be available in your school but that are used widely. Ask each student to choose one procedure and write a report about it. Collect the reports and collate them into a screening procedure booklet that can be used as a resource.

Materials Needed: outlines of screening procedures

Processing Questions:

1. What screening procedures are used in your school?

2. What occurs during each screening procedure?

Periodic health screening will aid a child's ability to learn.

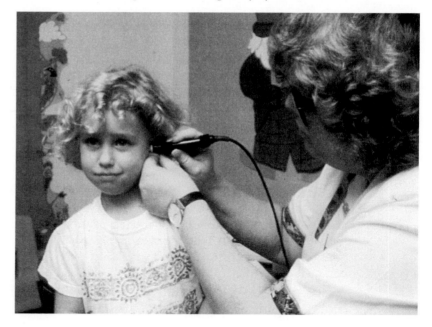

Experiments and Demonstrations/Body Systems

Body Drawings

Valued Outcome: The students will trace the outline of their bodies on a large sheet of paper. The students will weigh and measure their bodies.

Description of Strategy: Have the students pair off, and have the first student trace around the second student's body while the second student is lying down on a large sheet of paper. Then switch and repeat the process. Various body systems may then be drawn and colored by the students on their own body drawings. You may also wish to weigh and measure the students, and let them use the body drawings to keep up with these measurements throughout the school year.

Materials Needed: butcher paper, magic markers, scales, measuring tape

Processing Questions:

1. How is body weight determined?

2. How tall is each individual?

Body Systems Being

Valued Outcome: Students will participate in the construction of a "body systems being" to demonstrate an understanding of how each body system works and how they work together to maintain a healthy body.

Description of Strategy: An outline of a human form should be traced on a piece of butcher paper and pinned up so that the class can see it. This should be about the size of an average person in the class. Introduce the activity by explaining the following project goals to the class:

1. The class will construct an entire human model during the next nine class periods (or time modifications you need to make).

2. This model will have all the body systems that are needed for functioning.

3. All the body systems will be made out of construction paper and will fit inside the outline of the human form.

4. The organs should be shaped like the actual organs, and placed properly in the form.

5. The class will be divided into groups, and each group will be responsible for constructing one body system.

6. Each group will conduct research on their appointed body system. Resources should be available in the classroom, and students should be encouraged to do research outside of class as well.

7. Each group also will be responsible for creating a detailed presentation to the class about the body system. This should include how the system works, what it does, details about each organ in the system, and some interesting facts discovered during the research.

8. The final product should be a life-size model of the human body with all the systems placed over each other inside the form.

9. Each group will be responsible for deciding among its members all tasks necessary to construct the system and prepare the presentation for class.

10. Each of the classes will name their models, which will be on display in the room during and after construction.

11. The class will have a total of seven class periods to work on the group task of construction and presentation of their system.

12. A plan explaining how the group tasks will be divided should be agreed on during the first group meeting.

13. At the beginning of each class period, the class will meet as a whole during the first two to five minutes. During this time, the teacher will appoint a day leader for each group. Then each group will meet to discuss tasks for the day. During the last five to seven minutes of the class period, materials should be cleaned up and resources put back.

14. Each group member should report his or her progress to the day leader, who will record progress in the group activity log, "Duties of the Day Leader" (these should be posted and referred to daily):

   ○ to write down each of the group members and what they will be doing that day in the log
   ○ to keep group members on task
   ○ to report progress at the end of the period in the group activity log
   ○ to submit the group log to the teacher at the end of the period
   ○ to make sure the group has cleaned up well

The class should then be broken down into seven groups with approximately the same number of participants per group. The teacher will assign each group a body system. The teacher will appoint a day leader each day. Each group will be given a notebook to use as a group activity log. (This activity is an excellent way to incorporate cooperative learning in the classroom.)

Materials Needed: a large piece of butcher paper (approximately 3 by 6 feet); several reference books about the body systems; construction paper in a variety of colors; colored markers; scissors; glue and tape

Source: M. Bentley. 1995. The body systems being. *Journal of health education* 26(4): 245-247.

Digestive Tract Experiment

Valued Outcome: The students will see how important water is in the digestive tract.

Description of Strategy: The students will create a digestive tube by using the following method. A small amount of food is placed in a jar. Enough water is added to cover the food. The lid is screwed on tightly and the jar is shaken vigorously. If big chunks of food remain, a spoon can be used to simulate the crushing action of teeth. The digestive tube will be positioned in gentle bends to represent the true position in the body. Using an eyedropper, the food will be placed into the digestive tube. A peristaltic motion, the rhythmic contraction of the tube from top to bottom, will be used to help the food through the tube. Simulate this by squeezing the tube little by little. Add five droppers of water to the apparatus. Compare the ease with which it moves with the added water. A stopwatch will be used to record the start time (when food is introduced into the tube) and the time when the food reaches the other end. The activity will be repeated using ten and then twenty droppers of water. The times will be compared.

Materials Needed: stopwatch, flexible transparent aquarium tubing (approximately 4 feet per team—each foot of tubing equals 7 feet of intestine), eyedropper, jar with tight lid, water, paper towel, crackers, bread, or other soft food

Processing Questions:

1. Why do we need water?

2. How much water do we need to drink a day?

Source: D. Vaszily and P. Perdue. 1994. *Bones, bodies, and bellies.* Glenview, IL: Scott, Foresman, p. 73.

Dissecting a Heart

Valued Outcome: Students will further explore the structure of the heart by dissecting an animal heart.

Description of Strategy: Begin lesson by discussing any questions the students may have on the structure and function of the parts of the heart. Demonstrate the dissection of an animal heart. After you have finished with this, divide the class into small groups of four or five students. The groups should be small enough so that each student has the opportunity to handle the heart. Distribute to each group the student activity handout "Heart Dissection Procedure," and have students dissect their own specimens following the procedure outlined. Here are the answers:

1. Answers will vary.

2. It will feel slippery.

3. Answers will vary.

4. No, because the heart has stopped pumping.

5. These veins and arteries are tough and stretchable, and resemble a garden hose.

6. The pericardium is very thick, strong, and transparent. It looks very much like transparent plastic wrap.

12. The left side of the heart pumps blood to all parts of the body; it must work harder than the right side. The harder muscles work, the bigger they get.

13. The mitral valve strands are usually stronger and thicker.

15. To provide the heart with the oxygen and nutrients it needs.

After the students have finished with this experiment, explain to them that they have explored an actual heart to understand more completely the structure of the heart. Tell them they saw and felt the left side, which pumps blood to all parts of the body, and the right side of the heart, which pumps blood to the lung. Explain that the chart has an upper chamber that receives blood and a lower chamber from which blood is pushed out. The major function of the heart muscle tissue is to pump blood throughout our body. The heart muscle is an involuntary muscle that works twenty-four hours a day.

Materials Needed: student activity handout, one per student group; dissecting kits, one per student group; five-inch straws, one for each heart; paper towels, dampened with water, about 6 per group; newspaper or aluminum pie tins, one per group; sharp scissors or scalpel, one per group; animal hearts to dissect, one per student group

Processing Questions:

1. What was the most interesting part of the experiment?

2. List as many parts of the heart as you can remember.

3. Draw on a piece of paper the different parts of the heart you observed.

4. Where does the right side of the heart pump blood to?

Source: G. Ezell. 1993. *Healthy living,* sixth grade edition. Grand Rapids, MI: Christian Schools International, p. 120–121.

Feel Muscles in Motion

Valued Outcome: Students will demonstrate how their muscles work.

Description of Strategy: The muscular system allows our bodies to move. There are over 600 muscles in the body, of which the gluteus maximus muscles (buttocks) are the largest. Tell the students to stand up and put their hands against the sides of their outer thighs. Then have them slowly bend their knees and feel the muscles move in their legs. Next have them put their hands on their abdomens and quickly blow air out, saying, "Heh-heh-heh." Their abdominal muscles will quickly squeeze in and relax. Tell your students to make some funny expressions in front of mirrors. Tell them to note how their cheek and jaw muscles, eyebrow, and forehead muscles move as they make their faces. Muscles work by contracting, and each muscle contracts in only one direction. The contraction of a muscle results in a pull; muscles cannot push. When a muscle contracts and then relaxes, it goes through a full cycle of movement. This is what makes our hearts beat: a contraction and a relaxation. So, to move our extremities, two muscles work in opposition at every point. Your students can understand this by bending their arms to tighten their biceps. Tell them to keep their biceps tightened and at the same time to straighten their arms; it's impossible. Pair the students and tell them to stand facing each other and to hold hands. Tell one student in each team to pull his hands backward, taking his partner's hands with him. Then tell all the students to relax, letting their arms drop back to the starting position. Then the other student in each pair will pull his arms backward. Our muscles work this way: the biceps, for example, pull the wrist toward the shoulder, while the triceps pull the arm back down.

Materials Needed: mirrors

Processing Questions:

1. What is the importance of the muscular system?

2. What are some muscles in the body?

Source: K. L. Siepak. 1995. *Body systems and organs,* Step-by-Step Science Series, Grades K-3. Greensboro, NC: Carson-Dellosa, p. 11.

Bone Transformation

Valued Outcome: The students will familiarize themselves with the bones and how they can be used.

Description of Strategy: To begin this activity, the teacher will discuss the shape of the bones and the purpose of that shape, using real bones. The teacher will hand out to each student a copy of a drawing of a bone and have them cut it out. The teacher will then have the students place the bone in any position on their paper. Then have the students get in groups of three or four, and have them discuss and list many, different and unusual things bones could become. Each student will then illustrate a bone transformation on his or her own piece of paper. When the students are done with their transformations, they will discuss it and share them with class. The students will discuss how bones could be used and sum up this lesson with this discussion.

Materials Needed: real bones for examples, copies of a drawing of a bone for each student, pencils, crayons, drawing paper

Processing Questions:

1. Why do bones have to be certain shapes?

2. Why is the shape of the bone important?

What Does the Heart Do?

Valued Outcome: Explain the concept of circulation: Blood is pumped through tubes (blood vessels) through the body and back to the heart.

Description of Strategy: Ask them, "What does the heart pump?" Ask "Where does the heart pump blood?" Draw a large figure 8 on the chalkboard or on chart paper. Put an X in the middle where the lines cross each other. Give children pieces of chalk or markers and let them take turns tracing the figure 8, beginning at the X in the middle. Children may also trace the figure 8 pattern on their own bodies. Ask the children where they started tracing the figure 8 and when they finished tracing the figure 8. Point out that the heart is like the X on the figure 8. Trace the figure 8 again while explaining that blood goes from the heart to the lungs, back to the heart, from the heart to the body, and back to the heart. Expand the figure 8 to include a box labeled "Body" at the bottom. Then trace the path—heart, lungs, heart, body, heart—several times and ask children to name the parts as you trace. Explain that the heart, lungs, and blood vessels are the main parts of the circulatory system and that the heart is the pump that pushes the blood through the system. Display the dishpan filled with water, the measuring cup, and the pieces of rubber tubing. Let children take turns using the measuring cup to pour water through the tubes and into the dishpan. Explain that just like the water in the rubber tubes, blood goes to all parts of the body through tubes. These tubes, called *blood vessels*, are also part of the circulatory system.

Materials Needed: chalk, several 12-inch lengths of rubber tubing, dishpan, measuring cup, water

Processing Questions:

1. What are the three main parts of the circulatory system?

2. Which part of the circulatory system pumps blood?

Source: American Heart Association (AHA). 1996. *Heart power*, Kindergarten through Second Grade Manual. Dallas: AHA, p. 37.

Brain Viewing

Valued Outcome: The students will compare the parts of an animal brain to that of a human brain.

Description of Strategy: Obtain the brain of a sheep or cow. Have students compare the parts of the animal brain to those of a human brain, using a model of the human brain for the comparison.

Materials Needed: sheep or cow brain, model of human brain

Processing Question: Compare the animal's brain to the human brain with regard to size, function, shape.

Heart Rate

Valued Outcome: The students will take a one-minute pulse before and after exercise.

Description of Strategy: Have the students feel for their own pulse by placing their index and middle finger of the same hand on the inside of the neck. Have them count the beats for one minute and record the number (resting heart rate). Then have them jog in place for at least two minutes and record the heart rate for another minute. Wait an additional one minute and have them count the heartbeats to see how close it is to the original resting heart rate.

Materials Needed: clock, or watch with timer

Processing Questions:

1. What is the importance of knowing your resting pulse rate?

2. What affects the pulse rate?

Nerve Messages

Valued Outcome: The students will demonstrate how nerve impulses work.

Description of Strategy: Another simple demonstration to show how nerve cells work can be done by having students slightly touch a hot light bulb, then relate to the students how the nerves in the fingers send messages to the brain and then to the limbs.

Materials Needed: lamp with bulb

Processing Question: How does the nerve send messages to the brain and then to the limbs?

Experiments and Demonstrations/Personal Health ───────

Teeth Problems

Valued Outcome: Students will demonstrate proper dental hygiene.

Description of Strategy: Discuss with students problems that could occur from not taking care of their teeth, such as cavities, root canals, loss of enamel, false teeth, and so on. Discuss the proper steps for taking care of their teeth:

1. Brush teeth after every meal.
2. Use dental floss after brushing teeth.
3. Rinse mouth with mouthwash.
4. Take regular trips to the dentist.
5. Limit the amount of sugar you consume.

Have each student copy these steps as a reminder of the proper dental hygiene procedures. Distribute toothpaste and a toothbrush to each child.

Materials Needed: paper, pencil, toothpaste, and a toothbrush for each child

Processing Question: What are the proper steps for good dental hygiene?

Teeth and Digestion

Valued Outcome: The students will identify the role teeth, saliva, and digestive enzymes play in chewing.

Description of Strategy: Give each student a saltine. Have them chew it without swallowing and note what takes place. Explain that the teeth grind the food. At the same time, saliva and digestive enzymes in the mouth act on the food. Children should note how the taste of the cracker sweetens as this happens. The chewed cracker is being changed to a moist bolus so that it can be swallowed easily.

Materials Needed: crackers

Processing Question: What significant part do the teeth play in digestion?

Shadow Play

Valued Outcome: The students will demonstrate the difference between proper and improper posture.

Description of Strategy: The purpose is to gain an understanding of various postural defects and practice posture improvement. The materials you will need are a shadow screen (a bed sheet may be used), lights, and equipment necessary for the demonstration. This is an excellent way for children to compare and dramatize good and bad posture. A narrator, chosen by the group, discusses various aspects of maintaining good posture while standing, sitting, walking, and reading. As the narrator discusses each posture, a pupil standing behind the screen will demonstrate poor posture; and at the same time another will demonstrate proper posture. The positions of narrator and shadow casters can be changed so that all children participate.

Materials Needed: shadow screen (bed sheet), lights

Processing Questions:

1. What part does posture play in overall personal health?

2. How does poor posture affect the function of internal organs?

Properties of Skin

Valued Outcome: The students will examine the skin of the foot and note the different properties of the skin.

Description of Strategy: Ask each student to take off a shoe and sock so that one foot is bare. Have the students feel the difference between their skin and the sock covering the other foot. Let them notice the cooling reaction, and ask them why one foot feels cooler than the other. Then dab the foot with alcohol, demonstrating the evaporation principle. Ask the students how perspiration relates to this principle. Also have students pull on the skin covering their foot. Ask them if some places are tighter than others on the foot. Why does this matter? Ask them if some places are more sensitive than others. What does this tell us about skin?

Materials Needed: shoe, sock, alcohol

Processing Questions:

1. Why does the skin perspire?

2. How does the body lose heat through the feet?

Fingerprints

Valued Outcome: The students will compare fingerprints and recognize the different configurations of each.

Description of Strategy: Provide students with white paper and a stamp pad. Have them place their fingertips on the pad and then make an impression on the paper. Ask students to label the prints with their names. Then let them compare each other's prints to see that no two patterns are exactly the same. Discuss the anatomy of the skin ridges that form fingerprints (and footprints).

Materials Needed: stamp pad, white paper

Processing Questions:

1. Why do we have ridges on the fingertips?

2. Why do we each have unique fingerprints?

Pupil Dilation and Constriction

Valued Outcome: The students will describe the difference light plays on the dilation and constriction of the pupil of the eye.

Description of Strategy: Pair students and have them face one another so they can see their partner's eyes. Tell them to look at the partner's pupils for a few seconds, and observe their size. Then, at your signal, ask all students to close their eyes and not to reopen them until you tell them. Explain that on your signal, they are to open their eyes and look quickly at their partner's pupils. Give the signal after about 45 seconds, and have the students note the constriction of the pupils on being exposed to light.

Materials Needed: none
Processing Question: What is the purpose of the dilation of the pupil?

Sound Localization

Valued Outcome: The students will identify the location of different sounds while blindfolded.
Description of Strategy: Pair students. One student is blindfolded, sitting in a chair. The other student, who acts as the "tester," stands nearby and taps a pencil against a glass. The blindfolded student points to the direction he or she believes the sound is coming from. Have the tester move to several locations throughout the room, sometimes holding the glass high above the floor and sometimes holding it low. Repeat this with several other students to note differences. Also do the experiment with several blindfolded students who have one ear plugged, to note differences in sound localization ability.
Materials Needed: material that will serve as blindfolds
Processing Question: How does sight enable the sense of hearing?

Sleep Needs

Valued Outcome: The students will identify different needs for sleep with regard to age groups.
Description of Strategy: To demonstrate the varying needs for sleep at different ages, have students interview several people of different ages, (such as siblings, peers, parents, grandparents). Instruct them to write down the names and ages in chronological order by age. Have them report on the different needs for sleep for people of different ages.
Materials Needed: none
Processing Questions:

1. How much sleep does the student need?
2. Why do sleep needs vary at different stages of life?

Puzzles and Games/Body Systems

Body Parts Puzzle

Valued Outcome: The students will correctly put together a puzzle of body parts made of construction paper.
Description of Strategy: Divide the students into groups. Provide each group with a sealed package containing body parts made of construction paper. Each packet should contain identical parts. Separate the groups, and provide each with a large piece of paper that has the outline of the human body on it. At your signal, groups open their packets and place the body parts where they should be on the paper. The group to finish first wins. Time each group so that a few days later the same game can be played, with teams trying to improve their previous time score so that they are competing against the clock rather than against each other.
Materials Needed: construction paper, package, butcher paper
Processing Question: What is the correct placement of body parts within the body?

The Human Body

Valued Outcome: The students will identify vocabulary words that pertain to the human body.
Description of Strategy: During a unit of study on the human body systems, students will complete a word search by finding and circling such words as *genes, nerves, vein, uterus, lungs, aorta,* and so on. The word search will serve as a reinforcement activity.
Materials Needed: The Human Body word search worksheet for each student
Processing Question: none

Source: K. G. Zipprich. 1989. *Health education puzzles and puzzlers.* Portland, ME:J. Weston Walch, p. 3.

Figure 7.1

*Human Body
Word Search*

Name: _____   Date: _____

The Human Body

Directions: Find the words in the puzzle and circle them. The words are spelled horizontally, vertically, diagonally, forward, or backward.

Words to find:

AIDS	children	genes	lymph	semen
alimentary canal	diet	glands	mouth	senses
aorta	digestion	health	muscles	sight
balance	ear	heart	nerves	taste
birth	egg	hormones	nutrition	touch
blood	emotions	identity	organ	ureter
bones	endocrine	intestine	ovary	uterus
brain	eye	life	penis	vein
calcium	fetus	liver	posture	waste
cells	food	lungs	retina	x ray

© 1989 J. Weston Walch, Publisher.

Source: K. G. Zipprich. 1989. *Health education puzzles and puzzlers.* Portland, ME:J. Weston Walch, p. 3.

Body System Scramble

Valued Outcome: The students will exhibit their knowledge of the different body systems and their parts.

Description of Strategy: Prior to this lesson, the students will have already learned about body systems. This lesson is meant for a review. Give the students several scrambled words (list follows) to unscramble. Then have students place them underneath the appropriate heading. The unscrambled word will spell a scientific name for another part in the body.

OTMHU (MOUTH)	SERNNUO (NEURONS)
RIBAN (BRAIN)	LAAUCPS (SCAPULA)
TRSAEEIR (ARTERIES)	ALCECVLI (CLAVICLE)
RLVIASYA ADLSNG (SALIVARY GLANDS)	OSAMHTC (STOMACH)
LBFAIU (FIBULA)	LEILAASPICR (CAPILLARIES)
AISNLP RCDO (SPINAL CORD)	UMRHESU (HUMERUS)
ETRHA (HEART)	PRANESAC (PANCREAS)
SGSPEHUOA (ESOPHAGUS)	EVRIL (LIVER)
EVENRS (NERVES)	INSEV (VEINS)
APLTALE (PATELLA)	UEELCBRLME (CEREBELLUM)
RETVEREAB (VERTEBRAE)	RTNSEUM (STERNUM)

Categories: Digestive System, Skeletal System, Central Nervous System, Circulatory System
Materials Needed: pencil and paper
Processing Questions:

1. What are the four different body systems?

2. What are some examples of each?

Source: D. Vriesenga. 1994. *The human body*, Whole Language Theme Unit. Grand Rapids, MI: Instructional Fair, p. 3 .

Body Organs Game

Valued Outcome: Students will be able to describe the organs of the body and their functions.
Description of Strategy: The students will study the organs in a human body focusing on their functions. The teacher will then conduct a game similar to a spelling bee. The students will stand as the teacher goes around the room in order. The student will be given a body organ and asked to tell the function, or vice versa. If the answer is wrong, the student will sit, if not he or she will keep standing and stay in the game. The game will end when only one person is left standing.
Materials Needed: none
Processing Question: What are the major body organs, and what are their functions?

The Paper Race for the Respiratory System

Valued Outcome: Students will test their abilities to control their breathing.
Description of Strategy: In an open floor space, mark a finish line on the floor using masking tape or rulers. Have several children line up beside each other, rather than in back of each other.

Instruct each to put a ball of wadded-up (crumpled) paper on the starting line, and be sure every-one knows where the finish line is. Tell them to blow through the straws to move the papers from the start to the finish. If they touch the papers with anything—the straws, their hands, or any-thing else—they have to go back to the starting line and start again. The person who blows his or her paper across the finish line first is the winner. Repeat the activity with different students until everyone has had a chance to participate in a race. If you have table tennis balls, let the children try racing them after the paper race. The balls will be harder to control but still a lot of fun.

Materials Needed: wadded pieces of paper, clean straws, table tennis balls, masking tape or rulers

Processing Questions:

1. What is the importance of the respiratory system?

2. Why were some students able to finish faster than others?

Source: K. L. Siepak. 1995. *Body systems and organs,* Step-by-Step Science Series, Grades K-3. Greensboro, NC: Carson-Dellosa, p. 26.

The Body Systems Game

Valued Outcome: Students will comprehend health promotion and disease prevention concepts. *Description of Strategy:* Teacher will print the names of the body systems in red on the cards and the parts that belong under these body system in green. Begin activity by defining the system names. Use the terms *body system, circulatory system, digestive system, respiratory system, nervous system,* and *skeletal system.* Tell them that also included in the body system are the bones, knees, ribs, and the skull. Review these five body systems with the students before playing the game. After these terms are defined and reviewed, tell the students they are going to play "The Body Systems Game." Explain to students they will form a single line with one on each side of you. When they come to you, they are to turn their back so that you can tape a card with the name of a body sys-tem or the name of a part of that body system on their backs. Explain that they will not know what part of the body system is taped on their backs. One of the objectives of this game is for stu-dents to guess what is printed on the card on their backs. They are to do this by approaching other students. When they approach other students, they are to turn their backs so the person can read the card. Then the person will turn and ask a question. However, only a question that receives a yes or no response can be asked. For example, a student cannot approach another student and ask, "Am I above or below the waist?" After receiving an answer, the student must then approach another person. Explain that only one question can be asked of each person. Explain that when the word on the back is correctly identified, that student is to tape the card in the front of his or her body. This indicates to other students that that particular student guessed what was printed on his or her card. The student who has already guessed his or her card may still help others who have not guessed what is on their backs. After all the students have guessed their cards, explain to the students they are to remain nonverbal, and assemble themselves into the groups to which they belong. Each one belongs to one of five groups. Tell them to have their groups spread out so each one is distinct. After they have done this, explain to students they are going to look at ways to care for the body system their group represents. They can introduce any health facts they desire, but these facts must be presented as lyrics to a song. They must have a title to their song and a name for their group. Once students have shared their songs, use this information to review facts about the care of the different body systems.

Materials Needed: twenty-five 3" x 5" index cards; tape; one red marker; one green marker; pen-cil or pen

Processing Questions:

1. Write five facts about one of the body systems, and include at least one way to care for that body system.

2. Name two items that are found in the respiratory system.

3. What system is responsible for carrying out appropriate responses to stimuli from the extemal environment?

4. Name one thing you have learned from this game.

Source: L. Meeks, P. Heit and R.Page. 1996. *Comprehensive School Health Education*, 2nd ed. Blacklick, OH: Meeks Heit Publishing, p. 50.

Sense of Sight

Valued Outcome: Students will associate the sense of sight with the eyes. Students will identify ways to protect eyes from injury.

Description of Strategy: The lesson on sight will begin with a lively game of "I See" where the class will move to music and when stopped, the students will freeze and stare straight ahead. Ask one student, "What do you see?" The child answers by describing one thing in his or her line of frozen vision. The rest of the students have three tries to guess what the object is. After a few times, change from an object to what color they see. After several rounds of the game, have the students sit in a circle and discuss why we have eyes. Allow the students to respond. Compare our eyes to windows and explain that our eyes are our windows on the world. Identify some things our eyes help us do. Include ways our eyes keep us safe (for example, see oncoming traffic, obstacles, traffic lights). Work with the class to make a chart of ways to protect our eyes from injury. Note that our eyes are made in such a way that they would protect themselves with eyelids and eyelashes. Draw simple pictures on the chart to illustrate the safety rules. Include the following rules:

1. Carry sharp objects such as scissors and pencils in a point down position.

2. Don't point sharp things at others.

3. Don't run with sharp things.

4. If you get something in your eye, get help. Don't rub your eye.

5. Sometimes our eyes need eyeglasses to help them do their work.

Materials Needed: music to accompany the game "I See," chart paper
Processing Questions:

1. What do we see with?

2. How do our eyes help to keep us safe?

3. What are some ways to take care of our eyes?

Source: G. Ezell. 1992. *Healthy living, Kindergarten: God's Healthy Child*. Grand Rapids, MI: Christian Schools International, pp. 83, 84.

Memory Game

Valued Outcome: The students will repeat a sequence of movements to test their memory skills.

Description of Strategy: This game allows the students to see how the brain can store and use information. Divide the class into teams. The teacher reads several body actions, such as "Touch your nose," "Touch your toes," "Clap your hands." Each team will take turns to see how many actions can be followed in the sequence the teacher read before members of the team become disorganized.

Materials Needed: None

Processing Question: How does the brain function in order to store information?

Bean Bag Toss

Valued Outcome: The students will identify endocrine glands and their hormones while tossing a bean bag through holes in a cardboard box.

Description of Strategy: Cut several holes in the bottom of a very large cardboard box. Label each hole so that it represents a different endocrine gland and secure the box against the wall. Let each student have three chances at tossing a bean bag into the holes. Score one point for getting the bag into the hole and two points if the student can name one function of the gland or one of the hormones it secretes, just so long as that function or hormone has not already been named by another student. Tally scores and announce the winners. Repeat this game periodically, being sure to change the order, so that students who were first during the previous game have to go last, and vice versa.

Materials Needed: cardboard box, bean bags

Processing Questions:

1. What is the function of each gland in the endocrine system?

2. What is the function of the hormones secreted by these glands?

Blood Jeopardy

Valued Outcome: The students will play a game by matching parts of the blood with statements about the circulatory system.

Description of Strategy: Using an overhead projector and transparencies, write short statements about various parts of the blood and/or circulatory system. The students (divided into teams) guess which part of the blood that the statement applies to. Various amounts of points can be awarded according to the difficulty of the statement.

Materials Needed: overhead projector, transparencies

Processing Question: What are the various functions of the blood?

Puzzles and Games/Personal Health ───────────────

Take Time for Personal Health

Valued Outcome: The students will list different roles, functions, and health practices associated with various components of personal health.

Description of Strategy: Divide students into groups and assign each group a different component of personal health, such as care of the hair, skin, teeth, eyes, or ears, and the need for exercise, sleep, and relaxation. Allow the groups two minutes to list as many roles, functions, or health

practices associated with that component as they can. Read each list for accuracy and determine which group won the round. Play several more rounds, explaining that each time listings must be different. See not only which group can list the most per round, but also which group is able to list the most at the end of the game.
Materials Needed: none
Processing Questions:

1. What are the roles and functions of the hair, skin, teeth, eyes, and ears?

2. What are the personal health habits needed for each of these organs in order for the body to work efficiently?

Other Ideas/Body Systems

Respiratory System Travelogue

Valued Outcome: The students will learn the parts of the respiratory system by being guided through an imaginary trip of that system.
Description of Strategy: Draw a diagram of the respiratory system on a chart or overhead transparency. Take the class on an imaginary trip through the respiratory system. You are the tour guide. Use props and tour guide dialogue. This activity can be used for any body system.
Materials Needed: chart or transparency, various props to represent the lungs and body systems
Processing Question: How is air moved through the body by the respiratory system?

Body Builders

Valued Outcome: The students will construct Popsicle-stick figures simulating bones, muscle, and skin.
Description of Strategy: Craft time with Popsicle sticks, yarn, and cloth scraps will allow each student to make a character with "bones," "muscles," and "skin." Popsicle sticks provide the frame. Yarn wrapped around sticks represents muscles. Cloth scraps serve as skin. Additional features can be added to give each model some unique characteristics.
Materials Needed: Popsicle sticks, yarn, and cloth scraps
Processing Question: How do the bones, muscles, and skin work together to make the body more efficient?

Other Ideas/Personal Health

Dressing for the Weather

Valued Outcome: The students will understand that dressing appropriately for the weather can prevent illness.
Description of Strategy: Make an extra-large boy paper doll and an extra-large girl paper doll along with an accompanying and varied wardrobe for all kinds of weather. Let the students take turns each day dressing the dolls appropriately for the day's weather, or for different seasons.

Materials Needed: paper dolls, doll clothes
Processing Question: How can we dress appropriately for weather in order to prevent illness and/or discomfort?

Immunization Record

Valued Outcome: The students will list their immunization records.
Description of Strategy: Have each student make a chart listing his or her immunization record. Suggest that students should be proud to know that they have contributed to their own health by undergoing these immunizations.
Materials Needed: paper, pencil
Processing Questions:

1. Why is it important to maintain an immunization record?

2. Why is it important to get immunizations?

Exercise Health Fair

Valued Outcome: The students will set up a display using an exercise or an activity.
Description of Strategy: Let the students plan a health fair to which their families are to be invited. The students should choose exercises or activities to be in the fair. Let the students research the activity in the library, and write a report to be placed in a booklet given to all the health fair attendees. The students can set up and design displays regarding the activity for the fair.
Materials Needed: materials for health fair activities
Processing Question: none

References

Agency for Instructional Technology (AIT). 1985. *A teacher's guide to well, well, well with Slim Goodbody*. Bloomington, IN: AIT.

American Heart Association (AHA). 1996. *Heart power*, Kindergarten through second grade level. Dallas: AHA.

Being healthy. 1990. teacher's edition. Orlando, FL: Harcourt Brace Jovanovich.

Bentley, M. 1995. The body systems being. *Journal of health education* 26(4): 245–247.

Bruess, C., and G. Richardson. 1994. *Healthy decisions*. Madison, WI: Brown & Benchmark.

Christen, N., and D. Peppk. 1994. *Body systems*, Science Mini-Unit. Grand Rapids, MI: Instructional Fair.

Ezell, G. 1992. *Healthy living 2: Healthy and growing*. Grand Rapids, MI: Christian Schools International.

Ezell, G. 1992. *Healthy living, Kindergarten: God's Healthy Child*. Grand Rapids, MI: Christian Schools International.

Ezell, G. 1993. *Healthy living*, sixth grade edition. Grand Rapids, MI: Christian Schools International.

HBJ Health. 1983. Teacher's edition, Level 5. Orlando, FL: Harcourt Brace Jovanovich.

Health for life. Grade 1. 1990. Glenview, IL: Scott, Foresman, p. 141.

Meeks, L. & P. Heit. 1996. *Totally awesome health*, Sixth grade manual. Blacklick OH: Meeks Heit.

Meeks, L., P. Heit, and R. Page. 1996. *Comprehensive school health education*, 2nd ed. Blacklick OH: Meeks Heit.

National Center for Health Education (NCHE). *Growing healthy*. New York: National Center for Health Education.

Siepak, K. L. 1995. *Body systems and organs*, Step-by-Step Science Series, Grades K-3. Greensboro, NC: Carson-Dellosa.

Tillman, K., & P. R. Toner. 1990. *How to survive teaching health*. West Nyack, NY: Parker.

Toner, P. R. 1993. *Consumer health and safety activities, just for the health of it*. West Nyack, NY: Health Curriculum Activities Library, The Center for Applied Research in Education.

Vaszily, D., & P. Perdue. 1994. *Bones, bodies, and bellies*. Glenview, IL: Scott, Foresman, p. 73.

Vriesenga, D. 1994. *The human body, whole language theme unit*. Grand Rapids, MI: Instructional Fair, p. 28.

Zipprich, K. G. 1989. *Health education puzzles and puzzlers*. Portland, ME,: J. Weston Walch, p. 3.

Resources

Suggested Readings

Agur, A. M. R., and M. J. Lee. 1991. *Grant's atlas of anatomy*, 9th ed. Baltimore: Williams & Wilkins.

Guyton, A. C. 1992. *Human physiology and mechanisms of disease*, 5th ed. Philadelphia: Saunders.

Hahn, D. B., and W. A. Payne. 1997. *Focus on health*, 3rd ed. St. Louis: Mosby.

Hole, J. W., Jr. 1993. *Human anatomy & physiology*, 6th ed. Dubuque, IA: Brown.

Marieb, E. N., and J. Mallatt. 1992. *Human anatomy*. Redwood City, CA: Benjamin/Cummings.

Memmler, R. L., B. J. Cohen, and D. L. Wood. 1992. *Structure and function of the human body*, 5th ed. Philadelphia: Lippincott.

Miller, D. F., S. K. Telljohann, and C. W. Symons. 1996. *Health education in the elementary & middle-level school*, 2nd ed. Madison, WI: Brown & Benchmark.

Thibodeau, G. A., and K. T. Patton. 1992. *Anatomy & physiology*, 2nd ed. St. Louis: Mosby.

Videos

The following videos are available from Sunburst Communications, 101 Castleton Street, P.O. Box 40, Pleasantville, NY 10570.

The New Improved Me: Understanding Body Changes
Gives young teens and preteens a supportive explanation of male and female body changes to help them accept puberty as an exciting and important event in their lives and a normal, healthy part of growing up.

Looking Good, Feeling Good: Healthy You
Using catchy songs and fast-paced visual effects, shows students that when they eat a variety of wholesome foods, get enough exercise and rest, and take proper care of their skin, hair, and teeth, they not only improve their personal appearance, but grow in confidence and self-respect.

CD-ROMs

The following CD-ROMs are available from IVI Publishing, 7500 Flying Cloud Drive, Eden Prairie, MN 55344.

Welcome to Bodyland
Join Ricki and Hiccup, her funny parrot friend, on an adventure through Bodyland theme park. Kids can learn about their skeletons as they stroll down Bony Boulevard. By visiting Dream Land, they'll understand why we dream at night.

Features:

- Fun and challenging games and activities
- Thirteen unique lands to explore

- Teaches fundamentals of the human body
- Ages five to eleven
- Original musical themes at every destination
- A challenging quiz game reinforcing learning

Welcome to Bodyland is available for both Windows and Macintosh platforms.

The Virtual Body
A virtual exploration of the human body—a journey of exploration and discovery inside the human body

- Cross sections and closeups of the human body
- Answers to fifty-two of the most frequently asked questions
- Invaluable homework helper
- Tested by students, adults, and educators
- Ages ten and up

Follow blood as it circulates. Watch nerve cells firing. See the senses in action. Even the most complex workings of the human body—from genetics to circulation to brain development—are explained in *The Virtual Body*—children 10 and up.

Features: The Virtual Body answers some of the most frequently asked questions about the body, such as:

- What is DNA?
- How are egg and sperm cells made?
- How does a cut heal?
- Why is blood red?
- What is cancer?
- How does skin feel pain and heat?

The Virtual Body is available only for the Windows platform.

Web Sites

General Health

Resources for School Health Educators
http://www.indiana.edu/~aphs/hlthk-12.html

CDC Prevention Guidelines Database
http://wonder.cdc.gov/wonder/prevguid/prevguid.htm

Developing Educational Standards
http://putwest.boces.org/standards.html

Adolescent Health On-Line
http://www.ama-assn.org/adolhlth/adolhlth.htm

See particularly the Adolescent Health Links
http://www.ama-assn.org/adolhlth/gapslink/gapslnk2.htm#ADOL

PE Central
http://infoserver.etl.vt.edu/~/PE.Central/PEC2.html

Kathy Schrock's Guide for Educators
http://www.capecod.net/Wixon/health/fitness.htm

Health Education Forum
http://libertynet.org/~lion/forum-health.html

Education World—Subjects: Physical Education
http://www.education-world.com/db/phys-gen.shtml

The Life Education Network
http://www.lec.org/

American Cancer Society
http://www.cancer.org

Physical Activity and Health: A Report of the Surgeon General
http://www.cdc.gov/nccdphp/sgr/sgr.htm

American Social Health Association
http://sunsite.unc.edu/ASHA/

Adolescence Directory On Line (ADOL)
http://education.indiana.edu/cas/adol/adol.html

AIDS NOW! For Teens
http://www.itec.sfsu.edu/aids/aids.html

National Health & Education Consortium (NHEC)
http://www.nhec.org/

About Health
http://www.abouthealth.com/

National Parent Information Network
http://ericps.ed.uiuc.edu/npin/npinhome.html

Healthy People 2000
http://odphp.osophs.dhhs.gov/pubs/hp2000/default.htm

Exercise/Physical Fitness

Fitness Issues
http://www.inect.co.uk/nsmi/

FitnessLinks to the Internet
http://www.fitnesslink.com/links.htm

Fitness World
http://www.fitnessworld.com/fitnews/news.html

The Physical Activity and Health Network (PAHNet)
http://www.pitt.edu/~pahnet/

American College of Sports Medicine
www.a1.com/sportsmed

CDC National Center for Chronic Disease Prevention and Health Promotion
www.cdc.gov/nccdphp/nccdhome.htm

President's Council on Physical Fitness and Sports
www.dhhs.gov/progorg/ophs/pcpfs.htm

Physical Education

American Alliance for Health, Physical Education, Recreation, and Dance (AAHPERD)
http://www.aahperd.org

British Columbia Physical Education Specialists Association
http://www.etc.bc.ca/~dsamulak/

The Canadian Intramural Recreation Association
http://activeliving.ca/activeliving/cira.html

Worldguide Forum on Health and Fitness
http://www.worldwide.com/Fitness/hf.html

Educational and Community-Based Programs

CDC National Center for Chronic Disease Prevention and Health Promotion
www.cdc.gov/nccdphp/nccdhome.htm

Health Resources and Services Administration
www.hrsa.dhhs.gov

Healthy Cities Online
www.healthycities.org

Office of Minority Health Resource Center Washington State Department of Health
www.doh.wa.gov

Oral Health

American Association of Dental Schools
www.aads.jhw.edu

American Dental Association
www.ada.org

American Dental Hygienists Association, Consumer Information Center
www.adha.org/consumer.html

CDC National Center for Chronic Disease Prevention and Health Promotion
www.cdc.gov/nccdphp/nccdhome.htm

NIH National Institute of Dental Research
www.nidr.nih.gov

Surveillance and Data Systems

Agency for Health Care Policy and Research Data and Methods
www.ahcpr.gov:80/data

CDC National Center for Health Statistics
www.cdc.gov/nchswww/nchshome.htm

CDC Scientific, Surveillance, and Health Statistics, and Laboratory Information
www.cdc.gov/scientific.htm

CDC WONDER
wonder.cdc.gov

Health Care Financing Administration, 1996 Statistics at a Glance
www.hcfa.gov/stats/stathili.htm

General Sites

American Medical Association
http://www.ama-assn.org

MedicineNet
http://www.medicinenet.com

Medscape
http://www.medscape.com

Oncolink
http://www.oncolink.upenn.edu

ParentsPlace.com
http://www.parentsplace.com

Thrive@ pathfinder
http://pathfinder.com/thrive

Links Only

Hardin Meta Directory of Internet Health Sources
http://www.arcade.uiowa.edu/hardin-www/md.html

Medical Matrix
http://www.5lackinc.com/matrix

Chapter Eight

Mental Health and Stress Reduction

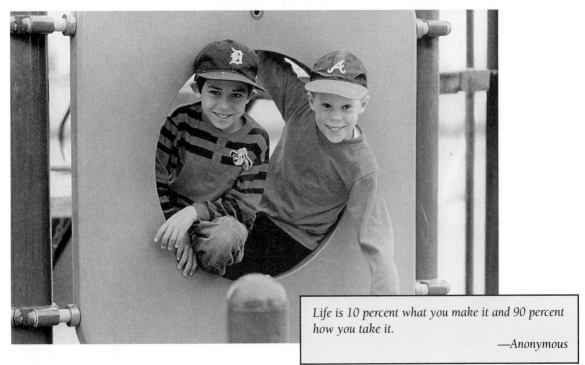

> *Life is 10 percent what you make it and 90 percent how you take it.*
>
> —*Anonymous*

Valued Outcomes

After reading this chapter, you should be able to

- ○ define mental health
- ○ identify the characteristics of mental health
- ○ describe how psychosocial factors contribute to mental health
- ○ discuss problems associated with latchkey children or children from separated/divorced families
- ○ identify the means of dealing with children who have experienced a death of a pet, grandparent, parent, or sibling
- ○ define the terms *stress* and *stressor*
- ○ describe the detrimental health effects of prolonged stress
- ○ discuss the problems of depression and suicide in the school-age population

○ briefly discuss each of the rules for fostering good mental health

○ identify strategies for dealing with stress

○ discuss the role of the family in maintaining a child's emotional health

The Importance of Mental Health

There is probably no area more vital than that of helping students to develop sound mental health practices. We need only look at the rates of alcohol and drug use among our nation's youth, the suicide rates for adolescents, the reported depression among youth, or the number of school-age children who run away from home each year to realize the importance of helping students achieve and maintain good mental and emotional health. Without the sense of inner peace and balance that comes with good mental health, no individual can be considered completely healthy. The links between mental and physical health are clear. Yet the goal of good mental health is in many ways more elusive than that of good physical health. If an individual receives proper nutrition, exercises on a regular basis, gets plenty of relaxation and sleep, and follows good personal health practices, he or she has a high probability of remaining physically fit. Unfortunately, there is no easy prescription for good mental health. There are, however, identifiable characteristics of people who are mentally healthy. Experts have defined **mental health** as the ability to perceive reality as it is, to respond to its challenges, and to develop rational strategies for living (Hales 1992, 25). A component of mental health is *emotional health,* or the ability to deal constructively with reality, regardless of whether the actual situation is good or bad (Greenberg and Dintiman 1992, 20).

Implied in these two definitions is the concept that emotionally healthy people are in touch with their feelings and can express those feelings in a proper fashion. This chapter provides information about mental health principles that will help your children develop sound mental health. Topics discussed include human needs and the development of self-esteem, behavior and the expression of emotions, stress and its relationship to mental health, values and patterns of decision making, and the role of the family in the development of mental health.

Characteristics of the Emotionally Healthy

If mental health is defined as the ability to perceive reality and to respond to the challenges of life, then what are the characteristics of an emotionally healthy individual? Although their list is not definitive, Mullen and her associates provide some traits of an emotionally healthy person, to use as points of reference (Mullen et al. 1993).

○ *The mentally well are real.* The concept that "what you see is what you get" is what is implied. Individuals can respond in a genuine, spontaneous fashion and feel no need to censor their words or actions for social approval.

○ *The mentally well are realistic.* They recognize what is and what ought to be and have the ability to change in light of new evidence.

○ *The mentally well are able to satisfy their needs.* There is a development of a sense of meaning and affirmation of life. They know they are not helpless, and they do not pretend to be.

○ *The mentally well are free and responsible.* There is autonomy and a feeling of control over one's life.

Health Highlight

Sensitivity to Multicultural Diversity

In society today there is a wide diversity of peoples and cultures. These differences have arisen because of the need to accommodate unique physical, demographic, and economic situations (Garcia 1991). The elementary teacher must strive to view all children of various cultures from students' perspectives rather than from his or her own cultural perspective. This means the classroom facilitates a climate of understanding and sensitivity to diverse cultures, ethnicities, and races.

To understand multicultural sensitivity and diversity, several terms must first be understood. Page and Page (1993, 91) define *culture* as a set of values, attitudes, and practices held in common by a group of people, usually identified by ancestry, language, and geography. *Ethnicity* refers to a portion of a population or subgroup having a common cultural heritage. *Race* denotes a population distinguished by genetically determined physical traits, such as hair texture or color, skin color, eye shape, and body shape.

The elementary teacher can develop multicultural sensitivity in several ways. He or she should strive to develop personal skills, such as showing warmth, respect, sincerity, concern, and caring for people of all cultures. It is imperative that the teacher understand the communities from which the children come. In addition the teacher must be culturally sensitive to how different ethnic groups learn and solve problems. Part of this is understanding learning style, communication patterns, and such factors as eye contact, body language, and physical closeness.

○ *The mentally well are open to new experiences.* New experiences are welcomed. All experiences, good and bad, are viewed as having potential for growth. Humor can help defuse unpleasant situations.

○ *The mentally well are capable of intimate relationships.* They have the ability to be unselfish in serving or relating to others. There is an increased depth and satisfaction in intimate relationships.

○ *The mentally well are tolerant and accepting of others.* People are judged on their individual merits. No one is expected to fit within narrow limits.

○ *The mentally well are capable of reacting in a wide variety of ways.* The person may lead as well as follow. One should be able to judge and empathize, to act as well as to yield.

○ *The mentally well are capable of joie de vivre.* One should be able to enjoy life, job, family, and community.

○ *The mentally well are self-accepting.* Probably the most crucial characteristic of the mentally healthy is a positive self-concept and high self-esteem. Most of all the previous points are predicated on this factor.

There is no one ideal for emotional health. Certainly the lack of any one characteristic does not indicate an emotionally unhealthy person. Probably no one has all these characteristics, and most

Teachers must be aware of possible depression in children.

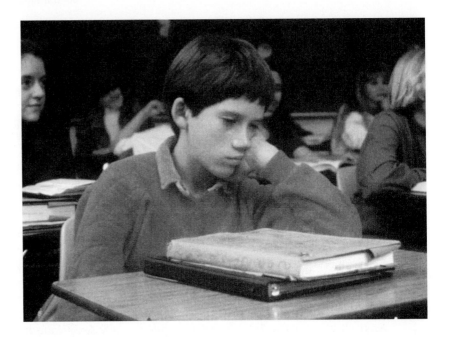

of us fall short at some time, but the list can provide a benchmark for how well we are achieving or moving toward being emotionally healthy.

This process of achieving mental wellness is a lifelong process and begins the moment we are born. How we interact with our siblings, how our parents relate and interact with us, and our perceptions throughout life influence our mental wellness. The experiences each child undergoes while in the elementary school are very important. The perceptions of success, feelings of acceptance by peers and teachers, and the supportive emotional climate in the classroom all contribute to the emotional well-being and the development of self-esteem of the child. The process begins when the child enters school each morning and continues until he or she leaves in the afternoon. The information learned each day, each year, year after year, eventually shapes self-perception and molds us into what we perceive ourselves to be. The home, family, and other institutions also help develop our perceptions, but none impacts as strongly as each teacher with whom we have contact during our elementary school years. The elementary teacher can provide confidence, appreciation, praise, fairness, security, approval, friendship, and acceptance. Through modeling, developing decision-making skills, and being in a success-oriented situation, the children learn to accept themselves and others.

What Children Need to Achieve Emotional Health

The fulfillment of basic emotional needs such as love, affection, acceptance, and a feeling of importance are essential to children developing a self-identity and their self-esteem. All people need to receive love and affection. Everyone needs to feel a sense of acceptance and importance from others. If these basic needs can be fostered, the child's potential for successfully interacting with others, meeting individual needs for independence and self-expression, and resolving personal and social conflicts are clearly enhanced. The child is freer to pursue higher human goals,

Health Highlight

Fostering a Positive Classroom Atmosphere

Here are several guidelines developed by Page and Page (1993) for fostering an emotional climate conducive to mental wellness.

1. Quickly learn the names of students, call them by name, become familiar with their interests and talents, and show respect for each student.
2. Be well prepared and enthusiastic. Make learning fun and subject matter relevant and challenging to students.
3. Begin each class promptly. Develop and maintain routines for taking attendance, opening class, and so on.
4. Remember the three Fs of good discipline: *Firm*, *Fair*, and *Friendly*.
5. Expect no problems: don't be looking for them. Expect students to be competent, capable, and eager to learn. It is better to be proven wrong than to have students live up to negative expectations.
6. When problems arise, handle them immediately and consistently before they escalate into larger ones. Don't use "major artillery" for minor infractions.
7. Avoid sarcasm, ridicule, and belittling remarks, and help students do likewise.
8. Avoid all suggestions of criticism, anger, or frustration. It is better to make personal corrections in private conferences with students.
9. Be alert for indications of latent skills and interests in students and encourage them in their development.
10. Listen nonjudgmentally to student comments, and create an atmosphere where students feel at ease.
11. Arrange for a high ratio of successes to failures in academic tasks.
12. Involve students in the setting of individual academic goals.
13. Avoid encouraging competitiveness between students in your grading practices and learning activities.
14. Demonstrate the characteristics of effective teachers: warmth, friendliness, fairness, a good sense of humor, enthusiasm, empathy, openness, spontaneity, adaptability, and a governing style that is more democratic than autocratic.

culminating with what Maslow (Hamrick, Anspaugh, and Ezell 1986) calls *self-actualization needs*. Maslow's hierarchy of human needs is shown in Figure 8.1 and applies throughout our lives and certainly in the early developmental years of the elementary child.

Self-Esteem and the Development of Emotional Health

The foundation of emotional health for the elementary child is self-esteem. *Self-esteem* can be defined as how worthy and valuable a person considers her- or himself. Development of positive emotional health requires that an individual be immersed in an open and nonthreatening environment that nurtures and supports feelings of self-worth and security.

Self-esteem is necessary for developing self-expression and independence. A person with a feeling of self-worth is also better equipped emotionally to show concern for others. As the individual begins to develop meaningful relationships with others that recognize and reward his or her unique qualities of expression, independent thinking flourishes. A strong sense of self-worth permits open and honest communication with others because rejection or disapproval are not feared as great risks. The establishment of self-esteem is a lifelong process. This lifelong quest is more easily attainable if the nurturing of emotional and social well-being has been emphasized in infancy and childhood, thus promoting a sense of security, identity, autonomy, and intimacy early in life.

Self-esteem is the result of three factors: (1) how children perceive themselves, (2) how they want to be, and (3) what expectations they perceive others have for them. The foundation of positive self-esteem is shaped in early childhood, primarily by the interaction with the parents and other family members. Positive comments and attitudes toward the child contribute to his or her sense of competency and shape the perception of self.

When children enter school, teachers can help them to develop positive self-esteem by observing the points mentioned in the Health Highlight on achieving a positive emotional climate in the classroom. Teachers also can help children view themselves realistically and as being unique and lovable. Children need to know they are valued and accepted regardless of intellect, appearance, dress, or other social criteria.

Values and Patterns of Decision Making

Central to the establishment of self-esteem, the expression of emotions and resulting behavior, and the ability to cope effectively with distress are the decision-making patterns that children learn in order to make life adjustments in harmony with their value system. When decisions about a particular issue reflect actions and attitudes that are in agreement with strongly held values, a person is left intact emotionally because personal behaviors and values remain compatible. If deci-

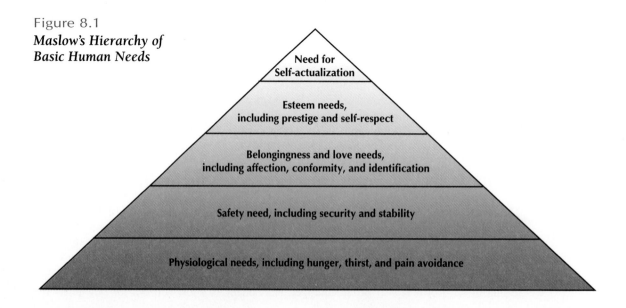

Figure 8.1
Maslow's Hierarchy of Basic Human Needs

Need for Self-actualization

Esteem needs, including prestige and self-respect

Belongingness and love needs, including affection, conformity, and identification

Safety need, including security and stability

Physiological needs, including hunger, thirst, and pain avoidance

sions produce behaviors that contradict a person's value system, self-esteem is diminished, emotions are exhibited in an unhealthy fashion resulting from lack of resolution over inner conflicts, and stress increases. Decision-making patterns can serve as valuable clues to the way individuals perceive themselves, their relationships with others, and the world around them. Children's actions tell much about their underlying value system, which in turn mediates many of the decisions made about life adjustments. Learning to make decisions following clarification and consideration of values can help each child sustain and enhance the emotional balance crucial to good mental health.

Behavior and the Expression of Emotions

The most obvious indicator of a child's emotional health status is behavior. Psychologists state that there is always a reason for behavior. Admittedly, the reasons may not be immediately apparent either to the child or to others; nevertheless, there are underlying motives for all behavior. Much of a child's behavior, both conscious and subconscious, is centered around fulfilling basic emotional needs. Such behavior patterns are often shaped by the ways in which these needs were satisfied or reinforced early in life. Thus, if a change in behavior is desired, the child must learn new, and perhaps more healthy, ways of fulfilling basic needs. Everyone experiences feelings of sadness, anger, joy, fear, depression, and apprehension, but the manner in which these emotions are expressed varies from individual to individual. Usually the emotional expression of these feelings becomes labeled as the individual's "behavior." Therefore, a better understanding of emotions may lead to greater understanding of a child's behavior and overall emotional health. The way in which children express their feelings is largely determined by the way the child perceives, either consciously or subconsciously, the situation that triggers the feeling. In other words, two children who are exposed to the same situation, say, disagreement with a teacher over an answer to a test question, may react quite differently, based on different individual assessments of the situation. Such assessments are based in part on how the situation affects fulfillment of basic needs or efforts aimed at attaining autonomy, identity, or other personal goals. In many cases, the situation is perceived as having little impact and therefore elicits minimal emotional expression. Situations that are perceived as having great influence tend to elicit stronger, more overt expression. Thus, emotions are displayed in varying modes of expression as well as varying degrees of intensity. A child is considered more emotionally healthy when emotions are exhibited in a positive way and with an intensity proportional to the situation's impact. Children who consistently display either minimal emotional expression about circumstances generally viewed as having major importance (intimacy with others, successful completion of a difficult task, death of a family member or pet) or intense emotional expression about events that are not generally viewed as having major importance (having to redo a homework assignment, misplacing an article of clothing, losing a football game) are considered less emotionally well adjusted.

It is not the emotion itself that determines mentally healthy or unhealthy behavior, but rather the degree and frequency of the emotion expressed. All children have on occasion allowed their emotions to run out of control or be expressed in ways that were not as appropriate, positive, or desirable as they could have been. This type of behavior is a problem only when it becomes a consistent pattern. Often such a pattern of emotional outburst is a result of inner anxiety due to stress originating from conflicts between unconscious drives or needs and conscious values that have been imposed. All people (adults as well as children) share the same emotions. A feeling or emotion is neither inherently "good" nor "bad" but can be expressed in ways that either promote well-being or detract from it. Mentally healthy behavior largely stems from an individual's ability to recognize, analyze, interpret, and communicate feelings in a consistent, balanced, and positive manner.

Defense Mechanisms

A defense mechanism is any behavior a person uses to avoid confronting a situation or problem. Children learn and use the various mechanisms very early in their elementary school years. Although defense mechanisms can be helpful in dealing with the stresses of life, some children can use them to the extreme. When defense mechanisms are used inappropriately, they can hinder the child's emotional health. Examples of common defense mechanisms are provided in Table 8.1.

Table 8.1

Common Defense Mechanisms

Defense Mechanism	Definition
Compensation	Making up for weakness in one area by emphasizing strengths in another area. *Example:* A child is unsuccessful as an athlete but is a musician, consequently, emphasis is placed on music.
Daydreaming	Escaping from frustrations, boredom, or unpleasant situations through fantasy. *Example:* Faced with a divorce of the father and mother, a child creates a mental image of the perfect family.
Displacement	Transferring feelings concerning one situation or person to another object, situation, or person. *Example:* Unable to respond to anger toward a parent, the child goes home and abuses a younger child.
Idealization	Holding someone or something in such high esteem, that it becomes perfect or godlike in the eyes of the child. *Example:* A star athlete that is held in such high regard that his or her human characteristics or shortcomings are overlooked.
Identification	Taking on the quality of someone that is admired. *Example:* Performers are often so admired that children attempt to talk, walk, and act as they perceive their idol to do.
Projection	Shifting the responsibility of one's behavior onto someone else. *Example:* The child blames the teacher because a test grade was poor rather than accept the responsibility for not studying sufficiently.
Rationalization	Providing plausible reasons for behavior that are not the real reasons. *Example:* A child states she does not like birthday parties and refuses to attend when she really just feels insecure.
Regression	Childish, inappropriate behavior by an adult or a return to former, less mature behavior when under stress. *Example:* Becoming extremely angry when unable to attend movie or social event. A regressive response may be to cry or throw something.
Repression	Attempting to bury or repress unpleasant or upsetting thoughts. *Example:* The child is unable to remember a psychologically painful event, such as the death of a grandparent.
Sublimation	Turning unacceptable thought or actions into socially acceptable behaviors. *Example:* An aggressive child turns to athletics to redirect his or her energies.

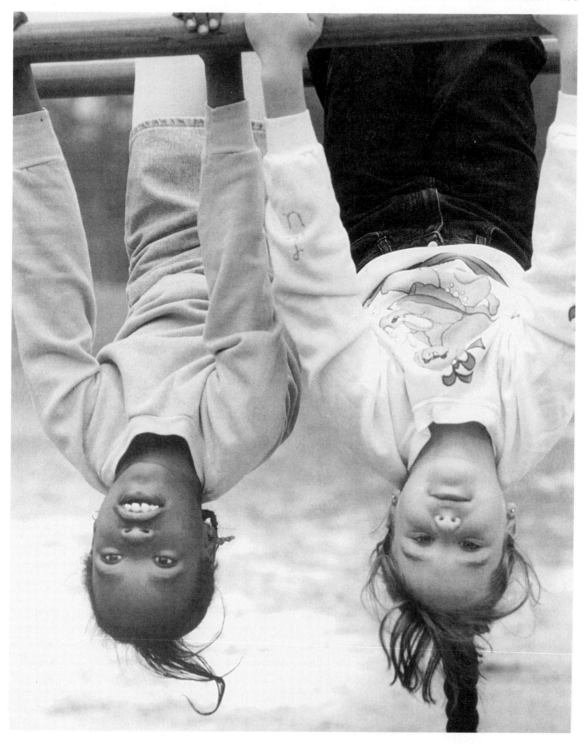

Happy, well-adjusted children have a greater chance of growing up to be contented adults than do unhappy, insecure children.

Latchkey Children

The term **latchkey children** describes any child regularly left without direct adult supervision before or after school. Indications are that over 7 million children under age thirteen are either left to go to school or return home without adult supervision. Kids left in these situations may be either the result of both parents working or of divorce. The end result is that many children leave home without breakfast, return home to care for themselves, with the possible consequences of fear of someone breaking into their home, fear of being alone, fear of older siblings, and greater likelihood of being lonely and bored (Stroher 1986). Fear and boredom can lead to involvement with gangs or simply to a greater chance of trouble resulting from just being alone or with friends or siblings. Undersupervised children may experience significantly more personality problems and a higher incidence of depression in adolescence and adulthood (Page and Page 1993).

Obviously latchkey children are expected to assume a great deal of responsibility for their welfare. Stroher (1986 16) has suggested ways in which teachers can help latchkey children:

1. Carefully structure homework assignments, because these children do not have adults around to help them complete assignments correctly. Consider the possibility of establishing a telephone hotline to help students with homework.

2. During the school day, allow time for children to discuss their personal concerns with the teacher. Latchkey children particularly need time to discuss or talk with adults.

3. Establish streamlined, workable procedures for contacting the parents in emergency situations involving the child.

4. Develop both before- and after-school day care programs. Children do better with continuous adult supervision in school-based programs than when left to their own resources.

Divorce and Separation—The Effects on Children

Almost half the children in the United States will spend some portion of their childhood in a single-parent situation. Over 1 million divorces occur each year, over 49% of second marriages result in divorce. Over 12.5 million children are living in a family where divorce has occurred (USDHHS 1994, 93). The net result is that teachers are having to deal with more emotional/psychological problems than ever before. These problems are represented by deliquency, psychological disturbance, hostility, low self-esteem, low evaluation of the family, poor self-restraint, and social adjustment (Fuhrmann 1986).

The reactions of children may depend on age. Preschoolers may become frightened about the separation or divorce because they see themselves as being abandoned. A child of this age may not want to attend or may fear attending school. Such children may regress in their behavior, with lapses in toilet training or become unable to dress themselves (Ricci 1982). They may use dolls, teddy bears, and blankets as security objects. Among children six to eight years of age, the most common feeling is sadness. This is manifested through crying, sobbing, and a desire to be with the missing parent. Children nine to twelve are likely to respond with vigorous activity. Older children may align themselves with one parent and want little or nothing to do with the other (Wallerstein and Kelly 1981). School-age children may blame themselves for causing the divorce.

The teacher may be the one source of stability and security the child has in a divorce or separation. This can be emphasized by the fact "that only 45 percent of children do well after divorce; 41 percent are doing poorly, worried, underachieving, self-deprecating, and often angry; and 14 percent are strikingly uneven. Girls consistently adjust better to divorce than boys, both socially and academically. This would imply that boys may be suffering more from the absence of their fathers" (Stepfamily Foundation, 1996). The teacher may be able to assure such children that the separation/divorce was not their fault and they are still loved, and help them discuss their feelings of fear, anger, and guilt. Encourage the child to be honest concerning feelings. In addition, be watchful for signs of academic failure, overaggressiveness, lack of concentration, nervousness, or becoming isolated from peers, which may require informing the parent or the school counselor.

Death and Children

In today's society, most children do not directly experience the trauma of death. The concept of death is alien to many children. The effects of death on children are discussed in greater detail in Chapter 22 on death and dying. Most children develop a sequence of understanding concerning death, beginning with total unawareness in early childhood to a developmental point where death is conceptualized as final and universal (Fredlund 1984).

For many children, initial contact with death may be the result of a pet dying. Children feel significant pain and need extra support to deal with their feelings of loss and grief, even for the death of a pet. There are several points to keep in mind when dealing with a child who has experienced the death of a pet, grandparent, parent, or sibling, or who may be facing his or her own death:

○ Help children learn how to mourn. Help them be touched by the positive memories, deal with any guilt they might feel, and to deal with the anger they may feel over the loss.

○ Help them mourn small losses, such as animals, so that they can better deal with the larger loss of grandparents, parent, sibling, etc.

○ Help children gain information about a death. When they are not informed and they see their parents upset, they may invent their own explanations or blame themselves.

○ Help children see the finality of death. Because abstract thinking may be difficult for many children, they may use the terms "went away" or is "asleep."

○ Help children say good-bye to the deceased by allowing them to be part of funerals or viewing, even only for a few minutes.

○ Provide opportunities for the child to deal with their feelings and perceptions of death through talking, dramatic playing, reading books, or expressing themselves through the arts.

○ The parents should assure the children that they (the parents) probably won't die until after the children are grown. It is equally important that children understand that almost all children grow up and live to be old.

○ Help children understand that everyone will die someday.

○ Allow children to show their feelings: to cry, become angry, or even laugh—try to empathize with their feelings.

○ Answer their questions honestly and in a fashion they can understand. (Butler 1984)

Depression and Children

Depression in children parallels that in adults with minor differences due to developmental considerations (Magg and Forness 1991). A condition characterized by loss of interest and feelings of extreme or overwhelming sorrow, sadness, and debility, depression is a symptom of underlying conflict, tension, or anxiety and may be exhibited in varying degrees for varying lengths of time. The same criteria used to identify depression in adults is used for diagnosing the condition in children. The American Psychiatric Association has stated that at least five of the following criteria must be present for a diagnosis of depression (APA 1987):

○ depressed mood

○ loss of interest or pleasure in all or almost all activities significant

○ weight loss or weight gain

○ insomnia or excessive sleeping

○ psychomotor agitation or retardation

○ fatigue or loss of energy

○ feelings of worthlessness or excessive or inappropriate guilt

○ diminished ability to think or concentrate; indecisiveness

○ thoughts of suicide or suicide attempts

The Causes of Depression

There are no simple answers to why children become depressed. Patros and Shamoo (1989) estimate that three to six million children and adolescents suffer from depression in the United States. They also state that most children with depression go untreated. Most experts now believe there are multiple reasons for depression. Obviously, not all the reasons apply to children, but some of the situations presented hold implications for the development of depression in children. Some possible factors include the following (Chandler and Kolander 1989, 4–5):

1. *Heredity:* Studies show some depressive disorders are hereditary. For example, manic-depression has been linked, in some cases, to a genetic defect.

2. *Environmental:* Environment can also contribute to the onset of a depressive disorder. Research has shown that stressful life events, especially those involving a loss or threatened loss, often precede episodes of depressive illness. Examples include the death of a loved one, a divorce, the loss of a job, a move to a new home, physical illness, the breakup of an important relationship, or financial problems. In most instances the loss induces feelings of sadness and anxiety and often guilt or shame. Less commonly, depression follows the achievement of a desired position—the so-called success depression. In this case, the loss typically associated with depression is the loss of a future goal.

3. *Background and personality:* People with certain psychological backgrounds or personality characteristics appear to be more vulnerable to depression. Many specialists believe that some depressive disorders can be traced to a troubled childhood; they attach particular importance to disturbed relationships between a child and his or her parents. Also, people who have low self-esteem, who consistently view themselves and the world with pessimism, or who become easily overwhelmed by stress tend to be more prone to depression.

4. *Biochemical factors:* Some types of depression may result from abnormal chemical activity within the brain. These chemicals play a role in the transmission of electrical impulses from one nerve cell (neuron) to another. These chemical "messengers," called *neurotransmitters*, set in motion the complex interactions that control moods, feelings, and behaviors. They also regulate pain, learning, and memory as well as the desire to eat, drink, and sleep. Three neurotransmitters—dopamine, norepinephrine, and serotonin—have been associated with depressive illnesses. Research suggests that episodes of depression or mania may be related to an improper balance of neurotransmitters. Do biochemical factors cause depression, or does depression cause the biochemical disturbance? No one knows with certainty. Some experts theorize that a genetic vulnerability combined with prolonged stress, physical illness, or some other environmental condition or event may bring about the chemical imbalance that results in depression.

5. *Physical illness:* People with chronic medical illnesses are at high risk of psychiatric illness, especially depression. Some diseases, such as hypothyroidism (underactive thyroid gland) or arthritis can bring on a depressive reaction. Depression also may follow a heart attack or stroke. It may be an early sign of a serious underlying disease such as cancer of the pancreas, a brain tumor, parkinsonism, multiple sclerosis, or Cushing's disease, among others. Also, depression can be an undesirable side effect of certain prescription medications—especially steroids (cortisonelike drugs), some antihypertensive medicines, antiparkinsonian agents, and, less commonly, oral contraceptives.

   Women frequently experience depressive symptoms with varying levels of severity preceding their menstrual periods (premenstrual syndrome), following childbirth (postpartum depression), or during menopause. Many specialists suggest there may be hormonal causes, but the biological mechanisms involving hormones and depression have yet to be discovered.

   As stated previously, not all of the above causes are considerations for depression in children. However, Patros and Shamoo (1989) have identified several indicators of childhood depression:

○ lack of interest—daydreams, withdrawn, poor schoolwork, disruptive

○ change in appetite—picks at food, gives away food, increase in appetite

○ changes in sleep pattern—falls asleep in class, listless, tardy, poor attention in class

○ loss of energy—tired or restless behavior

○ blaming self inappropriately—self-critical, cries quickly, upset by surprises or changes

○ negative feelings of self-worth—critical of others, socially withdrawn, doesn't stand up for herself/himself

○ feelings of sadness, hopelessness, and worry—sad, unhappy, feels defeated, withdrawn, acts frightened, poor peer relationships

○ inability to concentrate—does not complete work or takes a long time, forgets, appears not to listen

○ morbid thoughts—talks or writes about death, overreacts to someone's death

○ aggressive or negative behavior—picks on others, talks back, low frustration level

○ increased agitation—cannot sit still, short attention span, makes noise, talks under breath

○ increased psychosomatic complaints—frequently complains of headaches, stomach aches, or vague physical symptoms

○ decreased academic performance—drop in grades, poor concentration, messy work area, poor test performance

○ poor attention and concentration—cannot stay on task, frequently interrupts, disruptive behavior.

Suicide in Children and Adolescents ───────────────

Each year more than 5,000 young people between the ages of fifteen and twenty-four kill themselves. Each day over 1,000 people in this age group attempt suicide. For every individual who is successful at committing suicide, 100 more will attempt the act and fail. Statistics also reveal that children as young as five or six are committing suicide (Grollman 1988). Children and adolescents who commit suicide feel cut off, alienated, and isolated. They truly believe that living is useless and more than they can tolerate.

Although the overall rate of suicide in the United States has remained fairly constant in recent years, the rate of suicide among young children has increased. The numbers might even be higher if the current social stigma against suicide did not cause many adolescent suicide cases to go unreported. Ten percent of the children in any public classroom may be considered suicidal (DeSpelder and Strickland 1987).

Adolescents are most likely to commit suicide when they experience overcrowded conditions, a broken family, or feelings of rejection, hopelessness, or loss. Some wish to escape from a difficult situation, gain attention, or punish people who caused them to have negative feelings; therefore, they may view death as an acceptable alternative. Further, an adolescent is at higher risk for suicide if a significant adult role model attempts or commits suicide or if violence is commonplace in the child's environment (either in the home or through the media) (DeSpelder and Strickland 1987).

Most childhood suicides are preceded by changes in behavior, some subtle and some more overt. Nelson and Crawford (1991) found that elementary students who experienced thoughts of suicide reported that family problems were significant contributors. Such things as divorce, separation, and parental alcoholism were the main factors. Peer acceptance and academic pressures also contribute to elementary children's suicide attempts.

They may lose interest in school and friends, experience an increase of illnesses, become very sad for increasing periods of time, and quit eating or sleeping well. Other observable signs of suicidal behavior are

○ saying such things as "I wish I were dead" or "I'd be better off dead"

○ giving away prized objects

○ lacking direction or goal-setting behavior

○ exhibiting depression, withdrawal, weight loss, or apathy

○ showing a sudden lack of academic progress

○ communicating feelings of hopelessness

○ using drugs and alcohol

○ withdrawing from friends, family, and normal activities

○ undergoing a radical personality change

○ exhibiting violent, hostile, or rebellious behavior

○ revealing a preoccupation with death through a school composition

○ mutilating the self

○ running away from home

Other signs could probably be added to this list. Every teacher must be cognizant of these signs and symptoms if suicide is to be prevented. It is imperative that children suspected of suicidal thoughts receive help from professionals trained to deal with the situation.

Health Highlight

Common Myths About Suicide

U.S. society harbors many misconceptions concerning suicide. To help clear up some of the myths, the following list has been developed:

Myth: People who talk about suicide won't commit suicide.

Fact: Statistics indicate that eight out of ten individuals who commit suicide give definite warnings of their intentions.

Myth: Suicidal people are fully intent on dying.

Fact: Most suicidal people are ambivalent about living or dying. They are often willing to gamble with death in order to get the attention or help they desire.

Myth: Once an individual attempts suicide, he or she is suicidal forever.

Fact: People are usually suicidal for only a short period of time.

Myth: Improvement following a suicide attempt means that the crisis is over.

Fact: Most suicides that follow attempts occur within three months from the beginning of "improvement,"

or the initial lessening of the threat of suicide. The appearance of improvement may mean that the individual now has the energy to put suicidal thoughts into action.

Myth: Suicide occurs most often among the poor.

Fact: Suicide is neither the curse of the rich nor the disease of the poor. It is represented proportionately throughout all strata of society.

Myth: Suicide is inherited and runs in families.

Fact: Suicide is an individual pattern and does not run in families.

Myth: Suicidal people are mentally ill, and the act is a psychotic one.

Fact: Although suicidal people are extremely unhappy and depressed, they are not necessarily mentally ill.

Myth: Asking whether a person is considering suicide will lead him or her to make an attempt.

Fact: Asking a person directly often minimizes the suicidal feeling and acts as a deterrent to the act.

Source: M. Hamrick, D. Anspaugh, and G. Ezell. 1986. *Health.* Columbus, OH: Merrill, p. 191.

Rules for Developing and Maintaining Mental Health —————————————

Children should be encouraged to practice positive mental health habits in the same way they are taught to practice sound personal health habits. Just as children can take responsibility for their own physical well-being by following health "rules," they can also foster high levels of emotional well-being by following similar mental health "rules." By internalizing certain guidelines and incorporating them into daily living, each individual can promote good mental health and effective life adjustment. Positive mental health can be taught each day of every school year. Teachers must realize that they are directly responsible for establishing the emotional tone of their classrooms, as well as the foundation of children's self-worth. When each child leaves elementary school, she or he needs to have developed the positive self-esteem and perceptions of living that foster the following rules:

1. Teach the children to like themselves. Help them discover their unique qualities, skills, and talents and be proud of who they are.

2. Teach the children to be good to themselves. Encourage them to reward themselves periodically with "strokes"—emotional or material favors.

3. Help the children learn to be introspective, to examine motives for behavior, and to be insightful about their own conduct.

4. Help each child accept her or his limitations. Think in terms of competency levels rather than in terms of "success" or "failure."

5. Help the children deal with a problem or crisis as it arises rather than allowing pressures to mount by worrying about "what if's."

6. Help each child establish realistic goals, both short term and long term, and work toward accomplishing them.

7. Help the children express their emotions in terms of how the emotion makes them feel rather than in terms of how others make them feel. "I feel angry for having to do a homework assignment over the weekend" is healthier than "Ms. Barnes, you make me angry. You shouldn't assign a homework assignment over the weekend."

8. Encourage the children to involve themselves in diversified activities and cultivate many interests. Encourage them to not center their life around one person, place, or activity.

9. Encourage children to develop a sense of humor. Help them learn to laugh and enjoy life.

10. Teach the children to be optimistic.

The Role of the Teacher in Promoting Mental Health —————————————

There are many other ways in which the teacher can promote positive emotional characteristics. Each child should be dealt with as a unique individual. It is important for the teacher to offer personal observations or words of praise that let a child know he or she is performing well on a given task or is progressing well. Encourage children to hone their individual talents by providing opportunities for them to do so during the normal course of classroom activity. The chance to work on a special project of personal interest or contribute ideas and opinions without being ridiculed or rejected may enhance autonomy and initiative. Learning experiences that both challenge and provide success will reinforce children's feelings of competency and mastery.

The teacher is most important in establishing a positive classroom atmosphere.

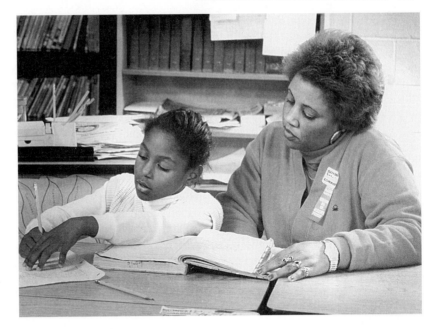

Teachers can provide activities that help children consider how they want to live their lives and what their goals should be. For example, a teacher can ask them to write down things they hope to accomplish in the near and in the distant future, and then can help them develop ways of achieving these goals. This method of clarifying important goals will help students keep minor problems in perspective (Olsen, Redican, and Baffi 1986). Furthermore, teachers need to help children place their inability to meet goals in the proper perspective, so that feelings of doubt, embarrassment, or inadequacy do not result.

It is important for a teacher to become an effective listener and a skilled observer. Children regularly need opportunities that let them express their feelings and thoughts openly. A teacher can become an active listener by paraphrasing the student's comments to let the child know the message was understood. Such active listening will demonstrate to children that the teacher genuinely cares about them.

The role of the teacher in promoting student mental health is crucial. The attitudes teachers demonstrate during their daily interactions with students affect the emotional climate of the classroom. One of the best things a teacher can do to promote emotional health in students is to help them learn to accept responsibility for their own behavior. A common mistake we all make is to try to shift the blame for something we did onto someone else. Children must be taught that a crucial element of emotional development is the ability to accept responsibility and live with mistakes. Further, the type of rapport that is established between teacher and student conveys many messages that influence children's perceptions about acceptance, trust, support, self-esteem, competency, and independence.

The Role of the Family in Developing Emotional Health

An individual's emotional health status can be gauged by assessing how much the basic emotional needs for love, acceptance, and support from others contribute to the individual's feelings of self-worth. It is helpful also to determine the degree of balance with which behaviors are expressed and the ways in which people face and resolve situations through use of decisions that are compatible with personal values. All these foundations of positive mental health are first learned and cultivated within the family. As a result, it is crucial that all teachers have some notion of how family structure, interaction, and values influence the behavior and attitudes of students in the classroom.

The high numbers of single-parent families that currently exist may greatly affect a child's view of self as well as the world in general. Some children also face the task of having to be incorporated into two different family structures that produce different sets of stepparents and stepsiblings. Teachers must be sensitive to these differences in living arrangements and family structure.

Family interaction also contributes greatly to the development of children's mental health. Communication patterns between parents, parents and their children, and between siblings are all important factors. Communication should allow for intimacy—that is, sharing of one's innermost fears and concerns—without reprisal or rejection. Interaction patterns between family members set the tone for all other social interaction. Within the family, children develop a sense about what they can do or accomplish, what their roles in life should be, and what types of behaviors are appropriate, acceptable, and desirable. Criteria for sharing, completing expected tasks, being praised or punished, and many other things are learned through family modeling and values. The family sets guidelines for all behavior by means ranging from types of discipline to ways of expressing love and affection. As a result, attitudes, habits, and emotions reflect family attitudes, habits, and emotions.

Stress and Its Relationship to Mental Health

Because of its influence on behavior and the expression of emotions that may result, the topic of stress should be included in any discussion of mental health. Everyone, young and old, is exposed to daily stress that must be accommodated to ensure emotional stability. Therefore, people of all ages must realize that many situations produce feelings of anxiety or apprehension that cause the same types of fluctuation in levels of mental wellness as those experienced in physical wellness. The key is to learn to reduce anxiety and tension as they arise so that levels of stress are more easily managed.

Stress is the nonspecific response of the body to an unanticipated or stimulating event. Stress can accompany a pleasant or unpleasant event. Hans Selye (1975) has described stress resulting from a pleasant event as **eustress.** This type of stress comes from events such as getting something new, changing from one school to another, or being selected as a class officer. Although anxiety is produced, this type of stress helps us be more effective in physical, social, and psychological functioning. **Distress** is stress generated from a negative or unpleasant event. Prolonged distress can have a negative or debilitative effect on health. Unchecked distress interferes with physiological and psychological functioning (Selye 1975).

Anything that elicits a stress response is called a **stressor** (see Figure 8.2). A stressor can be an event or situation. What one person may perceive as stress may be totally nonstressful to someone else. For example, skydiving would be terrifying for many people, yet others may view it as a relaxing recreational activity.

It is both impossible and undesirable to live in a stress-free environment. Stress does occur and cannot be totally avoided. From a positive perspective, stress can enhance ability, act as a motivator, and be a means of self-protection. Unfortunately many children live in highly stressful situations. Factors such as poverty, crowding, and exposure to drugs, abuse, and domestic and street violence can all contribute to stress.

Figure 8.2
Possible Sources of
Stress in Children

1. Death of a parent
2. Death of a brother or sister
3. Marital separation of parents
4. Divorce of parents
5. Death of grandparent

6. Hospitalization of a parent
7. Remarriage of a parent to a stepparent
8. Birth of a brother or sister
9. Loss of job by father or mother

The General Adaptation Syndrome

Any event or circumstance that upsets the body's physiological balance is a stressor. The body is constantly striving to maintain a physiological balance or *homeostasis*. Regardless of the type of stress that occurs, eustress or distress, when an individual perceives a stressor, the body automatically responds with a three-stage process known as the general adaptation syndrome (GAS) (Selye 1975). (See Figure 8.3.)

The first phase of the general adaptation syndrome is referred to as the alarm phase. The brain interprets an event or situation as a stressor and immediately prepares the body to deal with it. Sometimes this initial response is called the "fight or flight" syndrome because the body literally reacts as if it is either going to stand and fight or run away. The emotional response causes physical reactions such as muscle tenseness, increased heart rate, dry mouth, or sweaty palms. The second stage of the GAS is resistance. During this phase the perceived stressor is dealt with through increased strength and sensory capacity. Only after meeting the demands of the stressful event can the body return to normal.

When stress is chronic, sufficiently pervasive, or traumatic enough, the third stage of exhaustion is reached. At this point the body must restore itself and rest or rather serious health problems are potentially possible. Adverse effects of mismanaged or long-term stress include heart problems, stomach problems, high blood pressure, and/or achy muscles and joints.

All the stages in the GAS are the result of chemical messages in the form of hormones. For example, during the alarm phase the pituitary gland releases a hormone (ACTH) that stimulates other endocrine glands to also release hormones, resulting in the fight-or-flight response. Hormonal messages increase blood volume and blood pressure. The hormones epinephrine and norepinephrine initiate a variety of physiological responses, including increased heart rate and increased metabolic rate. They also stimulate the release of other hormones called *endorphins*, which serve to diminish pain.

Obviously, the continual hormonal stimulation caused by chronic stress doesn't let the body return to homeostasis. Fortunately, the effects of most stressors can be partially or completely reversed with adequate stress management techniques. Early use of these techniques can reduce the adverse effects of stress.

Effects of Chronic Stress

Chronic stress can cause problems in several areas of a child's life. Psychosomatic illness, such as headaches and physical injuries, may result from an abnormal response to stress. A child may

Figure 8.3
The General Adaptation Syndrome

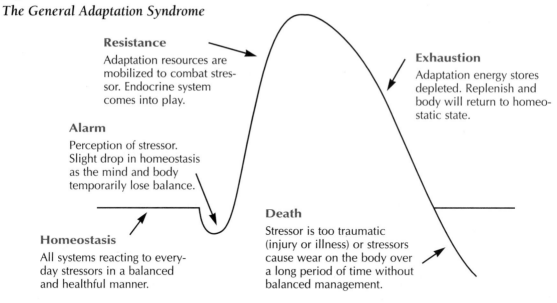

Resistance
Adaptation resources are mobilized to combat stressor. Endocrine system comes into play.

Exhaustion
Adaptation energy stores depleted. Replenish and body will return to homeostatic state.

Alarm
Perception of stressor. Slight drop in homeostasis as the mind and body temporarily lose balance.

Homeostasis
All systems reacting to everyday stressors in a balanced and healthful manner.

Death
Stressor is too traumatic (injury or illness) or stressors cause wear on the body over a long period of time without balanced management.

---

withdraw emotionally from others and experience feelings of worthlessness, apathy, loneliness, anger, hostility, and low self-esteem. Behavior problems such as hyperactivity, accident susceptibility, truancy, substance abuse, and low academic achievement may also result from stress. Low self-esteem and anxiety may lead to a lack of concentration and a disrupted capacity to process information (Jones 1985).

Other behaviors that could indicate that children are under too much stress are

○ frequent headaches

○ sighing

○ diarrhea/constipation

○ nausea

○ faintness

○ hair twirling

○ clenched fists

○ nervous cough

○ fast or excessive talking

○ fingernail biting

○ back-and-forth rocking

○ depression

○ anger

○ continual boredom

- ○ lip biting
- ○ crying
- ○ proneness to errors
- ○ nightmares
- ○ persistent (compulsive) itching

Dealing with Distress

It is important to determine which sources of stress arise from intrinsic stimuli, such as being inwardly driven to reach a goal, and which ones arise from extrinsic stimuli, such as pressure from a teacher to turn in a homework assignment, parental separation, or death of a grandparent.

It is also beneficial to attempt to determine whether the source is regular, routine, or consistent, as in the case of a daily conflict or being self-conscious with peers. Sources of stress that are regular, routine, or consistent generally have a greater potential for creating long-term negative effects if not dealt with because they wear on the individual constantly and may therefore demand more time to resolve. Sudden, isolated sources of stress tend to be crisis situations that first require a return to some degree of normalcy and may later involve a more lengthy process of conflict resolution.

Putting the stress-producing situation in realistic perspective is helpful in objectively evaluating its impact. To do this, the teacher should help the student mentally classify events as they arise and to decide which situations can be personally handled after careful consideration of the possible alternatives. Those events involving either deeper inner conflict or interaction with others may require the assistance of a third party or outside expert. After putting the cause of the stress into perspective and outlining possible courses of action, children should be helped to select the course of action that seems likely to produce the most healthful, positive, or desirable results. The child should then be aided in carrying out the course of action and evaluating its effectiveness to determine whether similar courses of action should be repeated for similar circumstances or whether modifications need to be considered.

Stress Management in Children

Stress management and stress reduction skills can help children cope with life's stresses and increase their potential for reaching and maintaining high levels of emotional health throughout life. There are a variety of healthful ways to reduce the adverse effects of stress. Examples include exercise, relaxation techniques, and deep-breathing exercises. Some children can use hobbies, arts and crafts, and reading activities as alternative forms of stress reduction.

Exercise

One of the most natural methods of relieving the body of the effects of stress is exercise. Aerobic exercise activates the hormones, fatigues the tense muscles, and allows the stressed child to return to a pleasantly tired, but relaxed, state. Activities such as walking, jogging, cycling, and swimming all directly reduce adverse symptoms of stress.

Health Highlight

The Mental Health Needs of Elementary School Children

A study has indicated some very revealing findings about the emotional needs of elementary children. For example, the most frequent behaviors/characteristics identified by respondents as not receiving adequate attention in the schools and thus representing unmet needs are

○ has poor decision-making/problem-solving skills
○ has poor self-image; makes negative self-statements
○ exhibits low self-confidence; avoids the difficult
○ is unable to resolve interpersonal conflicts

○ appears depressed, unhappy
○ is overly influenced by peers; has poor refusal skills
○ cannot concentrate; is inattentive

About 80 percent of the causes of these behaviors were directly parent or home related, whereas school-linked problems account for less than 5 percent of responses. To the contrary, only about 20 percent of proposed solutions to the problems directly involved parents, whereas the majority of the proposed solutions were school based.

This study provides strong justification for giving high priority to mental health as a major goal of schools, teachers, and parents.

Source: Adapted from L. Goodwin, W. Goodwin, and J. Cantrill. 1988. The mental health needs of elementary schoolchildren. *Journal of school health* 58(7):282–287.

Relaxation Techniques

Several kinds of relaxation techniques may be used to combat the ill effects associated with stress. These techniques include but are not limited to progressive relaxation, meditation, and creative visualization. A child who is able to relax under very trying circumstances will experience fewer of the physical symptoms associated with poor stress management.

Progressive relaxation is one method that is especially useful for children. Progressive relaxation requires a quiet room and the space to assume a comfortable position. Instructions can be given on an audio tape or verbally by a teacher/facilitator in a classroom situation.

The key to progressive relaxation is to tense each muscle group as the command is given (typically for about 10–15 seconds); then when the signal is given, relax that muscle group immediately and completely (for approximately 10–15 seconds). This is a procedure that needs to be practiced, but once the method is learned, it can certainly help to reduce stress.

Deep-breathing exercises are very similar to natural relaxation. In fact, deep breathing uses the body's natural relaxation response. Children can be reminded that they often use deep breathing (sighing) when under stress without being aware of it. Deep-breathing exercises done in regular patterns can further help the student relax when experiencing stress.

Meditation can be approached from several perspectives. The purpose of the technique is to help the student temporarily "tune out" the world while evoking the relaxation response. During a meditation session, a word or phrase is concentrated on to help eliminate all outside distractions. While in a comfortable position on a couch, chair, or bed, the participant breathes deeply, slowly inhaling and exhaling. The word or phrase is focused on with each breath. This format can best be learned from an instructor or tape that can provide instruction.

Visualization (creative imagery) is a form of relaxation that makes use of the imagination. This is an excellent method to teach children. To use this technique, a comfortable position is assumed, the eyes are closed, and several deep breaths are taken. There are several variations of visualization that an individual can use. For example, a tranquil scene such as a beach or forests can serve as the focal point for the visualization. Visualization can be used to envision a goal or behavior change. There are a variety of tapes available that can aid the teaching of this technique.

Biofeedback is based on scientific principles designed to enhance awareness of body functioning. Sensory equipment is used to create awareness of subtle body changes such as increases or decreases in body temperature, muscle contractions, or brain wave variations. As people become more sensitive to fluctuations in functioning, they can learn to evoke the relaxation response by countering their automatic stress response as it occurs. A few sessions are usually required to recognize differences and then alter physiological responses. Equipment for biofeedback ranges from relatively inexpensive to quite costly.

Other Relaxation Techniques

Other techniques that require no special equipment or training but serve to help dissipate stress symptoms are humor, music, and effective time management.

Laughing is a powerful stress-reducing agent. Laughing or humor helps us to keep things in perspective, maintain a positive attitude, and realize that life is seldom perfect. It has been found that blood pressure and heart rate can actually decrease after a good laugh. Laughing or even smiling are excellent ways to alter a negative mood. Certainly one of the things that can be promoted in a healthy classroom environment is laughter. The laughter should not be based on racial or ethnic factors or at the expense of a student, but on the funny things that occur during the school day.

Quiet music serves to soothe the autonomic nervous system by easing tensions and lessening strong emotions. It is difficult to invoke the relaxation response if the music is inappropriate or irritating to the listener. Classical music affords exposure to the artistic beauty of life as well as evoking the relaxation response.

A perceived or actual lack of time is a major contributor to stress response. In children, effective time management can be fostered by helping them to establish goals and priorities in their daily lives. By learning effective time utilization at an early age, a great deal of stress can be eliminated as the child matures. Some suggestions for effective time management include teaching children to

○ not procrastinate

○ set realistic goals

○ establish priorities and write them down

○ learn to say no when necessary

○ build in relaxation time every day

○ visualize themselves completing their priorities

The Role of Effective Communication in Reducing Stress

People often experience a tremendous amount of stress when they feel others are controlling their lives. Anxiety results when a person feels exploited, humiliated, and/or a lack of respect. This anxiety and the accompanying stress can be reduced through a change in attitude toward oneself and through the use of effective communication skills.

Many times stress will result from children's inability to express feelings to others honestly. Individuals often refuse to express their feelings to others because they want to avoid confrontations or because they do not feel as important as the other person. Some do not wish to hurt anyone's feelings, yet this type of passive behavior causes a child to think less of himself and to be angry at the other person. Such a lack of respect for self increases stress because the person tends to store the anger internally. Conversely, aggressive behavior, in which a person physically abuses, insults, or criticizes the other person, can ruin relationships and thus increase stress.

Assertive communication—the type that communicates a respect for self as well as the other person—permits individuals to stand up for their rights without ignoring the rights of others. An important part of assertive behavior is a healthy self-concept in which people believe they are worthy individuals, capable of having their own feelings and beliefs. It also implies that people have a right to speak up if they have been treated unfairly, and they have a right to say no. Assertiveness involves making "I" statements; for example, I feel . . . I think . . . , which imply that a person takes full responsibility for his or her feelings. Assertive people are able to clearly and confidently say no and tell others what they think and feel without hurting others or putting them down. Teachers can help children learn how to communicate and be good listeners. Children can learn to speak with positive verbal and body language and yet be polite. Such communication is very effective in improving self-image and relationships with others and in dealing with stress.

Emotionally intimate communication with others also helps lessen the effects of life's stressors. This type of communication is more than just discussing the weather or other superficial topics. Teachers can facilitate such communication by allowing children to share their innermost feelings. Children should not be afraid to share their feelings with others for fear of being rejected. If a child bares his or her soul to the teacher, the teacher must empathize with the situation and provide emotional support. If the teacher demonstrates through words or behavior an unwillingness to give emotional support, anxiety, loneliness, and rejection can result. However, if children learn they are safe in sharing their intimacies, teacher–child relationships can become much stronger. Such intimate relationships add greatly to the child's quality of life, whereas the lack of such relationships contributes to discontentment, anxiety, and stress.

▤ *Summary*

The characteristics of good mental health include positive self-esteem, positive sense of self-worth, a concern for others, the ability to develop meaningful relationships, and the ability to make decisions.

○ Unexpressed emotions can lead to frustration, hostility, and resentment.

○ Mechanisms used to deal with feelings include compensation, daydreaming, idealization, projection, rationalization, regression, and sublimation.

○ Depression is the most frequently occurring emotional disorder and is a symptom of underlying conflict or tension.

○ Depression can be the result of heredity, personal background, personality, biochemical factors, and physical illness.

○ Depression can be a major cause of adolescent suicide.

○ Children should be helped to like themselves, be good to themselves, accept their personal limitations, deal with their problems, establish realistic goals, express emotions properly, develop their sense of humor, and cultivate an optimistic attitude.

○ Teachers must recognize the impact of familial socializations on the child entering the classroom and attempt to relate equally and objectively to children from diverse backgrounds and living arrangements.

○ Children with special emotional health needs include the latchkey child, children of separation, divorce, single parents, or a child experiencing a loss in the form of death of parent, grandparent, sibling, or pet.

○ How children relate to emotional situations and crisis tends to depend on their age.

○ Teachers need to listen and show their acceptance, support, encouragement, and concern for all children, especially for those experiencing special situations or crisis.

○ Stress is defined as the body's physical and/or psychological response to an unanticipated event.

○ Stress can be pleasant (eustress) or unpleasant (distress); prolonged distress has a debilitating health effect.

○ Anything that causes stress is called a *stressor*.

○ The body goes through three stages (called the general adaptation syndrome) in response to a stressful event—alarm, resistance, and exhaustion.

○ Children can be taught techniques for dealing with stress, such as exercising, deep breathing, meditation, visualization, biofeedback, humor, and effective time management.

○ Learning effective communication patterns is one of the best methods of protecting against negative stressful responses.

Discussion Questions

1. Describe the link between mental and physical health.
2. Discuss the relationship between a positive self-image and emotional health.
3. Discuss the importance of expressing one's emotions in a positive way.
4. Describe several causes of distress.
5. How are defense mechanisms used to cope with distress?
6. Discuss how the teachers can become aware of the multicultural nature of the classroom.
7. Discuss depression and suicide as they are experienced by children.
8. What are some possible signs of depression in children?
9. How can good decision-making skills help the child deal with distress?
10. What should teachers strive to teach children for promoting their emotional health?
11. What are the implications of divorce for children?
12. What potential problems may arise for latchkey children?

References

American Psychiatric Association (APA). 1987. *Diagnostic and statistical manual of mental disorders*. 3rd ed., rev. Washington, DC: American Psychiatric Association.

Bruess, C. E., and G. E. Richardson. 1994. *Healthy decisions*. Dubuque, IA: Brown.

Butler, A. F. 1984. Scratchy is dead. In *Death and dying in the classroom: Reading for reference*, ed. J. L. Thomas. Phoenix, AZ: Oryx Press.

Chandler, C., and C. Kolander. 1988. Stop the negative, accentuate the positive. *Journal of school health* 58(7):295–297.

———. 1989. Depression. *Mayo clinic health letter—Medical essay*.

DeSpelder, L., and A. Strickland. 1987. *The last dance*. 2nd ed. Mountain View, CA: Mayfield.

Epstein, M., and D. Cullinan. 1986. Depression in children. *Journal of school health* 56(1):10–12.

Fredlund, D. J. 1984. Children and death from the school setting viewpoint. In *Death and dying in the classroom: Readings for reference*, ed. J. L. Thomas. Phoenix, AZ: Oryx Press.

Fuhrmann, B. S. 1986. *Adolescence, adolescents*. Boston: Little, Brown.

Garcia, R. L. 1991. *Teaching in a pluralistic society: Concepts, models, strategies*. 2nd ed. New York: HarperCollins.

Goodwin, L., W. Goodwin, and J. Cantrill. 1988. The mental health needs of elementary schoolchildren. *Journal of school health* 58(7):282–287.

Greenberg, J., and G. Dintiman. 1992. *Exploring health—expanding the boundaries of wellness*. Englewood Cliffs, NJ: Prentice Hall.

Grollman, E. A. 1988. *Suicide*. Boston, MA: Beacon Press.

Hales, D. 1992. *An invitation to health*. Redwood City, CA: Benjamin/Cummings.

Hamrick, M., D. Anspaugh, and G. Ezell. 1986. *Health*. Columbus, OH: Merrill.

Jones, J. 1985. Promoting mental health of children and youth through the schools. Paper presented at the American School Health Association Convention, October, Little Rock, AK.

Levy, M., M. Dignan, and J. Shirreffs. 1987. *Life and health*. 5th ed. New York: Random House.

Magg, J. W., and S. R. Forness. 1991, September. Depression in children and adolescents: Assessment and treatment. *Focus on exceptional children* 24:14–19.

Mullen, K. D., R. S. Gold, P. A. Belcastro, and R. J. McDermott. 1993. *Connections for health*. 3rd ed. Madison, WI: Brown and Benchmark.

Nelson, R. E., and B. Crawford. 1991. Suicide among elementary school-age children. *Elementary school guidance and counseling* 25:123–128.

Olsen, L., K. Redican, and C. Baffi. 1986. *Health today*. 2nd ed. New York: Macmillan.

Page, R. M., and T. S. Page. 1993. *Fostering emotional well-being in the classroom*. Boston: Jones & Bartlett.

Patros, P. G., and T. K. Shamoo. 1989. *Depression and suicide in children and adolescents: Prevention, intervention, and postvention*. Boston: Allyn and Bacon.

Ricci, I. 1982. *Mom's house, Dad's house*. New York: Macmillan.

Selye, H. 1975. *Stress without distress*. New York: New American Library.

Stepfamily Foundation. 1996. World Wide Web. 333 West End Avenue, Newark, NY. URL: http://www.stepfamily.org/tensteps

Stroher, D. B. 1986. Latchkey children: The fastest-growing special interest group in the schools. *Journal of school health* 56(1):16.

U.S. Department of Health and Human Services (USDHHS). 1994. *Child health* USA 93. Washington, DC: U.S. Government Printing Office.

Wallerstein, J., and Kelly, J. 1981. *Surviving the break-up*. New York: Basic Books.

Wass, H., F. Berardo, and R. Neimeyer, eds. 1988. *Dying: Facing the facts*. 2nd ed. Washington, DC: Hemisphere.

Chapter Nine
Strategies for Teaching Mental Health and Stress Reduction

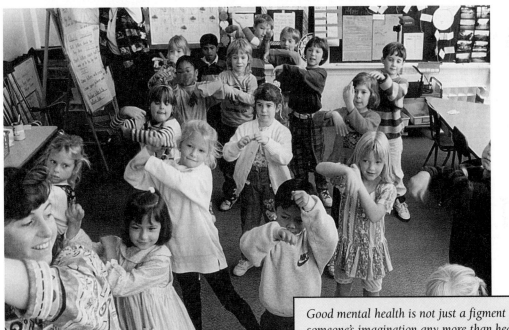

> Good mental health is not just a figment of someone's imagination any more than health is just a modern problem.
>
> —Phillip Rice (1992)

Valued Outcomes

After doing the activities in this chapter, the students should be able to express and illustrate the following guidelines:

○ Each person is unique and special, and everyone has many good qualities.

○ All people share basic human needs for physical safety, love, security, emotional support, and acceptance from others.

○ Personality development is affected by one's self-concept and self-esteem.

○ There are healthy and unhealthy ways to express any given emotion.

○ Mentally healthy expressions of emotion are consistent in frequency and intensity with the impact, influence, or importance of the event that triggers the emotion.

○ Positive interpersonal relationships with family and friends are vital to one's mental health.

○ Open and honest communication with others is a necessary part of mental health.

○ The attitudes, beliefs, and opinions that an individual has toward him- or herself determine self-concept, self-esteem, and feelings of self-worth. Strong feelings of self-worth are a necessary part of good mental health.

○ All people face stressful situations in day-to-day living.

○ Stressful situations can best be minimized by identifying the situation as it arises, putting the event into perspective, and altering or eliminating the situation if possible.

○ Learning to cope and deal with stressful situations successfully can enhance one's mental health.

○ Learning to relax and find pleasure in life activities on a day-to-day basis can help reduce stress.

○ Decisions about personal behavior and conduct are an integral part of an individual's mental health and are based on a learned set of values arising from social interaction and from expectations of the culture as a whole.

○ Decisions about personal conduct that are compatible with a person's value system can help balance individual drives, desires, and needs with family, community, and social expectations and therefore lead to a greater potential for emotional balance, unity, and inner peace.

○ The ability to apply problem-solving skills can help resolve individual and family conflicts.

○ Each person should accept responsibility for his or her own behavior.

Mental Health: An Integral Part of Life

Mental health is a very significant part of our overall health. Sometimes mental health is more difficult to maintain than our physical health. As teachers, we can enhance our children's mental health through the ways in which we interact with them. An open, accepting demeanor on the part of the teacher in a classroom can determine the effectiveness of the learning environment. Conversely, a regimented, pressure-filled atmosphere in the classroom will stifle students' creativity and interfere with their ability to learn. One of the most important aspects of mental health to teach elementary students is the acceptance of others. Teachers should emphasize that each individual is unique and that differences among individuals should make life more interesting, not more difficult. This concept of uniqueness is especially important to teach when a greater number of special students are mainstreamed into the "normal" classroom.

Another vital lesson to be taught in emotional health is the relationship between freedom and responsibilities. Elementary children struggle with ambivalent feelings toward dependence and independence. Sometimes they get angry when their parents treat them like little children, yet they are reluctant to accept the additional chores and responsibilities that accompany growing older. Students need to understand that growing older can mean greater freedom, in that they are allowed to do things younger children cannot do, but with the additional freedom comes the expectation to act prudently and responsibly.

Good relationships with others often begin with a healthy image of ourselves; therefore, a major goal in teaching mental health and stress reduction should be to foster self-esteem in children and to help them understand that in order to love others they must accept themselves. Healthy self-esteem can enhance effective communication with others, which in turn helps build good relationships and resolve conflicts with family and friends. Further, an important part of a relationship is being able to communicate assertively and listen effectively. Building good mental health must begin in infancy and early childhood. By the time children enter school, their mental health has been strongly influenced by family and peers. But effective learning strategies are also a powerful shaping influence. By helping children build feelings of positive self-esteem, developing good decision-making skills in harmony with their values, and learning to cope with the stressors in life, the teacher can guide children toward emotional well-being.

Cycle Plan for Teaching Concepts

Grade level Topic	K	1	2	3	4	5	6	7	8
Uniqueness	***	***	**	**	*	*	*	*	*
Human needs	***	**	**	***	*	**	***	*	*
Self-esteem	***	***	***	**	**	**	***	***	***
Emotion	***	**	**	***	*	***	**	**	**
Relationships	**	***	**	***	*	**	***	***	***
Communication	**	***	***	***	*	***	**	**	**
Stress	***	***	**	**	***	***	**	**	***
Decision making	**	**	*	**	***	***	**	***	***
Values	**	**	*	**	***	**	***	**	***

Key: *** = major emphasis, ** = emphasis, * = review

Value-Based Activities

Value-based activities are designed to help children develop their critical thinking skills, personalize information, and establish concepts conducive to high-quality wellness. Teachers can design a variety of activities that are value based, depending on the content being discussed. Some suggestions follow.

Valued Possessions

Valued Outcome: The students will be able to identify what is really important to them and their well-being.

Description of Strategy: This activity is designed to help children to determine what is important to them and to understand what we are expressing in our decisions are values or feelings concerning the type of life we wish to lead.

Value Question: Pretend that you are going on a trip in a spaceship. What three things would you take with you and why?

Processing Questions:

1. Why did you take your three choices?
2. Do these represent something you value?
3. How would you describe a value?
4. Do values reflect what we do and the decisions we make? Why/how?

Materials Needed: paper and pencils

Voting Questions

Valued Outcome: The students will examine their feelings for the various topics presented.
Description of Strategy: Voting questions are another way to help students establish their feelings on various topics. The teacher can develop a variety of questions that lend themselves to a particular topic. The questions should be read aloud. Ask students to raise their thumbs up if they agree with the question, thumbs down if they disagree, and to fold their arms if they are unsure or undecided. Some examples of potential questions:

How many of you . . .

. . . find it difficult to talk with your parents?

. . . feel scared to speak in a large group?

. . . have a friend to discuss problems?

. . . wish others would listen to you better?

Processing Questions:

1. What seem to be the areas that represent the biggest problems?
2. What are some ways we can deal with these problems?

Materials Needed: teacher or student prepared voting questions, paper, pencils

The Time of My Life

Valued Outcome: The students will be able to identify how they spend the hours of each day.
Description of Strategy: For this valued activity, have each student draw a circle and divide it into four sections on a piece of paper (see Figure 9.1). The circle represents a twenty-four-hour time span, with each quadrant equaling approximately six hours. From the categories shown, ask each student to divide the circle according to the amount of time that he or she thinks should be spent on these activities: with friends, with family, learning at school, for homework, for sleeping.
Processing Questions:

1. How do you like your time schedule?
2. Is there anything you need to change?
3. Why is how we use our time important?
4. Why do we tend to do those things we like best?

Materials Needed: paper to draw circle or have a prepared form for the class.

Name Tag Descriptors

Valued Outcome: The students will be able to name ways in which they are unique.
Description of Strategy: Each student should be provided with a piece of paper and crayons. Discuss how each person is unique. Instruct the student to make a name tag with a drawing that will show one of his or her interests. Cut the name tag out, and write the child's name on the tag. The class can then guess each person's interests.
Processing Questions:

1. How do the activities we like to do differ?

Figure 9.1
Time Circle

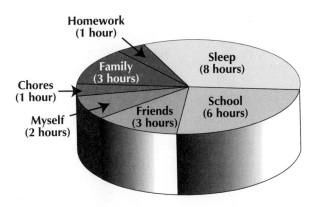

2. Is it OK that we all like different activities?

3. What are some ways that all of us are alike?

4. What are really important characteristics that we should all have?

Materials Needed: name tags, crayons or colored pencils

Friends Should Be . . .

Valued Outcome: The students will be able to name ways in which they are unique.
Description of Strategy: Using the following list, ask each student to rank-order within each grouping the characteristics most important to look for in a friend. Then group the students and ask them to decide, by consensus, rankings that are shared with all other groups.

A	B	C
____Smart	____Honest	____Loyal
____Popular	____Dependable	____Conscientious
____Funny	____Dedicated	____Trustworthy

D	E	F
____Open	____Quiet	____Healthy
____Discreet	____Bubbly	____Happy
____Closed	____Talkative	____Successful

Processing Questions:

1. What common characteristics did the various groups identify?

2. Were there differences between the boys' and the girls' choices of important characteristics?

3. What other characteristics would be important to you in a friend?

4. Of the important characteristics identified, do you feel you portray those characteristics?

Materials Needed: above list (may be expanded by the teacher/student), pencils

Children can be encouraged to think about their own and their peers' positive traits.

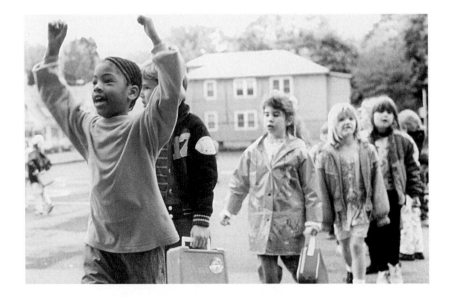

Relationship Collage

Valued Outcome: The students will develop insight into the many people who influence their lives.

Description of Strategy: This activity is designed to help students see the influence on them of the many relationships they have with peers, family, teachers, coaches, and so on. Have the children make a collage of their relationships. A picture of the child should be in the center of a piece of posterboard. Around his or her picture, the child puts other pictures or drawings that represent the many people he or she associates with.

Processing Questions:

1. Who are the most important people you are involved with?

2. What do these people do for you?

3. How do they influence you and your behavior?

4. Are there any negative influences from these people?

5. What can you do about the negative influences?

Materials Needed: paper and colored pencils

Decision Stories

Follow the procedure discussed in Chapter 4 for presenting decision stories, such as the following.

Where Did I Put Them?

Sally is getting ready for school. She cannot remember where she put her shoes. She looked under the bed, under the chair, and behind the door. Sally begins to cry because she thinks she will be late. *Focus Questions:* What could have been done to keep Sally from getting upset? What should Sally do now?

A Nasty Note

Sam was going to the lunchroom when he saw Fred sticking something in Peggy's locker. Later, Sam sees Peggy crying because she found the note, which made fun of her family.
Focus Questions: What should Sam do to help? How does Peggy feel?

I Dare You

Amy is new in her neighborhood and wants to make new friends. Jill asks her to take an unsafe dare in order to be accepted by the other girls in the neighborhood.
Focus Questions: What should Amy do? Is it worth placing yourself at risk to be accepted? How can Amy decide which is more important?

New Girl in School

Betty notices that the new student in class is being ridiculed by two of Betty's friends because the new student is the only one in class wearing glasses. They are talking with other girls and writing notes.
Focus Question: What should Betty do?

Handling Stress

John has just invited his friend, Alex, to play, but Alex replied, "I don't want to play with you anymore." John feels angry, frustrated, and rejected.
Focus Question: How can John handle the stress caused by this situation?

Other Strategies for Learning

Guess My Trait

Valued Outcome: The students will be able to express a specific personality trait through role-play.
Description of Strategy: Ask several children to role-play a personality trait that you have whispered to them. One child will act out the personality trait, and the rest of the class will guess the personality trait.
Materials Needed: none
Processing Questions:

1. What is one of your own personality traits?
2. Were all the traits demonstrated in the role-play situations desirable ones to have?
3. Differentiate between the desirable and the undesirable personality traits.

Truth and Consequences

Valued Outcome: The students will observe, discuss, and role-play consequences that result from taking specific actions.
Description of Strategy: Have a small group of volunteer students role-play the following situations and the resulting consequences:

1. Student decides not to do his homework.

2. Man speeds on the highway because he is late.

3. Girl receives a birthday gift and refuses to thank the person she received it from.

Afterward, discuss these questions: Did the person accept the responsibility involved? What results would occur if he or she had acted differently?
Materials Needed: none
Processing Questions:

1. What are the consequences of not doing your homework?

2. What are the consequences of disobeying laws or rules?

3. What action would you expect the girl who received a birthday gift to demonstrate?

Appropriate Personality Traits

Valued Outcome: The students will be able to demonstrate healthy ways to react to specific feelings.
Description of Strategy: Have class members role-play the following situations to illustrate healthy personality traits appropriate to the situation.

1. getting a poor grade on a test

2. losing your favorite toy

3. accidentally damaging someone else's property

Materials Needed: none
Processing Questions:

1. Is it OK to get angry? Why or why not?

2. What is one good way to handle anger?

3. Think of a situation in which you got angry. What did you do, and could you have reacted differently?

Body Language

Valued Outcome: The students will be able to identify ways in which a listener using positive or negative body language affects the speaker.
Description of Strategy: Group the class into dyads. One person is the listener, and the other is the speaker. The speaker talks about a teacher-selected topic, such as "My most embarrassing moment" or "What I want to do this summer." The listener responds nonverbally with positive body language, for example, nodding the head, eye contact, erect posture. Afterward, the class discusses the effects of positive body language on the speaker. This activity can be repeated with the listener displaying negative body language.
Materials Needed: none
Processing Questions:

1. Name two ways to demonstrate positive body language when listening.

2. Name two ways to demonstrate negative body language when listening.

3. Name one way the speaker reacts to each type of body language.

Role Playing: Emotional Reactions

Valued Outcome: The students will be able to explain how the same emotion can be expressed in different ways.

Description of Strategy: Role-play how one would act if one felt good about oneself or if one did not feel good about oneself, for example, after being disciplined in public by parents for inappropriate behavior. Ask two or three students to do this. Note how differently they role-play these emotions.

Materials Needed: none

Processing Questions:

1. Give an example of a wrong way to handle a specific emotion.
2. What might the consequences be of handling an emotion a wrong way?
3. Which way seemed to be the best way of dealing with the emotion and why?

Role Playing: Body Language

Valued Outcome: The students will be able to express emotions in both verbal and nonverbal ways.

Description of Strategy: Role-play how you can communicate the same thing with or without words. Have students use body language to express an emotion, and then have them verbally describe the same emotion.

Materials Needed: none

Processing Questions:

1. Give an example of a verbal statement to let someone know you care about them.
2. Name a nonverbal way to let someone know you care about them.
3. Give an example of a nonverbal expression of anger.

Hidden Messages

Valued Outcome: The students will be able to communicate in both verbal and nonverbal ways, identifying advantages and disadvantages to both ways.

Description of Strategy: Divide students into small groups. Ask half the groups to present a play with a hidden message or moral of their own making using dialogue, and ask the remaining groups to give their presentations nonverbally. After all groups have finished, ask for identification and interpretation of the messages, and discuss the advantages and disadvantages of verbal and nonverbal communication.

Materials Needed: none

Processing Questions:

1. Name one disadvantage of nonverbal communication.
2. Name one advantage of nonverbal communication.
3. Name one advantage of verbal communication.

Words Can Hurt

Valued Outcome: The students will be able to describe and discuss both tactful and rude ways to handle specific situations.

Description of Strategy: Ask the class as a whole to devise a hypothetical, open-ended situation in which communication could take the form of being either rude or tactful. Then divide the class into two groups. Ask one group to describe several tactful ways the situation could be handled. Ask the other group to describe several rude ways the situation could be handled. Follow by leading a discussion about students' views concerning each handling of the situation.

Materials Needed: none

Processing Questions:

1. What advantage does using a tactful answer have over using a rude response?
2. What might occur if a rude comment is used in response to a situation?
3. What might occur if a tactful response is used in a situation?

The Decision

Valued Outcome: The students will be able to demonstrate ways to handle emotions associated with rejection and family crisis situations.

Description of Strategy: Provide an open-ended hypothetical situation appropriate for the grade level that involves either rejection by a peer group or a family crisis. Then divide the students into three groups. Supply two of the groups with the ending they will enact. Ask the third group to devise their own scenario. Let each group dramatize its ideas and compare differences. If time and attention allow, provide additional situations and rotate tasks.

Materials Needed: none

Processing Questions:

1. What is one good way to handle rejection?
2. What is one bad way to handle rejection?
3. What is a helpful thing to do in a family crisis?

Pairing

Valued Outcome: The students will be able to demonstrate and discuss a variety of emotions associated with specific situations.

Description of Strategy: Pair students. Have one member of each pair draw a situation from a box full of hypothetical interactions between two people, such as making a new friend, responding to someone who has broken your favorite toy, or sharing ice cream with a playmate. Use imagination, creativity, and diversity in developing these situations, and focus on many areas of mental health. Allow each pair to act out its situation, and encourage class discussion after each enactment.

Materials Needed: none

Processing Questions:

1. What is a good way to respond to someone who has broken your favorite toy?
2. What is a bad way to respond to someone who has broken your favorite toy?
3. How would you go about trying to make a new friend?

Giving and Gaining

Valued Outcome: The students will be able to demonstrate an understanding of the necessity for compromise in specific situations.
Description of Strategy: Have several students role-play a situation where an individual's personal values must be compromised for the good of the group. Examples might include the mayor allowing an individual to make an unpopular speech, or a police officer enforcing a law he or she does not agree with. Follow with a discussion of why the person made the compromise.
Materials Needed: none
Processing Questions:

1. What is a situation in which it would not be good to compromise? Why?

2. Why is compromise necessary in some situations?

3. What might happen if no one ever compromised?

Getting to Know You

Valued Outcome: The students will be able to describe and discuss various aspects of their personalities.
Description of Strategy: Ask students to print the word *personality* as the heading on a sheet of notebook paper and have them write several phrases that describe their own personalities. Let volunteers share their papers with the class.
Materials Needed: none
Processing Questions:

1. What do you think is one of your most important personality characteristics, and why do you think it is important?

2. What personality trait do you find to be your least desirable?

3. If you could have any personality trait you wanted, what would you choose and why?

Question Box

Valued Outcome: The students will be able to identify personal fears, worries, or dilemmas.
Description of Strategy: Supply a large, colorful box, and encourage students to anonymously submit questions that they want to discuss regarding personal fears, worries, or dilemmas. Set aside about thirty minutes each week to discuss as many of these as possible.
Materials Needed: question box
Processing Questions:

1. What is your worst fear and why?

2. What specific things cause you to worry?

3. Who are some people you could talk to about your worries and fears?

Who Can I Turn To?

Valued Outcome: The students will be able to identify sources of help for specific situations.
Description of Strategy: Ask students to think about whom they can talk to when they need advice. Give the class a situation (a friend is making fun of you). Let the students decide whom they would go to for help in the situation.

Materials Needed: none
Processing Questions:

1. Whom do you feel you can go to about a problem you are having with peer pressure?

2. Whom do you feel you can go to about a problem you are having with a boyfriend or girlfriend?

3. Whom do you feel you can go to about a family crisis?

Ups and Downs

Valued Outcome: The students will be able to identify uplifting emotions and depressing emotions and associate them with specific circumstances.
Description of Strategy: Discuss emotions in terms of "ups" and "downs." What emotions make us feel up or down? Ask volunteers if they are feeling up or down today and what circumstances led to their feeling this way.
Materials Needed: none
Processing Questions:

1. Name two emotions that make you feel "up."

2. Name two emotions that make you feel "down."

3. Give an example of an event that caused you to experience emotions that made you feel "down."

We Are Different People

Valued Outcome: The students will be able to describe how they behave differently in various relationships.
Description of Strategy: Brainstorm examples of how one person can function in several relationships at one time, such as friend, sibling, child, student. Emphasize how we behave differently in various relationships.
Materials Needed: none
Processing Questions:

1. What is different about how you express anger at a parent and anger at a teacher?

2. What is different about the way you express love for a friend and love for a sibling?

3. Do you think we hurt the people we care about the most? Why or why not?

Picture the Emotion

Valued Outcome: The students will be able to identify the expression of specific emotions.
Description of Strategy: Photograph the students in a variety of situations. Post the photographs on a bulletin board, and ask the students to comment on the emotions being expressed in the photographs, such as happiness, love, sorrow, fear, and anxiety. This will help the students explore their emotions and the emotions of those around them.
Materials Needed: camera, bulletin board
Processing Questions:

1. What is the most common emotion depicted on the bulletin board?

2. Whose facial expression shows the most pain, and what are the circumstances surrounding this emotion?

3. Whose facial expression shows the most joy, and what are the circumstances surrounding this emotion?

Different Is OK

Valued Outcome: The students will be able to discuss the importance of being different and unique.

Description of Strategy: To emphasize the fact that all people are different and unique, discuss several categories or groups of plants and animals. Visual aids should be easy to obtain. For example, fruits come in many varieties, sizes, shapes, colors, and tastes, yet they are all fruits. People, too, are all different, but they are all people.

Materials Needed: plant and animal visual aids

Processing Questions:

1. Name two differences between you and your best friend.

2. Name two differences between your mother and your teacher.

3. Name two advantages of being different.

Caring

Valued Outcome: The students will be able to discuss ways in which he or she can help meet the needs of others by caring.

Description of Strategy: Discuss the different needs of a pet dog or cat. When the animal is hungry, we feed it. When it is lonely, we play with it and talk to it. When it is sleeping, we don't disturb it. People have needs that have to be met as well. Discuss how we can help meet the needs of others by caring.

Materials Needed: none

Processing Questions:

1. How could you help meet the needs of a sick parent?

2. How could you help meet the needs of an infant?

3. How could you help meet the needs of a grandparent in a nursing home?

Living by the Rules

Valued Outcome: The students will be able to identify reasons for rules.

Description of Strategy: Sometimes it is hard for young children to understand why it is necessary to follow directions or obey rules. Discuss several rules or laws and the reasons for each. For example, a traffic speed limit helps to prevent accidents, injuries, and deaths. It also helps to conserve fuel. Rules for a game help make the activity fair and fun. Discuss what happens when someone doesn't follow the rules of a game.

Materials Needed: none

Processing Questions:

1. Why are traffic laws necessary?

2. Why are rules necessary in games?

3. What are some possible dangers associated with not following parents' rules?

I'm Unique

Valued Outcome: The students will be able to compare differences and similarities among individuals.
Description of Strategy: Have children trace the outlines of each other's bodies on butcher paper. Compare the similarities and differences with other children in the class to emphasize that we are alike in many ways and yet unique.
Materials Needed: butcher paper, markers or crayons
Processing Questions:

1. What are some similarities that exist among students in the class?
2. What are some differences that exist among students in the class?
3. Name some advantages to being different.

Different Pictures of Me

Valued Outcome: The students will be able to identify unique characteristics of each stage of development.
Description of Strategy: Have students bring in pictures of themselves as an infant, as a toddler, and as a child. Have them note the unique characteristics of each stage of development.
Materials Needed: students' photographs
Processing Questions:

1. What unique characteristic did you have as an infant?
2. What unique characteristic did you have as a toddler?
3. What is a unique characteristic you now possess?

Which Emotion Am I?

Valued Outcome: The students will be able to draw facial expressions depicting specific emotions.
Description of Strategy: Give each child a paper plate and crayons. List several emotions on the chalkboard. Assign one emotion to each child, then have each child draw his or her face reflecting that emotion.
Materials Needed: paper plates, crayons
Processing Questions:

1. Describe the face that was drawn expressing anger.
2. Describe the face that was drawn expressing joy.
3. Can you always tell what someone is feeling by his or her facial expression? Why or why not?

Happy or Sad?

Valued Outcome: The students will be able to associate the emotions happy and sad with positive and negative situations.

The teacher can do much to foster each student's mental health by reinforcing special talents and allowing expression of feelings.

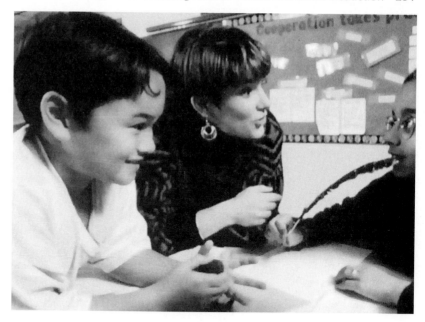

Description of Strategy: Let each child draw a happy face and a sad face on a paper plate. Attach these to Popsicle sticks. The teacher will give examples of positive and negative situations, and the students will hold up the face that indicates which face they would use in each situation.
Materials Needed: paper plates, crayons, Popsicle sticks
Processing Questions:

1. Can you give an example of a situation that made you feel happy?

2. Can you give an example of a situation that made you feel sad?

3. Happy and sad are two common emotions. What are some other emotions you have felt today?

Emotions Bag

Valued Outcome: The students will be able to describe personal emotional experiences as well as reactions in those situations.
Description of Strategy: Give each student a paper bag to keep for two days. Students should keep track of their emotions for that time period by writing a description about their emotional experiences and their reactions to those situations as they happen. Students will keep each description in their bag and then share them with class.
Materials Needed: paper bags, paper, pencils
Processing Questions:

1. What was an emotion you described that made you feel bad inside? What caused this emotion?

2. What was an emotion you described that made you feel good inside? What caused this emotion?

3. Did you experience the emotion anger? If so, how did you react?

Mental Health in Music

Valued Outcome: The students will be able to describe characteristics of healthy living.
Description of Strategy: Have students compose songs that describe healthy living. They can bring in tapes or CDs that describe a human relationship. Discuss the feelings depicted in the music. Pay attention to the tone of the music as well as the words of the song.
Materials Needed: students' tapes or CDs, tape or CD player
Processing Questions:

1. Can you name one characteristic of a healthy relationship?
2. What feelings are mentioned in the song you wrote?
3. Besides having healthy relationships, what are some other characteristics of healthy living?

Hearing Is Not Always Listening

Valued Outcome: The students will be able to demonstrate and discuss listening and observation skills.
Description of Strategy: Set up several "listening" and "observing" demonstrations to emphasize that these are learned skills. Here are some possible examples.

1. Prearrange with a student to share a hypothetical problem with several classmates during lunch or recess. They need to believe they are being told about the problem in confidence. The next day, reveal the setup to the class and ask each student involved about what he or she heard and understood to be the problem.
2. Prearrange with several students to get "lost" during recess. (Have them go to the library or other supervised area.) When the rest of the class returns, ask them to help with descriptions of each missing person. Also have them indicate anything they might have overheard during recess that might give a clue to why these students are gone. After the missing students return, discuss implications of the activity.
3. Tell students you are going to read a story and you want them to listen carefully. Read aloud a short story with several specific details about a main character's problem or situation and the succeeding events. Immediately following the story, ask each student to write a brief summary of the story, being as specific and accurate as possible. Let volunteers share their versions. Then read the original again. Compare listening skills.

Materials Needed: story, paper, pencils
Processing Questions:

1. What is the difference between hearing and listening?
2. How did the versions of scenario 1 differ, and why do you think this occurred?
3. What is the advantage of being a good listener?

Cartoon Personalities

Valued Outcome: The students will be able to identify personality traits of a cartoon character.
Description of Strategy: The teacher will ask the children to determine the personality traits of cartoon characters. The teacher will hold up a picture of a cartoon character and have the students describe the character's personality.

Materials Needed: pictures of cartoon characters
Processing Questions:

1. Which cartoon characters had undesirable personality traits, and what are these traits?
2. Which cartoon character had desirable personality traits, and what are these traits?
3. Do you have any of the same personality traits as the cartoon characters? Which ones?

Human Scavenger Hunt

Valued Outcome: The students will be able to identify human qualities that emphasize individual uniqueness.
Description of Strategy: Have students simulate a "scavenger hunt," but have them look for various unique human qualities, such as red hair, green eyes, friendliness, or quick-temperedness.
Materials Needed: none
Processing Questions:

1. What did you think was the most interesting quality you found in your scavenger hunt?
2. How many different qualities might one person have?
3. Do any two people have the same qualities? Why or why not?

Who Am I?

Valued Outcome: The students will be able to recognize the different and unique qualities of every individual.
Description of Strategy: Have students write a story and make a drawing about themselves. After they have completed the stories and drawings, take them up and read the papers aloud. Have students guess whose paper is being read.
Materials Needed: paper, pencils, crayons, or markers
Processing Questions:

1. Name as many favorite animals as you can that were mentioned by your classmates.
2. Name as many different hobbies as you can that were mentioned by your classmates.
3. What other interesting qualities were mentioned in your classmates' stories?

Feelings and Faces

Valued Outcome: The students will be able to associate emotions with facial expressions.
Description of Strategy: Hand out duplicated sheets of stylized emotions to the students. Have each student identify and label the emotion depicted on each face. Follow this activity with a class discussion.
Materials Needed: worksheet showing facial expressions depicting specific emotions
Processing Questions:

1. Which emotions are not showing a smiling face?
2. Which emotions are not showing frowns?
3. How do the eyes look on the face that shows surprise?

Costume Party

Valued Outcome: The students will be able to express personality traits through costume.
Description of Strategy: Ask each student to come to class in a costume that depicts as many of his or her personality traits as possible. The class as a whole lists what traits students think are revealed. A secret ballot vote is cast for costumes that are the most accurate, inaccurate, humorous, puzzling, and eye catching.
Materials Needed: costumes from students' homes
Processing Questions:

1. Explain why you chose the costume you were wearing.
2. Describe the costume and personality traits of your closest classmate.
3. Which classmate had the most humorous costume, and why?

Silent Steps

Valued Outcome: The students will be able to identify feelings experienced through a nonverbal group effort to reconstruct a jigsaw puzzle.
Description of Strategy: Divide students into groups of five to seven. Provide each group with a sealed manila envelope that contains a sheet of colored construction paper cut into five to seven shuffled jigsaw pieces. Each group should receive a different colored puzzle with differently shaped pieces of equal difficulty. Instruct each group member to randomly select a puzzle piece from the envelope. When you give the signal to start, students must reconstruct the pieces without saying a word. As each reconstructs the puzzle, have them raise their hands— they still cannot talk. When all groups have finished, allow the students to discuss their feelings during this activity.
Materials Needed: manila envelopes with jigsaw puzzle pieces
Processing Questions:

1. What feelings can result from nonverbal communication?
2. Discuss how the puzzle would have been solved if verbal communication had been used.
3. What are the advantages to verbal communication?

Steps to the Top

Valued Outcome: The students will be able to name a quality or rule for building mental health.
Description of Strategy: Have students trace their feet on construction paper. Inside the foot outline, ask each student to write a quality or rule for building mental health. These qualities can include self-love, self-respect, consideration of others, open communication, honesty, practicing what you preach, or sound decision making. Tack the footprints on a bulletin board in ascending steps to good mental health.
Materials Needed: construction paper, scissors, bulletin board
Processing Questions:

1. Explain how your footprint relates to building mental health.
2. Why is it important to have good mental heath?
3. What are some characteristics of poor mental health?

Health Highlight

Am I Stressed?

Stress is becoming a common cause for illness or other problems among students of all ages. Students need to be able to identify the causes of stress in their lives and their reactions to stressful events. There are several ways you can help them identify these.

1. Have the students determine stressful events that have occurred for a week by keeping a journal for one week. They should record stressful events and how they coped with the events. This will help them identify the coping mechanisms they are using. Keeping a journal will also allow them to identify their physical and emotional reactions. Let the students share their journals with each other and discuss the different ways they reacted.

2. There is a very good NBC video titled, "Stressed to Kill." This video is narrated by Connie Chung and contains experiments that explore the mind–body response to stress.

Coping with Stress

Valued Outcome: The students will be able to identify positive ways to reduce stress.
Description of Strategy: Divide students into four groups. Ask each group to create a bulletin board that focuses on positive ways to reduce stress. Bulletin boards should be redone each week for a month so that each group's message can be seen and discussed.
Materials Needed: construction paper, scissors, stencils, bulletin board
Processing Questions:

1. Name three positive ways to reduce stress.

2. What might happen to someone who is under too much stress?

3. How often should stress reduction techniques be used and why?

Facial Forecasts

Valued Outcome: The students will be able to draw a facial expression depicting a specific emotion.
Description of Strategy: Assign each student an emotion. Provide students with paper plates and crayons, and ask them to draw their own faces indicating the emotion. Have the students use mirrors if necessary. The plates may be used for colorful wall display.
Materials Needed: paper plates, crayons, mirrors
Processing Questions:

1. How did your face look when you expressed anger?

2. How did your face look when you expressed happiness?

3. Do people's facial expressions always indicate how they feel? Why or why not?

Refusal Skills

Valued Outcome: The students will be able to identify five refusal skills to use when responding to peer pressure.

Description of Strategy: Students will discuss the definition of peer pressure and how it is used by friends and others to influence their behavior. Specific techniques used by peers and others will be identified: name calling, acceptance, and so on. The teacher will solicit responses regarding the results of using poor judgment and giving in to peer pressure. The following questions will be asked:

1. How will you feel about yourself if you use poor judgment?
2. What kinds of trouble could you encounter as a result of your actions?
3. What physical effects will your action cause?

Explain and cite examples of the following refusal steps:

1. Ask questions.
2. Name the trouble.
3. Identify consequences.
4. Suggest alternatives.
5. Leave.

Students will practice refusal steps in an activity called "The Pressure Seat." Students sit in a circle with one student in the center of the group. The student chooses a peer pressure situation strip from the can. He or she reads the situation out loud and responds in one minute. The group is then called on to discuss the situation and tell if it agrees or disagrees with the decision made by the student. The student in the pressure seat then chooses another student to take his or her place until each group member has had a chance to sit in the pressure seat.

Materials Needed: chairs to form a circle

Processing Questions:

1. What are the five refusal steps?
2. What are some things that might occur if you are unable to effectively deal with peer pressure?
3. How did you feel about the decisions you made in the "pressure seat"?

Emotional Musical Chairs

Valued Outcome: The students will be able to associate emotions with facial expressions.

Description of Strategy: Students will discuss specific feelings they have had on specific occasions. Tell the students that everyone's feelings are important and should be respected. The students will participate in a game of musical chairs. Chairs are arranged in the same way as for the traditional game, however, no additional chairs will be removed during the game. Before the game, place pictures, each with a face showing a different emotion, in a box. Children will move around the chairs as the music plays and try to find a place to sit when the music stops. The child without a chair will draw a picture out of the box and show it to the other children. The child will then tell what emotion he or she thinks the person in the picture is feeling. All of the children will then tell what emotion he or she thinks the person in the picture is feeling. All the chil-

dren will then make faces and act out the emotion until the music starts again. The game will continue until all the emotions in the box have been acted out.
Materials Needed: chairs, pictures of faces showing different emotions, box, music player, music
Processing Questions:

1. What are some of the ways you express your emotions?
2. When do you share your feelings or emotions with others?
3. Discuss a time when you made someone else happy, sad, angry, and so on.

How to Handle Peer Pressure

Valued Outcome: Each student will be able to list two positive characteristics about him- or herself.
Description of Strategy: The teacher will solicit responses to the following questions:

1. Name a situation in which you were influenced by your friends in a decision you made.
2. Why do you think friends are able to persuade you to do things you know are wrong?
3. Why is it important to avoid the negative influence of your friends?
4. How can being influenced by your friends be dangerous to yourself and others? Give specific examples.
5. What are some positive ways peers can influence one another?
6. What is unique about you?
7. List four characteristics of your two closest friends.
8. List two physical and two personality characteristics of your two closest friends and discuss.

Emphasize the need for accepting who you are and being proud of your decisions.
Materials Needed: none
Processing Questions:

1. Why do we sometimes give in to peer pressure?
2. How are each of us different?
3. What are some dangers of peer pressure?

State of Mind

Valued Outcome: The students will be able to differentiate between positive and negative ways to express emotions.
Description of Strategy: Ask students to share with the class specific times when they felt happy, sad, mad, or some other strong emotion. Ask students to also share how they acted when they felt these emotions. Hand out copies of "Goofus and Gallant," a *Highlights* magazine cartoon series depicting two young boys, one who acts bad and one who acts good. The class will discuss why they think Goofus and Gallant acted as they did. Ask, "What will be the consequences of the good action?" Also call for a discussion of consequences of the bad action.
Materials Needed: photocopy of cartoon
Processing Questions:

1. Why is sharing our emotions with others so important?

2. Give an example of healthy ways to handle anger.

3. Give an example of unhealthy ways to handle anger.

Who Am I?

Valued Outcome: Each student will be able to identify and discuss unique qualities of his or her own and of others.
Description of Strategy: Lead a discussion emphasizing the uniqueness of every individual. Students will receive a worksheet to fill out about themselves. The teacher will then read one aloud and the students will guess who it is about.
Materials Needed: "Who am I?" worksheet
Processing Questions:

1. What does it mean to have a unique quality?

2. Will people have some different qualities even if they seem just alike? Explain.

3. What makes each person different?

Who Am I?

Listed below are several questions. After you are through we will share with the class to see if we can guess each others' identity.

1. My two favorite things to do are_____

2. My favorite food is_____

3. My favorite TV program is _____

4. My best subject in school is _____

5. I like best about myself _____

6. Friends should _____

7. If I could change one thing about me it would be _____

8. I am special because _____

9. I have brothers/sisters _____

10. My favorite activity is _____

11. Three words I would use to describe myself _____

Unique! That's Me!

Valued Outcome: Each student will be able to identify two ways in which he or she is unique in relationship to his or her classmates.

Description of Strategy: Ask students to discuss ways in which individuals are unique. The students will play a voice-guessing game to show how everything about a person, even the voice, is unique and special. A student will sing the words, "Voices never are the same. Can you guess what is my name?" to the tune of "Twinkle, Twinkle, Little Star." The rest of the class, with eyes closed, will raise their hands to guess the voice. Repeat the activity until everyone has had a turn to sing with students relocating around the room after each turn. Students will then examine their fingers and those of their classmates with a magnifying glass. Students will then be given fingerpaint ink and will make a thumb print on a paper star to be worn on their clothing.

Materials Needed: poster with song words, magnifying glasses, fingerpaint or ink, paper stars, safety pins for name tags

Processing Questions:

1. What does the word *unique* mean?

2. Is it good or bad to be unique? Explain.

3. In what ways are you a unique person?

Coping with and Controlling Stress

Valued Outcome: The students will be able to assess their stress level and use relaxation and self-management techniques in response to stressful situations.

Description of Strategy: Students will list three things they find stressful and want to discuss. List responses on the board. Ask, "Why are peer pressure, grades, and the need for acceptance such common stressors?" Lead a discussion on effectively dealing with these stressors, and explain the following techniques for handling stressful situations: quiet reflection, biofeedback, progressive muscle relaxation, and visualization. Students will then take a stress test to determine their current level of stress. Explain to students that they are to maintain a daily journal listing all stressful situations they encounter, how they react, and if there could be a better way to handle the stressor.

Materials Needed: stress test, paper and pencils for journal

Processing Questions:

1. What areas of your life create the most stress for you?

2. Describe one effective way of handling a stressor.

3. What are some advantages and disadvantages of stress?

Musical Compliments

Valued Outcome: Each student will be able to write positive statements about other students and will describe feelings in response to positive statements made about her or him.

Description of Strategy: Lead a discussion about self-esteem, asking the following questions:

1. How does it make you feel when someone says something nice about you?

2. Do you make it a point to compliment people when they do something good?

3. Do you try to note the good things about a person, even when there are things about them that you dislike?

4. Have you ever thought about your own good qualities and why people like to be around you?

Give each student a piece of paper cut into one of various shapes, such as a child, a musical note, or a heart. Have students write their names on the cutout they receive and pass them around the room while you play music. When the music stops, each child will write something positive about the person whose cutout they receive. Continue this until the students have written on several different cutouts. Give students a few minutes to sit quietly and read the comments written about them. Then ask students to write a paragraph telling how this activity made them feel.
Materials Needed: cutouts, markers, tape or record and player
Processing Questions:

1. Which comment on your card made you feel particularly special, and why?

2. How did it make you feel to write something nice about someone else?

3. Give an example of a compliment.

Emotions and Me

Valued Outcome: The students will be able to match facial expressions with emotions, identify emotions associated with specific situations, and discuss reasons for having specific feelings.
Description of Strategy: Ask who in the class is happy, sad, or angry, and why. Explain the importance of expressing emotions and understanding behaviors associated with specific emotions. Give students a worksheet showing different faces with different expressions (Figure 9.2). The worksheet will ask the students to match a word from the top of the sheet with its expression. Help students with this, asking what types of situations made the student feel each emotion. Students will then role-play different situations and discuss why the situation made them react the way they did.
Materials Needed: worksheet with faces and emotions, role-playing cards
Processing Questions:

1. What feelings make us feel good inside?

2. What feelings make us feel bad inside?

3. Why is it important to be able to express your feelings?

How Do I See Myself?

Valued Outcome: Each student will be able to describe and discuss differences and similarities between her- or himself and others.
Description of Strategy: Lead a discussion regarding differences and similarities among individuals, pointing out that many things that are similar have different qualities. For example, fruit includes all fruit, but a pear is not like an apple. Animals have many varieties, as do plants. Give students paper and crayons, and ask them to make their own name tags with drawings of things that describe them.
Materials Needed: visual aids of different fruits, animals, and plants; construction paper; crayons; safety pins for name tags

Figure 9.2

Worksheet for Emotions and Me

Emotions: Under each face, write the name of the emotion shown. The emotions are happiness, sadness, anger, excitement, kindness, and fear.

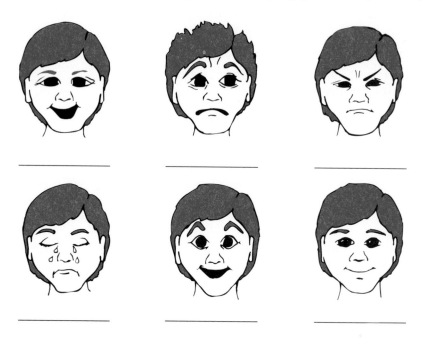

Processing Questions:

1. What are some positive aspects of individual differences?
2. What type of attitude should we have regarding other peoples' differences?
3. In what ways do you treat others the way you would like to be treated?

Self-Esteem

Valued Outcomes:

1. The students will be able to differentiate words and actions that give someone a positive feeling from those that give someone a negative feeling.
2. The students will be able to identify reasons to say no to drinking.
3. The students will be able to name some physiological effects of alcohol.

Description of Strategy: Read the IALAC story to the class. The class will participate by saying RIP every time a negative action affects Lou Ann, and a student will tear off a piece of her badge. When an action or word gives Lou Ann a positive feeling, the student will reattach a piece of the torn-off badge. Discuss the influence of the media on drinking, and explain some physiological effects of drinking.

Materials Needed: IALAC story, "How to Say No to a Drink" handout, Medical Hazards with Alcoholism brochure
Processing Questions:

1. In what ways do negative words and actions from others lower a person's self-esteem?

2. In what ways do positive words and actions from others raise a person's self-esteem?

3. List five good reasons to say no to drinking.

Stress Feelings

Valued Outcomes: The students will be able to define stress, identify five feelings they have that cause stress, and be able to use one breathing exercise to reduce stress.
Description of Strategy: Define stress, and lead students to think of times when stress has affected them. Discuss the advantages and disadvantages of stress. The students will list times when they have felt stress. Ask students to discuss the feelings and physical symptoms they have had in association with stressors. Demonstrate a breathing exercise effective in reducing stress. Have students keep a record of stressful events that occur at home and bring them back to class for discussion.
Materials Needed: poster showing common symptoms of stress for fifth graders, worksheets
Processing Questions:

1. Name two physical symptoms of stress.

2. Name two feelings that might be associated with stress.

3. Describe the breathing exercise demonstrated in class for stress reduction.

My Friends

Valued Outcome: The students will be able to describe qualities of an ideal friend.
Description of Strategy: Lead a discussion emphasizing the importance of having good friends. Students will participate in a game called "Hand Squeeze." Students will sit in a circle holding hands and pass a hand squeeze around the circle.

Ask students to compose an essay that begins with "A friend is someone who. . ." Essays may be placed on a bulletin board with a display about friendship.
Materials Needed: paper, pencils
Processing Questions:

1. Why does everyone need a friend?

2. What are some ways you can be a better friend?

3. What is a good way to initiate a friendship?

"Me" Poster

Valued Outcome: Each student will be able to identify personal interests, characteristics, relationships, goals, and other important aspects of his or her life.
Description of Strategy: The student will draw, bring in pictures, or write about their lives. They will then place items—possibly including baby pictures, birthday pictures, a list of future goals,

family members' pictures, or other important mementoes—on a poster to be displayed in the classroom. Set aside class time for the children to tell about their posters.

Materials Needed: glue, scissors, poster boards, essays, drawings, magazines, personal mementoes

Processing Questions:

1. Which things in your life make you feel proudest?
2. What has been the most important event in your life and why?
3. Who are the most important people in your life and why?

Facial Forecasts

Valued Outcome: The students will be able to identify signs, symptoms, and causes of stress and be able to describe effective coping mechanisms and resources for dealing with stress.

Description of Strategy: Lead a discussion about stress, including information dealing with signs, symptoms, and causes of stress. Students will use a mirror to observe their own facial expressions when they are under stress. Pass out paper plates and markers or crayons so they can draw their impressions of themselves under stress.

Materials Needed: photocopied pages of common stressors among children, danger signs of stress, ways of coping with stress, mirror, paper plates, markers, crayons

Processing Questions:

1. What are some signs of stress?
2. What is one thing you can do when faced with a stressor?
3. Who are people you can talk to about stressful events in your life?

Internet/WWW Activities

Valued Outcome: The students will investigate the Internet for information available on stress, mental health, or suicide among youth.

Description of Strategy: The student will conduct a search of the Internet for the topics that fall under the area of mental health and stress reduction. The teacher should review potential URLs (websites) for appropriateness for age group. Emphasize critical evaluation of the material found.

Processing Questions:

1. Was the information found good for your age group? Why or why not?
2. What is important for you to remember concerning your findings on the topic?

Resources

Books

Johnson, M. D. 1996. *Caring, sharing and getting along.* Santa Cruz, CA; ETR Associates.

Quirez, H. C. 1997. *Think, choose, act, healthy.* Santa Cruz, CA: ETR Associates.

Rice, P. L. 1992. *Stress and health.* Monterey, CA: Brooks/Cole.

Tillman, K. G., and P. R. Toner. 1990. *How to survive teaching health.* West Nyack, NY: Parker.

Pamphlets

Feeling Great! Self-Esteem for Kids (grades 4–6). Santa Cruz, CA: ETR Associates.
Encourages positive attitude and explains that a positive attitude is essential for believing in oneself.

Our Children's Self-Esteem—Thoughts for Parents and Teachers, Santa Cruz, CA: ETR Associates.
Provides important information about self-esteem and how it relates to children's abilities to develop a positive self-identity.

Internet/WWW, URLs

Mental Health:
http://www.apa.org

General Health Information:
http://www.yahoo.com/health

General Health Information:
http://www.ama-assn.org

General Health Information:
http://www.gen.emory.edu/medweb/medweb.consumer.html

Videos

Everybody makes mistakes (K–2).
Helps children understand that everyone makes mistakes. Helps students to see that you can learn from a mistake and that mistakes can be corrected. Sixteen-minute video available from Sunburst Communications, 101 Castleton Street, Pleasantville, NY 10570-0040.

I'm telling—A tattler's tale (K–2).
Helps children understand the difference between appropriate telling and inappropriate tattling. Fourteen-minute video available from Sunburst Communications, 101 Castleton Street, Pleasantville, NY 10570-0040.

I know how to listen (Pre-K–2).
Introduces children to paying attention, asking questions and listening for feelings at school, home, and at play. Fifteen-minute video available from Sunburst Communications, 101 Castleton Street, Pleasantville, NY 10570-0040.

Anger, rage, and you (grades 5–9).
Teaches students how to deal with anger before it gets out of control. Helps the student to identify and handle misplaced and suppressed anger. Twenty-three-minute video available from Sunburst Communicatins, 101 Castleton Street, Pleasantville, NY 10570-0040.

Kids and stress (grades 5–8).
Video looks at how stress affects kids. Discuss eating and sleeping disturbances, drug and alcohol use, mental illness, depression, and suicide. Twenty-eight-minute video available from Films for the Humanities and Sciences, P. O. Box 2053, Princeton, NJ 08543-2053.

Chapter Ten

Sexuality Education

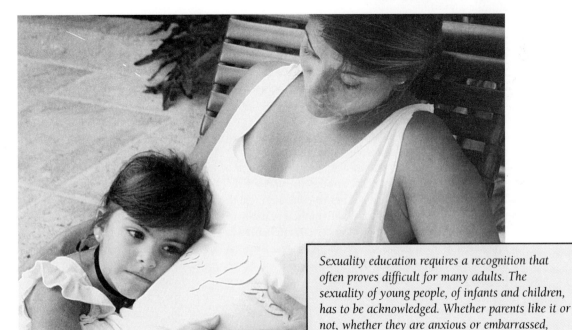

> Sexuality education requires a recognition that often proves difficult for many adults. The sexuality of young people, of infants and children, has to be acknowledged. Whether parents like it or not, whether they are anxious or embarrassed, their sons and daughters will learn about and experience sex.
>
> —Haas and Haas (1993)

Valued Outcomes

After reading this chapter, you should be able to

- ○ identify the goals of a sexuality education program
- ○ discuss the social aspects of sexuality and family living
- ○ discuss marriage, parenthood, and divorce
- ○ trace the psychological development of sexuality
- ○ describe the anatomy and physiology of the male and female reproductive systems
- ○ explain the problems of family abuse and violence

Sexuality education is among the most controversial areas facing teachers. Many people view inclusion of this subject as an attempt to teach sexual technique and lower the morals of today's youth. Based on these concepts, family life education would involve little more than teaching the act of coitus. Family life education does deal with sexuality, but this is not the same thing as sex. Sexuality involves one's total being and identity. An effective sexuality education program seeks to develop an individual's sexuality, which includes an appreciation for self and the opposite sex, the ability to develop fulfilling personal and family relationships, comfort with sexual roles (mother, father, sister, brother, friend, wife, husband), recognition of bodily functions as related to reproduction, understanding how emotions play a part in sexual behavior, maturing attitudes toward the function of sex in life, the responsibility of being a member of a family, and overall, a healthy attitude toward life.

The primary responsibility for teaching facts, attitudes, and values about sexuality should remain with the parents. However, there is frequently a gap between the education children receive about family life in their homes and their level of questioning, need, and interest. School is not the only source of information outside the home. Churches and other organizations can contribute significantly in this area. The school is an increasingly important contributor to education about family life. Before family life curriculum can be taught, parental approval must be obtained. Most communities will support such a program if the school administration and community understand what is to be taught. This is the most important first step, which cannot be ignored if sexuality education is to be successful.

The appreciation for self must start early in life and be built on each year if children are to feel comfortable with their sexuality through the preadolescent, adolescent, and adult years. As should be emphasized in all aspects of health education, children must recognize that they will eventually have to accept the responsibility of their sexuality.

If society is not willing to promote comprehensive sexuality education, then that component of a student's total being will be shortchanged. Personal and social problems such as unwanted pregnancies, sexually transmitted diseases, sexual unresponsiveness, and divorce will continue to plague society. A worthwhile educational effort in sexuality and family life must include social, psychological, moral, and biological components. In this chapter, these areas of concern are examined while providing the necessary overview of content for teaching sexuality education.

Implications for Sexuality Education

Few subjects in society evoke more discussion and controversy than sexuality education courses taught in our schools. It is amazing that one of the most significant aspects of our being is such a taboo topic. Humans are sexual from the moment they are born until well into old age. The adage that we are sexual beings from womb to tomb is certainly true. Although humans have learned a great deal about sexuality that can be taught in the educational process, we seek to repress and hide sex information and avoid discussing sexuality with our children. The mind-set of many people is that it is better to ignore problem pregnancies, the increasing rate of STDs, and the many misconceptions of the nation's youth.

There are groups opposed to sexuality education because they think the less adolescents know about sex the less likely they are to become involved. However, research has indicated that informing children concerning sexual matters has actually decreased premature and irresponsible sexual behavior. Some of the national groups opposed to teaching sexuality education are the American Family Association, American Life League, Concerned Women for American Life, Eagle Forum, and the National Association for Abstinence Education (Haffner and deMauro 1991).

It is important that a positive self-image be developed if children are to grow to adulthood with the ability to respect others.

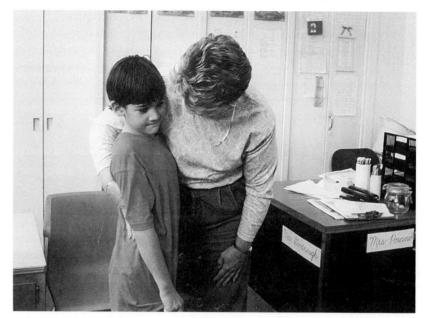

Parents greatly influence the views their children hold concerning sexuality. Parents provide the young child with a basic orientation by the verbal and nonverbal messages they send concerning nudity, masturbation, sex values, and so on. If the message is that sex is shocking, dirty, or disgusting, this is transmitted to the child. These types of messages are likely to interfere with enjoyable healthy sexuality in the adult years. It is important to note that when children learn about sex and sexuality from their parents, the information is more likely to be accurate and positive than that learned from peers. Children are more likely to view sex as "dirty" or something to be "ashamed of" if learned from peers. Research indicates that adolescents who report good communication with parents are more likely to use contraception than those adolescents who report poor communication. In addition, adolescents who receive sex education from their parents are more likely to behave in ways consistent with their knowledge.

One of the current dilemmas facing educators and schools is the teaching of abstinence versus responsibility. In question is whether schools should approach sexuality education from the perspective that all sexual problems can be avoided if students remain sexually abstinent, or if a more pragmatic approach should be followed, acknowledging that young people are going to be sexually active and that issues associated with such activity need to be discussed so sexual responsibility can be advocated. This latter approach fits well with the wellness approach and self-responsibility. However, since the early 1980s a variety of abstinence education programs have been adopted by several states. In these curricula, students are taught chastity is the only answer and that premarital sex can only lead to disease, pregnancy, and emotional turmoil. Opponents of such an approach point out that such views can cause extremely negative concepts concerning sex. In addition, issues such as preventing pregnancy, HIV, and other STDs are not discussed in abstinence programs. Omitting such information from sexuality education is actually dangerous to the welfare of students. Most educators favor a middle position on teaching sexuality education: Abstinence is encouraged, but with the realization that students do have premarital intercourse and that they do need to be informed and responsible for protecting themselves from unwanted pregnancies and possible infection with HIV or some other STD (sexually transmitted disease).

Sexuality education must include a open learning atmosphere, improved materials, and improved training of educators. In addition, the curricular planning process, the implementation of the curriculum, training of the teachers, audiovisual materials should all be open to parents/community for inspection and evaluation.

Teaching Sexuality Education

Teaching sexuality is different from yet has aspects in common with teaching any other subject. Like all teaching, sexuality education requires teachers who have effective communication skills; empathize with their students; understand the needs, interests, and characteristics of the various age levels; and believe in the need to develop the critical thinking skills of students. In addition, effective sexuality educators must be comfortable with their own sexuality and be able to overcome any embarrassment or self-consciousness they may feel. Another aspect of being an effective sexuality educator is using appropriate terminology. Kilander pointed out twenty years ago that using acceptable terminology helps children learn to respect their bodies, helps prevent negative connotations for body parts and functions, provides a common vocabulary for children, and makes children more comfortable when asking questions (Kilander 1968).

The acceptance of any program must involve the community in the planning process. People are more comfortable if they have opportunities to give input and to view the actual content, materials and activities associated with the curriculum. Successful sexuality programs were found to have a high degree of parental involvement, administrative efforts at teacher training, a cooperative relationship between a school and a family planning agency, and strong support from the school board (Scales 1984). However, the value system taught to each child should come from the family. The attitudes the students reflect are still the responsibility of the family to instill. The school can impact the student by providing knowledge, decision-making training, and opportunities for examining sexuality issues in a nonthreatening environment. At their best, family life programs in the school can strive to help students recognize and have insight into their own values. Their actual values should be drawn from the family and the institutions most important in their lives, such as the church or synagogue. What is important to remember concerning sexuality education is that even though opponents have received a lot of attention, most Americans support such education in the schools. As teachers we must take a stand for sexuality education and strive to make sure what students receive in the classroom is balanced and accurate. As Susan Spalt has suggested, every school professional should repeat the Serenity Prayer of Alcoholics Anonymous (Spalt 1996): "God grant the serenity to accept what I cannot change, the courage to change what I can, and the wisdom to know the difference."

Any teachers who teach in the sexuality education program at any level need to train in that area. Teachers also need to be objective concerning controversial issues and have the ability to appreciate the views of others. Of course, a sense of humor helps, as well as feelings of comfort with one's own sexuality. Finally, they need a broad base of knowledge concerning the biological, psychological, and social aspects of human sexuality (Byer and Shainberg 1994, 422).

If a school district does not have a curriculum or is considering a change in sexuality curriculum, an excellent source is *Sexuality Education Curricula: The Consumer's Guide*. This publication helps educators determine what is available in school-based sexuality curricula, provides evaluations of each curriculum by leading sexuality educators, and provides criteria with which local curriculum developer/evaluators can evaluate the various programs under consideration (Ogletree et al. 1994).

Health Highlight

A Sample Letter to Parents

Dear Parent/Guardian:

Our school is developing a program in family living, including sex education, following the guidelines recommended by the Steuben County Board of Education. Selected teachers have been trained in the program. The philosophy of the program stresses

○ the awareness and importance of family, religious, and moral values in making personal decisions

○ understanding the need for consideration, love, respect, and responsibility in family life

○ recognition of responsibilities to the school, the community and society

We recognize that you, as parents, have the major responsibility for the formation of desirable attitudes toward family living and sex education. The role of the school is to support your efforts. We have the professional resources to create a comprehensive, sequential, and up-to-date program that will assist your child in developing these important life attitudes. The course contents, books, and audiovisuals for this program have been carefully screened. Every effort is being made to meet the varied needs and interests of our children.

We invite you to join with us in developing our school program. Our first parent workshop has been scheduled for_____(date) at _____(time) in room_____. You are invited to review our course of study and the instructional materials. You are also welcome at any time to discuss this program with me.

Your interest and cooperation, as evidenced by the return of the tear-off form below, is very valuable to us. The response form also allows you the option of having your child excused from the program.

Sincerely,

Principal

_____

Please return to _____(school name) on or before_____(date).

_____I would like to have my child excused from the Sexuality Education program.

_____I can attend the parent workshop.

_____I cannot attend the parent workshop.

I would like an appointment to speak with _____my child's teacher   _____the principal

Parent/Guardian Signature:

_____   Date_____

Concepts to Be Taught in Sexuality Education —————————

Bruess and Greenberg (1994, 264–265) suggest that the following topics and concepts be taught in preschool through the upper elementary grades.

Preschool Sexuality Education

Preschool sexuality education should include

○ a recognition of the roles of family members
○ a recognition of the authority and concern of parents and others responsible for the care of preschool children
○ opportunities to make friends with children of both sexes
○ ways to cooperate with family members and others in work and play
○ an understanding that living things grow, may reproduce, and die
○ consideration of the behavior of babies

Early Elementary Grades

The concepts taught at the early elementary level will help prepare the students for materials taught in the upper elementary grades.

○ the basics of plant and animal (including human) reproduction
○ the similarities and differences in males and females
○ growth and development (physical changes and emotional feelings)
○ family roles and responsibilities
○ discussions of individual feelings about oneself and other people
○ an introduction to HIV/AIDS

Upper Elementary Grades

The emphasis in the upper elementary grades is predicated on the information presented in the preschool and early elementary years.

○ Biological information in greater depth
  ○ the endocrine system
  ○ menstruation
  ○ birth and pregnancy
  ○ nocturnal emissions
  ○ masturbation
  ○ body size differences (temporary and permanent)

- ○ response to sexual stimulation (contact, pictures, and reading)
- ○ birth control and abortion
- ○ physical abnormalities (this subject may seem peculiar, but at this age children are often hung up on the unusual rather than the usual)
- ○ Appropriate facts about HIV/AIDS

- ○ Interpersonal relations

  - ○ heterosexual feelings
  - ○ homosexual feelings
  - ○ how emotions affect body functions
  - ○ changing family responsibilities and privileges
  - ○ the need to use different approaches with different people
  - ○ different male and female feelings
  - ○ why brothers and sisters (mothers and fathers) fight

- ○ Self-concept

  - ○ how do people react to me?
  - ○ what kind of person am I?
  - ○ how do I feel about myself?
  - ○ why do people like me sometimes and not other times?
  - ○ why do I hate people sometimes?

Page and Page (1993, 135) have made similar recommendations concerning grade-level goals. They believe that the primary focus at kindergarten through third grade is to alleviate the children's fear of AIDS and to establish a foundation for discussion of sexuality in the upper grades. Their recommendations are

Grades K–3

- ○ Include information about AIDS in the larger curriculum on body appreciation, wellness, sickness, friendships, assertiveness, family roles, and different types of families.
- ○ Encourage children to feel positively about their questions about their bodies and to know their body parts and the differences between girls and boys. Teachers should answer their questions about how babies are developed and born.
- ○ Define AIDS simply as a very serious disease. Students should be told that young children rarely get it and that they do not need to worry about playing with children whose parents have AIDS or with those few children who have the disease.
- ○ Caution children never to play with hypodermic syringes found on playgrounds or elsewhere and to avoid contact with other people's blood.
- ○ Answer questions directly and simply; limit responses to questions asked.
- ○ Teach children assertiveness about refusing unwanted touch by others, including family members.

Health Highlight

Concepts and Topics in a Comprehensive Sexuality Education Program

Listed below are the main concepts and topics

Key Concept 1: Human Development

Reproductive anatomy and physiology

Reproduction

Puberty

Body image

Sexual identity and orientation

Key Concept 2: Relationships

Families

Friendship

Love

Dating

Marriage and lifetime commitments

Parenting

Key Concept 3: Personal Skills

Values

Key Concept 4: Sexual Behavior

Sexuality throughout life

Masturbation

Shared sexual behavior

Abstinence

Human sexual response

Fantasy

Sexual dysfunction

Key Concept 5: Sexual Health

Contraception

Abortion

STDs and HIV infection

Sexual abuse

Reproductive health

Key Concept 6: Society and Culture

Sexuality and society

Decision making

Communication

Assertiveness

Negotiation

Finding help

Gender roles

Sexuality and the law

Sexuality and religion

Diversity

Sexuality and the arts

Sexuality and the media

Source: Guidelines for Comprehensive Sexuality Education, 1991. New York: Sex Information and Education Council of the United States.

Grades 4 and 5

The same approach as for grades K–3, with emphasis on

○ affirming that bodies have natural sexual feelings

○ helping children examine and affirm their own families' values

○ providing basic information about human sexuality, helping children understand puberty and the changes in their bodies

○ answering questions about AIDS and AIDS prevention

Social Aspects of Sexuality and Family Living

Various cultural, historical, legal, religious, and other institutional factors influence families and the sexuality roles within the family. It is important to remember that many forms of the family can be found. With this in mind, some typical characteristics of the family will be examined.

Types of Families

The family fulfills a most important role in providing stability for the individual and society. The term *family* is used to describe two or more people living together who are related by blood, marriage, or adoption (Eshleman 1988). A *nuclear family* might be composed of a husband and wife, a brother and sister, one parent and a child or children, or both parents and one or more children. An *extended family* consists of a number of nuclear family groupings, often with blood ties. Extended family members can include uncles, aunts, grandparents, or cousins.

Because most people marry, they will be part of at least two different nuclear families, one in which they are born and one they start after selecting a marriage partner (see Figure 10.1). The nuclear family to which we are born is the first and most basic provider of socialization. The extended family also has an influence on our socialization.

The Changing Nature of the American Family

American youngsters in past generations generally grew up in one city or town, married someone from the surrounding area, and lived in the immediate locality. Chances were that members of the extended family, such as aunts, uncles, and grandparents, lived in the area also. In today's society, the nuclear family may be intact, but chances are that the extended family is not. For example, parents and grandparents may live in widely separate locations. As a result, grandparents may visit only on holidays or other special occasions. Thus, the interaction between these family members is not as frequent as in the past. The mobility of today's society and frequent job changes or transfers have served to separate the nuclear family from the extended family.

The advent, sometimes of necessity, of two-career households has brought about several changes as well. Families tend to have fewer children, and the care of the children may be left to day care centers or other individuals who are not family members. Consequently, children may come in contact with caretakers of various ages who influence the social/psychological and value system development of the child.

Divorce may also change children's perspectives and the roles and responsibilities they have to handle. Currently, one out of every five children lives with one parent, 90 percent with the mother. It has been estimated that by the end of this century, 50 percent of all children under the age of eighteen will have spent some time in a female-parent-only situation (U.S. Bureau of the Census 1988). It has been predicted that divorce leads to a significant increase in sexual problems, juvenile delinquency, and emotional and psychological maladjustment (Haas and Haas 1993, 320). See Chapter 8 on additional effects of divorce.

Technology has influenced the family. Easy access to transportation has enabled people to move throughout the country quite easily. Sometimes this has led to family members engaging in activities as individuals rather than as a unit. Television and other media have presented a variety of social values to children. In the past, the value system an individual initially accepted was a combination of beliefs fostered by the church, family, and school. Now, young people can witness a whole spectrum of values in a relatively short period of time by viewing, listening, or reading.

Individuals become socially, morally, and psychologically influenced by all the factors just described. Understanding the world is perhaps more difficult than ever before because of these transitions and because of a barrage of mixed signals. No wonder, then, that many young people are confused about their roles in society and the expectations of society.

The family is changing. However, it seems that people will always need others to whom they are bonded through closeness, sharing, and love. Such factors as the dual-career family, where both the father and the mother share child-rearing and household responsibilities, have required adjustments to the family model of the past. And divorce, separation, and death have made single-parent families very common today. Because the stigma of divorce is not as great as it once was and more opportunities exist for women to work, couples who in the past stayed together, often unhappily, now have the option of divorcing. An interesting aspect of divorce is that the fastest growing type of single-parent family is the male-headed household. Another outgrowth of divorce is the blended family, which brings together children from previous marriages. When divorced parents remarry, blending the children may well be the largest problem they need to overcome.

Another interesting change in family structure is the return of adults to the home of their parents because of divorce and/or lack of job opportunities. These adults are referred to as *boomerang children*, because they left the household once but now return to live with their parents. Situations where children return to the parents' home having once left can cause adjustment problems for all parties concerned. Issues of financial responsibility, privacy, and household responsibilities are all important.

Figure 10.1

U.S. Rates of Marriage, Divorce, and Remarriage

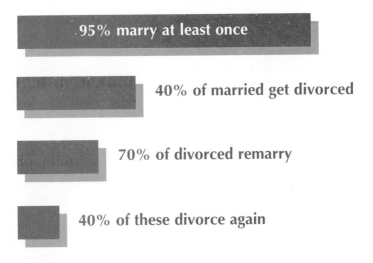

95% marry at least once

40% of married get divorced

70% of divorced remarry

40% of these divorce again

Another issue of the family is the growing elderly population. As family members live longer, caregiving for the elderly often falls to the family. In two-career families, this can create financial, as well as career-related challenges.

Even with the problems and issues facing families today, couples continue to marry, remarry, and have children. Whatever problems are faced by the family, the desire to give love, share love, and be a part of the family unit will continue to perpetuate the family.

Concepts of Love and Family

Children can discuss what they like in friends and begin to realize that the person they choose to spend their life with is a very important decision. Some concepts to discuss in relationship to family life are love and intimacy, courtship and marriage, parenthood, single parenthood, and divorce.

Love and Intimacy

From the socialization process, we learn that we are supposed to form relationships and "fall in love." Attempting to define love is a most difficult task. Love has been defined as "that condition in which happiness of another person is essential to your own" (Heinlein 1961, 345). This highly romantic definition of love can be seen in the popular songs we listen to, the scenario of Romeo and Juliet, and the reason Edward VIII left the throne to marry Mrs. Simpson. Certainly, the element of caring must be present. Without caring, what is thought to be love may be strong desire. The problem is determining what love really is. Erich Fromm wrote that caring and respect for another is central to love and that people can achieve a meaningful type of love only after they are secure in their own identity. Fromm goes on to define mature love as "union under the condition of preserving one's integrity, one's individuality" (1956, 17). Fromm suggests that a lover must feel, "I want the loved person to grow and unfold for his own sake and in his own ways, and not for the purpose of serving me" (1956, 24).

The English language is limited in that only one word is available to describe a wide variety of feelings and relationships called love. The ancient Greeks had several terms to describe more precisely the different kinds of love. *Eros* referred to passionate or erotic love. *Storge* meant affection such as the feelings parents have for their children. *Philia* indicated the type of love in friendships, and *agape* referred to a kind of love associated with the traditional Christian view of being undemanding, patient, kind, and always supportive. In our society, love has been defined in terms of romantic, rational, and mature love. Romantic love is an intense emotional experience that can totally captivate our existence. Another type of love is rational love, which is based on acceptance of the partner's imperfections as well as affections and is more likely to lead to fulfilling, long-lasting relationships. Mature love is maintained through communication and separateness of the partners. It involves respect, admiration, and the desire to help each other. Lovers who exhibit maturity in their relationship are best friends who are committed to each other and their relationship.

To help deal with the concept of love, Coutts (1973) has described five levels of love. The first is called *sentimentality*, which centers on one's own feelings, needs, fears, and insecurities. If people remain at this level, they become insensitive and exploitative in their relationships. The second level is *awareness*. Sharing and caring develop mutually between the partners, and an intimacy emerges based on facts, not impressions. The third level is *involvement*, in which the partner sees what is needed and works very hard at offering the support. The fourth level is *dedication*, in which the partners are willing to make sacrifices of their needs, safety, and comfort. The fifth level of loving is *commitment*. This is the most powerful of all love relationships. It encompasses intellect, emotions, body, lasting awareness, and involvement. As difficult as love is to define and identify, perhaps it will help to pose several questions to help distinguish between healthy and problematic love (Peele and Brodsky 1976, 83–84):

1. Do both lovers have a secure belief in their own value?
2. Are the lovers improved by the relationship?
3. Do the lovers maintain serious interests outside the relationship, including other meaningful personal relationships?
4. Is the relationship integrated into, rather than being set off from, the totality of the lovers' lives?
5. Are the lovers beyond being possessive or jealous of each other's growth and expansion of interest?
6. Are the lovers also friends? Would they seek each other out if they should cease to be primary partners?

As love develops, so does intimacy. Like love, intimacy needs time to develop and goes through several stages (Calderone 1972). Those stages are

1. *Choice:* Two people meet; they like each other and begin to become closer.
2. *Mutual:* Their desire for closeness is mutually shared.
3. *Reciprocity:* They give to each other and grow by confiding in each other. There is an equal sharing of confidences.
4. *Trust:* Their deepest feelings and thoughts are accepted.
5. *Delight:* They have unconditional acceptance of one another and delight in the relationship.

Dating helps in the processes of socialization, personality development, and learning to get along with the opposite sex.

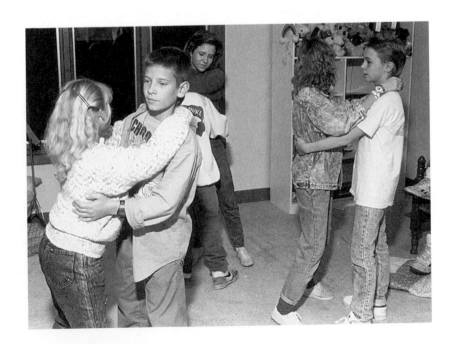

To be intimate means to be vulnerable. It means risking rejection or suffocation of one's self. However, compatible partners replace those risks with trust and satisfaction. Essentially, individuals must remain responsible for themselves yet help each other with their goals, problems, and desires. Enjoying, sharing, and caring should be the outcomes of living with someone with whom love and intimacy are shared.

Why People Marry

People marry for both personal and societal reasons. There is no single reason why people marry. Some marry because they do not want to be alone. They want someone to share confidences, and they want to give and receive affection. A happy marriage can offer intimacy, sharing, support, and stimulation for personal growth.

Some people marry for economic reasons. For example, they may wish to pool their incomes, or the husband may provide financial security to the wife and children, while the wife runs the home and cares for the children. Most people marry because they enjoy a person and can depend on that person in times of need. Marriage theoretically provides someone to share both joy and sorrow.

Marriage serves many functions for individuals, including establishment of a family, companionship, economic strength, emotional security, a sexual outlet, and children. The greater the success in meeting these needs, the greater the likelihood the marriage will remain intact. Because each year more than two million marriages take place in the United States, it seems safe to say that marriages exist to fulfill basic needs associated with the husband–wife relationship. For these individual needs to be met, each partner must be committed to the marriage, develop effective communication, and accept the responsibility to nurture and enhance the marriage.

Parenthood

When children enter a family, couples must assume new roles. The wife must become a mother and the husband a father. The exclusive attention of the partners toward each other as well as the time demands and interests of the couple must change. Parenthood is a most difficult task, yet couples are expected to fulfill this role automatically with little or no formal training. Parenthood is a lifetime commitment. Individuals can quit their jobs or divorce their mate, but there is no honorable way to withdraw from the role of father or mother. Many groups are now teaching parenthood education programs that promote parenting skills. These courses attempt to teach ways to facilitate communication between parents and children, improve methods of discipline, and develop appropriate behavior for parents and children.

Advantages and Disadvantages of Parenthood

The obvious advantage of parenthood is the opportunity to love and nurture another human being. The psychological pleasure from being part of a loving family and helping to direct its development can bring a couple closer together, with the long-term benefit of pride in having done so. Beside the extreme economic cost of having and raising children, parenthood usually requires an adjustment in the career of at least one of the partners. Further, a child takes away from the emotional sharing time of the couple. Much time is spent in guiding and showing affection to the child. Some personal activities must be changed or eliminated, and there is a constant need to transport the children to and from various activities and functions as they become older.

One of the greatest joys of parenthood is the opportunity to love and nurture another human being.

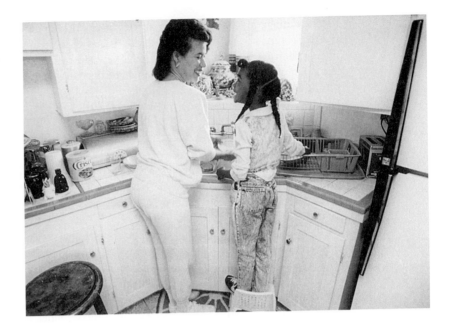

Single Parenthood

Parenthood is difficult when two partners share the nurturing and love that children require. It can become even more difficult if only one parent is present. Through death, desertion, or divorce, single-parent situations often arise. Some individuals cope quite successfully with single parenthood, whereas others struggle with the many roles and situations they face in raising their children.

A single parent may experience various problems. It may be difficult to meet the emotional needs of the child. There are a variety of ways to express love for children. Telling them they are loved and demonstrating that love with quality time serve to express love; however, the demands of working and maintaining a home may be so overwhelming that children's emotional needs may not be met adequately. It also may be hard for the single parent to provide proper supervision for the child. Making arrangements for the child's care and supervision is difficult and costly and may take a large share of the budget. In addition, because women tend to make less money than men, households headed by women can experience financial difficulties. Finally, the single parent may experience unfulfilled emotional and sexual needs. Unmet emotional needs can develop because of the lack of time to seek a relationship. Because most single parents wish to hide their sexual involvement, finding a time and place can present problems. Nevertheless, being a single parent does not have to be a disaster. It is important that single parents have sufficient financial, material, and emotional support to meet their own and their children's demands.

Divorce

The most frequent method for dissolving a marriage is through divorce. In 1992 there were 4.7 divorces per 1,000 people. Since the 1992 marriage rate was 9.4 per 1,000, this means that about half of all marriages are destined to end in divorce (Byer and Shainberg 1994, 450).

Divorce is usually viewed as a failure of the family system as well as a great personal crisis. However, it is also a way to end physical abuse and emotional tension. Personal factors most often given as reasons for divorce include financial problems, physical abuse, mental abuse, drinking, in-law problems, lack of love, adultery, and sexual incompatibility. Divorces can be obtained in most societies. Six social factors that seem to have contributed to the increased divorce rates are

1. *Changing family functions:* Outside sources may now fulfill functions that were once considered primary family responsibilities. These may include medical, religious, and recreational aspects of family life.

2. *Casual marriages:* Hasty and youthful marriages complicated by pregnancy are often unstable.

3. *Jobs for women:* With greater job opportunities available to a large number of women, a great barrier to divorce for many women was removed.

4. *Decline in moral and religious sanctions:* Although not all churches openly state it, most have taken a more liberal attitude toward divorce. Also, society does not attach the severe stigma to divorce that it once did.

5. *The philosophy of happiness:* If happiness does not materialize to the degree anticipated, divorce or separation is accepted as a way of dealing with the feeling.

6. *More liberal divorce laws:* The liberalization of divorce laws, including no-fault divorces, has made it easier to terminate a marriage.

The emotional impact of a divorce is most difficult. Anyone who has experienced a divorce will usually describe it as a painful, devastating experience. Problems with finances, personal adjustment, and children can create an extremely stressful situation. Children whose parents are divorcing may develop deep feelings of guilt, fear, anger, loneliness, and/or sadness. Many times children feel that they must take sides in the conflict, which only serves to enhance their guilt feelings. Because of the emotional conflict between the marriage partners, they may fail to recognize the worry the children feel concerning their own welfare. It is important to remember that despite the family fighting, the children will continue to love both parents. It is extremely important that children have sensitive parents and understanding teachers during and after a divorce. Many children will require counseling, which places an even greater burden on the teacher and school system.

Blended Families

Statistics indicate that about 80 percent of those who divorce will remarry. Many times children from previous marriages find themselves in a stepfamily or blended family situation. The transition and adjustment for both the parents and the children may be difficult. Dealing with sibling jealousy and new rules and striving for affection can put stress on the blended family.

Psychological Aspects of Sexuality and Family Living

Individuals have a wide variety of options for displaying their psychological and physiological traits. Also, in today's society there is greater flexibility in sex roles. This section deals with those psychological aspects of human sexuality and family life that help determine how people feel and react as individuals.

Gender Development

From birth, social expectations largely guide gender development. Parents consciously and unconsciously manipulate their children's gender development from infancy based on the sole criterion of sex. From dress and toys to behavior, the child learns to accept the parameters of being either a girl or a boy. By age two children know what sex they are and understand some of their society's expectations for that sex.

By the time children have reached school age, task orientation and emotional responses are based almost solely on what has been learned about gender. Children's activities are tied to traditional social images of adult roles. Boys are focused on achievement and sports, whereas girls are pointed toward personal beauty or the roles of wives and mothers. This is not to say that girls do not participate in sports or aggressive activities, but these activities are not stressed for girls to the extent they are for boys.

Throughout the school years, the student observes traditional concepts of adult roles. For example, most elementary teachers are female, whereas most administrators are male. Boys typically are encouraged toward achievement, competition, and occupational goals. Girls typically are encouraged toward compliance, dependence, and submissiveness of occupation and position to males.

Gender identification is a most important organizer of expectations and conduct. Society places a great deal of emphasis on socializing and maintaining gender differences. In some cases this process may be beneficial; in others, detrimental to the potential of both boys and girls.

Sex Roles

Since the 1960s, there has been a growing realization that both males and females have a right to expand their individual potential and not be held to traditional roles and stereotypes. Traditional

The family serves an important role by providing stability in the individual and society.

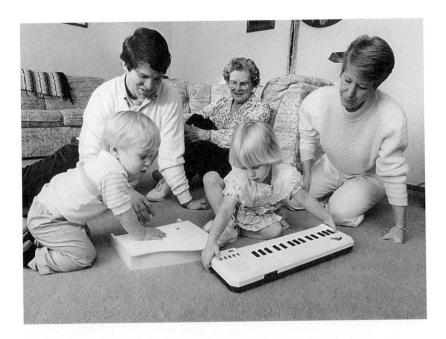

sex roles are learned in the same ways as is gender identity. The emphasis in sex roles should be on the humanness of people, not on their gender. Through such an emphasis, factors that inhibit the complete development of the individual can be discarded. Sharing household duties, child rearing, and economic responsibilities can all contribute to the personal development of both partners. Males need not always be expected to be aggressive, nor females always passive.

Overcoming traditional sex roles is not easy because they are established early in life and are constantly reinforced throughout the years. Self-evaluation and a sense of adequacy are linked to sex role performances as defined by parents and peers in childhood. Some say that sex roles are a natural part of growing and learning. However, it is important not to use "tradition" to psychologically lock people into sex roles that inhibit their growth as individuals.

Developing Sexuality

All aspects of human sexuality develop over a long period of time, from early childhood through the adult years. The groundwork for sexual values begins to develop in infancy, as children learn trust, initiative, and love. As they grow older, children try to achieve self-confidence in their interactions with parents, adults, and peers. Development of self-confidence is crucial to the development of the child's sexuality. If children grow up feeling at ease with themselves, they are more likely to appreciate themselves and members of the opposite sex.

Anything that affects a child's developing identity will eventually affect his or her sexuality as well. If the child learns to be defensive, unforgiving, or mistrusting in daily life, these attitudes will carry over into the sexual component of that individual's personality. Consequently, it is imperative that children learn to give and receive love and have a positive self-image if they are to be at ease with their sexuality later in life.

Biological Components of Sex Education

It is essential for all teachers to have a basic knowledge of the reproductive system and how it works. Obviously all the material presented in this section will not be presented in the elementary classroom, but teachers need the information for their own understanding of the reproductive system.

The Male Reproductive System

The male reproductive system, shown in Figure 10.2, is not as hormonally or endocrinologically complex as that of the female because men do not have sexual cycles. The major male sexual endocrine glands are the two testes, or *testicles*, which are contained and protected in a saclike structure called the *scrotum*. At puberty, the testes begin producing mature *sperm*, the male reproductive cells. Attached to the top of each testis is the *epididymis*. This structure consists of tightly coiled tubes through which the sperm pass to the *vas deferens*. The two vas deferens serve as storage areas for the mature sperm and are the means by which sperm move to the urethra. The two vas deferens eventually form into one structure called the *ejaculatory duct*. This tube connects with the *urethra*. The urethra is a tube that runs the length of the *penis*. The penis is the male organ for sexual intercourse and consists of spongy material called erectile tissue. The head of the penis is called the *glans penis*. This area contains many nerve endings and is very sensitive to sexual stimulation.

Figure 10.2
The Male Reproductive
System

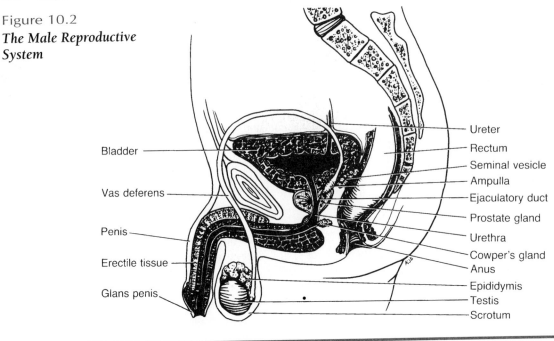

The *seminal vesicles*, the *prostate gland*, and the two *Cowper's glands* manufacture substances important to the sperm and ejaculate. The seminal vesicles produce a simple sugar, fructose, that adds volume to the ejaculatory fluid, called semen, and activates the movement of the sperm. The prostate gland provides a highly alkaline milky fluid that helps neutralize the highly acidic vagina, which facilitates the movement of sperm through that organ. The pea-sized Cowper's glands also produce an alkaline fluid that lubricates and neutralizes the urethra, which is also highly acidic. The Cowper's glands secrete this substance prior to ejaculation. The combined fluid produced by the seminal vesicles, prostate, and Cowper's glands, along with the sperm it contains, is *semen*.

It should be noted that the testes manufacture mature sperm on a consistent basis from puberty through old age. On release of interstitial cell-stimulating hormone (ICSH) into the bloodstream from the anterior lobe of the pituitary, the testes also secrete testosterone. Although it plays many diverse roles, testosterone is needed to trigger the male adolescent growth spurt, which is accompanied by the development of secondary sex characteristics.

The Female Reproductive System

The female reproductive system, shown in Figure 10.3, is composed of the external genitalia and the internal organs consisting of the *vagina, uterus, fallopian tubes,* and *ovaries.* The external genitalia are the *labia majora* (the outer lips) and the *labia minora.* The *clitoris* is a small structure at the top of the labia majora that facilitates sexual stimulation. The *vagina* is an elastic canal extending from just behind the cervix to the opening of the external genitalia. It serves as the organ for sexual intercourse and as the birth canal. The *uterus* is a pear-shaped organ, a cavity where the fetus develops. The uterus has three layers: the *perimetrium* (outer layer), the *myometrium* (muscular layer), and *endometrium* (inner layer). The endometrium is sloughed off during menstrua-

Figure 10.3

*The Female
Reproductive System*

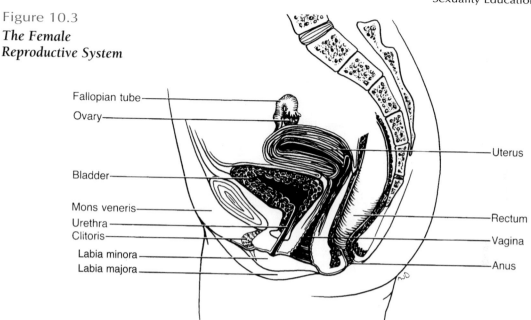

Fallopian tube
Ovary

Bladder

Mons veneris
Urethra
Clitoris
Labia minora
Labia majora

Uterus

Rectum
Vagina
Anus

tion. Two armlike projections called the *fallopian tubes* branch from the uterus. These tubes are three to five inches long and have *fimbria* (small fingerlike projections) at the far ends next to the ovaries. Through these tubes the eggs, or *ova*, pass. If fertilization takes place, it occurs in the upper third of one of the fallopian tubes. Two ovaries produce ova and secrete hormones that bring about the development of the female secondary sex characteristics, such as the rounding of the female figure, breast development, and pubic hair.

Each ovary contains 200,000 to 400,000 saclike structures called *follicles* that store immature egg cells. At the onset of puberty, due to the release of follicle-stimulating hormone (FSH) into the bloodstream from the anterior lobe of the pituitary gland, several follicles are activated in the ovary each month. Only one will evolve into a mature ovum. Simultaneously, estrogen is secreted by the follicle. Estrogen signals the womb, or uterus, to prepare for a potential pregnancy by filling its lining with blood and nutrients for nourishment of the embryo. As the maturing follicle and its ovum move to the surface of the ovary, with the follicle continuing to secrete estrogen, lutenizing hormone (LH), is released into the bloodstream from the anterior lobe of the pituitary. The production of LH causes the follicle to rupture and release the mature ovum into the fallopian tubes. This process is known as *ovulation* and usually occurs midway into the monthly reproductive cycle of twenty-eight days. This cycle is shown in Figure 10.4.

During ovulation, estrogen is at its highest level and causes cessation of additional secretions of FSH. At the same time, LH continues to be secreted and produces closure of the ruptured follicle. The empty follicle, now called the *corpus luteum,* and the mature ovum begin to produce another hormone in addition to estrogen called *progesterone.* Progesterone further prepares the uterus for implantation of a fertilized egg and continues to maintain the uterus during pregnancy. Simultaneously, the levels of estrogen begin to decrease.

From the moment that conception occurs, the woman's body begins to change. Through pregnancy a weight gain of 17 to 24 pounds is normal and looked on as desirable because this helps

Figure 10.4
The Monthly Reproductive Cycle

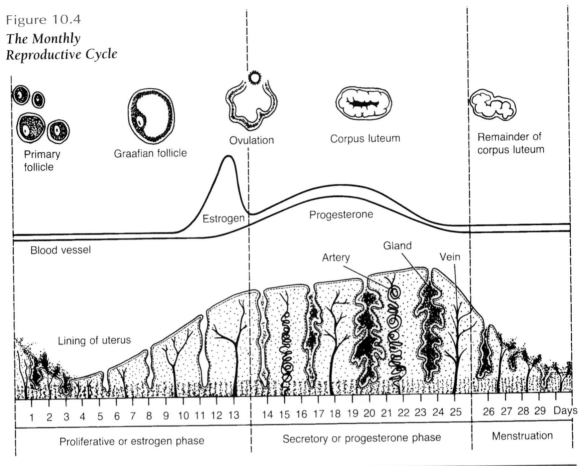

ensure adequate development of the fetus. The average fetus weighs approximately seven pounds at birth. Table 10.1 lists the development of the fetus through each trimester.

If the mature ovum is not fertilized within 24 to 48 hours after ovulation, it disintegrates, thus diminishing the amount of estrogen and progesterone in the bloodstream. Around the twenty-fourth day of the cycle, the corpus luteum also stops secreting progesterone and estrogen. As a result, several days later the uterus expels its blood-rich lining through the vagina. This process is referred to as *menstruation*. Following menstruation, the reproductive cycle begins again in preparation for possible fertilization and pregnancy. Menstruation begins with puberty. The onset of menstruation at this time is called *menarche*.

Conception and Pregnancy

Conception occurs when a single sperm fertilizes an egg to produce a zygote. Conception usually occurs in the upper third of the fallopian tube and must take place in the first or second day following ovulation. When a sperm enters an egg, the membrane thickens to prevent further penetration by sperm. To facilitate conception the sperm go through biochemical changes that enable penetration of the egg. This process is referred to as *capacitation* (Denney and Quadagno 1992, 132).

Table 10.1
*Development during
Pregnancy*

First-trimester development

A small mass of cells is implanted in the uterus.

Development into a fetus begins.

Major organ systems are present and recognizable.

During the fourth to eighth weeks, the eyes, ears, arms, hands, fingers, legs, feet, and toes develop.

By the seventh week, the liver, lungs, pancreas, kidneys, and intestines have formed.

By the end of the first trimester, the fetus weighs two-thirds of an ounce and is about 4 inches in length.

From this time on, development consists of enlargement and differentiation of the existing structures.

Second-trimester development

By the end of the fourteenth week, movement can be detected.

By the eighteenth week, a fetal heartbeat can be detected.

By the twentieth week, the fetus will open its eyes.

Around the twenty-fourth week, the fetus is sensitive to light and can hear sounds. It will also have periods of sleep and wakefulness.

Third-trimester development

Fat deposits form under the skin.

During the seventh month, the fetus turns in the uterus to a head-down position.

By the end of the eighth month, the fetus weighs an average of 5 lb, 4 oz.

At birth, the infant weighs approximately 7.5 lb and is 20 in. long.

Genetics

The human body is made up of trillions of cells that provide for various specialized functions. Each cell contains a nucleus. This nucleus contains genes that provide the hereditary information in smaller rod-shaped bodies called *chromosomes.* Twenty-two pairs of autosomal chromosomes account for individual facial features, hair color, height, body build, and a myriad of other characteristics. Gender is determined by the twenty-third, or sex-determining, chromosomal pair. One member of the pair is called an X chromosome. The other can be either an X or Y chromosome. If two X's pair, a female develops. An XY pairing produces a male offspring.

Mitosis is ordinary cell division. This process results in two new cells that each contain the full complement of forty-six chromosomes. *Meiosis* is the cell division by which sperm and ovum are formed. These cells are called *gametes* and contain only twenty-three chromosomes. When a male gamete (sperm) unites with a female gamete (ovum), the twenty-three pairs unite to determine gender. The ovum always contains the X chromosome, whereas the sperm can have either an X or Y chromosome. If a sperm with a Y chromosome fertilizes the egg, the baby will be a male, or XY.

The Embryonic Period

Immediately after conception, the zygote begins to divide to form other cells. It travels down the fallopian tube and within ten days attaches to the uterine wall. From the time it attaches to the wall until the eighth week, it is called an *embryo*. The embryo divides into three layers of cells from which the various body organs and systems develop. The innermost layer, the *endoderm*, becomes the digestive and respiratory systems; the next layer, the *mesoderm*, forms the skeletal, muscular, circulatory, and reproductive systems; and the *ectoderm*, or outermost layer, becomes the nervous system and skin. The head develops first, with the lower body developing last. After eight weeks, the embryo is called the fetus.

The *amnion* is a thin protective membrane that is filled with a fluid called the *amniotic fluid*. This fluid serves as insulation and protection for the embryo against shocks and blows to the mother's abdomen. The fluid also allows for changes in position as growth and movement occur. The *umbilical cord* connects the placenta and the embryo.

The *placenta* is the organ through which the embryo receives nutrients, vitamins, antibodies, and other substances such as drugs, alcohol, and diseases. The fetus also gives off waste products, such as nitrogen compounds and carbon dioxide, which are carried through the umbilical cord to be diffused through the placenta and given off in the mother's urine and through her lungs. This is accomplished even though there is no mixing of the embryo's and mother's blood. The placenta is expelled shortly following the birth of the child and is referred to as the *afterbirth*.

Multiple Births

Several factors contribute to multiple births. Heredity, age of the mother, and social factors seem significant (McCary 1984). Multiple births occur more often in certain families than in others. Women in their thirties are more likely to have multiple births than are women in their twenties.

Identical twins develop from a single fertilized ovum that divides to form two individuals. Such twins are always the same sex and look very much alike. *Fraternal twins* develop from two different ova. The ova are fertilized at about the same time. However, fraternal twins may not be of the same sex and look no more alike than any other siblings born to the parents.

Triplets usually involve two fertilized ova, one of which separates and then develops into twins. *Quadruplets* usually involve two fertilized ova that then divide and develop into two pairs of identical twins.

Childbirth

The process of birth occurs in three stages and is referred to as *labor* (see Figure 10.5). This process begins when the amniotic sac that has protected the fetus ruptures and the amniotic fluid flows from the vagina. Labor pains occur at regular intervals, usually fifteen to twenty minutes apart, with the cervix dilating three to four inches to permit the emergence of the fetus through the vagina. This first stage of labor may last twelve to sixteen hours (or even longer) for the first birth, but usually is shorter in subsequent births.

The second stage begins when the cervix has fully dilated and the baby's head enters the vagina. It ends with the birth of the baby. Contractions are quite severe and last from a minute to a minute and a half, with a two-to-three minute interval between contractions. The contractions serve to move the baby down the birth canal. Just before the head of the child appears, it rotates

Health Highlight

Calculating the Due Date

To find out when the baby is due, use the following formula:

1. Add 1 week to the first day of the last menstrual period.
   Example: January 1, 1994 + 7 days = January 8, 1994

2. Subtract 90 days.
   Example: January 8 – 90 days = October 8, 1993

3. Add one year.
   Example: October 8, 1993 + 1 year = October 8, 1994

Note: 60 percent of births occur within 5 days of a date calculated in this manner.

to the side to pass the pelvic bone. The neck and shoulders emerge, and the rest of the body follows rather quickly.

The third and final stage lasts only a few minutes and consists of the delivery of the placenta. The placenta separates from the wall of the uterus and is expelled as afterbirth. It is examined to determine that all of the organ has been delivered.

Occasionally, complications do arise during labor. For example, some conditions may require a *caesarean section.* When this procedure is used, an incision is made through the abdominal wall. Another incision is made in the uterus and the baby is removed. The reason for a caesarean section is usually a contracted pelvis, in which the baby is unable to pass into the vagina. Other reasons are that the baby is in a breech (buttock or leg presenting first) position; the placenta has prematurely separated from the uterus, causing a loss of oxygen; a vaginal infection is present; or the mother is incapacitated because of injury or trauma. To help identify potential complications, a fetal monitor may be used during the birth process.

Unwanted Pregnancies

The abortion issue is far from settled. Many states have circumvented the 1973 ruling allowing abortions by establishing laws that make abortions more difficult to obtain. The U.S. Congress has placed restrictions on government-paid-for abortions by prohibiting Medicaid funds from being used to pay for the procedure, except when the mother's life is in danger. The issues associated with abortion are now being more hotly debated than at any previous time. Both pro-choice and antiabortion groups are actively pursuing their goals. The outcome is yet undetermined and will probably not be settled in the next few years.

If the decision is made to not terminate a problem pregnancy, there are other options. The woman may choose to keep her child or place the infant up for adoption. In general, the younger the woman, the more difficult her decisions. Parenting is a most demanding job, and if the woman

Figure 10.5
The Three Stages of Birth

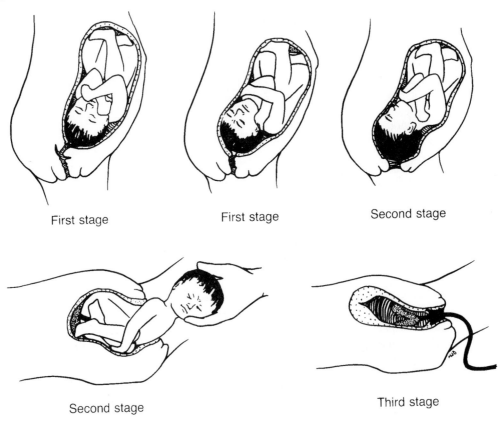

First stage

First stage

Second stage

Second stage

Third stage

is unwed, the difficulty is even greater. Many times she must rely on her parents or other relatives to aid in caring for the child. Unfortunately, too often the maturity necessary to be a good parent is lacking. The woman is faced with the difficulty of supplying a safe place for the child to grow and develop, providing adequate nutrition, developing sufficient economic resources, and having a secure, supportive environment. The options open to a single, young parent may be severely lacking from a social, educational, and economic perspective. Even if marriage occurs, the chances of a teenage marriage surviving is much less than if marriage occurs later in life.

Adoption is also a difficult decision, but many couples want to provide the love, closeness, and resources a child may need. Being an adoptive parent is virtually no different from being a natural parent. The same love, rewards, and frustrations are experienced by both parents and children.

Problems of Abuse and Violence

Child abuse is a particularly difficult problem to combat because the abuse usually occurs in the home and because there is often a public reluctance to intervene in and report what is thought to

Health Highlight

Indicators of Sexual Abuse

Psychological Signs

1. Fear of being alone with a specific person
2. Sleep disturbances, such as nightmares, fear of going to bed, and fear of sleeping alone
3. Irritability or short temper
4. Clinging to parent or parents
5. Unexplained fears
6. Changes in behavior and schoolwork or in relating to friends or siblings
7. Behaving like a younger child (regression)
8. Sexual sophistication or knowledge greater than age group
9. Fear of going home or running away from home

Physical Signs (Caused by Sexual Acts)

1. Difficulty in walking or sitting
2. Pain or itching in genital areas
3. Torn, stained, or bloody, underwear
4. Bruises or bleeding in external genitals, vagina, or anal areas
5. Sexually transmitted diseases
6. Pregnancy

Source: N. W. Denney and D. Quadagno. 1992. *Human sexuality.* St. Louis: Mosby Yearbook.

be a family matter. The National Center on Child Abuse and Neglect estimates that one million children are maltreated by their parents each year. Of these children, as many as 100,000 to 200,000 are physically abused; 60,000 to 100,000 are sexually abused; and the remainder are neglected. Each year, more than 2,000 children die in circumstances of abuse or neglect. It is estimated that 200,000 to 500,000 sexual assaults occur each year in the United States to females between infancy and thirteen years of age (Denney 1992). Other researchers have estimated that 27 percent of women and 16 percent of men are sexually molested before they reach their sixteenth birthday (Calderone and Johnson 1989, 161). Further statistics indicate that one in four women and one in seven men are abused during their lifetime.

Aside from the obvious physical effects, a child's psychological development can be seriously handicapped by abusive treatment. Many abused children are emotional cripples for the rest of their lives. A child who is abused in the home is one who loses the chance to be a child. Unable to understand why they are being punished, these children come to believe that they deserve such treatment because they are "bad." They see the world as cold and hostile and have little faith in themselves or in their ability to succeed in life. They learn that using force is an acceptable way to deal with others and, most tragically, often become child abusers themselves.

Many parents become physically or emotionally abusive because of their own history of abuse, failure to understand the needs of their children, or as a response to unmanaged stress. They

Health Highlight

Information for Teachers on Abuse

1. Child sexual abuse (molestation) involves the misuse of power by an adult or older child to engage a younger child in sexual activities to gratify the adult's needs.

2. Both touching and nontouching offenses are included in the category of sexual abuse. Examples of nontouching behaviors include showing children pornography or having children pose for pornographic pictures. Touching offenses include fondling and penetration.

3. Although the actual behavior involved in child sexual abuse varies, the following characteristics are common:

    a. It usually starts at an early age before children are aware of the inappropriate nature of the acts.

    b. The adult takes advantage of the child's need for approval, trust, and lack of knowledge.

    c. The behavior is surrounded with secrecy.

    d. The adult uses authority to threaten, bribe, or trick the child into complying.

    e. The child feels responsible for the abuse.

4. The child's reaction to the situation depends on his or her perception of the offense and the reactions of those important to him or her, rather than the legally defined severity of the offense.

5. Current information suggests that at least one in four girls and one in seven boys are physically molested by the age of eighteen. In 80 to 90 percent of the reported cases, the perpetrator (offender) is someone who is known to the child; in over 50 percent of the cases, the offender is a family member.

6. Most often, the perpetrator is someone the child knows well. The child may be emotionally tied to the individual and may even love him or her. Therefore, it should be emphasized that abuse can happen with someone we know or love; do not overemphasize danger from strangers.

7. Some children are aware of the inappropriateness of abusive behavior but are still unable to terminate it. Others are unable to recognize or respond appropriately to abusive or potentially abusive behaviors.

8. The educator should be sensitive to the manner in which material is presented and to the reactions of the students. Disclosure is often vague or indirect.

9. *Talking about Touching* by Harms and James and the *Personal Safety Curriculum* by Crisci are excellent curricula that contain lesson plans, resources, and activities for grades K–6. A list of audiovisual and written materials is provided after each section of the instructional sequence and in the annotated bibliography.

10. Define the subject according to the child's age. For young ones, explain that, although most adults are good and care, some do not make good decisions about touching children. They may try to touch children on private parts of the body for no good reason. A broader range of offenses and behaviors can be included when defining molestation to older children.

Health Highlight–cont'd

Use examples of touching and nontouching behaviors to make sure they understand the entire concept.

11. It is equally important for children to understand the characteristics of healthy interpersonal and familial relationships. Indicate that most adults do care and want to help children. Use examples of positive interpersonal relationships as well as negative ones in teaching the material.

12. Lessons for younger children need to stress developing the self-confidence and self-esteem needed to resist the attention and gifts often "earned" through participating in the abuse. Older children should begin to recognize characteristics of cooperative and exploitative relationships and relate these to their daily activities.

13. Touches can be categorized according to one's personal reaction to the touch. Good touches make one feet warm, secure, or happy; bad touches make one feel angry, hurt, or ashamed. Those touches that confuse are often sexual touches, or touches that are delivered in a contradictory manner that perplexes the child. Teachers can refer to resource materials, the local school district, or the state department of education for additional information.

14. Lessons should include opportunities to role-play and use the skills taught. For examples of assertiveness and decision-making activities, refer to the various resource materials available through state departments of education and local school districts.

typically do not have the self-confidence, ingenuity, and ability to cope with crises within the family. For them, any crisis presents a greater danger than for someone with better coping skills. Even a minor occurrence may be enough to lead to loss of self-control and an abusive attack on the innocent child. In many instances, abusing adults reverse roles with their children, requiring the child to love and care for them without providing the emotional support the child needs. With sexual abuse, abusers may actually convince themselves that they are doing a child a favor by showing the child the "facts of life" in a more loving way than an outsider would do (Office of the Attorney General 1985). There is hope for reeducation of the adult if the matter can be brought to the attention of the proper authorities. Successful therapy seems directly related to the perpetrator's willingness to change.

Every state has laws that make it mandatory for teachers to report suspected abuse. Not every bruise should be considered abuse, but if a pattern of injury is observed, teachers should report this concern. Proper authorities may be the state department of family and child services or a local health agency (see Health Highlight: "Indicators of Sexual Abuse").

▤ Summary

○ No area in health education is more controversial than that of sexuality education.

○ The vast majority supports sexuality education.

○ There are those who are very vocal and vehemently oppose sexuality education.

○ Schools can only provide the knowledge base and assist students in developing critical thinking skills, communication skills, self-esteem, and a solid knowledge base.

○ The family should provide the value base on which students base their decisions.

○ Sexuality education at the elementary level consists of many components, including the biological aspects, self-esteem, relationships, personal skills, social mores, and sexual health.

○ The family is the basic unit of society, although because of the increase in divorce the family has become an institution in transition, leading to many variations of family units, including single-parent and blended families.

○ Six factors contribute to the increased divorce rate: changing family functions, casual marriages, jobs for women, decline in moral and religious sanctions, the philosophy of happiness, and more liberal divorce laws.

○ Human sexuality develops over an extended length of time ranging from early childhood to the adult years.

○ The various structures of the male and female reproductive system are designed to enable human reproduction.

○ Unwanted or problem pregnancies are a continuing problem; the options available for consideration are keeping the child, planning for adoption, or terminating the pregnancy. For all three opinions, there are consequences that must be faced by the individuals involved.

○ Estimates are that about one million children are maltreated by their parents each year.

○ Every state has laws that require teachers to report suspected abuse.

Discussion Questions

1. What reasons are there for opposition to sexuality education?
2. What are some of the groups that oppose sexuality education, and what are their grounds for opposition?
3. What qualifications should a teacher have for teaching sexuality education?
4. Discuss the female and male reproductive systems.
5. What important functions does the family fill?
6. What factors should the classroom teacher be aware of when there are children of divorce in the classroom?
7. What are the shortcomings of inflexible gender roles?
8. Differentiate among and explain the different types of abuse.
9. What are some possible concepts that could be stressed in sexuality education at the preschool, K–3, and 4–6 levels?
10. What are the key concepts that a comprehensive family life and sexuality education program should contain?

References

Bossard, J. 1932, September. Residential propinquity as a factor in marriage selection. *American journal of sociology* pp. 219–224.

Bruess, C. E., and J. S. Greenberg. 1994. *Sexuality education—Theory and practice*. Madison, WI: Brown and Benchmark.

Byer, C. O., and L. W. Shainberg. 1994. *Dimensions of human sexuality*. Madison, WI: Brown and Benchmark.

Calderone, M. 1972. Love, sex, intimacy and aging as a life style. In *Sex, love, intimacy—Whose life styles?* New York: Sex Information and Education Council of the United States.

Calderone, M. S., and E. W. Johnson. 1989. *The family book about sexuality*. New York: Harper & Row.

Coutts, R. 1973. *Love and intimacy: A psychological approach*. San Ramon, CA: Consensus Publishers.

Denney, N. W., and D. Quadagno. 1992. *Human sexuality*. 2nd ed. St. Louis: Mosby Year Book.

Eshleman, J. 1988. *The family: An introduction,* 6th ed. Boston: Allyn and Bacon.

Fan, D. P., and C. L. Shaffer. 1990. Use of open-ended essays and computer content analysis to survey college students' knowledge of AIDS. *Journal of American college health* 38: 221–243.

Fromm, E. 1956. *The art of loving*. New York: Harper & Row.

Guidelines for Comprehensive Sexuality Education (GCSE). 1991. New York: Sex Information and Education Council of the United States.

Haas, K., and A. Haas. 1993. *Understanding sexuality*. St. Louis: Mosley.

Haffner, D. W., and D. deMauro. 1991. *Winning the battle: Developing support for sexuality and HIV/AIDS education*. New York: Sex Information and Education Council of the United States.

Harris, L., and Associates. 1988. *Public attitudes toward teenage pregnancy, sex education and birth control*. New York: Harris and Associates.

Hatcher, R. A. 1990. *Contraceptive technology*, 15th ed. New York: Irvington.

Heinlein, R. 1961. *Stranger in a strange land*. New York: Putnam.

Hyde, J. 1990. *Understanding human sexuality*, 2nd ed. New York: McGraw-Hill.

Insel, M., and W. T. Roth. 1991. *Core concepts in health*. Mountain View, CA: Mayfield.

Kephart, W. 1991. *The family, society and the individual*. Boston: Houghton Mifflin.

Kilander, F. H. 1968. *Sex education in the schools*. Toronto: Macmillan.

Kinsey, A., W. B. Pomeroy, C. E. Martin, and P. H. Gebhard. 1953. *Sexual behavior in the human female*. Philadelphia: Saunders.

LeBoyer, F. 1975. *Birth without violence*. New York: Knopf.

McCary, J. 1984. *Human sexuality*. New York: Van Nostrand.

McCary, J., and S. McCary. 1984. *Human sexuality*, 4th ed. Belmont, CA: Wadsworth.

Monahan, T. 1970. Are interracial marriages really less stable? *Social Forces* 48:461–473.

Office of the Attorney General. 1985. *Child abuse prevention handbook*. Sacramento, CA: Office of the Attorney General.

Ogletree, R. J., J. V. Fetro, J. C. Drolet, and B. A. Rienzo. 1994. *Sexuality education curricula—the consumer's guide*. Santa Cruz, CA: ETR Associates.

Page, R. M., and T. S. Page. 1993. *Fostering emotional well-being in the classroom*. Boston: Jones & Bartlett.

Peele, S., and A. Brodsky. 1976. *Love and addiction*. New York: New American Library.

Reiss, I. 1988. *Family systems in America*, 4th ed. New York: Holt, Rinehart & Winston.

Renshaw, D. 1983. *Incest: Understanding and treatment*. Boston: Little, Brown.

Scales, P. 1984. *The front line of sexuality education*. Santa Cruz, CA: Network Publications.

Schiller, P. 1973. *Creative approach to sex education and counseling*. New York: Association Press.

Spalt, S. W. 1996. Coping with controversy: The professional epidemic of the nineties. *Journal of school health* 66(9):339–340.

U.S. Bureau of the Census. 1979. *Statistical abstract of the United States*. Washington, DC: U.S. Government Printing Office.

———. 1988. *Marital status and living arrangements: Current population reports*. Washington, DC: U.S. Government Printing Office.

Woodward, K. L. 1978. Saving the family. *Newsweek* (May 15).

Chapter Eleven
Strategies for Teaching Sexuality Education

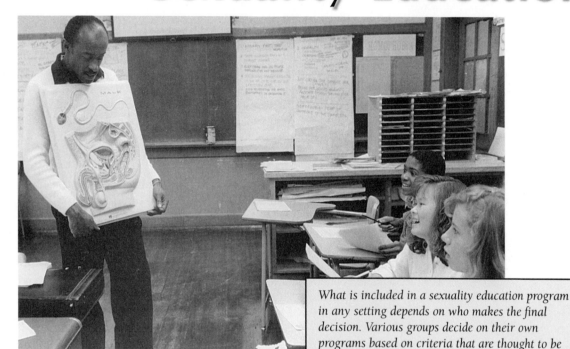

> *What is included in a sexuality education program in any setting depends on who makes the final decision. Various groups decide on their own programs based on criteria that are thought to be sound in their particular situations.*
> —Clint E. Bruess and Jerrold E. Greenberg

Valued Outcomes

After doing the activities in this chapter, the student should be able to express and illustrate the following guidelines:

- ○ There are many different types of families; not all families consist of a husband, wife, and children living together.
- ○ Each member of a family is important, and each has certain privileges and responsibilities.
- ○ Interpersonal skills are necessary for strengthening individual and family life.
- ○ Friends help one another feel good about themselves and provide support.
- ○ A positive self-image is necessary if we are to be at ease with ourselves.
- ○ Understanding of self and others is a foundation for successful adulthood.
- ○ Children have rights, and no one should be mistreated, taken advantage of, or abused by another person.

○ Heredity and environment influence growth and development.

○ Physical, social, and emotional growth occur over a long period of time; such growth differs in each individual.

○ Procreation is a function of both males and females.

○ Menstruation is a normal process that each female experiences.

○ Wholesome attitudes toward sexuality constitute a basic factor for happiness throughout life.

○ Sexual values and sexual responsibilities are often individual decisions.

Building Self-Esteem and Responsible Decision Making

Traditionally, the area of sexuality education has always been the primary responsibility of the family. The church and other social institutions have also played a significant role. For a complex variety of reasons, these sources are no longer always completely adequate. For children, the result is often confusion, misinformation, guilt, self-doubt, anxiety, and unhealthy adjustment. The schools, by supplementing, not replacing, traditional sources, can lessen this possibility by providing well-designed and tested sexuality education programs that can provide beneficial results for all concerned—children, parents, and society in general.

The classroom is a nonthreatening atmosphere where reliable and accurate information can be presented about sex and family matters. But sexuality education is more than just factual information. An effective program must be based on the development of self-esteem and responsible decision making. If children learn to feel good about themselves, they are less likely to need to exploit others and less likely to be open to exploitation in sexual and family functioning. Sexuality education strives to teach equality and respect between the sexes and an appreciation for self and others.

The suggestions in this chapter will help you work toward these goals. These learning opportunities will assist students in obtaining factual knowledge, developing their value systems, and growing psychologically as individuals.

Value-Based Strategies

Rights and Responsibilities

Valued Outcome: The student will be able to identify the factors that help families live in happy environments.
Description of Strategy: Have the class prepare parallel column lists of their rights and responsibilities as family members. Under the "Rights" column, they may list such things as being provided with food and shelter, having free time to play or watch television, being allowed to express their opinions on certain family matters, and spending their allowances as they wish. Under the "Responsibilities" column, students may list such things as keeping their rooms clean, taking out the trash, helping with housework, caring for a younger sibling, being honest in family matters, and accepting parental decisions. After the lists have been prepared, discuss the significance of the items listed. Ask questions such as the following:
Processing Questions:

1. Do you think your rights and responsibilities are equally balanced?

2. How have your rights and responsibilities changed as you have gotten older?

3. Do boys in a family have certain rights and responsibilities that girls do not have?

4. Do girls have certain rights and responsibilities that boys do not have?

5. How much say should children have about their rights and responsibilities?

6. If you made all the rules in your home, what changes might you consider? Why?

7. What do your rights and responsibilities suggest to you about your own level of maturity?

8. How would you feel if you had no responsibilities?

Attitude Inventory—How Do I Feel?

Valued Outcome: The student will identify feelings concerning family, friends, and themselves.
Description of Strategy: Prepare individual sheets like the one shown here, and ask the students to offer their opinion about each statement. Follow with a general class discussion.

How Do I Feel?

	Agree	Disagree	Not Sure
1. Each child is an important member of his or her family.	_____	_____	_____
2. Families do a lot of fun things together.	_____	_____	_____
3. Mothers should hug and kiss their children more than fathers should.	_____	_____	_____
4. Children who have no brothers or sisters are unhappy.	_____	_____	_____
5. Mothers and fathers should not hug and kiss each other in front of their children.	_____	_____	_____
6. The more I learn about myself, the better I like myself.	_____	_____	_____
7. Children who don't help with the housework should not get an allowance.	_____	_____	_____
8. The best way to learn about sex is to ask friends.	_____	_____	_____
9. I'd be too embarrassed to ask my parents about sex.	_____	_____	_____
10. Sometimes I dread becoming a teenager.	_____	_____	_____
11. I have trouble telling friends how I really feel.	_____	_____	_____
12. My friends often pressure me to do things I don't want to do.	_____	_____	_____
13. When a friend does something wrong, I usually tell the person how I feel.	_____	_____	_____
14. Children should be allowed to set some of the family rules.	_____	_____	_____
15. Adults are free to do what they want most of the time.	_____	_____	_____

Processing Questions:

1. Were there questions that were difficult to answer?

2. Why were the selections to some of the questions difficult?

3. What three things did you learn from your responses?

Getting to Know Me

Valued Outcome: The student will be able to list characteristics that make them special.
Description of Strategy: Prepare sheets or cards with the following statements or categories on them. Pass out a sheet to each student to complete, then collect and shuffle all the responses. Either as a class or small-group activity, see if students can identify each other by the responses. Have the students consider what this suggests about the unique individuality of each person.

Something that I do well: _____

Music that I like: _____

Three words that describe me: _____

If I could have a dream come true, it would be:_____

What I like to do in my spare time: _____

I'm looking forward to: _____

One thing I like about myself:_____

Who am I?_____

Processing Questions:

1. Were there any questions that were difficult to answer?
2. What were you proud of in your answers?
3. What would you like to change about your answers?
4. Did anything surprise you about your answers?

That's My Opinion

Valued Outcome: The students will develop insight into what boys and girls look for and expect from the opposite sex.
Description of Strategy: This activity is designed to help boys and girls understand the many misconceptions about qualities desired by the opposite sex. The class should be divided into males and females, with a recorder and spokesperson assigned for each group. Have each group respond to the questions "I like girls (boys) who . . ." and "I dislike girls (boys) who . . .." The recorder should keep a record of all responses and have the spokesperson read the response aloud (the teacher may wish to screen the responses first).
Processing Questions:

1. What did the boys seem to like about the girls? dislike?
2. What did the girls seem to like about the boys? dislike?
3. Why do you think there were differences between the two lists for both the likes and dislikes?
4. What do you think we can learn from the likes and dislikes of boys and girls?

Decision Stories

Present decision stories such as the following, using the procedures outlined in Chapter 4. The content of the stories that you present should be appropriate for the developmental levels of your students. The examples here range from stories suitable for the early elementary grades to the upper grades, but they are not identified as to grade level because appropriateness must be determined in the social context of your own group.

Am I Stuck with Me?

Kevin is overweight and not very good at sports. He is often chosen last in team sports and games, which bothers him a lot although he tries to make a joke of it. In fact, he makes a great many jokes because he wants the other kids to like him. And they do. They think Kevin is a lot of fun. But Kevin doesn't just want to be the class clown. He wants the other kids in class to respect him for what he is. He would like the girls in class to think more highly of him too.
Focus Questions:

1. What might Kevin do to feel better about himself?

2. Are there some things that he should not change? Why or why not?

The Crush

Jackie couldn't seem to stop thinking about the boy who lived down the street. He was a lot older than she was, and he thought she was "just a kid." Jackie went out of her way to be around him. She hoped that he would invite her out on a date, even though she wasn't really old enough to start dating. Then one day Jackie saw him with another girl—one closer to his own age. She felt terrible. How could he do this to her?
Focus Question: What should Jackie do next?

John's World

John's parents were divorced last year. John is living with his mother, but he sees his father regularly. One weekend, while John is staying with his father, he finds out that his father is going to get married again. "John," his father says. "This is Janet. I know that you're going to like each other." But John doesn't like his father's woman friend. He is still feeling bad about the divorce. Now this! Will this woman become his stepmother? What will happen to his real mother? What kind of a family will this be? John is confused, very angry, and deeply unhappy.
Focus Questions:

1. Should John pretend he likes this woman, or should he treat her badly so she will know how he feels?

2. What could John say to his father about this situation?

Stories or Facts?

One day after school, some of the girls are talking about how babies are made. Susan is listening with interest. Some of the things she hears are new to her. She has learned a little bit about sex education from her parents and in school, but she is still not sure about all the details. Now she is more confused than ever. She wishes that she knew which of these things were really true.
Focus Questions:

1. What can Susan do to get accurate information?

2. Who should she try to talk with?

3. Should she rely on her friends for information?

Fooling Around

Bob and his friend George are spending the afternoon together in George's home. It is raining, so they have to stay inside. George's parents are not at home. The two boys start to talk about sex. Then George suggests that the two of them "fool around" together and play with each other's bodies. Afterward, Bob feels that maybe he did something wrong. He feels guilty and frightened. The next day, he feels even worse about what happened. He is afraid to tell his parents what happened. *Focus Question:* What should Bob do?

The Party

Tina's friend Marie is having a party and has invited her. At the party, Tina knows only a few of the other guests. Everyone seems to be having a good time. There is music, and the boys and girls are dancing. Later, Tina notices that some of the couples are kissing and making out. A boy named Carl comes over to her. "Would you like to dance with me?" he asks. She is not sure. She doesn't really know Carl. What if he tries something? What could she do? She feels flattered that Carl is paying attention to her, but she is also unsure of herself in situations like this.
Focus Questions:

1. What should Tina do?

2. What are some possible reasons she feels uncomfortable?

3. What decisions does Tina have to make now and in the future?

Being Friendly

Sharon was playing in her backyard one day when Mr. Smith, the man next door, asked her if she would like to come over and have some ice cream. Mr. Smith had always been nice, so Sharon quickly accepted his invitation. Once inside his house, Sharon learned that Mrs. Smith was not there. Mr. Smith started putting his arms around Sharon and brushing up against her. That made Sharon feel uncomfortable. Sharon wanted to leave, but Mr. Smith was very anxious to have her stay.
Focus Questions:

1. Is Mr. Smith acting appropriately?

2. What should Sharon do in this situation?

3. Should she worry about hurting Mr. Smith's feelings?

4. How should Sharon react if the person touching her is her stepfather or another relative?

Health Highlight

What's Happening?

Martin Heesacker, in the book *Portraits of Adjustment* has stated, "Long-term studies indicate that many of the behavioral, psychological, and academic problems shown by children following divorce are traceable to conflict in the dysfunctional family prior to the divorce" (p. 254). Some of the research findings indicate that girls tend to act out less than boys; that eleven-year-old boys whose parents had divorced within the last year had 19 percent more behavioral and academic problems than 11-year-old boys living in an intact family; and divorces tended to generate their own problems, whether in reducing economic well-being or in further disrupting relations among parents and children.

Source: Heesacker, M. 1994. *Portraits of adjustment*. Boston: Allyn and Bacon.

Other Strategies for Teaching

Being My Own Perfect Friend

Valued Outcome: The students will be able to assess the qualities they desire in themselves and others who are friends.

Description of Strategy: Ask the students to make a list of five qualities they would like in a perfect friend. Have them describe each of these qualities in a sentence, such as "My perfect friend gives me good advice when I am not feeling happy" or "My perfect friend accepts me for who I am." Ask students to share their ideas in class, and prepare a master list on the chalkboard, poster board, or overhead projector.

Materials Needed: index cards or sheets of paper, pencils

Processing Questions:

1. How can each of you be your own "perfect friend"?
2. If you cross out "my perfect friend" in your sentences and substitute the word "I," what do you notice about the sentence?
3. How can each of us be more of a "perfect friend" to ourselves instead of sometimes being our own "worst enemy"?
4. What are the implications for ourselves and our friends?

Love, Love, Love

Valued Outcome: The students will verbally list nonsexual ways to express love toward others.

Description of Strategy: Have a "love discussion" where the class talks about all the different kinds of love (between them and brothers and sisters, parents and stepparents, relatives, friends, teachers). Have students list different appropriate ways of expressing love to family members by their words, the tone of their voices, body language, and actions toward each other.

Materials Needed: paper, pencils

Processing Questions:

1. How many different people do you love?
2. What are some ways in which you express your feelings to everyone you love?
3. How can you tell if someone loves you?

Solving Problems

Valued Outcome: The students will develop possible choices for solving problems they may encounter.

Description of Strategy: Divide students into an even number of groups of four or five each. One student in each group will be a recorder. Have each group write three problems that require a decision. Emphasize that these problems should be typical ones that their age group faces and should be about relationships or risky behavior. When finished, pair groups and have them exchange problems. Each group then writes possible solutions for the new problems. The recorders can report the results to the class.

Materials Needed: paper, pencils

Processing Questions:

1. Did any groups list the same problems?

2. Is it always easy to make positive decisions?

3. Does it sometimes help to get other opinions about what to do?

Growing Up

Valued Outcome: The students will complete sentences describing how they will respond to various situations associated with growing up.

Description of Strategy: The passage to adulthood can be an especially awkward and confusing time as young people struggle with new signals from their bodies and the maturing young men and women around them. Many will experience emotional changes, mood swings, feelings of uncertainty, and increased feelings of independence and sexuality. A positive and confident attitude can help them handle these changes better.

As students grow, fewer adults will be making decisions for them, but the pressure to be part of the peer group will increase. They will need to rely on their own values to help make the choices most appropriate for developing a positive and healthy life.

Have your students read the following statements and complete each sentence.

1. I want to drive my friend's car, but I don't have my license. I'm going to . . .

2. I know my girlfriend has cramps because she has her period. I'm going to . . .

3. My parents can use my help around the house more often. I think I'll . . .

4. I haven't developed physically as fast as my friends. This makes me feel . . .

5. I have acne on my face. I will . . .

6. My parents are going away next weekend. I'm going to . . .

7. Some of my friends like to talk about sex. This makes me feel uncomfortable. I should . . .

Materials Needed: Copy of questions listed below
Processing Questions:

1. Why are some of the questions more difficult to deal with than others?

2. Is a person's maturity indicated by what they say? Do?

3. Are there certain pressures to say or do certain things?   Give examples.

4. Can you identify some decisions based upon these questions that might (might not) indicate good decision making?

The Answer Is No

Valued Outcome: The students will gain experience in having to tell others they may not do something they want to do. The students will then report how it feels to be in the position of saying no.

Description of Strategy: Have the students divide into pairs of their own choosing. Explain that one student will play the part of a parent, and the other will play the part of that parent's child. The child will ask permission from the parent to go to a party where both boys and girls will be present. The student acting the part of the child will explain about the party—who will be there, where it will be, and so on. After listening, the student acting as parent refuses permission. The son or

In developing relationships, adolescents need to rely on their values and learn to communicate effectively.

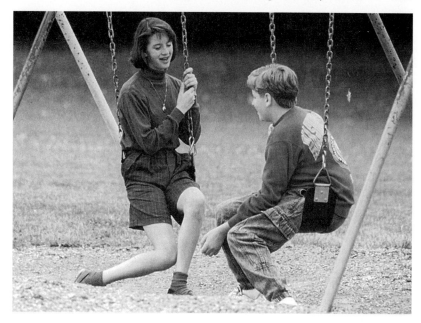

daughter argues for permission, but is still refused. Let several pairs of students act out the situation in front of the class, but do not require anyone to do so who does not wish to participate. Discuss how the different pairs of students handle the same situation. Then, without forewarning the class that you will do so, have selected pairs of students switch roles and repeat the activity. Use discretion in choosing which pairs of students to use for this second part of the activity.
Materials Needed: none
Processing Questions:

1. What differences do you note in individual roles when these roles were reversed?

2. What did you learn from this activity?

How Would You Handle It?

Valued Outcome: The students will act out commonly faced situations.
Description of Strategy: Divide the class into pairs, making sure that close friends are not paired. (There will be no role switching in this activity.) Have each pair act out situations such as the following:

1. asking for and getting a date

2. asking for and being refused a date

3. introducing a friend to one's parents (a third child should play the part of the friend)

4. telling a divorced parent that you don't care for the person the parent is dating

5. introducing yourself to a member of the opposite sex to whom you feel attracted

6. being polite to someone you don't like

7. handling rejection on being socially rebuffed

Materials Needed: none
Processing Questions:

1. Which of the preceding situations do you find the most difficult?

2. What is most important when attempting to convey a message to someone?

3. How many ways can you think of to handle each of the situations?

Understanding Others

Valued Outcome: The students will imitate personal characteristics that they do not have.
Description of Strategy: Not everyone is alike; some people are bossy and others are shy. Assign different roles to various children, such as Noisy Ned, Bossy Betty, Shy Sam, Iceberg Irene, Chatterbox Chester, Silent Sylvia, Blustery Ben, Whirlwind Wanda, Studious Stu, Laughing Larry, Somber Sarah, and Flighty Frank. Make sure that the children assigned to each role do not have the characteristics of the role they are to play. Have each child act out the part for a few minutes.
Materials Needed: none
Processing Questions:

1. How can you deal with these different personality types?

2. What do you find appealing about the characteristics of each personality type?

3. Why might others be put off by some of these characteristics?

4. Why is it good that all people are not alike?

Superkid

Valued Outcome: The students will list ways that life is difficult for everyone, no matter what talents or gifts they have.
Description of Strategy: Have the students divide into pairs. One student will play the part of Superkid and the other will be his or her press agent. Each pair will decide what abilities each Superkid will have. These abilities might include flying, speaking any language, singing or playing a musical instrument so well that the person is a superstar, possessing great athletic talent, and so on. First, the student playing the press agent introduces the Superkid and describes his or her abilities in the most glowing terms. Then, Superkid acknowledges his or her popular acclaim, but notes to the class that life is not perfect even for a Superkid. The student should then explain why being a Superkid isn't as completely wonderful as the press agent has said. If the person is described as an athlete, for example, he or she might explain the anxieties about getting injured on the field, the pressure of competition, and so forth.
Materials Needed: none
Processing Questions:

1. Does anyone have all their problems taken care of?

2. Is it possible that extreme talents can create more problems sometimes?

3. If you had one incredible ability, what would you like it to be?

4. What talents do you have that make you super in some way?

Me and My Self-Confidence

Valued Outcome: The students will recognize that many people are very successful even though they may not look perfect.

Description of Strategy: Discuss characteristics that can cause people to feel self-conscious, such as being overweight or underweight, being very short or very tall, having a large nose, or having skin problems. Note that some of these characteristics are either temporary or ones that can be changed while others are permanent or difficult to change. All characteristics can actually become an asset. Discuss famous individuals noted for unique or unusual physical features. These might include Barbra Streisand and her nose, or Dudley Moore and his shortness. Emphasize that each of these individuals relied on developed talent rather than inherited physical characteristics to achieve success and that self-confidence was often the key to success.

Materials Needed: none

Processing Questions:

1. Can you name some people you really admire that may have an unusual physical characteristic?
2. What physical characteristics do you have that you feel are less than perfect?
3. What characteristics and talents do you have that make you proud?

Opportunities for All

Valued Outcome: The students will recognize and name professions that were once male or female dominated but in which both genders now have increasing opportunity to participate

Description of Strategy: In years past, many occupations were considered as appropriate only for males or females. Today, this social attitude is changing, as are our conceptions of sex roles and sex stereotyping in general. After discussing this point with the class, have them divide into small groups to talk about and research individual instances of changing professions for the sexes. Some groups can look into changing occupational opportunities while others can look at changing social or familial roles. For example, many police officers in cities and towns throughout the nation are now women and some men now stay home and care for the children. Ask each group to compile a report on how changes in their area of research have resulted in greater opportunity for both men and women.

Materials Needed: none

Processing Questions:

1. Do you think females should be involved in all professions?
2. Do you think it is appropriate for males to engage in all professions? Why or why not?
3. What profession do you think you would like to be a part of when you grow up?

Information Please

Valued Outcome: The students will rank sources of information concerning sexuality questions.

Description of Strategy: Prepare a worksheet like the list here, giving possible sources of information on sexuality. Have each student rank the list from the source most likely to provide accurate information to the source least likely to provide accurate information. Then discuss the different rankings in class. Be sure to point out that even what might be considered the most informed source may not be able to supply information on a particular question without research. Avoid disparaging any valid source of information, but suggest that some are probably more useful than others. If appropriate, you might also note that sometimes more than one source should be consulted for more complete information.

Possible sources of sexuality information
Movies and television
Health teacher
Minister, priest, or rabbi
Friends
Parents
Books from the library
Physician (doctor)
Newspaper columns
Magazines
Textbooks used in schools

Materials Needed: worksheet
Processing Questions:

1. Can any one source answer all the questions you might have?
2. What should you do if a source is unsure of some of the information it gives you?
3. Should you ever consult more than one source about a question you have?

Legal Rights

Valued Outcome: The students will learn what sexual abuse is and what options they have if they are abused.
Description of Strategy: Unfortunately, many children in this country are sexually abused. Such abuse may come from other family members or from trusted adults or friends. Often, children are completely unaware of their legal and moral rights in such instances. After becoming informed on legal recourses, present an objective lecture on the subject to your class. It is very important that you preface your discussion by emphasizing that the child has no reason to feel guilty or ashamed for being a victim of sexual exploitation of any kind. Suggest sources that children can turn to for help if such exploitation is occurring. A good first choice is the school psychologist, counselor, or physician.
Materials Needed: none
Processing Questions:

1. Is it ever a child's fault if he or she is sexually abused?
2. If you are being treated in a way that makes you think you are being abused, what should you do?
3. Who are some people you could tell if you are being abused?

Families Are Different

Valued Outcome: Students will realize that any family structure can provide a loving and healthy environment for personal growth, even if it is not "typical."

Description of Strategy: Invite adults of your acquaintance to come to class to discuss different types of families in which they grew up. Include individuals from a wide variety of familial backgrounds, including traditional American nuclear families, extended family situations, single-parent families, and so forth. This is not an easy activity to do, but it can be a most valuable one. Your guests should not gloss over any difficulties they had growing up in their particular situation, but children should not get the impression that singular events are typical of any situation.

Materials Needed: guest speakers who can effectively address identified issues
Processing Questions:

1. Are all families the same?

2. Can you be a normal person if you do not live with your real mother and father?

3. Is growing up easy for anyone?

Individual Reports

Valued Outcome: The students will learn more about human development.
Description of Strategy. As appropriate for the developmental level of your particular students, assign individual report topics on aspects of physical and emotional growth. Have the students use your health textbook and other approved informational sources to research particular areas, such as the growth spurt that occurs in adolescence; puberty; menarche; first encounters with the opposite sex in social situations; and dating behavior in the early teen years. On a separate sheet of paper, have students list questions for which they did not find answers during their research. Consult with each student on an individual basis to assist in finding appropriate solutions to these questions. In doing this activity, rely on the advisory committee to your sexuality education program for appropriate responses to individual student questions or dilemmas.

Materials Needed: paper, pencils, or pens
Processing Questions:

1. What kinds of questions do you have for which you did not find answers?

2. What did you learn that you did not know before about human development?

Why Not?

Valued Outcome: Increase student awareness of possible consequences of some kinds of sexual behavior.
Description of Strategy: After discussion and approval of this activity by all members of the family life advisory committee, invite various representatives of sex education groups in your community to lecture to the class on the ramifications of certain sexual decisions that each individual must make, such as the decision to have intercourse outside of marriage. Make it clear before the activity that you as the teacher are not advocating any behavior that goes against general community norms.

Materials Needed: guest speakers who are screened carefully before talking to the group
Processing Questions:

1. Is it wise to make sexual decisions based on how you feel at a certain time?

2. What are some reasons for delaying some kinds of sexual behavior?

Dictionary with a Difference

Valued Outcome: Students will develop a page about themselves in a "human dictionary."

Description of Strategy: Have students make a "different dictionary" about themselves to be exhibited in the classroom. Each child has a page that is his or her dictionary entry. Included should be a picture, below which is the last name, first name, the phonetic respelling, and birth date. There should be a line telling the age and grade, a line listing identifying characteristics, a line for interests, and a qualitative statement (e.g., I am good at . . .).

Materials Needed: photos of students, paper, pencils or pens

Processing Questions:

1. What is something really special about yourself?

2. How are you different from last year?

Guppies

Valued Outcome: Students will recognize that birth and reproduction is a normal part of the life cycle of all living things.

Description of Strategy: After discussing the concept that all living things can reproduce, let students observe the birth process in live-bearing fish. Obtain some young female guppies and young male guppies. Raise them in separate aquariums. Point out to the class the physical differences between the females and the males. Note that the female guppy is larger and somewhat drab in coloration in contrast to the smaller, brightly colored male. Explain that in many animal species there are obvious differences between the male and female, as there are with human beings. When the fish are mature, place one or more males in the tank with the females. In a few weeks, one or more of the females will become pregnant. This will soon be obvious. With luck, birth may take place while class is in session. Have the children observe the birth process. Also point out differences in the birth process for different species, for example, many fish and all birds are egg layers. (As soon as the female guppies give birth, separate the adults from the young, as guppies are cannibalistic.)

Materials Needed: aquarium, guppies

Processing Questions:

1. Are all babies born alive? Which ones are not?

2. Were you born alive?

Baby Animals

Valued Outcome: The students will observe mammalian birth.

Description of Strategy: If appropriate, you may wish to breed white mice or other rodents in the classroom. After the female has given birth, have the children observe the offspring.

Materials Needed: mice, cage, food, nesting materials

Processing Questions:

1. How are the adults and children alike? How are they different?

2. How does the mother take care of her young? Why does she take such good care of her children?

3. Do all animals nurture their children?

4. Are animal families like human families? How? How are they different?

Genetics

Valued Outcome: The students will observe how offspring inherit different traits from their parents.
Description of Strategy: If you decide to breed mice or other animals in the classroom, you can also use the project to demonstrate inherited traits by using a male and a female with different physical characteristics, such as fur coloration. Observe how many of the offspring have inherited coloration traits similar to those of the male or those of the female. For upper elementary school children, discuss dominant and recessive traits.
Materials Needed: mice, cage, food, nesting materials
Processing Questions:

1. What traits did you inherit from your mother? What traits did you inherit from your father?

2. Can you give other examples of some traits you have observed in the offspring of pet cats or dogs?

Inherited Traits

Valued Outcome: Students will realize that some personal characteristics are inherited.
Description of Strategy: The human genetic code contains information about thousands of inherited traits. These include hair, eye, and skin color; shape of ears and nose; and general physique. Emphasize to your class that even individual rates of growth are to a large extent genetically controlled, which explains why some children grow more quickly than others. To demonstrate that some genetic traits are less obvious than others, ask the class to roll their tongues. Some children will be able to roll their tongues, but others will be unable to do so. This ability is a genetic trait.
Materials Needed: none
Processing Questions:

1. What are some other characteristics that you have that are unique?

2. Does having a certain genetic trait make you better or worse than anyone else?

Reproduction Systems Crossword Puzzle

Valued Outcome: The students will increase their vocabulary about reproduction.
Description of Strategy: Prepare crossword puzzle sheets as shown in Figure 11.1.

Word Hunt

Valued Outcome: Through a word hunt puzzle, the students will become more familiar with words associated with reproduction.
Description of Strategy: Duplicate Figure 11.2 and have the students find and circle each of the words listed. The words may read in any direction—up, down, across, or diagonally.

Figure 11.1

Reproduction Systems Crossword Puzzle

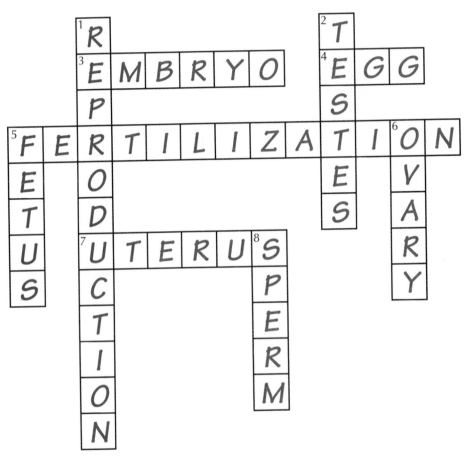

Down

1. the act of producing or recreating

2. the part of the male reproductive system where sperm are developed

5. the name given to the unborn child from about 2½ months till birth

6. the part of the female reproductive system where eggs are stored

8. the male sex cell

Across

3. the name given to the unborn child during the first stages of development

4. the female sex cell

5. the union of egg and sperm

7. the muscular organ of the female reproductive system that holds the baby before birth

Figure 11.2
Student Activity Sheet for Word Hunt on Reproduction

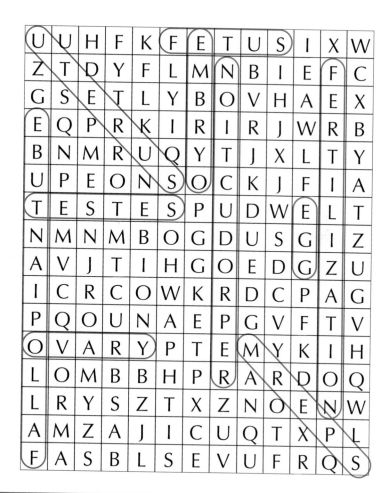

FETUS
EMBRYO
SPERM
FALLOPIAN TUBE
EGG
TESTES
OVARY
FERTILIZATION
REPRODUCTION
UTERUS

Scrambled Sentences

Valued Outcome: Students will review the reproductive system by unscrambling sentences.
Description of Strategy: Have the students unscramble each of the following sentences about the human reproductive systems.

1. canal acts birth as the vagina a   (*The vagina acts as a birth canal.*)
2. ova the hormones and ovaries produce   (*The ovaries produce ova and hormones.*)
3. tubes occurs in fertilization the fallopian   (*Fertilization occurs in the fallopian tubes.*)
4. begins females in at menstruation puberty   (*Menstruation begins in females at puberty.*)
5. in the fetus uterus the develops   (*The fetus develops in the uterus.*)
6. are cells the male sperm reproductive called   (*The male reproductive cells are called sperm.*)
7. testes produced in the cells sperm are   (*Sperm cells are produced in the testes.*)

8. fluids other and semen of made is up sperm   (*Semen is made up of sperm and other fluids.*)

9. puberty begin at sperm produced to be   (*Sperm begin to be produced at puberty.*)

10. at testosterone the triggers spurt male puberty growth   (*Testosterone triggers the male growth spurt at puberty.*)

Matching Parts and Functions

Valued Outcome: Students will review information on the reproductive system by labeling the parts.

Description of Strategy: Draw a large diagram of the female reproductive system on the chalkboard. Draw leader lines from each of the parts, and allow room for labeling. Prepare a similar diagram for the male reproductive system. Divide the class into two teams. Point to a part on either diagram and ask the first player to identify it. If the student knows the answer, he or she should come to the board and label the part. If the student does not know the correct answer, the first player from Team B gets a chance. Score one point for each correct answer. After a part has been correctly labeled, ask the next player to explain one function of that part. If the student knows the correct answer, she or he should come to the board and write the function next to the name of the part.

Materials Needed: blackboard, chalk

Processing Questions:

1. What were the most significant things we learned?

2. What were some of the most difficult questions to answer?

True or False?

Valued Outcome: The students will review information about human sexuality through team competition.

Description of Strategy: Divide the class into two teams and ask each player to decide whether a statement that you make is true or false. Score one point for each correct answer. Then write each of the true statements on the chalkboard. Review the true statements at the end of the game.

Sample statements might include the following:

1. Girls should not swim during menstruation. (false)

2. A wet dream is a sign that a boy is reaching puberty. (true)

3. Fertilization leading to pregnancy occurs when a sperm unites with an egg. (true)

4. The beginning of menstruation means that a girl can now become pregnant. (true)

Materials Needed: chalkboard, chalk, prepared list of statements

Processing Questions:

1. What were the most difficult questions to deal with?

2. What was most difficult to talk about?

Growing Up

Valued Outcome: The students will increase understanding of the growth process.
Description of Strategy: Have each student trace his or her hand on a sheet of paper. Ask the students to take their tracings home, and have one or both parents trace their hands over the child's tracing.
Materials Needed: paper, pens
Processing Questions:

1. Is your parent's hand larger than yours? Why?
2. How do body parts grow?
3. Will your whole body be larger when you are grown?

Family Activities Collage

Valued Outcome: Students will make a collage of activities they engage in with their families.
Description of Strategy: Have each student search through magazines to find pictures of family activities. These activities can include watching television together, going on trips or outings, working around the house, talking with one another, and so forth. Explain to the students that the pictures they choose need to represent a family activity. Thus, a picture of a television set by itself can represent watching television together, an airplane can represent a trip to relatives in another part of the country, and so on. Have each student prepare a colorful collage, and then explain to the class the meaning of each component.
Materials Needed: poster board, magazines, scissors, glue or glue stick
Processing Questions:

1. What activities do you do most often with your family?
2. What family activities are your favorite?

My Family Tree

Valued Outcome: Students will develop a family tree and discuss characteristics they might have inherited from other family members.
Description of Strategy: Distribute photocopies of Figure 11.3 and have each student prepare his or her family tree. Younger children may need the assistance of their parents to fill in the names of forebears. After the diagrams are completed, discuss each family tree. This may be an area where sensitivity will be needed if some children in the classroom are adopted. If approached carefully, this activity may provide an opportunity to discuss what adoption is, why people adopt, and which traits any of the adopted children in the class perceive they have that are similar to those of their adoptive parents.
Materials Needed: photocopies of the family tree
Processing Questions:

1. What physical features do you have in common with siblings, parents, grandparents, and so on?
2. Do you have any interest similar to your ancestors?
3. Which relative do you think you most resemble?

Figure 11.3
Family Tree

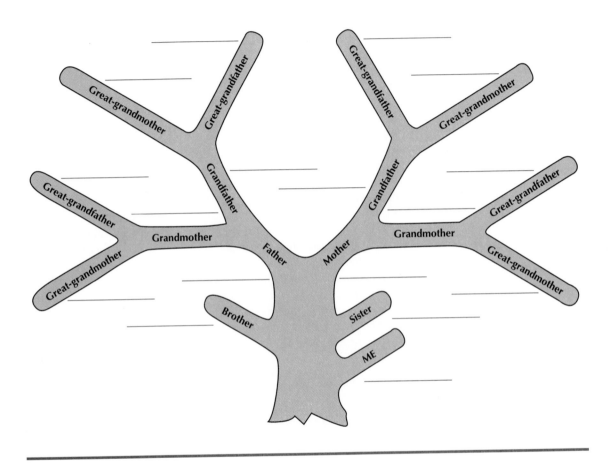

Caught in the Act

Valued Outcome: Students will observe and record classmates' behaviors.

Description of Strategy: What positive behaviors do you see your classmates use? Are they *responsible, cooperative,* or *courteous*? Read the following examples. See if you can catch your classmates in the act. Write in the names of the people who use these behaviors.

Being Responsible	Who Did It?
Returned something that was borrowed	_____
Admitted making a mistake	_____
Finished all schoolwork and turned it in on time	_____

Being Cooperative   **Who Did It?**

Followed the line leader   _____

Worked well with someone to get a job done   _____

Tried hard in a game or in physical education   _____

Being Courteous   **Who Did It?**

Helped someone who had a problem   _____

Waited for his or her turn in line   _____

Gave someone else a compliment for doing something well   _____

Materials Needed: worksheet

Responsibility

Valued Outcome: Students will list the different responsibilities family members have.

Description of Strategy: Write your name and your family members' names in the following spaces. Put an *X* in each column that tells a responsibility each person has in the home. Add other responsibilities if needed.

Family Member	Cooking	Washing Clothes	Doing Dishes	Paying Bills	Taking Out Trash	Cleaning Bathroom	Other
____							
____							
____							
____							
____							

Processing Questions:

1. What are the consequences of people not completing their responsibilities?

2. Do you always fulfill your responsibilities?

3. Do you have to be reminded to do your jobs around the house?

How My Decisions Affect Others

Valued Outcome: The students will list how they think their decisions to perform various tasks affects their family.

Description of Strategy: Use the following chart as an example. Students should consider different situations they may face and think about how the decisions they make affect their family.

What if I decided to. . .   **How I think my family would feel about my choice**

1.   . . . say no to a drug a friend offered me   _____

2.   . . . not clean my room after being told to do so   _____

3.   . . . try to do my best in math   _____

4   . . . do my homework for a week without being reminded _____

Processing Questions:

1. Do your actions affect the people around you?

2. Can you do things that will make life easier for your family?

Helping Others

Valued Outcome: The students will develop a list of ways that they can help their friends and family.

Description of Strategy: Using the following chart, have students compile a list of things they can do to help out family and friends. These acts of kindness need not be big chores or sacrifices. They can be little things that may make a difference in the day of the people they love.

Whom I can help	How I can help	How many times I've helped
Parents	_____	_____
Grandparents	_____	_____
Brother or sister	_____	_____
My teacher	_____	_____
My best friend	_____	_____

Materials Needed: worksheet
Processing Questions:

1. Was it difficult to think of ways to help any of the people on the list? Why?

2. Do you feel you have helped the people on the list as much as you should?

3. How does helping others make you feel?

Family Rules

Valued Outcome: Students will list various rules they are supposed to follow every day.
Description of Strategy: Discuss with the students the different kinds of rules they may be expected to follow every day. Two rules are given. Have the students discuss rules and then complete their own daily lists, placing an X in the columns of the days they successfully followed each rule.

	M	T	W	Th	F	Sa	S
Get up on time _____							
Brush my teeth _____							
_____							
_____							
_____							

Materials Needed: worksheet
Processing Questions:

1. Are some rules more difficult to follow? Why?

2. Why are there rules to follow?

3. What would happen if there was no rules? Would you really like that?

The Menstrual Cycle

Valued Outcome: The students will learn the different phases of the menstrual cycle.
Description of Strategy: About every twenty-eight days a new menstrual cycle begins in the female body. The cycle begins with the shedding of the lining of the uterus. This is called *menstruation* and takes about four or five days. For the next several days, the lining, or endometrium, is very thin, and an egg cell in an ovary begins to ripen. The lining starts to thicken, and, by the fourteenth day, a ripened egg is released into a fallopian tube. This is called *ovulation*. The endometrium continues to thicken as the egg moves toward the uterus. If the egg is not fertilized, it disintegrates and menstruation takes place, signaling the beginning of a new cycle.
   Figure 11.4 shows a 28-day menstrual cycle. Tell the students to put the letter of each phase on the blank spaces of the diagram in the correct order. Then tell them to indicate on the circle when ovulation takes place.
Materials Needed: worksheet (Figure 11.4)
Processing Questions:

1. What is menstruation?

2. Why is menstruation called a 28-day cycle?

Why Are They Like That?

Valued Outcome: Students will have an opportunity to ask questions about the behavior of the opposite sex.
Description of Strategy: Certain aspects of the behavior of boys is often a puzzle to girls and vice versa. Have each student write one question about some aspect of the "typical" behavior of the opposite sex that is puzzling or perhaps annoying. The questions should be unsigned. Collect all the questions and read those out loud that seem most germane to a discussion of behavior among boys and girls at your class's grade level. Have volunteers attempt to explain the point of view of the opposite sex that might shed light on a particular aspect of behavior. For example, girls may be more interested in boys at a certain age than boys are interested in girls. Maturational differences explain this fact. As a result, girls may be attracted to older boys, giving boys their own age the feeling that they are not seen as sexual peers. Act as moderator in the discussion, and provide factual information as necessary.
Materials Needed: slips of paper, pencils, or pens
Processing Questions:

1. Did you learn anything new about the opposite sex?

2. Do you think the behavior of the opposite sex makes any more sense than it did before?

3. Do males and females think the same way?

Figure 11.4
*Timing of the
Menstrual Cycle*

Start Here

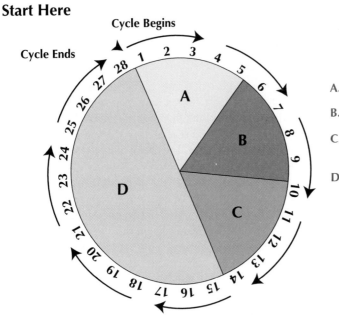

A. **Menstruation takes place.**

B. **Uterus lining is very thin.**

C. **Uterus lining begins thickening and
ovulation takes place.**

D. **Lining becomes thicker as egg travels.**

Source: Worksheet reproduced by permission of Tambrands, Inc., Lake Success, New York 11042 © 1989 Tambrands, Inc.

Advice Column

Valued Outcome: The students will ask questions about family and human sexuality.
Description of Strategy; With your assistance and supervision, have the class put together a newspaper advice column. First, have each student write a letter to the column asking for some advice about a sexuality or family life matter. Students may ask for simple factual information, such as "What is masturbation?" or for advice on handling a personal problem, such as "How can I ask someone for a date?" Collect all the letters, which should be unsigned or signed with something like "Puzzled" or "Wondering," and group them into categories. Restate a typical example of each category, writing this paraphrase on the chalkboard. Then have each student write an answer for the "column." Again using your discretion, collate the different suggestions offered and discuss them with the class. Properly handled, this activity can offer you important insights into the sexual development of students in your class. As "managing editor" of the advice column, however, you must make sure that topics covered stay within guidelines set up for your school's sexuality education program.
Materials Needed: paper, pencils or pens, chalkboard, chalk

Processing Questions:

1. What did you learn that you did not know before?
2. What do you think is the most important part of relationships with others?
3. Did you find out what you most wanted to know?

Reference

Bruess, C. E., and J. S. Greenberg. 1994. *Sex education: Theory and practice.* Dubuque, IA: Brown and Benchmark.

_____. 1995. *Puberty and reproduction—teacher/student resources.* Santa Cruz, CA: ETR Associates. (Grade 5–9)

_____. 1996. *Abstinence—Health facts.* Santa Cruz, CA: ETR Associates. (Grade 5–9)

_____. 1996. *Family relationships.* Santa Cruz, CA: ETR Associates. (Grades 5–9)

Ogletree, R. J., J. V. Fetro, J. C. Drolet, and B. A. Rienzo. 1994. *Sexuality education curricula—the consumer's guide.* Santa Cruz, CA: ETR Associates. (Teacher)

_____. 1994. *Family life education.* Santa Cruz, CA: ETR Associates. (Grades 4–6)

Pamphlets

101 Ways to Say NO to Sex. Santa Cruz, CA: ETR Associates. Suggestions on how teens can say no to sex. (Grades 6-12)

Male Facts. Santa Cruz, CA: ETR Associates. Provides basic information about male reproductive anatomy and physiology. (Grade 5–8)

Female Facts. Santa Cruz, CA: ETR Associates. Gives young women important facts and information on the menstrual cycle and how hormones control. (Grades 5-8)

CD-ROMs/Computer Software

A.D.A.M. essentials. Available in both Macintosh and Windows. Contains all body systems including the reproductive systems of males and females. (Grades 7–9)

Human sexuality. Relationships, communication, and decision-making are discussed. IBM- and Macintosh-compatible. Allows students to consider sexuality in the larger context of values, relationships, and communication. (Grades 6 & up). Available from NASCO, 901 Janesville Avenue, P.O. Box 901, Fort Atkinson, WI 53538-0901.

Internet/WWW, URLs

General Health Information:
http://www.ama-assn.org

General Health Information:
http://www.yahoo.com/health

Explicit Questions and Answers on Sexuality (Site referred to as Go Ask Alice!: Sexuality:
http://kwaziwai.cc.columbia.edu/cu/healthwise/cat6.html

Sexuality Information and Education Council of the United States (SIECUS)
http://www.siecus.org/

Videos

Kids and divorce. Provides insights into kids and divorce through children's first-hand accounts of their feeling about parents, and the breakup of their families. Twenty-minute video available from Sunburst Communications, 101 Castleton Street, Pleasantville, NY 10570-0040. (Grades 2–5)

Growing up! For girls. Provides the facts on becoming a young woman. Information on changes, good health and hygiene, and promoting of self-confidence in girls. Takes a realistic look at the responsibilities of adulthood. Fifteen-minute video available from NASCO, 901 Janesville Avenue, P. O. Box 901, Fort Atkinson, WI 53538-0901. (Grades 4–6)

Growing up! For boys. Information on physical and psychological changes that are a part of growing up. Seeks to foster self-esteem. Fifteen-minute video available from NASCO, 901 Janesville Avenue, P. O. Box 901, Fort Atkinson, WI 53538-0901. (Grades 4–6)

We're growing up!. Designed for mixed audiences and covers a review on male/female anatomy, sexual development, and provides an emphasis on responsible choices during adolescence. Fifteen-minute video available from NASCO, 901 Janesville Avenue, P. O. Box 901, Fort Atkinson, WI 53538-0901. (Grades 5–8)

When mom and dad break up. Helps children work through the confusion and pain of parents' divorce. Thirty-two-minute video available from the National Center for Elementary Drug and Violence Prevention, 117 HWY. 815, P. O. Box 9, Calhoun, KY 42327-0009. (Grades K-6)

Chapter Twelve

Substance Use and Abuse

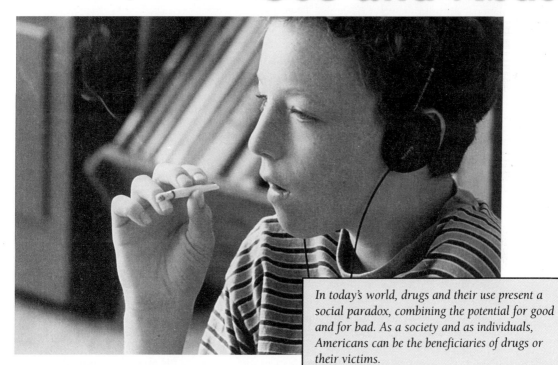

> In today's world, drugs and their use present a social paradox, combining the potential for good and for bad. As a society and as individuals, Americans can be the beneficiaries of drugs or their victims.
>
> —Levinthal (1996, xiii)

Valued Outcomes

After reading this chapter, you should be able to

○ define substance use, misuse and abuse

○ identify reasons that people abuse substances

○ describe the various effects of different drugs on the body

○ describe how tobacco advertising influences youth to use tobacco products

○ list recommendations for schools to reduce alcohol, tobacco, and other drug abuse problems among their students

○ give examples of the signs and symptoms of substance use and abuse

○ describe the most effective drug abuse education and prevention programs

: or Drug Abuse

For too long, a wide use of illicit drug use has afflicted America's young people, robbing many of life itself and preventing many more from fulfilling their hopes and dreams. Drugs have torn apart America's families, corrupted the nation's values and devastated countless communities. Drugs have affected all parts of our society, sparing no one—no social class, no region, no neighborhood, and no school.

Over the past decade, however, substance abuse has begun to recede. Fewer young people now are abusing some illegal drugs than at any time since 1975. Young people deserve much credit for turning away from drugs, and their hardening attitudes toward drugs have been documented in national attitudinal surveys (Levinthal 1996, 13).

Still, far too many young are abusing alcohol and other drugs—drugs that pose serious health hazards to young people. For example, alcohol-related traffic accidents are still the leading cause of death among young people. For this reason, the work of educators is not yet done in reducing substance abuse among young people.

For many people, the word *drug* is an emotionally charged term associated with such substances as heroin, cocaine, marijuana, and LSD. These substances are drugs, of course, but so are antibiotics, aspirin, the caffeine in a cup of coffee, and the alcohol in a glass of table wine. All these substances have in common the ability to bring about a change, and if taken under a physician's orders can help combat stress in a specific situation. However, if a person uses tranquilizers that have been prescribed for someone else, that is misuse. If an individual relies on tranquilizers as an emotional crutch, that is abuse. Likewise, many people enjoy a glass of wine with a meal, but drinking a glass of wine while under the influence of a drug such as an antihistamine or a sleeping pill is misuse. Drinking a quart of wine a day constitutes abuse. Drug misuse is the inappropriate use of medicines, whether intentional or not, and includes not following directions for proper medication, "lending" prescribed medicine to other people, and using old medicines for current problems. To some degree the difference between use and abuse is a value judgment. More objectively, substance abuse can be defined as the ingestion of any substance that leads to deleterious effects, either physically, psychologically, or both. Drug education is one of the more controversial aspects of health education. There are many differences of opinion as to how the subject should be approached. In fact, some parents would prefer that the subject not be approached at all.

In this chapter, we examine those substances that are commonly abused or misused. Some of them have little or no therapeutic value but can be purchased by adults for their personal use. Over-the-counter drugs, such as cough medicines, can have beneficial effects when used carefully. Because many people wrongly consider these drugs to be essentially harmless, however, misuse and abuse are common. Prescription drugs, such as tranquilizers, are more closely controlled, but these substances are also widely abused. Finally, we look at illegal substances, such as heroin, hallucinogens, cocaine, and marijuana.

Reasons for Substance Abuse

Individuals misuse or abuse drugs for a variety of reasons. Young people are especially likely to do so for the following reasons:

Curiosity. There exists in all of us an intrinsic desire to experience the unknown, and this desire is especially pronounced during the ages of strong peer influence, when many of a youngster's friends are experiencing drugs.

Low Self-Esteem. Many people have poor opinions of themselves. By using drugs, these individuals attempt to avoid coming to grips with their own feelings of inadequacy. Drugs thus serve as a coping mechanism.

Peer Pressure. Particularly during adolescence, individuals have a strong need to belong to "the group." If peers are abusing drugs, there is strong pressure on the part of all members of the group to do likewise.

Adult Modeling. Young people want to feel grown up, and they view drug taking as a form of adult behavior to be emulated. Smoking tobacco or marijuana, drinking alcohol, or taking pills may all result from adult modeling.

Mood Alteration. Some people take drugs simply to change their psychological state. The mellow feeling or the excitement produced is the motivation for this behavior.

Boredom. Many young people, especially during the teenage years, are at loose ends about their place in society. The activities of childhood no longer interest them, but they are not yet able to engage in adult activities. As a result, they feel bored with life.

Alienation. Some individuals feel that they have little or no power to control their destiny. They may also feel unwanted and unloved. Often, such people have few friends and view themselves as misfits in society. Drugs provide an outlet for the expression of such feelings of alienation.

Youth at Risk for Substance Abuse

The National Household Survey on Drug Abuse and the national High School Senior Survey provide insight as to trends in youth substance abuse. For example, males are more frequent users of drugs; most young people have their first alcoholic drink at twelve years old; whites are more frequent abusers than other races; junior and senior high school students consume about 35 percent of all wine coolers sold in the United States; at least half of all people arrested for major crimes in the United States—including homicide, theft, and assault—were using illegal drugs at the time of their arrest; and drug users report greater involvement in crime and are more likely than nonusers to have criminal records. Typically, youth at high risk for illegal substance and alcohol abuse include the economically disadvantaged; children of substance abusers; school dropouts; pregnant teens; victims of physical, sexual, and psychological abuse; runaways or the homeless; and youth who have committed a violent or delinquent act (Carroll 1996, 18–22).

Symptoms of Possible Substance Abuse in Youth

Several indicators can alert adults that a young person might be involved in substance abuse:

○ sudden or gradual changes in grades
○ absence from classes
○ school suspensions
○ withdrawal from family and other social functions
○ breaking curfew or lying
○ playing one authority figure against another
○ an increase in arguments with others

- a persistent and nagging cough
- weight loss
- difficulty sleeping
- vagueness about new friends and what they do together
- associating with an older crowd (Hunton 1991, 1)

Effects of Drugs on the Body

Drugs are chemicals that work in predictable patterns. First, a drug substance either mimics, facilitates, or antagonizes the body's normally occurring functions. Second, a drug substance can have one of four effects on a cell: It can increase activity, decrease activity, increase sensitivity, or disrupt the cell so that normal activity is sporadic. Third, the effect obtained from a drug substance depends on the concentration of the drug at the site of the action (Ray and Ksir 1996, 103). The effects of drugs result from their biochemical actions. This action depends on the substance reaching the desired site and on the body's chemistry. Other factors include the route of administration, distribution, dosage, expectations of the user, and frequency of use.

Route of Administration

Drugs can be taken orally in the form of pills, capsules, or liquids. They may be injected intravenously (directly into the bloodstream through a vein), intramuscularly (into a muscle), or subcutaneously (under the skin). Certain substances may be inhaled. Another method of administering a drug is topically, that is, by the external application of the substance to the skin or mucous membranes.

The amount of time required for a drug to take effect after use largely depends on the technique employed to administer it. The method of administration yielding the strongest and most rapid effect is intravenous (IV) injection. This procedure is considered the most dangerous because the risk of infection, vein collapse, or overdose is extremely high. Overdose is a significant problem with IV injection because chemicals enter the circulatory system rapidly and without intervening or protective factors. Smaller amounts of a drug are needed than for any other form of application.

Intramuscular injection works most rapidly in the deltoid muscle and least rapidly in the buttocks, because the poorer blood supply is found in the buttocks. Subcutaneous injection can be extremely irritating to the tissue. Topical administration is usually short acting and may damage the skin or mucous membrane because the chemical being administered often serves as an irritant.

Even oral ingestion creates problems. This technique requires the drug to enter the bloodstream by passing through the stomach, where it may be destroyed or altered to an inactive form. Then the substance must be lipid (fat) soluble in order to cross cell membranes and target the problem. Lipid-soluble products tend to be retained by the body and show cumulative effects. If water soluble, the substance is rapidly excreted by the body. Last, substances absorbed in the digestive tract go to the liver before being absorbed into general circulation; the function of the liver is to break down chemicals for excretion. Ultimately, oral ingestion creates difficulty in controlling the actual dosage absorbed by the body.

Distribution

Drugs are carried to body parts through the bloodstream. Some drugs are absorbed and then excreted quickly. Aspirin is an example of a drug that is excreted within a few hours. Other drugs are cumulative and are excreted very slowly. It may take several days to build up the level of the drug in the body to produce the desired therapeutic effect. Once built up, only maintenance doses are needed to maintain the drug's level. Certain heart medications are of this type.

Dosage

Dosage is the amount of a drug that is administered. The dosage serves to determine the effect of the substance on the body, or the dose–response relationship. The larger the amount taken, the greater the probability of several different effects. The *threshold dose* is the minimum amount required to produce a therapeutic effect. The dose in which maximum effect is obtained is called the *maximum dose*. The *effective dose* is the dose needed to produce a desired effect. A *lethal dose* is the amount that will produce death. The ratio between the effective dose and the lethal dose is the *therapeutic index*. This is obtained by dividing the amount of a lethal dose by the amount required for an effective dose. The higher the index, the lower the chance of a given dosage being lethal.

Another important concept concerning dosage is the *potency*, or the difference in effective doses between drugs that are used for the same purpose. For example, substance A may require twice the dosage to achieve the same effect as substance B. Therefore, substance B is a more potent drug. The time required for the substance to produce an effect after the body receives it is called the *time–action response*. As a general rule, the more quickly an effect appears, the shorter its effectiveness.

The presence of more than one drug can produce what is called *synergism*, in which the combined action of the drugs is greater than the sum of the effects of any one of the drugs taken alone. For example, some drugs *potentiate*, or increase the effect of another drug. The effect of one substance may be enhanced because of specific enzymes or formation of more potent metabolites or unknown reasons. It is frightening that pesticides, traces of hormones in meat and poultry, traces of metals in fish, nitrites, nitrates, and a wide range of chemicals used as food additives have been shown to interact with and potentiate some drugs. The classic example of synergism causing a dangerous potentiation is that a safe dose of alcohol mixed with a safe dose of a barbiturate can become lethal by depressing respiration. Conversely, a drug that acts as an antagonist blocks or interferes when used in combination with another drug, or it may inhibit a normal biological compound, such as a hormone.

Expectations of the User

The mood of the user and the setting in which the drug is taken may also affect the reaction to the drug. If the person expects the substance will help a problem or produce a particular effect, then the probability of that effect actually occurring is greater. The effect may occur even when the substance administered is only a placebo, or inert substance. The placebo effect is quite common. If the environment is such that particular results are expected from the drug, then these results are more likely, because of the drug, not expectations. Friends, soft lights, and music may help create an environmental setting for particular drug effects.

Placebos are often effective against pain because of an individual's belief that a drug will help. This effect was not understood until the endorphins and enkephalins were discovered. Both are peptides (biochemical chains of two or more amino acids) produced by the body and have an action similar to morphine. Enkephalins were first isolated from the brain and endorphins from the pituitary gland. Research has shown that endorphins and enkephalins alleviate pain. Physicians are just beginning to realize the importance of the mind in controlling disease and pain. It is clear that there is some biochemical process that is mobilized when a belief system, or the power of suggestion, is strong enough to have physical manifestations (Fishbein and Pease 1996, 73).

Frequency of Use

When some drugs are used frequently, larger dosages are required to maintain the effect. This is called *tolerance*. There are several forms of tolerance: disposition tolerance, cross-tolerance, pharmacodynamic tolerance, and reverse tolerance. *Disposition tolerance* concerns the rate at which the body disposes of a drug. Certain drugs tend to increase the rate of action of enzymes in the liver and, consequently, the deactivating of the drug. Alcohol and barbiturates are examples of drugs that cause the liver to produce the metabolic enzymes. Another important point is that these enzymes are not very discriminating; therefore, tolerance to one substance may lead to tolerance of other drugs that are pharmacologically similar. This effect is called *cross-tolerance*. Usually a heavy drinker will exhibit tolerance to barbiturates, tranquilizers, and anesthetics.

Evidence indicates that a considerable degree of central nervous system tolerance to certain drugs may develop independent of changes in the rate of absorption, metabolism, or excretion. This is called *pharmacodynamic tolerance* and occurs when the nervous tissue or other target tissues adapt to the substance so that the effect of the same concentration of a chemical decreases. In the case of reverse tolerance, users will have the same response to a lower dose of a drug that they had with initial higher doses. *Reverse tolerance* is believed to be primarily a learning process and does not result from a physiological response. However, it is possible for some drugs, such as marijuana, to be stored in the fat cells and released later as the fat cells are broken down. The fact that drug products remain in the body for extended periods of time may account for some of the reverse tolerance effect (Ray and Ksir 1996, 128). Usually, tolerance to a substance that requires increasing amounts of a chemical to maintain normal body functioning will lead to a physical dependence.

Some drugs, such as aspirin, cause neither tolerance nor dependence. Psychological dependence, or habituation, occurs when a person has a strong desire to repeat the use of a drug either occasionally or continually for emotional reasons. With psychological dependence, there is a feeling of satisfaction or psychic drive that requires repeated administration of the substance to produce an effect or avoid discomfort (Carroll 1996, 78–79).

Substance dependence, either physiological or psychological, appears to be synonymous with substance abuse. The model of addiction-producing drugs is based on the opiates, which require the development of tolerance, along with physical and psychological dependence. Opiates, alcohol, and barbiturates are examples that fit the traditional addiction model.

Over-the-Counter Drugs

Drugs that can be purchased without a prescription and that are used for self-medication are called over-the-counter (OTC) drugs. There are thousands of OTC drugs. These include aspirin and other analgesics, cold remedies, antihistamines and allergy products, vitamins, laxatives, antacids, and mild sedatives.

Most OTC drugs are somewhat effective in relieving the symptoms of the mild illnesses and disorders for which they were developed, as long as they are used according to directions. However, despite regulation by the Federal Trade Commission and other government agencies, advertising claims for many OTC products are often misleadingly optimistic. As a result, when the product fails to produce instant relief, some individuals may be tempted to exceed the recommended dosage in hopes of additional or faster aid. This sort of misuse can create health hazards.

Individuals should also recognize that there is some risk involved in using any medication, including aspirin, even when the directions are carefully followed. First, there is a possibility of allergic reaction. In rare cases, such reactions can be fatal. Second, relief provided by an OTC drug may mask symptoms of another illness or underlying disorder. For this reason, self-medication should only be attempted when the problem is minor and obvious, as in the case of a mild cold.

Another risk in using OTC drugs comes from *synergism*. As mentioned earlier, if two or more drugs or medications are taken at the same time, one substance can cause an increase or decrease in the potency of another. This synergistic reaction can have harmful and even fatal results.

As with any drugs, OTC drugs can have a stronger effect on children than on adults. Recently, for example, children's aspirin, formerly thought to be safe, has been identified as a cause of a severe reaction that can lead to death under certain conditions.

Depressants

Drugs that slow down, inhibit, or depress the nervous system are classified as depressants. The most commonly used depressant drug is alcohol. There are dozens of other depressants, most of which are prescription drugs. Whether obtained legally or illegally, however, depressants are among the most common of misused and abused drugs.

Depressant drugs have four main effects on the body. As sedatives, they can produce relaxation. As tranquilizers, they can reduce anxiety and act as muscle relaxants. As hypnotics, they can promote sleep. As anesthetics, they can create a loss of sensation. Various depressant drugs differ in their potencies, but in sufficient amounts they can all produce these four effects.

The sedative-hypnotics include barbiturates and tranquilizers. Examples of barbiturates by trade name include Amytal, Nembutal, and Seconal. Commonly prescribed tranquilizers include Valium, Librium, and Miltown. Both of these types of drugs are usually taken orally, although some can be given intravenously as a general anesthetic.

Alcohol

The use of alcohol by youth still remains a problem, despite declining levels of use and increased awareness of the dangers of these substances. Over 25 percent of eighth graders, almost 40 percent of tenth graders and over half of twelfth graders report drinking alcohol in the last thirty days (Langton 1996, 21). Further, alcohol use among young people appears to stimulate a progression to other drug use. The use of alcohol and tobacco among youth is correlated with other health problems, including adolescent suicide, homicide, school dropout, delinquency, early sexual activity, sexually transmitted diseases, problem pregnancy, and motor vehicle crashes. Alcohol-related traffic crashes are the leading cause of death and spinal cord injury for young Americans. Young adults are unlikely to develop alcohol problems if the age of first use is delayed beyond childhood and adolescence.

Alcohol is used in a variety of social and recreational settings in our society.

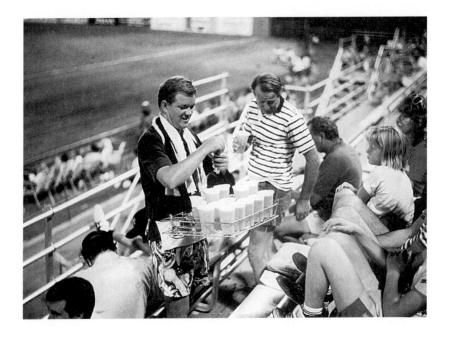

Many teachers says that alcohol use is at least a moderate problem in their schools, according to a report published by the National Center for Education Statistics (Appalachian Educational Laboratory 1992). In surveying 1,350 elementary and secondary school teachers nationwide, the report finds that 54 percent of secondary teachers reported that alcohol use is a concern. Twenty-four to 30 percent of these secondary school teachers said that prevention programs and policies for reducing alcohol use are either not very or not at all effective.

Ethyl alcohol is the active ingredient in beer, wine, and distilled beverages such as whiskey. Ethyl alcohol is not as toxic as are some other forms of the chemical, such as methyl alcohol, which is used as rubbing alcohol. In this discussion, we use the term *alcohol* to refer to ethyl alcohol. Alcohol is a colorless, flammable liquid formed by the fermentation of fruits, juices, or cereal grains. Alcoholic beverages contain varying amounts of alcohol, depending on the type of beverage. Beer usually contains from 5 to 7 percent alcohol. Wines may vary from 11 to 20 percent. Distilled beverages have the highest alcohol content. This content is measured by the proof of the beverage, which is a number that is twice the alcohol content. For example, a 100-proof whiskey contains 50 percent alcohol, whereas a 90-proof one contains 45 percent.

Effects of Alcohol

Alcohol is a central nervous system depressant. In small doses, the substance has a mellowing or tranquilizing effect. The individual may feel relaxed and free from tension. As a result, behavior may become less inhibited, leading to the misconception held by some that alcohol is a stimulant. Actually, what appears to be stimulated, or at least animated, behavior results from the anesthetic, depressant effect that alcohol has on the cerebral cortex area of the brain.

The effects of alcohol on the body corresponds with the amount of alcohol in the system. The amount of alcohol can be measured by the percentage of the blood that is composed of alcohol. In large amounts, alcohol impairs brain activity, muscular control, coordination, memory, reaction time, and judgment. Heavy intake over a short period of time can bring about a dulling of the senses. Continued heavy drinking can result in coma and death.

Consumption of alcohol over a long period of time can result in damage to the brain and liver. The brain may be damaged to the extent that memory, judgment, and learning deteriorate. Cirrhosis of the liver is a potentially fatal condition caused by damage to that organ by alcohol. Cirrhosis of the liver does occur in nonalcoholic drinkers, but this is rare. Recently, the harmful effects of even moderate amounts of alcohol consumed by pregnant women have become known. The alcohol can have a deleterious effect on the developing fetus, resulting in a condition known as *fetal alcohol syndrome*. A child born with this condition may suffer permanent impairment. Characteristics of the condition include low birth weight, smaller head circumference, abnormal formation of the nose, small fingernails, smaller stature, poor joint movement, ear abnormalities, and mental retardation.

In moderation, alcohol does not seem to harm the body permanently. However, if an adult decides to partake of alcoholic beverages, care should be exercised. Alcohol should be consumed slowly, with adequate food in the stomach. Individuals should also recognize that tolerance to alcohol builds up. More of the substance may be required to produce the pleasant, mellow effect associated with its use. Drinking without recognizing the potential dangers of alcohol can lead to tragedy.

Why Do Youth Begin Abusing Alcohol?

Children are naturally curious—exploring new ideas, behaviors, and relationships. They feel the need to take risks, to exercise their judgment and their independence. In the process, some become users of alcohol and other drugs. Schools, families, and friends need to support them in channeling their curiosity away from using alcohol. Adults, who have a direct impact on the alcohol-using behavior of young people, are unaware of how their own behavior influences kids. Some ways in which adults may, unknowingly, contribute to childhood alcohol use are

1. the extent of the legal recreational use of alcohol by the parent in the home
2. the poor quality of parenting
3. the misuse and abuse of other drugs by the parents—either in the past or currently (Langton 1996, 21–28).

Consequences of Alcohol Use

Alcohol can interfere with a child's motivation to do well in school, become involved in useful activities, or form healthy relationships—ones that do not revolve around alcohol and other drug use. As a result, intellectual growth, social skills, and self-confidence are compromised. Most young people who consistently use alcohol lack social skills and have poor parenting. They often want desperately to belong, even to the extent of doing things that go against their better judgment. Because alcohol can reduce inhibitions, youngsters (already concerned with being popular) who use alcohol are more likely to become involved in risk-taking behaviors.

Drinking and Accidents

Alcohol remains the primary cause of automobile accidents among drivers. Alcohol is involved in 50 percent or more of all fatal traffic accidents. Without question, drinking and driving don't mix. Two of the many groups who are keeping the drunk driving issue alive by making people aware of the problem are MADD (Mothers Against Drunk Driving) and SADD (Students Against Drunk Driving). MADD also serves to mobilize the public to help individuals modify their drinking habits and protests the judicial system when someone with a history of drunk driving is allowed to continue to drive. MADD has been successful in reducing the legal blood alcohol concentration (BAC) in various states and has initiated several effective programs to limit drinking and driving. The purpose of SADD includes helping students save their own lives and the lives of others; to educate students on the problem of drinking and driving; to develop peer counseling among students about alcohol use; and to increase public awareness and prevention of alcohol abuse everywhere. An important feature of the SADD program is the "Contract for Life," a teenager–parent contract in which the teenager agrees to call the parent for advice and/or transportation at any time from any place if the teenager or if his/her driver has had too much to drink. The parent in return agrees to transport the teenager in such a situation, and also agrees to seek sober transportation for him- or herself in a similar situation. SADD has chapters in over fifteen hundred colleges and has an offshoot called Student Athletes Detest Drugs geared toward the problem of drug use by athletes (Avis 1996, 261).

Alcoholism and Alcohol-Related Problems

Perhaps the area for greatest concern among substance abuse professionals is alcoholism among young people. According to the National Council on Alcoholism, alcoholism is the number one drug problem among the nation's youth. Forty percent of children have tasted alcohol by age ten. The average age for a first drink is just under thirteen. Nearly 30 percent of teenagers have experienced negative results from abuse of alcohol. These range from auto accidents to arrests to detrimental effects on schoolwork and others mentioned earlier in this chapter. Ironically, 42 percent of fourth-graders failed to recognize alcohol as a drug. Only 72 percent of children in the upper grades realize it is a drug, and, therefore, dangerous.

Definitions of this term, *alcoholism*, vary from source to source. In general, the disease alcoholism can be described as when a person is unable to choose whether he or she will drink and is unable to stop drinking. Alcoholics use the substance in such a way that their personal, social, and occupational behavior is interfered with or totally disrupted. The problem is common among ministers, homemakers, politicians, factory workers, musicians, police officers, and retired people. Both rich and poor, young and old, are susceptible. As many as 10 million Americans have a serious drinking problem.

Alcoholism is best characterized as a disease. The causes of alcoholism are not completely understood, but research has established biological factors that may differentiate alcoholics from nonalcoholics (Levinthal 1996, 272). Recent studies provide strong evidence that genetics plays a role in some cases of alcoholism. Some people—for example, about half of all Far East Asians—produce low levels of an important enzyme that helps metabolize alcohol; these people cannot tolerate even small amounts of alcohol. However, the absorption rates of alcohol in the intestinal tract may predispose some Native Americans to alcoholism (Hahn and Payne 1997, 193).

Regardless of how important the heredity factor is, social and psychological factors also influence the development of alcoholism. Because alcohol is generally accepted in our society, many individuals feel free to use it. Too often, however, use leads to misuse, and alcoholism is the result. The drug becomes a crutch for dealing with everyday problems, until the individual can no longer get along without it.

Alcohol-related problems are all too well known in our society. Aside from the thousands of traffic deaths and injuries that occur each year because of alcohol abuse, alcohol is also related to the high divorce rate, job absenteeism, crimes of violence, suicide, and social disorder.

Alcoholics and their families can receive help from many sources, including such nonprofit groups as Alcoholics Anonymous (AA). AA is a support group of fellow alcoholics designed to help each other remain sober. There are also many commercial alcoholic treatment programs. These can be expensive, but many insurance companies now pay for such treatment. Al-Anon, Alateen, and Alatot are groups specifically established to assist the families of alcoholics. Al-Anon is a group for spouses, relatives, and friends of alcoholics. Alateen and Alatot are groups that are designed for children of alcoholics. These groups are designed to help these friends and relatives understand the alcoholic and thereby better cope with the alcoholic's lifestyle. Further, these groups help the individuals learn from each other (Witters, Venturelli, and Hanson 1992, 207). These groups also help the family members understand the roles they play as codependents—that is, the behavior of family members that sometimes enables the alcoholic to continue his or her lifestyle. For example, if a spouse calls her alcoholic husband's employer and tells the employer that her husband will not be at work because he is sick, this action enables the alcoholic to continue his behavior.

Barbiturates

Barbiturates have historically represented one of the nation's biggest drug abuse problems. Generally known as downers, barbiturates are often taken as a way of escaping from the problems of daily living. Abusers of this type of drug "fog out" and feel removed from the cares of existence. The potency of such drugs is increased by combining them with alcoholic intake, which often results in fatal overdoses that cause cardiorespiratory failure. More commonly, barbiturate abuse results in mental confusion, dizziness, and loss of memory.

Barbiturates are highly addictive. Physical, as well as psychological, dependency can quickly develop. Withdrawal from barbiturate dependency can be life threatening and should be undertaken only under close medical supervision.

Tranquilizers

Tranquilizers are classified as major and minor. The major tranquilizers, such as Thorazine, are used to treat psychosis. Minor tranquilizers, such as Valium and Librium, are prescribed for stress and anxiety. They are also useful as muscle relaxants. However, partly because they are so widely prescribed, such tranquilizers are often abused. Physical and psychological dependency can result. Symptoms of physical dependency include drowsiness and slurred speech. Psychological dependency may be characterized by increased irritability and irrational fear. As in the case with barbiturates, withdrawal from tranquilizers can be highly traumatic.

Cross-Tolerance and the Depressant Drugs

Tolerance to depressant drugs can be developed fairly quickly. Then higher and higher doses of the drug must be taken to produce the desired relaxing effect. Tolerance to one kind of depressant drug also produces tolerance to other types of depressant substances that are not even being taken. This phenomenon is known as *cross-tolerance*. The danger of cross-tolerance may not be as obvious to drug abusers as it should be. Once tolerance to one depressant drug has developed, the individual may decide to switch to another depressant in hopes of achieving the same desired effect. However, because of cross-tolerance, the outcome is not as hoped. A higher dose may then be resorted to. If the new drug is more potent, a fatal overdose may result.

Narcotics

Narcotic drugs are produced for the most part from opium and its derivatives, although some are synthesized substances. Such drugs act on the central nervous system and gastrointestinal tract. They are excellent painkillers, but they can be highly addictive, both physically and psychologically. Opium is derived from the opium poppy. Morphine, codeine, and heroin also come from this source. Morphine is a potent painkiller used primarily to relieve severe pain such as acute sickle cell crisis and heart attack.

Codeine is often used in conjunction with acetaminophen to relieve moderate pain. In addition, codeine is effective in suppressing the cough reflex. Heroin is not used for medical purposes.

Heroin is one of the most dangerous drugs abused. Much heroin is produced illegally in foreign countries in Asia and smuggled into the United States. The drug can be smoked, swallowed, injected under the skin, or injected directly into a vein. The latter method is used most often by heroin addicts because the drug reaches the bloodstream most quickly this way. The desired effect is a sudden rush of euphoria, followed by a dreamy state of complete relaxation. This period may last up to several hours, depending on a variety of factors, including the strength of the dosage. "Street" heroin is always sold in an adulterated state, usually mixed with milk sugar, so that the actual percentage of heroin is small.

Although considered physiologically "clean," in the sense that it does not damage organs, heroin is extremely addictive, and a user soon may live for no other reason than to inject more heroin. Tolerance also quickly develops, leading to a need for higher and higher or more frequent doses of the drug. The result is too often a fatal overdose, which results in death because of cardiorespiratory failure.

Withdrawal from heroin is agonizing. It is characterized by chills, fever, diarrhea, and vomiting. However, painful as it is, heroin withdrawal is seldom life threatening. Still, most heroin addicts, even when they would like to quit, find it almost impossible to do so because of the craving they have developed for the drug.

The dangers from heroin use are manifold. Aside from weight loss, lethargy, sexual inadequacy, and the constant problems of withdrawal that require regular doses of the drug, injection of heroin can lead to other health problems, including hepatitis and AIDS because of dirty needles and anemia caused by disregard for proper nutrition. Toxic adulterants in heroin sold on the street can also kill.

After heroin was outlawed in 1914, heroin addiction declined steadily to a low point during World War II. Heroin addiction peaked in the early 1950s, but it dropped again to another low point in the early 1960s. The upsurge in marijuana and other hallucinogenic drug use was accompanied in the 1970s by another rise in heroin abuse. By the mid-1970s, the estimates of the number of addicts were in the four to five hundred thousand range. Now, there is an increase in heroin use by young people through smoking (Ray and Ksir 1996, 344–349).

Stimulants

Stimulants are drugs that stimulate, or speed up, the nervous system. Physiologically, the stimulant drugs increase heart rate, blood pressure, and amount of circulating blood sugar. They also constrict the blood vessels and dilate bronchial tubes and the pupils of the eyes. Some can produce a temporary euphoria.

Caffeine

The most common stimulant is caffeine, which is contained in coffee, tea, cola drinks, and even chocolate. Caffeine is a mild stimulant that is often abused. Nonetheless, it is a drug and should be recognized as one that can lead to health problems.

Caffeine is absorbed rather quickly into the bloodstream and reaches a peak blood level in about 30 to 60 minutes. It increases mental alertness and provides a greater feeling of energy. However, high doses of caffeine can overstimulate and cause nervousness and increased heart rate. Caffeine can also cause sleeplessness, excitement, and irritability. In some cases, high doses of caffeine can induce convulsions.

Coffee or cola drinking, let alone chocolate eating, cannot be considered drug abuse by most commonly accepted standards, but some individuals seek out caffeine for its own sake, in OTC products and in illegal substances to produce a caffeine "high." Because it is not considered a dangerous drug, the opportunities for caffeine abuse are often overlooked.

Amphetamines

Amphetamines represent a more serious stimulant drug abuse problem. These drugs have limited legitimate and useful medical applications, but because of their wide availability, they are often abused. Examples of commonly prescribed amphetamines include Benzedrine, Dexedrine, Methadrine, Ritalin, and Narodin. Because of the possibility of dependency, the uncertainty of side effects, and the questionable nature of some applications, use of amphetamines has come under closer scrutiny in the last few years. For example, although amphetamines do suppress hunger, they are no longer recommended as "diet pills" by most doctors. Recently, national surveys have shown that there is an alarming rise in the number of adolescents that abuse amphetamines. It is feared that this increase is the beginning of a pattern of escalating amphetamine abuse (Hanson and Venturelli 1995, 264).

The general street name for such drugs is "speed," because of the way these substances seem to speed up the nervous system. Amphetamine pills are also known as "uppers." Abusers of amphetamines pass into an extremely excited state and may feel omnipotent until the drug begins to wear off. A depressed period, called a "crash" by abusers, then follows, leading to a craving for more amphetamines.

As with many drugs, a craving for amphetamines often undermines a person's regard for good personal health practices. Because appetite is inhibited by such drugs, poor nutrition leading to weight loss often results. Once the stimulating effects diminish, chronic users frequently enter into periods of depression that are sometimes severe (Fishbein and Pease 1996, 188–189).

There is debate as to whether amphetamines result in true physical dependency, but there is no doubt that strong psychological dependency soon develops. Long-term use of these drugs can result in heart, liver, and kidney damage. Speech problems and facial twitches may also be apparent. In high doses, amphetamines can cause hallucinations, delusions, and disorganized behavior. Withdrawal from amphetamines is not life threatening, but the process does result in depression and anxiety. Professional treatment is often necessary.

Cocaine

Known on the street as "snow" or "coke," cocaine is an illegal drug that continues to rise in popularity. Currently, cocaine trafficking and consumption represent the most significant drug problem in the United States. The groups most vulnerable to cocaine use include adolescents and young adults who demonstrate higher than average levels of tobacco, alcohol, and especially marijuana use. The risk of becoming a cocaine user does not decrease after the teen years. Initiation to cocaine use occurs anytime from adolescence to adulthood.

According to the 1993 National Household Survey on Drug Abuse, over 23 million Americans above the age of twelve used cocaine at some time in their lives. About 1.5 million Americans over the age of twelve reported using cocaine twelve or more times during the past year. On a positive note, the use of crack among high school seniors has declined since 1987, the perceived risk of using cocaine (especially crack), has continued to increase among high school seniors and young adults, and there has been a decrease of perceived availability of cocaine in the last few years (Fishbein and Pease 1996, 159–161).

Cocaine is legal and useful for limited medical purposes. Because of its vasoconstrictive and anesthetic properties, cocaine is used as a local ingredient in Brompton's cocktail, a preparation for treating severe pain in individuals with a terminal illness. Cocaine is taken to produce a feeling of intense euphoria and boundless energy. As this fades, depression—sometimes severe—follows, along with the strong desire for another dose, or "hit." Although physical dependence is not seen with cocaine, psychological dependence is common and can be very potent. Withdrawal symptoms from cocaine are limited to mild depression and anxiety with limited use. Paranoid thinking, hallucinations, and psychosis can occur with heavy, extended use.

Cocaine is most often found in the form of a white powder, which is usually sniffed or "snorted" up the nostrils or smoked. The drug enters the bloodstream through the nasal membranes when sniffed or snorted. The cocaine concentration in the blood rapidly increases for about 30–40 minutes, then gradually declines for three or more hours after use (Hanson and Venturelli 1995, 275–277).

Following intravenous administration, the total amount of cocaine enters the bloodstream in a few minutes. Within seconds after injection, cocaine users experience an incredible state of euphoria. The "high" is intense but short lived; within 15–20 minutes, this "high" is followed by a depression that may last 10 to 40 minutes (Hanson and Venturelli 1995, 277). Oral use is not common in the United States, but the high is comparable to other forms of use.

A process used for purifying or refining cocaine is called *freebasing*. This method produces a more potent form with an accelerated and intense high. The drug is heated to a high temperature and mixed with other substances, some highly volatile, resulting, on occasion, in explosion. The resulting mixture is then smoked in a water pipe.

Recently, a new form of cocaine has become popular. "Crack" or "rock" gets its name from the sound made by the crystals when heated, or the rocklike appearance. Crack may be 90 percent pure, compared to 15 to 25 percent purity in regular cocaine. The drug is smoked in a glass water pipe, resulting in rapid absorption into the blood. Crack reaches the brain in less than 10 seconds, with the high lasting from five to seven minutes. Following this intense rush, crashing depression may occur and may last two to three times longer than the high.

Many people perceive smoking to be less dangerous, but this route provides direct absorption via the lungs, into the blood, and to the brain in less than 10 seconds. The speed with which crack acts and the purity it displays make it very dangerous. Crack is widely available for about $5 a hit, erasing the notion that cocaine is an upper-class drug.

Cocaine's action on the body most directly affects the cardiovascular system. The heart rate increases, and small blood vessels constrict, resulting in increased blood pressure. This sudden increase in cardiac activity, coupled with vasoconstriction, leads to an elevated risk of cardiac ischemia, resulting in heart attack or rhythm disturbances. These risks can occur when using small amounts, either by sniffing, snorting, smoking, or IV use. In addition, the absence of an underlying heart condition does not make one immune from cardiac consequences.

Treatment of cocaine dependence varies for different programs. From 30 to 90 percent of the patients who persist in outpatient treatment programs are considered successful, but these figures may be misleading since they do not take into account the patients who drop out of programs (Hanson and Venturelli 1995, 281).

Tobacco

Tobacco has been known and used for hundreds of years. It can be snuffed, chewed, placed between the gum and lips, or smoked. The most popular method of tobacco use is smoking. Cigarettes became popular in the early 1900s. Before then, tobacco was usually chewed or smoked in a pipe.

Since the U.S. Surgeon General's first warning about smoking and cancer, heart disease, and other health problems, the nation's smoking rate has fallen dramatically. In the mid-1960s, an estimated 40 percent of the adult population smoked—53 percent of men and 32 percent of women. Now the rate of cigarette smoking is the lowest ever reported, with just 28 percent of men and 23 percent of women classified as regular smokers. Only 20 percent of these regular cigarette users are estimated to smoke every day. However, 12 million Americans—most adolescent males and young adults—use smokeless tobacco (Carroll 1996, 173).

Cigarette smoking remains the single, most important preventable cause of death in our society (Levinthal 1996, 299). Smoking is directly responsible for about 390,000 deaths each year in the United States; thus, we can fairly blame smoking for more than one of every six deaths in our country.

About 90 percent of adult smokers began their addiction as children or adolescents, and these young smokers will account for many health problems in the future. The younger a person is when he or she starts to smoke, the more likely he or she is to become a long-term smoker and to develop smoking-related diseases. Preventing youngsters from taking up smoking is far more cost effective than treating the addiction later in life, and far less expensive than treating the resulting diseases.

Effects of Tobacco Smoking

According to the U.S. Surgeon General, cigarette smoking is the primary avoidable cause of death in our society and the most important health issue of our time. Cancer is the second leading cause of death in this country, and smoking accounts for nearly one-third of all cancer deaths. Prevention of smoking in young people is a critical goal, particularly in view of the limited success that many smokers have in quitting (Langton 1996, 218).

The primary drug in tobacco is nicotine. A typical filter cigarette contains between 1 and 2 mg of nicotine, with about 90 percent of this amount being absorbed when inhaled. Smoking results in the constriction of the blood vessels, which decreases the skin temperature. Nicotine acts as a stimulant on the heart and nervous system, causing an increased heartbeat and elevated blood pressure. In addition, the blood decreases in its ability to carry oxygen because of the carbon monoxide in tobacco smoke, which is more easily picked up by hemoglobin.

Cigarette smoke also contains chemicals known collectively as *tars*. These substances have been identified as carcinogens, or cancer-causing agents. Smoking is a major cause of lung cancer

Health Highlight

The Report of the Surgeon General: Preventing Tobacco Use among Young People

The U.S. Surgeon General's report entitled *Preventing Tobacco Use among Young People,* reached the following conclusions:

1. Nearly all first use of tobacco occurs before high school graduation; this finding suggests that if adolescents can be kept tobacco free, most will never start using tobacco.

2. Tobacco is often the first drug used by those young people who use alcohol, marijuana, and other drugs.

3. Adolescents with lower levels of school achievement, fewer skills to resist pervasive influences to use tobacco, friends who use tobacco, and lower self-images are more likely than their peers to use tobacco.

4. Community-wide efforts that include enforcement of minors' access laws and school-based tobacco use prevention programs are successful in reducing adolescent use of tobacco.

Source: P. Langton. 1996. *The social world of drugs.* Minneapolis: West, 218.

and may contribute to other forms of malignancies as well. Smokers not only run an increased risk of developing cancer, but they also have much higher rates of coronary heart disease. Emphysema, a breathing disorder that results from deterioration of lung tissue, is also associated with cigarette smoking, as are many other respiratory diseases.

The relationship between a mother's smoking and harmful effects on a developing fetus has been established. It has been estimated that in the United States approximately one-third of the women of childbearing age are smokers. Furthermore, only 5 to 10 percent of these women quit smoking during pregnancy. Some of the most important findings related to smoking and pregnancy are

1. Cigarette smoking during pregnancy causes a reduction in infant birth weight. The mean birth weight of infants born to mothers who smoke during pregnancy is 7 ounces less than that of infants born to nonsmoking mothers.

2. Cigarette smoking is related to significantly higher fetal and neonatal mortality.

3. Cigarette smoking is associated with an increase in spontaneous abortions (Fishbein and Pease 1996, 217).

Both male and female current cigarette smokers experience more workdays lost, days of bed disability, and long limitation of activity due to chronic diseases than do people who never smoked. In addition, current and former smokers report more hospitalization than nonsmokers in the year before being interviewed in research studies. Even though most studies show a reduction in the risk of mortality among former smokers, data on disability and illness often show continued high risk among former smokers. All measures of smoking disability are dose related; that is, the more smoking there is, the greater the likelihood of developing a disability or disablement (Carroll 1996, 194).

Although cigarette smokers run the highest risk, use of tobacco in other forms can also lead to serious problems. For example, pipe smoking is related to cancer of the lip. Both pipe and cigar smokers run a higher risk of developing cancer of the mouth, larynx, and esophagus. Snuff dippers, or people who use smokeless tobacco, have a higher incidence of cancer of the gums than do nonusers.

Why People Smoke

People begin smoking for some of the same reasons that apply to drinking. Adult modeling and peer pressure are certainly factors. The appeal produced by cigarette advertising also plays a part. According to Schlaadt and Shannon (1990, 130–131), once a person has developed a smoking habit, one or more of the following reasons may apply:

Stimulation. Smokers claim that smoking helps wake them up, organize their intellectual activity, and enhance their energy level.

Relaxation or Tranquility. Smokers say that smoking helps promote and enhance pleasant feelings. Smokers also believe that smoking reduces negative feelings.

Stress Reduction. Smokers use cigarettes in times of stress or personal discomfort. Smoking is seen as a tranquilizer, again helping to reduce negative feelings.

Physiological and/or Psychological Dependence. The smoker is dependent on cigarettes; there is a psychological and possibly physical dependence on cigarettes.

Habit. Smoking is done simply out of habit, although the smoker gets very little pleasure from smoking. The person may have minimal awareness of the act of smoking, sometimes lighting one cigarette while another one is still burning.

A very forceful motivation for smoking is advertising. Cigarette manufacturers spend more than $3.2 billion each year promoting cigarettes and the acceptance of smoking. Cigarette advertising reveals very few facts about cigarettes, but rather appeals to individual needs, a memory of good feeling, the universal need for companionship, and a desire for escape and adventure. Cigarette ads also are designed to reduce one's anxieties about growing old, being alone, losing one's health, or one's sex drive. According to the U.S. Centers for Disease Control (1990, 264), cigarette advertising and promotion may increase cigarette consumption among children and adolescents by encouraging them to experiment with and initiate regular use of cigarettes. Also, the promotional activities of tobacco companies are designed to result in the trial and/or purchase of tobacco products. Free samples may encourage initiation of tobacco use among children and adolescents, especially when distributed at youth-oriented events, such as concerts. Cigarette sponsorship of sporting events allows cigarette brand names to be shown or mentioned on television (even though cigarette commercials are prohibited in the broadcast media), and cigarette sponsorship of televised sporting events is reported to increase cigarette brand recognition among children.

The impact of such advertising on potential smokers (young people) is substantial (Levinthal 1996, 303). A recent poll indicated that Joe Camel (a character used in Camel cigarette ads) was one of the two most recognizable media cartoon characters among young children, tieing with Mickey Mouse. In response to this poll, the current U.S. Surgeon General called for Camel to remove Joe Camel from its ads. A U.S. senator was recently quoted on the television news as stating that any company who marketed a product that killed off its clientele (such as tobacco companies) must advertise strongly to attract new customers (young people).

Advertising of tobacco products to girls and women has been successful. By the late-1990s, the percentage of women who smoke is expected to exceed that of men who smoke. The explanation is not only that more girls than boys have taken up the habit in the past decade but also that fewer girls quit. The targeting of girls and women in advertising tobacco products is made easier by the fact that smoking artificially and temporarily holds down body weight, and societal pressure for girls and women to be slender is intense. Weight control is one of the most important reasons girls start smoking, and one of the biggest barriers preventing them from quitting. Since youth are very concerned about body image and since adolescent girls are prone to low self-esteem, they are particularly vulnerable to tobacco advertising (Mintz 1991, 592). The effects of the resulting tobacco use among girls and women have been devastating. Lung cancer has overtaken breast cancer as the number one cause of cancer death among women, and lung cancer death rates among women continue to increase at an unrelenting pace. Other smoking-related disease, such as heart disease and emphysema, also are exacting a terrible toll on women. For example, women who smoke are more than three times as likely to have a heart attack as women who have never smoked (Sullivan 1990, 2).

A study by the Centers for Disease Control and Prevention (CDC) shows that antismoking strategies needed in childhood to counteract the effects of advertising. Findings from CDC's latest Youth Risk Behavior Survey indicate that students who smoke their first cigarette at less than twelve years of age are more likely to become regular and heavy smokers than students who begin smoking at a later age. In addition, students who participate in sports activities smoke less than students who do not participate. These findings suggest that antismoking education should be available during childhood before smoking becomes a problem. Also, since another study showed that few youth who smoke receive counseling about nicotine addiction, smoking cessation education should be available to youngsters who do smoke (CDC 1993, 1391–1395).

Secondhand and Sidestream Smoke

Although an individual may choose not to smoke, being in an enclosed area with smoking forces him or her to smoke involuntarily. Sidestream smoke is the smoke that comes from a burning cigarette. Secondhand smoke is exhaled from the smoker. This smoke has much higher concentrations of some irritating and hazardous substances than mainstream, or inhaled, smoke. Carbon monoxide is especially significant with secondhand smoke. With several people smoking in an enclosed area, the Environmental Protection Agency's safe limit recommendation can be exceeded. Most standard air filtration systems do not remove carbon monoxide gas from the air. Only dilution with fresh air can lower carbon monoxide levels.

Nicotine from sidestream smoke generally settles out of the air, with only small amounts being absorbed from heavily polluted air. Other carcinogens are absorbed in small amounts, but the carcinogenic effect is not known. Other substances from sidestream smoke probably are not hazardous, just irritating to nonsmokers. People with cardiovascular disease or bronchopulmonary disease can be adversely affected. Children of parents who smoke are more likely to have bronchitis, pneumonia, and reactive airway diseases during the first year of life and as youth.

Reducing the Hazards of Smoking

The best way to avoid the hazards of smoking is simply not to smoke. This means not beginning in the first place or giving up the habit if smoking has already begun. People who smoke should also recognize the possible harmful effects of secondhand smoke on others. Inhaling smoke produced by a smoker can aggravate respiratory conditions and may even be the cause of such conditions in a nonsmoker. Those who refuse to stop smoking can lower the risk they run by choosing a brand of cigarettes with less tar and nicotine, by smoking fewer cigarettes, by taking fewer puffs and not inhaling so deeply, and by not smoking the cigarette all the way down to the end.

Smokeless Tobacco

Advertising claims have made it appear that smokeless tobacco is a safe alternative to smoking tobacco. Evidently this effort has been successful, because smokeless tobacco is the only type of tobacco product whose use has increased in recent years. Advertisements for this product feature athletes and run in adventure and sports magazines, thereby appealing to young people, and adolescents have gotten the message. Nearly 12 million try smokeless tobacco every year, and 6 million are regular users (Ray and Ksir 1996, 276).

Smokeless tobacco comes in three forms: loose leaf, snuff, and plug. Chewing tobacco is sold as either loose leaf or a plug. Snuff is finely ground tobacco that is placed between the cheeks and gums. This method of use is called *dipping*. Sometimes the snuff is placed on the back of the hand and sniffed up the nose. A plug is solidly formed, like a brick, and must be cut with a knife. The plugs of tobacco are then placed between the teeth and gums, causing the person to salivate.

The Surgeon General's report indicates the following health risks associated with the use of smokeless products:

○ The risk of cancer of the cheek and gum may be fifty times higher for snuff users.

○ Smokeless tobacco can lead to the development of leukoplakia (white patches) in the mouth, particularly where the tobacco products have been placed. These white patches represent a precancerous condition.

○ There are many carcinogens (cancer-causing) agents in smokeless products, such as nitrosamines, hydrocarbons, and polonium.

Other problems associated with smokeless tobacco have been identified by Carroll (1996, 189–190):

○ an association with cancer, especially of the oral cavity

○ an association with gingival recession, or receding gums

○ increased number of dental caries

○ a strong dependence on nicotine

○ a supporting role in the origin of coronary artery disease and peptic ulcers

○ darkening of the teeth, resulting in bad breath

Preventing and Reducing Tobacco Use

As stated earlier in this chapter, about 90 percent of adult smokers began their addiction as children or adolescents, and these young smokers will account for many health problems in the future. The younger a person is when he or she starts to smoke, the more likely he or she is to become a long-term smoker and to develop smoking-related diseases. Preventing youngsters from taking up smoking is far more cost effective than treating the addiction later in life, and far less expensive than treating the resulting diseases. As with so many other health issues, tobacco addiction should be attacked with prevention measures, and this implies a vigorous effort to discourage children and youth from ever starting to use tobacco (Sullivan 1990, 3).

The Healthy Youth 2000 Initiative states that a carefully planned, comprehensive school health education program can make a big difference in preventing the onset of smoking. The United States has launched an initiative to reduce and/or prevent tobacco use among children—that of improving the enforcement of state laws against smoking by minors. As a result of a study by the U.S. Department of Health and Human Services (DHHS), Sullivan reports that children in this country can easily buy cigarettes virtually any time they want to, in violation of the law. However, DHHS also found that where state and local officials take their responsibilities seriously, and devise enforcement tools that are workable and effective, these laws can be successfully enforced.

Preventing the use of tobacco products will do more to enhance the length and quality of life in the United States than any other step that could be taken.

Inhalants

Substances that are inhaled to produce altered states are called *inhalants*. These substances are classified as volatile solvents and aerosols. Common chemicals inhaled are fingernail polish remover, lacquer thinners, glue, gasoline, and liquid paper. Inhalation is a rapid means of ingesting substances, equivalent to intravenous injection in the time required to reach the brain. Altered consciousness can be achieved within one to two minutes of inhaling a large concentration, and five to ten minutes with low doses. Inhalants can also be ingested through the mouth. This method is called *huffing*, and it is not as prevalent as inhaling.

Most volatile substances are classified as depressants, although some may exhibit hallucinogenic characteristics. The effects of inhaled chemical include initial nausea with some irritation of airways causing coughing and sneezing. With low doses there is often a brief feeling of light-headedness, mild stimulation followed by a loss of control, lack of coordination, and disorientation accompanied by dizziness. Chronic use can result in permanent brain damage, impairment of motor behavior, severe psychological problems, and damage to lungs, kidneys and liver (Hanson and Venturelli 1995, 357, 359).

There has been a recent disturbing increase of inhalant abuse by younger kids. Almost 20 percent of eighth graders in the United States report having used inhalants (Hanson and Venturelli 1995, 359).

Designer Drugs

Designer drugs are substances produced synthetically by underground chemists and sold under the false assumption that they are some other drug. Compounds are altered in order to give the appearance of the original drug, and to some extent, the effects, but they contain only legal substances. They are often called *look-alikes*. The most familiar designer drugs were amphetamine look-alikes that contained caffeine, ephedrine, and phenylpropolamine—the same ingredients as in many over-the-counter diet and cold compounds. Designer cocaine may consist of powdered sugar and a topical anesthetic such as benzocaine. The user experiences sinus numbing, but the cocaine rush is absent. Naive users may be fooled, but experienced coke snorters quickly recognize the impostor.

In addition to differing in chemical makeup, some designer drugs are more dangerous than the drugs they imitate. They may contain very dangerous drugs that can be lethal in very small amounts. The user injects his or her usual dose, which may result in death. Other effects such as brain damage and paralysis have occurred. Designer drugs are banned in the United States by a bill passed in 1986.

Hallucinogens

Hallucinogens are substances that occur naturally or are produced synthetically that distort the perception of reality. Such drugs cause sensory illusions that make it difficult to distinguish fact from fantasy. Perhaps the most widely known hallucinogen is LSD (lysergic acid diethylamide), which was first synthesized in 1938. Although still occasionally used in medical research, the drug has no commonly used therapeutic applications. Even a tiny amount is enough to cause hallucinations, which manifest themselves in intensified colors, individualized sound perceptions, and bizarre visions, which may be pleasant or extremely frightening.

In mentally unstable individuals, LSD can produce psychotic reactions. There is also a danger of so-called flashbacks, where an individual will suddenly have hallucinations even weeks after having last ingested the drug. LSD does not cause physical dependency or seem to result in brain damage or birth defects, as once supposed. However, a "bad trip," or unpleasant experience while under the influence of the drug, can have long-lasting psychological effects.

Other hallucinogens are either derived from peyote, a kind of cactus that grows in Mexico and the American Southwest, or made synthetically. Most have effects similar to those produced by LSD, but some are particularly dangerous because of unpredictable side effects. One of the more common of these illegal drugs is PCP (phencyclidine hydrochloride), known as "angel dust." Originally synthesized as an animal tranquilizer, PCP is a relatively easy chemical to manufacture illegally. The drug is usually mixed with tobacco or marijuana and ingested by smoking.

PCP produces perceptual distortions, feelings of depersonalization, and changes in body image. Apathy, sweating, and auditory hallucinations may also result. High doses produce a stupor and overdose coma that can last for several weeks. This period can be followed by weeks of a confused mental state. In some individuals PCP also has been reported to precipitate extremely violent behavior, including murder.

Marijuana

After alcohol and nicotine, marijuana is the third most popular recreational drug in the United States—in other words, it is the dominant illicit drug. Over 35 percent of American high school seniors report having used marijuana in their lifetime, and 16 percent report using it during the past month. The percentages of eighth graders in 1993 who reported smoking marijuana significantly increased over comparable data collected in 1991 (Levinthal 1996, 14, 219–220).

Marijuana is a prepared mixture of the crushed leaves, flowers, small branches, stems, and seed of the hemp plant, *Cannabis sativa.* Hashish is a more potent resin derived from this plant. Marijuana is a hard drug to classify. Depending on various factors, including the amount of drug taken, the type of drug, the setting, and the mood of the user, cannabis intoxication may resemble the effects of alcohol, a sedative, a stimulant, or a hallucinogen. Marijuana in low to moderate doses causes a sedative effect. However, at higher dose levels marijuana produces effects quite similar to the mind-expanding psychedelics. Like the powerful psychedelics, there is little cross-tolerance for marijuana and, for example, LSD. In average doses, it acts much like alcohol. In addition, there is distortion of time, increased heart rate, increased appetite and thirst, dilation of the blood vessels in the eyes, and perhaps muscular weakness. Some individuals may act emotionally unstable or anxious, or experience sensory distortions. The ability to think, in terms of short-term memory, seems to be reduced. The ability to drive a car effectively is hindered by reduced perception and motor coordination.

The health effects from long-term marijuana use are still under investigation. Several major problems can result from intense marijuana abuse. It is assumed from current research that chronic bronchitis, cancer, and emphysema will result from long-term marijuana smoking—in fact, the risks of these diseases is greater from marijuana than from tobacco because marijuana smoke goes into the body unfiltered. There have also been reports suggesting that marijuana smoking adversely affects the body's ability to fight off disease.

Marijuana affects the reproductive system in various ways. It affects the sympathetic nervous system, increasing vasodilation in the genitals, and thus delays ejaculation. Chronic marijuana use has been shown in some studies to reduce testosterone (male hormone) levels and lower sperm counts, but results are not consistent (Hahn and Payne 1997, 167).

Although marijuana tolerance can develop, the frequent user may actually require less to gain the effects of the drug over time. Physical dependence seems to be rare. There is a danger of psychological dependence, however.

For some time, marijuana has been under investigation for possible medical use. In fact, marijuana has been used for numerous medical purposes since the ancient Chinese first employed the cannabis plant as a therapy. It is possible that some patients not helped by conventional therapies could be treated successfully with marijuana. In addition, cannabis might be combined effectively and safely with other drugs to produce a treatment goal. According to Carroll (1996, 260–261), marijuana has been used medically in the following ways:

Glaucoma: Marijuana has been found to reduce the vision-threatening intraocular pressure of glaucoma. However, older patients experience undesirable physical and psychological side effects. Despite its beneficial effects for some patients, marijuana neither prevents glaucoma nor improves vision.

Chemotherapy-Caused Nausea and Vomiting: Because cancer chemotherapy can produce increased survival in patients with certain cancers, the nausea and vomiting that interfere with a person's ability or willingness to continue therapy become life-threatening side effects. The U.S. government has established a program to make marijuana available through capsules and cigarettes through specified pharmacies to physicians who want to use the drug in their chemotherapy patients. Marijuana has been proven effective in controlling nausea and vomiting. Some patients, however, report anxiety. Also, some other patients find that marijuana does not reduce their nausea and vomiting.

Appetite stimulant: Research now suggests that there may well be a stimulating influence on food intake in advanced cancer patients who use marijuana in conjunction with chemotherapy.

Antiasthmatic effect: Long-term marijuana smoking constricts the airways. However, short-term smoking has actually produced a bronchodilation effect in patients with bronchial asthma; therefore, it is considered useful in the treatment of asthma.

Muscle relaxant action: Limited studies suggest that marijuana is effective in relieving the muscle spasm common in patients with multiple sclerosis.

Analgesic action (pain relief): Some test subjects in research studies did attest to marijuana's pain-relieving effects; however, they also tended to experience "mental clouding" and other undesirable pharmacological effects. Marijuana, therefore, is not considered any more effective than currently available analgesics.

Treatment for drug abuse: Research has failed to find marijuana useful in treating alcoholism. Also, there is no evidence that marijuana is more effective than currently available treatment for opiate withdrawal.

Should marijuana become an accepted drug? Marijuana is an unstable substance that has a poor shelf life. It will probably be found to contain over a thousand chemicals, of which only about 400 are known now because it hasn't been researched very long. It contains dozens of things that may not be useful in treating a specific problem. At best, marijuana is a controversial drug. Although it may not be as harmful as some researchers report, it certainly is not harmless. Any use of THC (tetrahydrocannabinol) for medical purposes does not stand as an endorsement for the recreational aspects of the drug.

Drug Education

Evaluation research on drug education prevention programs done over the last thirty years indicate that these programs have not been effective. In fact, the findings state that these programs essentially had no effect on the drug problem. Although studies of the more recently developed programs are more optimistic, the findings still do not provide strong evidence of highly effective programs. The goals of these programs has been to affect three basic areas: knowledge, attitudes, and behavior. The programs have had some success in increasing knowledge and, to a lesser extent, attitudes toward drugs; however, increases in knowledge and changed attitudes do not mean much if the actual drug behavior is not affected. In fact, those programs that only increase knowledge tend to reduce anxiety and fear of drugs, and may increase the likelihood of drug use. For example, one approach in the past was to provide students with complete information about all the possibilities of drug abuse, from the names of every street drug, to how the drugs are usually ingested, to detailed descriptions of possible effects of the drugs and possible consequences of an overdose. Given the inquiring nature of children, such an approach could well amount to a primer on how to take drugs, not how to avoid them.

The only effective approach to drug education is one in which children come to see that drug taking constitutes unnecessary and self-abusive consequences of drug abuse. Teachers must provide alternatives and realistic ones. Too often, the real appeal of such drugs as marijuana or alcohol is dismissed by asking children to take up a sport or go bike riding or learn to play a musical instrument. Such suggestions are fine as far as they go, but they often fail to take into account the personal problems that children are experiencing that may tempt them into drug abuse.

The social influence education programs show the most promise in reducing or delaying onset of drug use. Psychological approaches in which social influences and skills are stressed are more effective than other approaches. The most effective programs in influencing both attitudes and behavior were "peer programs" that included either refusal skills—with more direct emphasis on behavior—or social and life skills, or both.

Something appears to be working to reduce drug abuse problems—whether better educational programs, media campaigns, or other programs. Almost all the indicators of drug abuse showed a significant decrease in the 1980s. It may be magazine and television campaigns, school-based or community-based prevention programs, or various treatment programs. Also, the general reduction in drug use in U.S. society may be the result of changes in social norms and an informal control system unrelated to conscious and deliberate prevention, treatment, or law enforcement efforts (Akers 1992, 179–183). The National Commission on Drug-Free Schools (1990) echoes this sentiment of optimism in stating it has witnessed signs that the drug battle is being won. In its investigations, it finds that students in schools and colleges have taken leadership roles in peer programs to prevent alcohol and other drug abuse on their campuses; parents have organized party safe-home networks;

School-based prevention programs appear to be helping to reduce drug abuse problems.

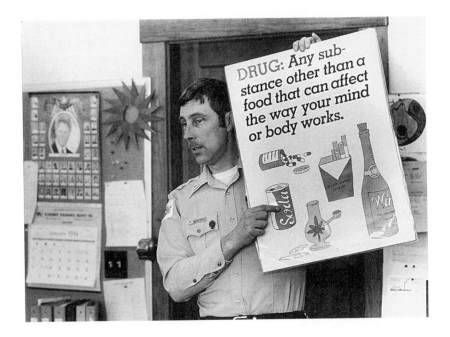

schools in a variety of communities have developed programs for high-risk students who need help with drug abuse and other problems; law enforcement officers and public housing residents have kicked drug gangs out of their areas.

As a teacher, you must become aware of the drugs that are commonly being abused in your community so that you can act and react appropriately. Your knowledge of abused drugs should include street names of the substances, symptoms of their use, and possible consequences of abuse.

Combatting Substance Abuse in Schools

The Western Regional Center for Drug-Free Schools and Communities has identified the following as characteristics contributing to effective prevention programming:

1. Target multiple systems (youth, families, schools, workplaces, community organizations, and media), using multiple strategies (provide accurate information, develop life skills, create positive alternatives, and change community policies and norms).

2. Target the whole community in prevention efforts.

3. Target all youth as opposed to only "high-risk" youth.

4. Programs that are part of a broader, generic prevention effort focused on health and success promotion. This is true because substance abuse is part of a constellation of interconnected problem behaviors, such as delinquency, truancy, school failure, and precocious sexuality, which share common antecedents.

5. Provide long-term duration with interventions beginning early and continuing through life stages.

6. Provide a sufficient quantity of prevention. One-shot prevention efforts do not work.

7. Integrate activities into family, classroom, school, and community life.

8. Build a supportive environment that conveys high expectations and encourages participation and responsibility (Benard 1993, 1).

A drug education program is not an easy undertaking. For every strategy that has been proposed, there have been critics with good and plausible arguments as to why that strategy is the worst one possible. There are even those, including many parents, who feel that the best approach is no approach at all. This is the concept that if adults don't mention drugs, then the problem doesn't really exist. This latter view seems out of touch with reality, and yet it is understandable considering how so many drug education programs have led to unfortunate results.

The use of scare tactics in any health education program, including drug abuse education programs, are counterproductive. Children soon learn to recognize the difference between fact and possible fiction. Attempts to equate the dangers of marijuana with those of heroin, suggestions that any drug can kill or permanently impair an individual, and other dire warnings, no matter how true, are often disregarded as propaganda.

Teachers must never lie about the dangers of drugs, either one way or the other, or play down the problems that children are facing that may make drugs seem to be an appealing way to cope. Effective drug education walks a fine line, one that requires teachers' sensitivity to the environment in which children must live and function. It is always important to point out that, no matter what the circumstances, each individual has a choice and must make a choice about substance use or abuse. Drug education must be a part of a comprehensive mental health education program. Only when children realize that drugs are not the answer to a problem, but part of the problem, can instruction be considered successful.

≣ Summary

○ A drug is any substance that alters bodily functions.

○ Drugs can be used or abused.

○ Reasons for substance abuse include:
low self-esteem
peer pressure
adult modeling
mood alteration
boredom
curiosity
alienation

○ Drugs act on the body by stimulating or depressing cellular activity.

○ Even when drugs are prescribed for medical purposes, there is a possibility that substance abuse can result.

○ Over-the-counter drugs are usually safe when taken as directed, but ingestion of any drug, no matter how mild, can cause health hazards.

○ Advertisements for OTC drugs can often lead people to believe that they are safer and more effective than the compounds actually are.

- Particularly dangerous drugs include barbiturates and amphetamines, known commonly as "downers" and "uppers."
- Barbiturates are depressants, and amphetamines are stimulants. If abused, these drugs can cause serious health problems or death.
- Alcohol is one of the most commonly used and abused drugs.
- Alcohol can easily lead to psychological and physical dependency, sometimes resulting in alcoholism, a disease that can wreck lives.
- The disease of alcoholism can and does occur to youth.
- Alcoholics and their families can receive help from many sources, such as Alcoholics Anonymous.
- A stimulant drug that is currently one of the most dangerous we have in our society is cocaine, known as "snow" or "coke" or "crack."
- Crack is cheap and readily available, and is smoked and absorbed into the bloodstream in less than 10 seconds.
- Most crack-related deaths result from brain hemorrhage, blocking of the heart's electrical system, lung failure, or associated heart and vessel complications.
- Smoking tobacco is also a serious health problem.
- Smokers often become psychologically and physically dependent on tobacco.
- Tobacco companies' advertising and promotional activities have led many children to start smoking and to use smokeless tobacco.
- Smoking is a difficult habit to break, but failure to do so can lead to a variety of serious diseases, including cancer and emphysema.
- The sidestream and secondhand smoke from the end of a cigarette can cause similar problems to nonsmokers who live and/or work with smokers.
- Smokeless tobacco can lead to similar problems as smoking tobacco.
- Narcotics are in some ways much more dangerous than barbiturates.
- The narcotics class of drugs includes opium, morphine, and heroin.
- Heroin is extremely addictive, and can lead to psychological breakdowns and irrational acts.
- As with any street drug, the user can never be sure of just what is contained in the dose sold.
- The hallucinogens include such drugs as LSD and PCP.
- Although not physically addictive, hallucinogens can lead to psychological breakdowns and irrational acts.
- Marijuana, for various reasons, is in a class by itself.
- Although not particularly dangerous, marijuana use can lead to personal and social harm.
- The stronger derivatives of the cannabis plant, including hashish and hashish oil, are more potent and can lead to even greater harm than marijuana.
- Ongoing research is determining the medicinal effects of marijuana.
- Substance education is a difficult topic, one where there are no easy answers as to the correct course.

○ Factual information must be provided, and yet substance education must not be allowed to become a primer on how to take drugs.

○ Effective drug abuse education programs are needed to change not only knowledge and attitudes, but behavior as well.

○ Community mores and lifestyles must be considered so that information and advice given are realistic and practical.

○ The best course is to build self-esteem in students so that drugs are not seen as a viable alternative for coping with personal problems.

Discussion Questions

1. What is the definition of a drug? Give examples of substances that qualify as drugs under this definition.

2. List six common reasons for substance abuse, especially as these reasons apply to young people.

3. What factors contribute to the misuse and abuse of OTC drugs?

4. Describe the effects of alcohol on the body at various blood alcohol concentration levels.

5. List six reasons that contribute to the habit of smoking tobacco.

6. Discuss the adverse effects of smokeless tobacco.

7. Discuss cocaine and the various forms of the drug.

8. Why is marijuana considered to be a harmful substance? How can it effectively be used medicinally?

9. What approach to substance education is the most effective, and why?

10. What are the characteristics of a good substance abuse prevention program in the schools?

References

Akers, R. L. 1992. *Drugs, alcohol, and society: Social structure, process, and policy.* Belmont, CA: Wadsworth.

American Medical Association. 1990. *Healthy youth 2000.* Chicago: Author.

Appalachian Educational Laboratory. 1992. *R&D notes,* (Charleston, WV) 6(10), 2.

Avis, H. 1996. *Drugs & life,* 3rd ed. Madison, WI: Brown & Benchmark.

Benard, B. 1993, Spring. Characteristics of effective prevention programs, *CenterPage* (Southeast Regional Center for Drug-Free Schools and Communities, Louisville, KY) 2(1), 1.

Carroll, C. R. 1996. *Drugs in modern society,* 4th ed. Madison, WI: Brown & Benchmark.

Fishbein, D. H., and S. E. Pease. 1996. *The dynamics of drug abuse.* Boston: Allyn and Bacon.

Hahn, D. B., and W. A. Payne. 1997. *Focus on health.* St. Louis: Mosby.

Hanson, G., and P. J. Venturelli. 1995. *Drugs and society,* 4th ed. Boston: Jones and Bartlett.

Hunton, H. T. 1991, November. Is your child using drugs? *Alternatives,* p. 1.

Langton, P. A. 1996. *The social world of drugs.* Minneapolis: West.

Levinthal, C. F. 1996. *Drugs, behavior, and modern society.* Boston: Allyn and Bacon.

Mintz, M. 1991, May 6. The nicotine pushers: Marketing tobacco to children, *The Nation,* p. 592.

National Commission on Drug-Free Schools. 1990, September. *Toward a drug-free generation: A nation's responsibility.* Washington, DC: Author.

Ray, O., and C. Ksir. 1996. *Drugs, society, and human behavior,* 7th ed. St. Louis, MO: Mosby.

Schlaadt, R., and P. Shannon. 1990. *Drugs,* 3rd ed. Englewood Cliffs, NJ: Prentice Hall.

Sullivan, L. W. 1990, May 24. *Statement before the Committee on Finance,* U.S. Senate, Washington, DC.

U.S. Centers for Disease Control (CDC). 1990, April 27. *Current trends: Cigarette advertising—United States 1988,* (Atlanta, GA) 39(16), p. 264.

U.S. Centers for Disease Control and Prevention (CDC). 1993. Youth risk behavior survey. *Journal of the American Medical Association,* 269 (11), pp. 1391-1395.

Witters, W., P. Venturelli, and G. Hanson. 1992. *Drugs and society,* 3rd ed. Boston: Jones & Bartlett.

Chapter Thirteen
Strategies for Teaching about Substance Use and Abuse

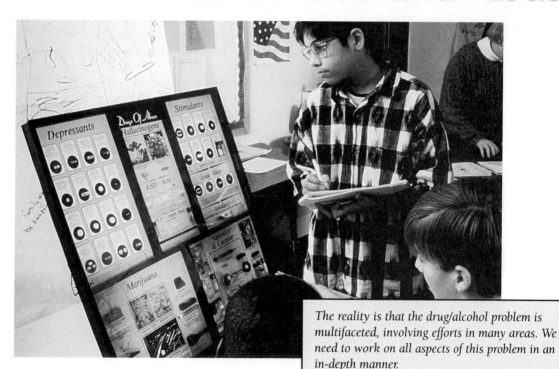

> The reality is that the drug/alcohol problem is multifaceted, involving efforts in many areas. We need to work on all aspects of this problem in an in-depth manner.
>
> —R. Fields (1995)

Valued Outcomes

After doing the activities in this chapter, the student should be able to express and illustrate the following guidelines:

○ Dealing effectively with personal problems is important in preventing substance abuse.
○ Poor self-image increases the potential for substance abuse.
○ Drugs should be taken only when a doctor prescribes them and only in the amount prescribed.
○ People use and abuse drugs for physical, emotional, and social reasons.
○ Certain drugs can be legally purchased only with a doctor's prescription.
○ Some drugs, called *over-the-counter (OTC) drugs,* can be purchased without a doctor's prescription.
○ Smoking is dangerous to health.
○ Tobacco smoke can be harmful to those who do not smoke as well as to smokers themselves.

- ○ Alcohol is a drug.
- ○ Misuse of alcohol can cause physical, emotional, and social problems.
- ○ Alcoholism is a disease.
- ○ Alcoholism can lead to many health problems.
- ○ Barbiturates can cause both physical and psychological dependency.
- ○ Cocaine and crack are very dangerous drugs and should not be used under any circumstances.
- ○ Amphetamines, like barbiturates, can be dangerous if abused. Illegal drugs, including narcotics and hallucinogens, can have unpredictable and serious health consequences.

The Challenge of Substance Abuse Education

Elementary school children need to be provided with learning experiences that will help them develop attitudes and values that build self-esteem and respect for the body so that drug taking is not seen as a way of coping with life. They must be taught to accept responsibility for their own behavior so that they will know how to deal with the problem of drugs in society.

The challenge of drug education is not to make every child a drug expert, nor to frighten children with scare tactics. Instead, it is to help children recognize that there is no need for them to misuse or abuse any drug, regardless of what reason they may have for being tempted to do so.

It is important for teachers to realize that there are almost as many reasons for drifting into substance abuse as there are different kinds of drugs. A youngster may wish to start smoking for an entirely different reason from the reason a youngster might begin amphetamine abuse. The temptation to take a particular drug may not stem from any self-destructive impulse, although sometimes it does. The problem is that the resultant behavior is always self-destructive, in varying degrees, regardless of the motivation. If children recognize this fact, and if they are on their way to building a strong self-image, then substance abuse is far less likely to occur in later years.

Value-Based Activities

Smoking and the Law

Valued Outcome: The students will be able to describe the variables involved in making a decision about smoking.
Description of Strategy: After you have discussed the definition of a drug, point out that tobacco qualifies under the definition. Note that although smoking is known to be hazardous to health, tobacco products can be purchased legally by adults. Ask students to consider the implications of this fact. Point out that each individual must make a decision about smoking. Then have the students consider the following question:
    Should laws be passed that prevent people from smoking in certain public places?
Materials Needed: none
Processing Questions:

1. What are some reasons to be considered in making such laws?
2. Should cigarettes be made illegal? Why or why not?

3. What legal rights should smokers have?

4. What legal rights should nonsmokers have?

5. How do you feel about laws regulating smoking?

Smoking and You

Valued Outcome: The students will be able to list reasons why a person might decide not to start smoking.

Description of Strategy: Have each student prepare a list with two columns. In the first column, ask the students to write reasons why they think a person might want to start smoking. In the second column, have them list reasons why a person might decide not to start smoking. Talk over the various reasons that the students list in a general discussion. Which reasons in each column are rational ones? Which are irrational ones?

Materials Needed: paper and pencil

Processing Question: What are the emotional and social reasons a person would start smoking?

Living without Drugs

Valued Outcome: The students will be able to describe alternative ways to alleviate various health problems.

Description of Strategy: Have students bring in drug advertisements from magazines and newspapers. Look especially for ads that deal with stress ailments, such as headaches, backaches, insomnia, diarrhea, and so forth. After comparing the ads and discussing them, have the students brainstorm alternative ways to deal with these problems. Alternatives to medication may include taking time to talk to a friend or loved one, listening to soft music, eating properly, exercising, drinking plenty of water, or doing something special.

Materials Needed: none

Processing Question: Why is our society so drug dependent?

Living with Drugs

Valued Outcome: The students will be able to explain the connection between societal problems and substance abuse.

Description of Strategy: Have students collect and bring in magazine articles and newspaper clippings about accidents, domestic problems, violence, suicide, and crime. Discuss the clippings and the role drug or alcohol use may have played. Have the class members consider reasons why these things might have occurred and what kinds of actions can be taken to avoid them in their own lives (alternatives to destructive behavior).

Materials Needed: newspapers and magazines

Processing Question: Why is there such a positive correlation between substance abuse and violence/crime?

Where Do You Stand?

Valued Outcome: The students will be able to clarify their values regarding substance abuse.

Description of Strategy: Draw a chalk line on the floor. Explain to your students that the line is a continuum on how they feel about various decisions. One end of the line represents complete disagreement with a position, and the other end represents complete agreement. Or the line could represent degrees of willingness or unwillingness.

Then ask for volunteers to demonstrate where they stand on a variety of questions that you put forward. Try to keep the questions nonthreatening and nonincriminating. Questions that you might ask include the following:

1. Where do you stand on smoking cigarettes?
2. Where do you stand on drinking alcohol?
3. How willing would you be to tell a friend who takes drugs that you do not approve of that behavior?
4. How dangerous do you think it is to take a drug that you yourself don't know anything about?

Sentence Completion

Valued Outcome: The students will be able to complete statements with their own values-related answers.
Description of Strategy: Ask the students to complete statements such as the following with values-related answers:

1. For me, smoking is . . .
2. If I saw another student using drugs, I would . . .
3. Some people start drinking alcohol because . . .
4. Drugs are . . .
5. To me, substance abuse means . . .
6. The best reason for not taking any drugs is . . .
7. One thing I don't believe about drugs is . . .
8. If I made the laws about drugs, I would . . .
9. I was surprised to learn that drugs . . .
10. People who take drugs . . .

Materials Needed: handouts with the preceding questions and writing instruments
Processing Question: What factors in your background influence your values regarding substance abuse?

The Family's Influence

Valued Outcome: Students will describe ways in which families help influence decisions.
Description of Strategy: The teacher should cut out pictures of families engaged in healthful activities out of an old magazine. The teacher should show different kinds of families. The teacher will then show the pictures to the class and have the students tell what the families are doing to enjoy themselves. Explain to the students that family members have a responsibility to keep each other safe and that parents or guardians help protect their children from harm. The teacher will explain that is why parents want their children to stay away from strangers and never take anything from them. The parents want to keep you safe but a stranger may want to harm them. The teacher should then give each student a piece of paper and some crayons. The students will draw

a picture that shows them with one or more family members doing something fun and safe. After students are done, have them share their drawings and explain what they are doing.
Materials Needed: old magazines, crayons, paper
Processing Question: Why is it important to stay away from strangers?

Source: L. Meeks, P. Heit,. & R. Page. 1995. *Drugs, alcohol, and tobacco: Teaching strategies.* Blacklick, OH: Meeks Heit, 276.

Drug Rating Scale

Valued Outcome: The students will express their opinions about drugs.
Description of Strategy: The students will complete a rating scale on their beliefs about drugs. Then there will be a classroom discussion about why they feel the way they do. The rating scale is 1 = strongly agree, 2 = agree, 3 = don't know/neutral, 4 = disagree, 5 = strongly disagree

1. It is okay to smoke marijuana every once in a while.
2. Crack cocaine is the worst drug a person can take.
3. Nicotine in cigarettes is a drug.
4. Smoking cigarettes is not good for your health.
5. Tripping on acid only affects you once, and then you never feel the effects of the drug again.
6. The best thing I can do when asked to take drugs by someone is to say no and walk away.
7. Drinking alcohol is not the same as taking a drug.
8. Alcohol won't hurt you.
9. I can smoke now and then quit when I get older and it won't hurt me.
10. The only kind of people who take drugs are those who are bad students who are always getting in trouble.

Materials Needed: paper and pencils
Processing Questions:

1. Why do we want to say no to drugs?
2. What happens when people take drugs?
3. If a person takes drugs, will it affect him or her the rest of his life?

Effects of Drugs on the Fetus

Valued Outcome: The students will learn about the harmful effects of alcohol and other drugs on fetal development.
Description of Strategy: Prepare for this lesson by reviewing normal fetal development. Discuss the importance of the first trimester of pregnancy, when the developing fetus is at greatest risk of malformation due to drugs. Then ask students to identify drugs that could adversely affect the developing fetus (examples: alcohol, marijuana, cocaine, tobacco, caffeine, prescription drugs). Give each student a copy of the handout "Harmful Effects of Drugs on the Fetus," and have the class read it. Discuss the following questions:

○ Which drugs cause withdrawal symptoms?
○ Which drugs cause seizures?

❍ Which drugs cause low birth weight?

❍ Which drugs cause physical handicaps?

❍ Which drugs cause learning disabilities and behavior problems?

❍ Which drugs affect men's and women's reproductive system?

❍ What could happen to your family as a result of drugs?

Discuss the myths, "I'll quit (smoking, drinking, taking drugs) when I get pregnant" and "Stopping when I get pregnant will be soon enough to prevent problems." (A woman usually doesn't know she is pregnant until six weeks into pregnancy, by which time the damage may already have been done.) Divide the class into pairs and have the students practice asking a friend or relative who is pregnant, or wants to be pregnant, to give up tobacco, alcohol, or other drugs. Have the students share what they learned with the rest of the class.
Materials Needed: "Harmful effects of drugs on the fetus" handout
Processing Questions:

1. What can be learned from discussing and practicing myths?

2. Why is it dangerous to experiment with drugs when you or your girlfriend is pregnant?

3. What happens as a result of a pregnant mother taking drugs?

Source: C. Flatter and K. McCormick. 1990. *Learning to live drug-free: A curriculum model for prevention.* National Clearinghouse for Alcohol and Drug Information, Ninth-twelfth grades. U.S. Department of Education, Washington, DC, p. 13.

Decision Stories

Present decision stories such as the following, using the procedures outlined in Chapter 5.

Want a Smoke?

Mark always walks home from school with a group of friends. One day, two of his friends light up cigarettes. Mark is surprised because he didn't know that they had started smoking. "Want a smoke?" his friend Jim asks. "They're real mild," his other friend George says. "Try one." Mark can see that Jim and George are trying to look grown up. He wants to look grown up, too. The other two boys in the group are not smoking. However, Mark wonders what he should do.
Focus Question: What should Mark say to his friends?

Problems at Home

Michael's problems at home are getting worse, and he feels he has nowhere to turn. He is very lonely and frightened about what is happening in his life. His parents are always fighting. They don't seem to have any time for him anymore. He wants so much to have someone show him love and concern. He also wishes that he could just leave his problems behind him.
Focus Questions:

1. What are some methods of coping that Michael might try?

2. What might be the consequences of each of these methods?

Slumber Party

Sally is throwing a slumber party at her home. Her parents respect Sally's judgment and ask her to make sure that the party does not get out of hand. Sally doesn't think it will. But after her parents have gone to bed, some of Sally's friends start passing some pills around. They tell her that these pills are fun to take and are not dangerous. They also say that Sally doesn't have to try the pills if she doesn't want to. But they ask her not to spoil the party for them.
Focus Question: What should Sally do?

Drugs in the Neighborhood

Darlene knows that some of the older kids in her neighborhood are using and selling drugs. They don't seem to care that Darlene sees what they are doing. "It's none of your business," one of them told her. But Darlene is not so sure. A couple of her friends bought some of these drugs and have started using them. Darlene doesn't know what will happen in the neighborhood next.
Focus Question: What can Darlene do about the drug problem in her neighborhood?

Mom Drinks Too Much

Often, when David arrives home from school in the afternoon, his mother is sitting in the living room with a glass or a bottle beside her. Sometimes she is very loving, and other times she seems very angry at him. Sometimes she is asleep on the couch, and he has trouble waking her up. Sometimes Mom can't fix supper for David and his younger sister. David knows that his mom uses alcohol more than she should. She is frequently depressed and upset. David is afraid of how his mom will act when he comes in every day, and he is afraid that she will get hurt. He also worries about who is taking care of his sister when he is not there. David constantly worries about what will happen to his family if his mom doesn't stop drinking.
Focus Questions:

1. What actions should David take?
2. Who does he need to talk to about his problems?
3. Who might be able to help David, his sister, and his mom?

Sleepover

Leah was looking forward to tonight. It was her tenth birthday and she was having a sleepover party in her backyard. Her parents were letting her and her two friends, Casey and her sister, Allison, sleep in her tent. The girls had eaten sandwiches and were about to play cards when Casey pulled out a pack of cigarettes from her coat pocket. "Hey, let's light up," she said. Casey and Allison both took out a cigarette. Casey offered the pack to Leah. "No, I don't want to," she said. "What's the matter, big baby? Are you scared?" asked Casey. "We didn't know we were sleeping over with such a baby. Maybe we'd better go home." Leah had been having lots of fun, but she did not know that her friends smoked.
Focus Question: What should Leah do?

Dramatizations

Drug Court

Valued Outcome: The students will be able to dramatize various drug-related court actions.
Description of Strategy: Have the students role-play various drug-related court actions. In this court, the class acts collectively as judge and jury. Various students come before the court acting the part of the arresting officer. They explain to the court that they have arrested an individual on a drug charge and then describe the offense. In each case, the defendant has already pleaded guilty to the charge. It is up to the court to decide what sentence or decision to make. The class must come up with a consensus on each offense. Follow each decision with general discussion. Also note to the students what the penalty might have been in an actual court.
Materials Needed: none
Processing Questions:

1. Why is it illegal to use/abuse certain drugs?
2. What penalties are given to those who illegally use/abuse drugs?

Public Service Messages

Valued Outcome: The students will be able to devise a one-minute message on substance education.
Description of Strategy: Divide the class into small groups. Have each prepare a 60-second public service message for television broadcast about substance education. Encourage imagination. Some students may wish to write and sing a song bearing their message. Others may wish to act out a skit. Still others may opt for a panel format. Have each group give its "televised" presentation in front of the class. Each presentation must be one minute long. After the presentations, have the class discuss each. You may wish to have the students vote for the most effective presentation.
Materials Needed: none
Processing Questions:

1. How can antidrug messages best be given to the public?
2. What should these messages include?

What Would Happen If . . . ?

Valued Outcome: The students will be able to simulate various activities while pretending to be under the influence of certain kinds of drugs.
Description of Strategy: After discussing the effects that various kinds of drugs can have on the body and brain, have students role-play situations in which a person attempts an activity while under the influence of a certain kind of drug. For example, what would happen if an airline pilot tried to land a plane while under the influence of alcohol? What would happen if a surgeon tried to operate while under the influence of a hallucinogen? Have one student play the affected person. Another student, at the last minute, steps in and saves the day. After the activity, emphasize to the class that sometimes no one can keep a tragedy from happening. Bring this point home by discussing drunk-driving statistics or other examples from the news.

Materials Needed: none
Processing Questions:

1. What effects do drugs have on the body?

2. How can the effects of drugs affect one's job performance?

I'm No Dummy

Valued Outcome: The students will be able to to demonstrate refusal skills.
Description of Strategy: Have the students use hand puppets to act out skits about drug use and abuse. One puppet, for example, might be offered drugs by other puppets. "I'm no dummy," the first puppet replies, and then gives reasons for refusing.
Materials Needed: paper lunch bags or cloth for making puppets, markers
Processing Question: What is the best way to refuse the offer of drugs?

Peers Helping Other Peers

Valued Outcome: The students will be able to persuade a peer to prevent drug abuse.
Description of Strategy: Have the students role-play a drug-related incident. Pick four students who are willing to participate in the role playing. Without the class hearing, explain to the four students that they are at the mall and see a couple of friends. They watch their friends walk around to the back of the mall. Deciding they want to see what their friends are up to, they follow them. Little did they know their two friends were doing drugs. Once approached, they started acting really funny. The good students are to tell their friends the effects of the drugs on their body and to help them understand that what they are doing is wrong. Have them role-play this. Explain to the students they are to use their prior knowledge from the unit on substance abuse to persuade the students to quit. After this is accomplished, ask the class to tell the four students what they did wrong or what they did right. Follow this with discussion on what they could have done to prevent the drug use.
Materials Needed: none
Processing Questions:

1. What can you do as a student to keep your friends off drugs?

2. What would you do if approached with a harmful substance?

3. What can you do for the community to cut down substance abuse?

Drugs in the Real World

Valued Outcome: Students will understand the consequences of drug-related behavior.
Description of Strategy: The students are invited to engage in a bit of hyperbole. Although the dramatization is an exaggeration for the purpose of the demonstration, the inappropriate use of alcohol can lead to "real world" devastating consequences. To start the activity, use the chalkboard to draw a continuum that indicates the range of emotions that humans experience. At one end is "euphoria"—the ultimate positive emotion. Euphoria can be described as a feeling of vigor, well-being, or high spirits. Ask the students to describe situations that might elicit euphoria. Examples might include successfully completing a class, becoming a parent, winning an award, or receiving a special prize. Although euphoria is a positive emotion, students should recognize that among emotionally healthy people it is a temporary state.

At the other end of the continuum, write "depression." This is the antithesis of euphoria. As before, ask the students to demonstrate or express situations of depression. Examples might include the death of a loved one, having a friend move away, or failing a class. As with euphoria, among emotionally healthy people depression is also a temporary state.

In the center of the continuum, write "normalcy," and explain that this is where people's emotions are located most of the time. Point out that neither euphoria nor depression can be maintained for extended periods of time in healthy people. Rather, emotions soon "swing" toward the central area of the continuum—as one attains normalcy.

Having described the continuum, ask a volunteer from the audience to come forward to present "euphoria." Give them a wildly designed shirt in which to dress for effect. Ask your "Euphoric Emma" (or "Eugene" as the case may be) to actively demonstrate "euphoria." Jumping up and down, shouting, and general enthusiasm are appropriate here. Lead this person over to the end of the continuum where "euphoria" is listed.

Ask for another volunteer, and indicate that you want him or her to display "depression." Provide the most dreaded-looking, forbidding shirt you have. Have this student demonstrate what depression looks like by practicing a very sullen and sad look. Direct "Depressed Duke" (or "Daisy" as the case may be) toward the depression end of the continuum.

A third volunteer is required to represent normalcy. This person is given a buttoned-down oxford shirt. "Normal Norma" (or "Norman" as the case may be) is asked to stand near the normalcy area. When "Normal Norma" is in place, have each of the persons along the continuum demonstrate their designated emotions.

The next volunteer will be the "star" of the show and the centerpiece of conversation for the next few minutes. Ask the class to imagine that this person is a "typical" sixteen-year-old (for this example, imagine that our volunteer is a female), and have the crowd describe this "typical" teenager.

Once the class has described this "typical" teen, put her in the "normal" area on the continuum. Describe a typical day at school. The instructor (acting as another teen) invites her to a party this weekend. Ask her what she might do to prepare for the party, what she would tell her parents concerning the party, and what she would say if she were asked to drink at the party. While having a good time at the party, a fellow party-goer (the instructor) convinces "Typical Teen" to have a drink of alcohol. It may take some coaxing, but once she succumbs, slowly slide her over to the euphoria extreme. This euphoria is the result of a social environment in which she is feeling comfortable, and not necessarily from intoxication. (However, it should be noted that the feelings expressed here by "Typical Teen" are not "etched in stone." A twinge of remorse may have dampened her spirit.) When the party is over, she may still be euphoric, but soon (within the next few hours) she moves back toward normalcy. Explain that "Typical Teen" wasn't drunk—she had just one drink.

As the activity progresses, indicate to the class that "Typical Teen" has been partying consistently and has begun drinking more often. In fact, the police crash the next party. Naturally, since she is underage, her parents are contacted. Bummer! Her parents are furious! (The instructor can then simulate an angry parent.) "Typical Teen" begins the inevitable descent into depression, which may not pass as quickly as her first bout of remorse. Indicate to the class that this, from an emotional aspect, is an example of drug abuse. In this case, being caught by one's parent is depressing. However, we do not expect this depression to be of the long-lasting variety (despite the punishment her parents give her). "Typical Teen" will eventually arrive at normalcy once again.

A few more weeks have passed in the life of "Typical Teen." Things are going downhill rapidly for our heroine as she misses homework assignments, gets into deeper trouble with her parents, and becomes constantly depressed. Her friends may see a change in her. Throughout these few minutes, you as the instructor discuss how "Typical Teen" is in search of the "never-ending party." As this progresses, she has more problems with her family, school, friends, and work due to her alcohol consumption. As a result, "Typical Teen" stays in the depressed range of emotions longer and longer. No longer does drinking bring her pleasure or euphoria. Eventually, she "needs" to drink, just to feel "normal." Explain the concept of dependency at this point.

Now ask the class to describe the current status of "Typical Teen." Chances are she has changed many of her goals and outside interests. She may even be cultivating a new group of friends (those that enable her to continue drinking without feeling remorse or noticing the consequences of her habit).

Source: M. Barnes, K. DeBarr, and M. Kittleson. 1996, July–August. Teaching the emotional aspect of drug use, abuse, and dependency. *Journal of health education* 27(4), 261–262.

Hidden Messages

Valued Outcome: Students will see and understand the hidden messages in tobacco or alcohol ads.
Description of Strategy: Show the students some examples of tobacco or alcohol ads in the magazines or on the television. Then discuss with the students the hidden messages that many ads are trying to convey. Have students get into groups of three or four and make up their own dramatization of a commercial that helps the watcher of television understand these hidden messages. Students should give a positive outlook on not smoking or drinking in their ad. Have students think about what they could say on television that might make at least one person stop drinking or smoking (that is something they might want to say in their ad). They should make it clear in their ad that the commercials about tobacco and alcohol are not always true and that many of them hold hidden messages.
Materials Needed: magazines, videotape of tobacco or alcohol commercials
Optional: poster board, markers (for visual in their commercial)
Processing Questions:

1. What are the hidden messages in television and magazines?

2. How can the commercials convince my peers to try their product?

Source: Derived from: G. Ezell. 1993. *Healthy living, Building blocks for health,* Grade 3. Grand Rapids, MI: Christian Schools International, p. 172.

Asserting Yourself to Refuse Substances

Valued Outcome: Students will be asked to recognize the power of asserting themselves when confronted with possible substance abuse.
Discussion of Strategy: The students will have a lengthy discussion on how to stand up to peer pressure. They will discuss the effects of illegal drugs, alcohol, and smoking. The class will discuss the dangers of each and how to handle a situation when faced with a decision. Then the class will be read three dramatizations and discuss the proper responses to each.

Situation 1: Charlie was roving the neighborhood with his friends one Saturday morning. On any other Saturday, Charlie, Lee and Tommy would have lots of things to do. However, on this particular Saturday the boys were not quite sure what they were going to do. Tommy gave a sly grin and said, "I've got something that could be very interesting to try." With that, he pulled out a pack of cigarettes along with a book of matches from his coat pocket. What should Charlie and Lee say and do?

Situation 2: Liz was visiting her new neighbor, Julie, after school one day. They were putting a jigsaw puzzle together in Julie's room. Liz could smell a strong, burning odor. It was like tobacco smoke, but not quite the same. She asked if Julie could smell it too. Julie casually said it was her older brother smoking marijuana in his bedroom. "It's no big deal," Julie said. "Would you like to smoke some?" What should Liz say and do?

Situation 3: Frank and Jerry were walking home from school when they came on several older boys who were drinking something out of a dark colored bottle hidden in a paper bag. One of the older boys dared Frank and Jerry to have a drink of beer. "Come on you two, you are not little babies, now, are you?" Jerry looked at Frank and asked, "It could not hurt us, could it? Not just a little bit?" What should Frank say or do?

In each situation, the class will act out the appropriate responses and discuss why these drugs are dangerous and should be avoided.

Materials Needed: none, unless props are available for the various characters
Processing Questions: What should you do when confronted with smoking cigarettes? Marijuana? Drinking beer?

Source: M. Fisher. 1996. *Health and safety curriculum.* Grand Rapid, MI: Instructional Fair, p. 39.

Using Medicines Safely

Valued Outcomes: Students will identify reasons for using medicine, describe prescription and over-the-counter medicines, and apply what they have learned to specific situations.
Description of Strategy: Begin the lesson by stating that everyone gets sick sometime. Engage students in a conversation about how it feels to be sick. Note that sometimes we get better by getting lots of rest and drinking fluids, but sometimes we need medicine. Write the word *medicine* at the top of the chart. Ask, "How does medicine help us?" Allow answers to this question from the class. Sum up the discussion, and write the main points on the chart. Include the following ways:

1. Medicine helps us feel better. It controls our symptoms. For example, taking medicine such as aspirin for a headache or cough syrup for a cough.

2. Medicine helps fight sickness. For example, pills for curing sore throats; ointments for eye infections; drops for ears or nose.

3. Medicine helps prevent sickness. For example, immunizations to prevent measles and other illnesses. Immunizations are often shots, but sometimes they are in liquid form to be taken orally.

Have students act out situations related to using medicine safely. Divide students into groups and suggest or assign a situation to each group. Suggested situations:

○ Children are playing doctor at a friend's house. The friend takes medicine from the bathroom cabinet to use for the "game."

○ A group of children find a bottle of medicine on a bench in the park or at the mall. Several want to "try" it.

○ A child who has a stomachache decides to use a sister's medicine. The child knows the medicine was prescribed for stomachache, and now he or she also has a stomachache.

○ A younger brother or sister doesn't feel well and wants a sibling to give aspirin or other medicine to feel better.

○ Children playing together decide to take cough syrup or other medicine because it tastes like candy. Make sure the danger of each situation is clear. Guide the groups to stress the best way to deal with each situation. If necessary, reenact the scene to show safe behavior.

Materials Needed: chart
Processing Questions:

1. Why is medicine good for us?

2. How can it be bad for us?

3. What should you do if you feel you are getting sick: take medicine on your own, or go to an adult?

Source: G. Ezell. 1992. *Healthy living, Level 2: Healthy and growing.* Grand Rapids, MI: Christian Schools International, pp. 178, 179.

Making Substance Abuse Decisions

Valued Outcome: Students will learn the scientific method through role-playing decisions about drugs.

Description of Strategy: Outline the fundamentals of the scientific method, and discuss how these concepts can be applied to an experiment related to drug research (example: the effect of smoking on the lungs). Explain that people can solve everyday situations and problems using steps similar to those in the scientific method:

1. Ask yourself what the problem is *(problem)*.

2. Decide on your goal *(hypothesis)*.

3. Stop and think of as many solutions to the problem as you can *(analysis)*.

4. For each solution, think of all the things that might happen next *(data, observations)*.

5. Choose your best solution *(conclusions)*.

6. Rethink it once more *(just to be sure)*.

Divide the class into teams of four, and explain that each group will be acting out situations that will require careful thinking to arrive at a decision on which everyone agrees. Give each group a situation to enact. Explain that members of each group, using the modified scientific method, must decide together the best way to handle the situation. Two group members are responsible for role-playing the situation, while the other two members identify and record the steps the group takes in reaching consensus. The role-playing is over when the group arrives at a decision on which everyone agrees. Have each group present their role play and explain their conclusions, using the steps of the problem-solving method. Review similarities between the scientific method and the problem-solving model. Emphasize that, although the problem-solving model most often is a mental process, it must be practiced if people are to make effective decisions.

Materials Needed: role-playing cards
Processing Questions:

1. How are the two methods similar?

2. Why is it important to role-play decisions?

3. What are some ways to make decisions easier to make?

Source: C. Flatter and K. McCormick. 1990. *National clearinghouse for alcohol and drug information,* Seventh–ninth grade. Washington, DC: U.S. Department of Education, p. 21.

Discussion and Report Strategies ─────────────────

Mock Supreme Court

Valued Outcome: Students will seek out important information concerning health issues.

Description of Strategy: Set up a mock Supreme Court with nine class members sitting on the bench. Divide remaining students into two groups: those who are in favor of the legalization of marijuana and those who are not. Have both groups gather evidence to support their argument and present it to the Court. Conclude by having the Court render its decision.

Materials Needed: "evidence" to be gathered by the students

Processing Questions:

1. What facts are we basing our decision on?

2. Do these facts lead to a just decision?

3. What effect will our decision have on the people if it is enforced?

Source: D. Read. 1980. *Creative teaching in health*, 3rd ed. Prospect Heights, IL: Waveland Press, p. 137.

Presentation by Health Professionals

Valued Outcome: The students will learn numerous facts about substance use and abuse from a professional in the field.

Description of Strategy: With permission from your school administration, invite an official from a substance abuse program to speak to your class about substance use and abuse. Talk with your guest alone before the presentation, and emphasize that no scare tactics should be used. The presentation should be factual and objective. Allow time for a question-and-answer session afterward.

Materials Needed: none

Processing Questions:

1. What types of treatment are given in substance abuse programs?

2. How effective are these programs?

The Question Box

Valued Outcome: The students will be able to identify personal problems and write them on an index card.

Description of Strategy: Have each student write on an index card a problem he or she is concerned about personally. No names or other means of identification should be included. Then have the students place their cards in a large ballot box. Allow them to place questions in the box for a week. After class, open the box and screen out any cards that inadvertently reveal any problems that would lead to identification of the student involved. The next day, distribute the remaining cards to the students on a random basis and have them tell how they would deal with the problem. Allow other students with different opinions to add comments.

Materials Needed: index cards, pen

Processing Question: What type of problems in relationships or school could lead to a substance abuse problem?

Sharing

Valued Outcome: The students will be able to relate personal positive experiences to each other in the class.

Description of Strategy: Have the students sit in a large circle on the floor. Each student then shares one positive experience that happened to him or her in the last month. Sharing may relate to home, school, athletics, play, and so on. No one is to interrupt or ask any questions until every student has had an opportunity to share. Follow the activity with a discussion. Ask the following questions: Was it hard to find something to share? What were the similarities among the things shared? Did people share more as the activity progressed? What does this indicate?

Materials Needed: none

Processing Question: What types of positive activities can serve as effective alternatives to substance abuse?

Dealing with Problems

Valued Outcome: The students will be able to identify personal problems and then share solutions with each other in class.

Description of Strategy: Have the students, in groups, complete these four sentences:

1. I have a problem . . .

2. This is what happened . . .

3. My feelings were (or are) . . .

4. I need your help to . . .

Have each group discuss or role-play for the rest of the class a real problem for them personally. Then let the group present their ideas for positive solutions and get the class response.

Materials Needed: pen and paper

Processing Questions: If you find effective solutions to problems, can that keep you from using/abusing drugs?

Who Influences Your Decisions?

Valued Outcome: The students will learn about decision making and how those decisions may affect others.

Description of Strategy: Talk with students about how all people make decisions every day. Some decisions affect our lives more drastically than others. There are easier decisions to make, such as which shoes to wear to school on a particular day, and there are much more difficult decisions, such as what to do if a friend wants to copy your test answers. It is important to know where to go for help when making important decisions. Whom you consider when making your decisions reflects your personal value system. Have students brainstorm a list of people, places, and institutions that are important considerations when they make a decision. Influences might include family, TV, friends, church, teachers, and so on. Have each child decide who or what he or she considers to have the greatest influence on his or her own life. Students then can create collages about all the many different influences that affect their thinking and decisions every day.

Materials Needed: none

Processing Questions:

1. What is the most effective way to make a wise decision?

2. How can effective decision making help prevent a substance abuse problem?

Peer pressure can be a positive or negative influence in a person's life.

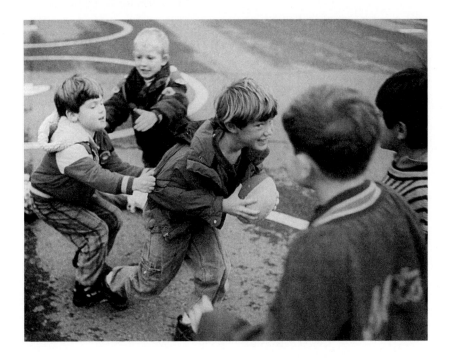

What Would Happen If . . . ?(II)

Valued Outcome: The students will be able to identify consequences that follow certain actions.
Description of Strategy: Consequences are the results of our actions. All actions have some kind of consequences. Although it is impossible to always know what all the consequences of a particular action will be, it is important to attempt to figure out logical consequences of important decisions. Have students title a paper "What would happen if . . ." and provide them with some situations such as

- ○ You helped a friend with a chore.
- ○ You cheated on your homework.
- ○ You cleaned the house for your mother before she got home from work.
- ○ A friend asked you to do something you felt uncomfortable doing, such as stealing from a store.
- ○ You become angry and hit a friend.
- ○ You get up too late on a school morning and drive to school too fast so you won't be late.

Students may want to contribute their own ideas for actions they confront every day.
Materials Needed: pen and paper
Processing Questions:

1. Why is important to consider the consequences of all our actions?
2. How can this type of consideration prevent a substance abuse problem?

The Space Colony

Valued Outcome: The students will be able to originate a drug policy and drug laws for a new planetary settlement.

Description of Strategy: Tell the class that they are about to travel to a new planet by spaceship. On this planet there are as yet no governments or laws. As a group, the class must decide on the drug policy and drug laws for the new planetary settlement. The class, acting as a committee, must decide what drugs, if any, are to be taken to the new planet and how such drugs will be distributed or made available. Have the class keep in mind that drugs include useful medications, but that such medications can be abused. Laws relating to the misuse of drugs on the new planet must also be discussed. After thorough discussion, have the class come to a consensus about drug policy on the new planet. Write their conclusions on the chalkboard. Then have each student prepare an individual report, including any dissenting opinions. Such opinions must be backed up with reasons.

Materials Needed: chalk, chalkboard

Processing Questions:

1. Why are drug laws needed?
2. Are these laws effective in preventing substance abuse?

Individual Reports

Valued Outcome: The students will be able to initiate research and prepare a report on a drug-related problem.

Description of Strategy: Ask students to do further research on a drug-related problem and prepare individual reports on what they find. Topics can include "Smoking and Health," "Alcohol Abuse and Accidents," "Drugs and the Law," and "Dangers of Substance Abuse."

Materials Needed: none

Processing Questions:

1. What is the relationship between smoking and health?
2. What are the dangers of substance abuse?

Saying No to Drugs

Valued Outcome: Students will demonstrate drug awareness.

Description of Strategy: Discuss with the students what drugs are. Explain to them that the drugs will hurt them badly, and it is not good to use them. More than likely the students will be able to tell the teacher the names of some of the drugs. Tell the students it is all right to say no to using drugs. Tell the students that people who want you to try the drugs are not their friends. Allow the children to talk about the topic of drug abuse. Advise them on the right and wrong thing to do. Tell them about famous people who have died from drug abuse. After the discussion is finished, give each student a piece of drawing paper and some crayons. Give the students suggestions to draw campaign signs against using drugs (for example, "Just Say No"). Tell them to make the signs as colorful and noticeable as possible. The signs will be hung throughout the school as a reminder to the rest of the students that drug abuse is not welcome to our students.

Materials Needed: crayons, paper

Processing Questions:

1. What should you do if someone offers you drugs?

2. What is drug abuse?

3. Are drugs good for your body?

Researching Substance Abuse

Valued Outcome: Students will learn more about different drugs and know the effects that drugs have on the human body.

Description of Strategy: Discuss with the students different types of drugs. Allow the students to share anything (within reason) they know about the different drugs and the effects they have on the human body. This project will take some time to complete. Have a set of encyclopedias and manuals on drugs or drug abuse in the classroom, accessible to the students throughout the entire time they are working on the project. Allow the students to pick a topic on which to do research. They should pick a drug or type of drug, and then describe it and the effects it will have on the human body. The first step the students should work on is research. This can be started on the first day of the assignment. Tell the students to document their information. The second step is a rough draft. This should be approximately six pages, and they should skip every other line. It will be hand written. The third step is to correct the rough draft and turn in the final copy. It should be three pages handwritten or one and a half pages typed and double spaced. These papers will be read orally in class.

Materials Needed: paper, pencil, encyclopedias, drug abuse manuals

Processing Question: What types of drugs are there?

Effects of Drug Use

Valued Outcome: The students will become aware of the effects of drugs on the body.

Description of Strategy: To begin this activity, the teacher will define the word *drug*. Discuss how some drugs can be helpful and others harmful. The class will discuss how some drugs that are helpful can be harmful if used wrongly. The teacher will have certain situations printed on index cards. The teacher will have the students get in groups of four and have them decide which drugs are harmful and which drugs are helpful. When the groups are done, they will share with the class what their group has decided. The teacher will write *harmful* and *helpful* on the board and list the situations where the class indicates. To close this activity, the teacher will summarize why it is important to know how and what drugs are used for. The teacher will also discuss a few helpful things that drugs do and a few harmful things.

Materials Needed: index cards and chalkboard

Processing Questions:

1. Why is it important to know about effects of drugs?

2. How can people abuse helpful drugs and make them harmful?

Substance Abuse Problem Solving

Valued Outcome: Students will demonstrate problem-solving skills relating to substance misuse.

Description of Strategy: Prepare poster-sized paper with the following situations written on them. These are then taped to the walls around the room. Explain to the students that it is their right and responsibility to refuse to do things that can harm them. However, saying no is not always easy. Knowing why they need to refuse can make it easier to say no. Having a plan can also help them get out of a difficult situation. Divide the class into groups of five, and have the groups circulate around the room and use markers to list answers to the following questions:

1. What are three reasons you need to refuse drugs?
2. One day after school you meet a classmate with whom you would like to become friends. The classmate asks you to share a marijuana cigarette. How could you refuse?
3. You are at your best friend's house. Your friend starts to get soft drinks out of the refrigerator for the two of you. Your friend finds two cans of cold beer and dares you to drink the beer instead. How can you refuse?
4. Peer pressure can make refusing drugs hard to do. You might be afraid people will laugh at you when you refuse. You might not want to hurt your friends' feelings by saying no. What can you do when the peer pressure is hard for you to handle?

Follow this activity with a class discussion of what answers were given and what they mean to the students. Allow time for questions and answers.

Materials Needed: poster-sized paper, markers, masking tape

Processing Questions:

1. What values must I have in order to make the decision to refuse drugs?
2. How do self-esteem and a positive self-image contribute to my refusal skills?

Source: L. Olsen, R. St. Pierre, and J. Ozias. 1990. *Being healthy,* Teacher's Edition. Orlando, FL: Harcourt Brace Jovanovich, p. 273B.

Community Resources

Valued Outcome: Students will participate in an activity that will increase awareness of the location of drug treatment centers in their community and what information may be available to people in need of help for problems associated with drug use.

Description of Strategy: Explain to students that drug treatment centers are found throughout the United States. Have each student write to or call the nearest center to obtain information on current methods of treating the use of illegal drugs. Have each student share the information with the class in a short oral report.

Materials Needed: a phone book for your local community

Processing Question: What types of drug treatment facilities are available to the members of my community?

Source: L. Olsen, R. St. Pierre, and J. Ozias. 1990. *Being healthy,* Teacher's Edition. Orlando, FL: Harcourt Brace Jovanovich, p. 273.

Paying for Substance Abuse

Valued Outcome: To analyze the effects of tobacco, alcohol, and other drug use on crime rates and the economy.

Description of Strategy: Explain that drug use costs the United States billions of dollars every year. Much of this money is spent on law enforcement, rehabilitation, and prevention education. Point out that a portion of taxes that students' parents pay goes to support institutions involved in fighting the drug war (military, police, prisons, hospitals) and in preventing drug use (schools, social services, research institutions, and others). As a class, have the students discuss the following:

○ How do students feel about their families' having to pay for the effects of drug use?

○ How else could this money be used? (Examples: youth programs, educational loans, scientific research.)

○ How else could the United States get money to deal with the drug problem? (Examples: raise taxes, use money confiscated from drug sellers.)

○ How would the students solve the drug problem?

Materials Needed: none
Processing Questions:

1. What can be learned from the statistics regarding substance abuse?

2. What as students can you do to change the relationship between drugs and crime?

3. How does drug use hurt the user and society?

Source: C. Flatter and K. McCormick. 1990. *National Clearinghouse for Alcohol and Drug Information,* Seventh–ninth grade. Washington, DC: U.S. Department of Education, p. 11.

Tobacco Advertising

Valued Outcome: Students will be able to identify the real theme of cigarette advertising and will be able to identify to whom the message is directed and tell the class how they came to this conclusion.

Description of Strategy: Ask each student to select a cigarette advertisement from a magazine, cut it out, and bring it to school for discussion. Ask the students to study their advertisement, and be ready to explain to the class to whom they think the message is directed and how they came to this conclusion. After all students have presented their ad, ask students to form groups of three. Ask the groups to create an advertisement that would encourage elementary school children not to smoke. The students will present these advertisements to the class, explaining their ideas behind their ads.

Materials Needed: magazines, white paper, construction paper, scissors, glue, markers
Processing Questions:

1. Why do you think cigarette companies want to target young people?

2. Do you think cigarette commercials should be banned?

3. What do you think could be done to discourage young people from smoking?

Source: B. J. Gray and D. J. Merki 1977. *Classroom strategies in health education.* Minneapolis: Burgess, p. 155.

Debating Drug Abuse

Valued Outcome: The students will be able to explain the pros and cons of taking drugs.

Description of Strategy: Split up classroom into two groups. Half the class should be on one side of the room, and the other half should be facing them. One side should be side A, and the other side should be side B. Tell the students on side A that they are against taking drugs and cannot stand to be around those who do. Tell side B that they all take drugs and they think all drugs should be legal. These two sides are both given the question of "Should all drugs be legalized?" Side A should detail the facts of the effects of drugs and side B should give excuses about those facts and excuses that people taking drugs would make. Then discuss the harm that drugs do have and the exceptions of the drugs that are legal for medicinal purposes only.

Materials Needed: none

Processing Questions:

1. Should drugs be legalized?

2. Is it that dangerous to take illegal drugs without a prescription?

Defending Yourself from Pressure

Valued Outcomes: The students will see that the media do not always portray life accurately, and will see the harmful effects of legal/illegal drugs.

Description of Strategy: The class will be lectured on the effects alcohol, smoking, and illegal substances may have on the body. The class will be asked for examples they know of where drugs have had an ill effect on someone. Then the class will discuss why people become involved in such things. The instructor will lead the class to discuss what is cool, peer pressure, and the effects of the media. The class will discuss how to defend themselves from such pressures. The class will talk openly and honestly about the problems they may have faced and the best way to avoid the situation. An assignment will be given at the end of the discussion. The students are to make a collage of advertisements from magazines concerning substance abuse. They will develop a theme such as "just say no to false advertisement" to put on their collage. The students will be expected to explain their slogans and collage clippings. They should tell how the pictures apply to the slogan. They will be graded on (1) doing the project and doing it well, (2) originality, (3) time and effort put into it, and (4) explanation of collage. When the task is done, the collages will be placed in different areas around the school such as the cafeteria to remind other students of the misrepresentations in the world.

Materials Needed: poster board, magazines for clippings, construction paper or markers for slogan, glue, scissors

Processing Questions:

1. How do magazines misrepresent the information?

2. How can you avoid an awkward situation with drugs?

Saying "No!"

Valued Outcome: Students will recognize the power in asserting themselves when confronted with possible substance abuse.

Description of Strategy: This lesson in assertiveness is accompanied by a physical demonstration of how assertiveness strengthens itself with repetition. Students are encouraged to develop an arsenal of assertive responses telling why they won't indulge in a harmful substance. The more they practice their responses, the more powerful their will becomes. Sample responses might include "No! That is harmful, and I won't become involved with it." Or "I've seen (heard) what can happen by using that. It's not for me." Or "I respect my body too much to do that to it." Assertive behavior includes more than just a set of words. Encourage students to be firm and quick with their rejections of the substance. In fact, the more directly the offer is rejected, the faster the situation is dealt with, and the easier it becomes for the student to turn his or her back on the solicitation. Help students realize that anyone who would tempt them to harm themselves in such a way is definitely not a friend, no matter how long he or she may have known them. Hold one dowel length out in front of you with both hands (thumbs extended toward the middle of the rod). Explain to the class that the dowel represents willpower and the ability to say "No!" to using harmful substances such as cigarettes, drugs, or alcohol. Tell the students if they are tempted by someone to try such a harmful substance for the first time (slowly and firmly place pressure on the center of the dowel by pulling the ends in toward you), their will is being tested just as the strength of the dowel is being tested. Ask the students, if a person has never said "No!" to this substance before, do they think that person's will could withstand the temptation? (Allow students to offer responses. Their answers may vary.) Continue the even pressure until the dowel breaks in the middle. Explain to the students that since some people never learn to say "No!" their will could break easily the first time. Now take four dowels and stack two on top of the other two. Secure the grouping of dowels at either end with rubber bands. Hold them out in front of you as you did earlier. Explain that these four dowels represent someone who has said "No!" several times before. Ask the students if they think it will be easier or harder for their will to be broken. (Allow for student responses.) Again, with the thumbs extended toward the middle of the bundle of four dowels, attempt to pull back on the ends (holding the dowels away from students). More than likely, it will be rather difficult to break this bundle. Explain to the class that putting the four dowels together is as if someone had been able to say "No!" four times to the offer of a dangerous substance.

Materials Needed: wooden dowels, each approximately 18 inches long
Processing Questions:

1. What are some good responses when confronted with drugs?

2. What is likely to happen to someone who has never said *no* before?

3. Is it easier to say *no* after you have said it once before?

Trafficking Ticket

Valued Outcome: Students will demonstrate an understanding about the role that drug use and drug trafficking play in increasing the risk of violence.

Description of Strategy: Have students design and complete a "traffic ticket" on a 3- x 5-inch index card stating a specific offense associated with drug use or drug trafficking and a penalty for the offense. For example, the trafficking ticket may cite a person for selling cocaine. The penalty might be a prison term, an assignment to a drug rehabilitation program, a fine, and several hours of community service. After students have completed their traffic tickets, have them share their citations and penalties with the class. If possible, invite a law enforcement officer to class to discuss local laws regarding drugs and penalties for drug offenses. Have students prepare questions in advance, and have them take notes so they will have a record of the visit from the law enforcement officer.

Materials Needed: 3- x 5-inch cards, markers

Processing Questions:

1. What are different forms of drug trafficking?

2. What are some ways that a person involved with drugs might be guilty of breaking the law?

Source: L. Meeks and P. Heit. 1995. *Violence prevention: Totally awesome teaching strategies for safe and drug-free schools*. Blacklick, OH: Meeks Heit, pp. 341–342.

Effects of Smoking

Valued Outcome: Students will discuss the negative components of smoking cigarettes and the effects smoking has on the lungs.

Description of Strategy: Discuss with the students the effects of cigarette smoke on the human lungs. Have students find statistics of smoking related to the human body. Show the students pictures of a human lung affected by cigarette smoke and one without any effects. Have the students divide into small groups, and make a list of positive and negative effects of smoking. Then the students will discuss and compare their lists with the rest of the class.

Materials Needed: paper, pencil, resource material and statistics on smoking, pictures comparing lungs

Processing Questions:

1. What is the job of our lungs?

2. What are the effects of smoking cigarettes?

3. What do statistics show is the proper thing to do regarding smoking?

Hitting the Target

Valued Outcome: The students will be able to detail the effects of cocaine on various body parts.

Description of Strategy: Write the initial effects of inhaling cocaine from the nose to the heart and the areas in between. What are the long-term effects?

	Initial Effects	**Long-Term Effects**
Nose:	_____	_____
Brain:	_____	_____
Eyes:	_____	_____
Lungs:	_____	_____
Heart:	_____	_____

Materials Needed: None

Processing Question: Why do we need to be concerned with long-term effects of drugs versus short-term effects?

Adapted from: P. Gerne and T. Gerne. 1991. *Substance abuse prevention activities for secondary students*. Englewood Cliffs, NJ: Prentice Hall, pp. 13–18.

Make a Change

Valued Outcome: The students will be able to accurately complete sentences about the effects of drugs.

Description of Strategy: Have the students complete the following sentences:

1. Fetal alcohol syndrome is the leading cause of _____.
2. Pregnant women should check with a doctor before taking any _____.
3. AIDS can be transmitted to the baby through _____.
4. Marijuana use during pregnancy may produce defects similar to _____.
5. The organ of the body that oxidizes drugs is the _____.
6. Smoking slows down delivery of _____ to the fetus.
7. _____ amount of alcohol can affect the unborn baby.
8. Babies born to a woman who is addicted to alcohol or other drugs can be born _____.
9. The most abused drug in our society is _____.
10. When the body needs more and more of the drug to get the desired effect, that response is called _____.
11. The organ of the body most sensitive to alcohol is _____.
12. The unpleasant physical and emotional symptoms that result when the drug is stopped are called _____.
13. _____ is the greatest roadblock to accepting help.
14. Nicotine only initially _____ the central nervous system.
15. The Surgeon General says there are no _____ cigarettes.
16. Cigarette smoking is the major single cause of _____ cancer.
17. The poison found in tobacco is called _____.
18. Regular users of tobacco become _____ on it.
19. The use of tobacco causes the teeth to _____.

Materials Needed: handouts with the preceding questions for each student
Processing Question: How can the preceding information help you make a wise decision about substance abuse?

Adapted from: P. Gerne and T. Gerne. 1991. *Substance abuse prevention activities for secondary students.* Englewood Cliffs, NJ: Prentice Hall.

Experiments and Demonstrations ─────────────

Smoking Machine

Valued Outcome: The students will be able to become aware of what cigarette smoking does to the body.
Description of Strategy: The purpose of this demonstration is to show the effect of cigarette tars on the human body by way of analogy. You will need a large glass bottle, a two-hole rubber stop-

Figure 13.1

Smoking Machine
Apparatus

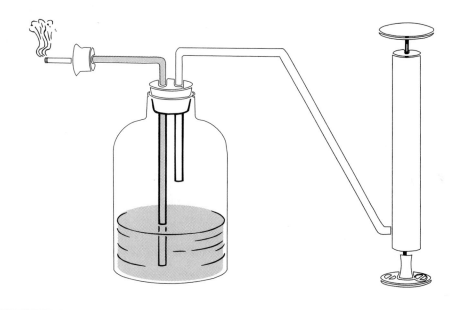

per, glass delivery tubes, a cigarette holder, cigarettes, and a small hand pump. Most of this equipment can be found in a school chemistry lab or can be obtained from a scientific supply house. Set up the apparatus as shown in Figure 13.1 Fill the bottle halfway with water. Place a cigarette in the holder and light it. Operate the pump to draw smoke from the cigarette into the bottle and water. Continue to pump until the cigarette is burned completely. Burn additional cigarettes as necessary until tars can be seen in the water. Then have the students examine the water, and note the distinct smell. Tars may also collect in the glass tubing. Ask students how this demonstration illustrates what happens when a person smokes a cigarette.

Materials Needed: water, a large glass bottle, a two-hole rubber stopper, glass delivery tubes, a cigarette holder, cigarettes, and a small hand pump

Processing Questions:

1. What happens to cigarette smoke when it enters the body?

2. What are the short-term and long-term health effects of cigarette smoking?

Goldfish Demonstration

Valued Outcome: The students will learn about the toxic qualities contained in cigarette smoke.
Description of Strategy: This demonstration illustrates the toxic qualities contained in cigarette smoke. Before you begin, explain to the class that there are more than three hundred chemical substances in cigarette smoke. These substances include nicotine, cyanide, formaldehyde, lead, arsenic, and carbon monoxide—all poisons. Set up a smoking machine apparatus like that shown

in Figure 13.1 This time, first add two or three goldfish to the water in the bottle. Then process three or more cigarettes by using the pump. The fish will begin to lose their equilibrium as they are affected by the chemicals in the cigarette smoke. As soon as this begins to happen, remove the fish by pouring the water into a net. Place the fish into a bowl of clean water. Do not pour the contaminated water into the clean water as you do this, or the fish will die from continued exposure to the contaminants.

Materials Needed: water, a large glass bottle, a two-hole rubber stopper, glass delivery tubes, a cigarette holder, cigarettes, and a small hand pump

Processing Questions:

1. What are some of the chemicals in cigarette smoke?

2. How does the body react to these chemicals when they enter the body?

Breathometer Demonstration

Valued Outcome: The students will be able to learn the dangers of drinking and driving.

Description of Strategy: Invite a local police officer to class to demonstrate how a breathometer works. This device is used to test the amount of alcohol in a driver's bloodstream. Have the police officer explain the dangers of drinking and driving. The person should note that even a small amount of alcohol has a deleterious effect on driving ability.

Materials Needed: none

Processing Questions:

1. What are the effects of alcohol on the body?

2. Why do police officers have to test drivers' blood alcohol concentration?

Effects of Smoking on the Lungs

Valued Outcome: Students will recognize tar as the sticky, brown, poisonous substance found in cigarettes.

Description of Strategy: In preparation, cut the opening in the nozzle of a squeeze bottle large enough to snugly insert the end of a cigarette. Unscrew the top and stretch the cotton ball across the top and around the threads like a filter. Secure the cotton ball by screwing the cap back on the bottle. Insert the (filter) end of the cigarette into the opening of the bottle's nozzle. After having discussed the hazards of smoking with the class, show the class a clean cotton ball. Explain that for purposes of the upcoming demonstration, the cotton ball will represent the healthy tissue of a nonsmoker's lungs. Allow the students to handle, observe, and pass around the cotton ball. While the cotton ball is being passed around, bring out the "smoker's lung" device. Explain that this contraption will represent a smoker. The cotton ball inside is the lungs. The smoker will smoke one cigarette, and then the class will have the opportunity to observe the damage to the lungs. Light the cigarette. (Be sure to keep the matches out of reach of the students. Also, it is best to do this demonstration near an open window so that the cigarette smoke will be leaving the room.) Squeeze and release the bottle in a methodical fashion to draw air into the cigarette and thus "smoke" it. Use the jar lid as a makeshift ashtray. After the cigarette has been "smoked" to within about an inch of the bottle nozzle's opening, put the cigarette out by crushing it in the jar lid. Allow the remnants of smoke to escape out the window. Allow students to gather around in a central location for purposes of observation. Unscrew the bottle's nozzle and remove the cotton ball (alias "lung tissue"). Allow the students to personally inspect the stained cotton ball.

Materials Needed: an empty squeeze bottle (may have contained mustard, ketchup, etc.), two cotton balls, cigarette (filterless, if possible), book of matches, lid from a jar
Processing Questions:

1. How is this cotton ball different from the cotton ball passed around earlier?

2. What damage might tar cause in your lungs?

Source: M. W. Fischer. 1996. *Health & Safety Curriculum,* Primary manual. Grand Rapids, MI: Instructional Fair/TS Denison, p. 40.

Learning How to "Just Say No"

Valued Outcome: Students will be able to convince their peers to stay off drugs.
Description of Strategy: Cut a regular piece of poster board in half. Have students write the letters "Just Say No" down the side of the poster board. Instruct students to write a sentence, with each letter, that they could say to another student to help keep that student off drugs. The students should use their own creativity to color and make the poster presentable to the class. They should prepare a presentation for the class. After they have made their poster, choose a few students or volunteers to present their poster to the class and explain what they have written. Allow other students to provide feedback.
Materials Needed: poster board, markers, magazine cutouts
Processing Question: How can I help my peers stay off drugs?

Source: Derived from G. Ezell. 1993. *Healthy living, Building blocks for health,* Grade 3. Grand Rapids, MI: Christian Schools International.

Emphysema Simulation

Valued Outcome: The students will experience one of the harmful effects associated with smoking.
Description of Strategy: This demonstration would be presented in conjunction with other information on the harmful effects of smoking. The instructor will distribute one drinking straw to each student in the class. She or he will then instruct the students to put the straw in the mouth and hold their noses. The instructor will tell the students to breathe only though the straw, while she or he times them for thirty seconds. The instructor will then tell the students that this is what people with emphysema feel like when they breathe.
Materials Needed: enough drinking straws for each student to have one, and students' own writing materials
Processing Question: The instructor will ask the students to write down what it felt like to breathe through the straw for thirty seconds. They can share their answers with the class.

Source: L. Meeks and P. Heit. 1990. *Merrill health: focus on you,* Fourth Grade Teachers' Edition. Columbus, OH: Merrill.

DUI Demonstration

Valued Outcome: Students will demonstrate what takes place in a DUI arrest and what happens to a DUI offender by dramatizing the procedure.
Description of Strategy: The teacher will arrange prior to class for a police officer to come and talk regarding drinking and driving. During the class, the officer and the students will act out a

true-to-life DUI conviction. The officer will treat the students (preferably only one or two, so the rest of the students can observe what takes place) as if they had actually committed this crime, using all the correct questioning and procedures. The classroom will turn into the crime scene, the police station, and the jail cell. Class participation will be the key for the lesson to come across to the students. The students should know the statistics of death-related accidents due to drinking and driving. Also, the students should understand the problem with drinking under age and driving as well.

Materials Needed: classroom space, police officer (arrangements should be made prior to class)

Processing Question:

1. Should anyone drive after consuming alcohol?

2. What are the procedures someone who has been convicted of drinking and driving must go through?

Responsible Use of Medicines

Valued Outcome: Students will analyze the short-term and long-term consequences of safe, risky, and harmful behaviors in relation to substance use.

Description of Strategy: Discuss the responsible use of prescription and over-the-counter drugs. Explain drug interactions. Demonstrate an addictive effect. Pour one cup of water into a glass. Then pour a second cup of water into the same glass and have students observe the level of the water. Explain that one cup of water plus one cup of water produced two cups of water. Demonstrate a synergistic reaction. Place one cup of vinegar in a glass. In a separate container, dissolve two tablespoons of baking soda in one cup of water. Tell students that the vinegar represents alcohol. The water solution represents barbiturates. Now you will add the water and baking soda to the vinegar in the glass. Make sure you have a bowl below the glass or are holding the glass over a sink when you mix the two. When you mix the ingredients from the two glasses, the ingredients will overflow.

Materials Needed: two glasses, water, vinegar, baking soda

Processing Questions:

1. What types of drug interactions can occur?

2. What makes prescription drugs different from over-the-counter (OTC) drugs?

3. What information is contained on an OTC label?

Source: L. Meeks and P. Heit. 1996. *Totally awesome health,* Sixth grade manual. Blacklick, OH: Meeks Heit, p. 111–112.

Alcohol and Coordination

Valued Outcome: Students will experience a simulation of one of the effects that alcohol has on coordination.

Description of Strategy: On a sheet of paper, have each student write in cursive his or her first and last name. Then have each student do the same thing, but with the opposite hand—the hand with which they do not normally write. Have the students describe what it felt like to write with the opposite hand. They will share that they did not feel as comfortable and it was not as easy. They will indicate that their handwriting was more sloppy and that they wrote more slowly than when they used their usual hand. Explain that alcohol affects the body in many different ways. In a way, this activity simulates having a drink of alcohol.

Materials Needed: pencils and paper
Processing Questions:

1. How might alcohol use create dangerous situations?
2. What other effects does alcohol have on the body?

Source: L. Meeks and P. Heit. 1996. *Totally awesome health,* Fourth grade manual. Blacklick, OH: Meeks Heit, pp. 97–98.

Puzzles and Games

Drugs Spell Trouble

Valued Outcome: The students will be able to match the names of drugs with clues about those drugs.
Description of Strategy: Prepare individual worksheets as shown in Figure 13.2. Have students write the name of the drug that answers each clue given in the letter spaces provided. The completed puzzle spells out vertically a message about substance abuse, as shown in Figure 13.2.
Materials Needed: worksheets, pen/pencils
Processing Question: What clues about drugs can identify those drugs?

Figure 13.2
"Drugs Spell Trouble"
Puzzle

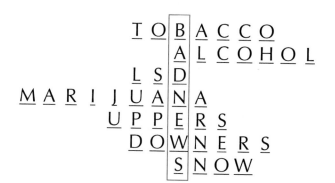

1. What cigarettes are made of.
2. The drug in beer, wine, and whiskey.
3. Three letters for a substance that causes hallucinations.
4. Substance made from the cannabis plant.
5. Street name for amphetamines.
6. Street name for barbiturates.
7. Street name for cocaine.

Smoking Crossword Puzzle

Valued Outcome: The students will be able to use their knowledge of the detrimental health effects of smoking to complete puzzles.
Description of Strategy: Prepare individual puzzle sheets as shown in Figures 13.3 and 13.4. After you have discussed smoking in class, distribute the sheets and have the students complete the puzzles. In these examples, the correct answers have been provided.
Materials Needed: puzzle worksheet, pen/pencils
Processing Question: What are the detrimental effects of smoking?

Let's Play Tic-Tac-Toe

Valued Outcome: The students will be able to distinguish facts from misconception with regard to several substance abuse-related statements.

Figure 13.3
Word Search on Drugs

CAN YOU FIND THESE WORDS?

emphysema
cigarette
cancer
smoke
chemicals
incurable
hashish
counselor
stimulants
pharmacy
dosage
dependence
withdrawal
tolerance
hangover
tar
caffeine
hallucinogens
narcotics
depressant
overdose
marijuana
alcoholic
cirrhosis

Find each of the words and circle them. The words may read in any direction—up, down, across, or diagonally. The words may even intersect.

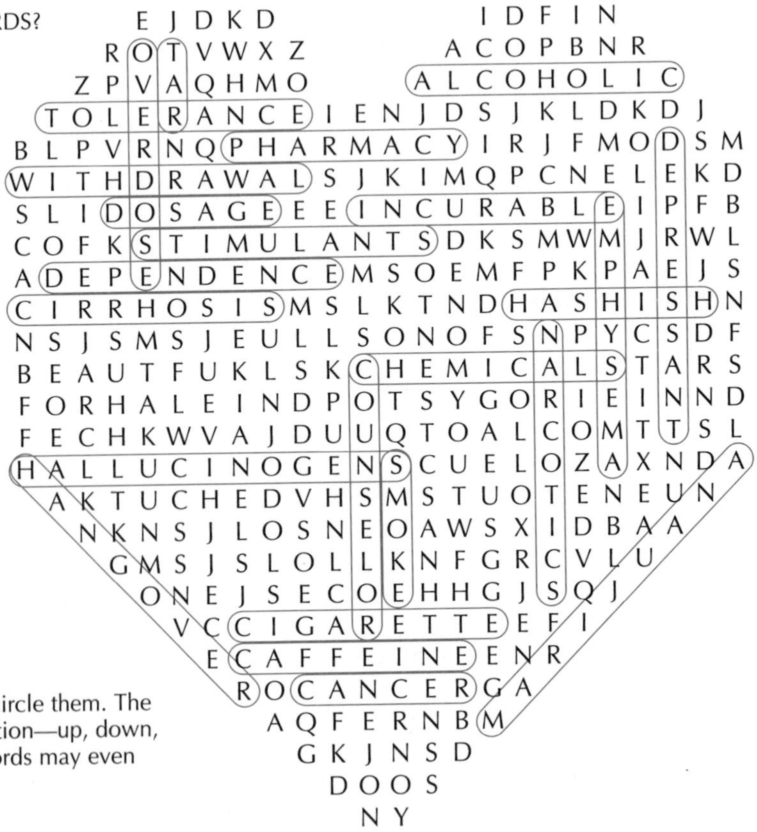

Figure 13.4
*Smoking Crossword
Puzzle*

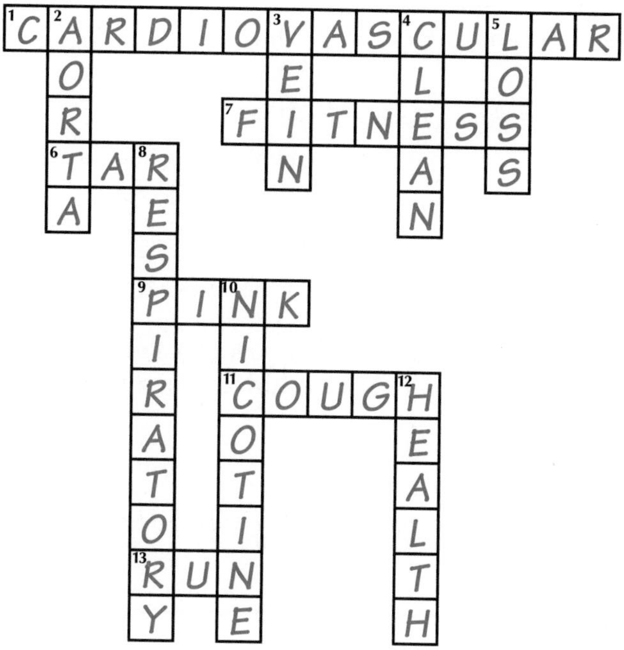

```
 1      2        3      4      5
 C  A  R  D  I  O  V  A  S  C  U  L  A  R
    O           E        L        O
    R          7F  I  T  N  E  S  S
 6T  A  8R        N        A        S
    A     E                N
          S
         9P  I 10N  K
          I        I
          R    11C  O  U  G 12H
          A        O        E
          T        T        A
          O        I        L
        13R  U  N           T
          Y     E           H
```

ACROSS

1. The _____ system contains the heart and blood vessels.
6. The cancer-causing substance in tobacco smoke is _____.

7. Cigarette smoking can lower your physical _____.
9. Normally, the lungs are a _____ color.
11. Many smokers awake every morning with a _____.
13. Cigarette smoking may cause you to be more breathless when you _____.

DOWN

2. The blood vessel that carries blood from the heart to the rest of the body is an _____.
3. The blood vessel that carries blood back to the heart from the body is a _____.
4. Non-smokers have a right to breathe _____ air.
5. When a person develops emphysema, there is a definite _____ of lung function.
8. Smoking is also bad for your _____ system.
10. A substance in tobacco that causes blood vessels to get smaller is _____.
12. Warning: The Surgeon General Has Determined That Cigarette Smoking Is Dangerous To Your _____.

Description of Strategy: Tell the students to place an O in the squares with true statements, then to place an X in the squares with statements that are not true.

○ The family does not cause the drug-dependent person to take drugs.

○ Drug dependency does not occur in "good" families.

○ Talking to someone you trust about a drug problem is helpful.

○ Family members of drug-dependent people never need help.

○ Drug-dependent people may be unable to stop taking drugs unless they get special help.

○ Family members can make drug-dependent people stop taking drugs by being good and by doing nice things.

○ A drug-dependent person has an illness.

○ "Bad" children cause their parents to drink.

○ Drug-dependent people do not love their families.

How many scored tic-tac-toe? Have students change some of the *false* statements to *true* so they can be winners.

Materials Needed: tic-tac-toe sheets, pen/pencils

Processing Questions:

1. Why are there so many misconceptions about substance abuse?

2. How can we reduce the amount of misconceptions about the public about substance abuse?

The Magic Gumball Machine

Valued Outcome: The students will be able to discuss healthy activities as alternatives to substance abuse.

Description of Strategy: Prepare individual sheets as shown in Figure 13.5. Pass them out and have students complete the activity. Follow with a discussion of activities your students enjoy.

Materials Needed: worksheets

Processing Questions:

1. What are some activities you enjoy?

2. How can healthy activities serve as alternatives to substance abuse?

Figure 13.5

The Magic Gumball Machine

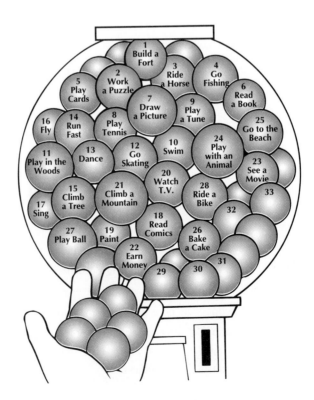

Safe Use of Medicines

Valued Outcome: Students will learn to identify the safe use of several common over-the-counter medicines.

Description of Strategy: In preparation, make an enlarged transparency of the front side of a flattened box or wrapper, for use on an overhead. Repeat this for each package. Cut a piece of construction paper to cover the flattened box. Then cut this paper into four or five interlocking shapes, creating a sort of jigsaw puzzle. Number each piece according to its difficulty from 1 to however many total pieces are used to cover the image. (The most obvious puzzle piece clues would have the higher numbers on them. Place number 1 over the directions.) Use a little bit of tape to hold each cover piece to the transparency.

Divide students into groups. Explain to the class that on the overhead is the image of a common over-the-counter medicine with which they may be familiar. It is presently covered by several pieces of a jigsaw puzzle. Each group in rotation will be asked a true/false question about the safe use of medicine. If the group answers the question correctly, the students ask to have a specifically numbered piece of the puzzle removed. They then have ten seconds to see if they can identify the mystery medication. If no one correctly guesses the product, the puzzle piece is replaced on the overhead, and the second team is offered a true/false question with the possibility of removing a puzzle piece and correctly identifying the hidden product. When a correct identification of the hidden product is given, that team obtains a point value equal to the sum of the numbered puzzle pieces left on the transparency. If the puzzle originally had four pieces and only pieces number 1, number 2, and number 4 were left on the transparency, that team would score 7 points. Continue the game until either all the true/false questions have been covered or all the images have been identified. The highest score wins. As a review, have each student complete the worksheet.

Materials Needed: the outer boxes or wrappers of several well-known over-the-counter medicines—aspirin, nasal spray, acetaminophen, eye drops, etc.; transparency sheets (one for each product); overhead projector; several sheets of construction paper (one for each product); true/false questions; clear tape; a copy of "review" worksheet for each student

Processing Questions:

1. Can an over-the-counter drug be bought without a doctor's prescription?

2. What should you do before taking an over-the-counter drug?

Get That Word

Valued Outcome: Students will review substance use/abuse concepts.

Description of Strategy: Review material on substance use and abuse by playing the game "Get That Word!" Follow these steps:

1. First, teach or review words on game cards. Tell students they'll have to know these words to play the game. Discuss any words the students do not understand.

2. Second, divide the class into two teams. Have the students sit in a circle. The teacher should sit in the middle. Distribute the word cards, one to each student. Each team should have a set of the word cards. (One student on each team needs a word card to correctly complete each sentence the teacher will read.) As you pass out the cards, students should read their words silently. Make sure students know their words.

3. Explain how to play the game. The teacher reads one of the incomplete statements. The student on each team who has the correct word brings the card up to the teacher. The first person to bring the correct word wins a point. If the students don't understand the statement, reword it or give additional clues.

Play the game until all the statements have been used. The team with the highest score wins. If time permits, have students write scrambled messages warning about the use of drugs. They can trade messages with partners (or team members) and then enjoy deciphering the code.

Conclude by stressing that what the students have learned about drugs and their effects can help them make safe and healthy choices as they grow up.

Note: The statements and word cards can be modified to fit what you've covered in class.
Materials Needed: student activity game cards and teacher statements
Processing Questions:

1. What other statements can we use for these words?

2. Have the students prepare or suggest additional statements for clues.

Source: G. Ezell. 1992. *Healthy living, Level 2: Healthy and growing.* Grand Rapids, MI: Christian Schools International, p.106.

Smoking Cessation

Valued Outcome: Students will participate in a game to increase their knowledge of the complexity of smoking cessation.
Description of Strategy: Using masking tape, form a three-foot square box on the floor. Select a student to stand inside this square. Explain to this student that this is called the "Pool of Tobacco." Explain that this is a different kind of pool. This pool takes them inside and makes it difficult for people to get out. To make an analogy, when a person uses tobacco products, that person will have difficulty trying to stop using these products because tobacco causes dependence. Dependence is a need for a particular drug.

Ask another student to stand away from the pool. Have this person hold one end of a string and the person inside the pool hold the other end of the string. Explain that the person on the outside can pull the person away from tobacco if this person is given enough support. Explain that the support is to come from the class in the form of statements about the dangers of tobacco products. Students are to tell dangers of tobacco use one at a time. With each danger, the person outside the pool will tug the person inside the pool slightly.

After students have named about seven dangers of tobacco products, the student in the pool should be towed to the outside. Explain that once this person is free of tobacco, this person should not attempt to use tobacco products again, because it will be easy to become trapped in the pool again. The dangers of tobacco use should be enough to keep people on safe ground and to avoid areas of danger.
Materials Needed: masking tape, a piece of string about 10 feet long
Processing Questions:

1. How does tobacco harm the body?

2. What is the difference between tobacco and smokeless tobacco?

3. What signs may be apparent in those who use tobacco?

Source: L. Meeks and P. Heit. 1996. *Totally awesome health,* Fourth grade manual. Blacklick, OH: Meeks Heit, p. 99–100.

Other Ideas

Dealing with Peer Pressure

Valued Outcome: The students will be able to describe how peer pressure can be a positive and/or negative factor with regard to substance abuse.

Description of Strategy: Divide the class into groups of six to eight students. Have each group form a circle. Place pieces of candy in the center of each group. Give five members of each group a slip of paper stating that they are to eat the candy and attempt to get anyone not eating to do so. Give the remaining students in each group a slip of paper stating that they should not eat the candy and should resist all attempts to get them to do so. Let this interaction go on for about five minutes. Then ask the students to take their regular seats. Ask the following questions:

○ What were you feeling when you were doing this exercise?

○ What do you think the purpose of this exercise was?

○ What is peer pressure?

○ Why is it important to know about peer pressure?

Materials Needed: paper, pieces of candy
Processing Questions:

1. What is peer pressure?

2. How can peer pressure be a positive factor in your life?

3. How does negative peer pressure lead to substance abuse?

Slogans

Valued Outcome: The students will be able to develop a list of slogans against drug use.
Description of Strategy: Have the students develop a list of slogans used by tobacco, alcohol, and OTC drug manufacturers. Discuss what the slogans are attempting to convince the consumer to do. Discuss the irrational appeal often used in this advertising approach. Then have the students come up with counterslogans that seek to convince the consumer to do the opposite.
Materials Needed: poster board, butcher paper
Processing Question: How can antidrug messages convince the public not to abuse drugs?

Affirmations

Valued Outcome: The students will be able to describe how support from friends can prevent substance abuse problems.
Description of Strategy: Have each student come up to the front of the class and say, "Sometimes I don't feel so good about myself." Then have the student turn his or her back to the class. Have other students then volunteer to affirm one fine quality about that individual. Every student should get three affirmations from the class. These may refer to being a loyal friend, being kind, being a good student, being fair, being friendly, and so on.
Materials Needed: none
Processing Questions:

1. How can young people offer moral support to their friends through praise?

2. How can such praise prevent substance abuse problems?

Be a Friend to Yourself!

Valued Outcome: The students will be able to discuss the importance of having good relationships with friends.

Description of Strategy: Pose the following questions to your students:

○ If you had a best friend who was very special to you, how would you act toward that person?

○ Would you say nice things to him or her?

○ What kind of nice things would you say?

○ Would you let your friend know that you liked him or her?

After class members have shared their ideas, follow up with these points: You do have a best friend. You are your own best friend. The most important person for you to be a friend to is yourself. Being a friend to yourself means saying nice things about yourself and doing things for yourself.

Materials Needed: none

Processing Questions:

1. What are some nice things about you that you like about yourself?

2. What are some special things you can do for yourself?

Keeping Physically Fit

Valued Outcome: The students will be able to relate how exercise can help prevent substance abuse.

Description of Strategy: Invite to your classroom some older people who keep physically fit. Let the children talk to them and ask questions about their diet and exercise program. Afterward, design a survey that includes (1) things the students do to keep fit, (2) how often they exercise, and (3) reasons why they do or do not exercise.

Materials Needed: poster board, butcher paper, markers

Processing Questions:

1. Why is it important to remain physically fit?

2. How can keeping physically fit prevent substance abuse?

Source: Join Together. 1994, Winter. Second national survey: Coalitions want policy changes. *Strategies,* 2(4).

References

Barnes, M., K. DeBarr, and M. Kittleson. 1996, July–August. Teaching the emotional aspect of drug use, abuse, and dependency. *Journal of health education.* 27(4).pp. 261–262.

Ezell, G. 1993. *Healthy living, building blocks for health*, Grade 3. Grand Rapids, MI: Christian Schools International.

Fields, R. 1995. *Drugs in perspective*, 2nd ed. Madison, WI: Brown & Benchmark.

Fischer, M. 1996. *Health and safety curriculum.* Grand Rapids, MI: Instructional Fair.

Flatter, C., and K. McCormick 1990. *National clearinghouse for alcohol and drug information:* Ninth-twelfth grades. Washington, DC: U.S. Department of Education.

Gerne, P. and T. Gerne. 1991. *Substance abuse prevention activities for secondary students.* Englewood Cliffs, NJ: Prentice Hall.

Gray, B. J., and D. J. Merki. 1977. *Classroom strategies in health education.* Minneapolis: Burgess.

Join Together. 1994, Winter. Second national aurvey: Coalitions want policy changes." *Strategies,* 2(4).

Meeks, L., and P. Heit. 1990. *Merrill health focus on you: Fourth Grade, Teachers' Edition*. Columbus, OH: Merrill.

Meeks, L., and P. Heit, 1995. *Violence prevention: Totally awesome teaching strategies for safe and drug-free schools*. Blacklick, OH: Meeks Heit.

Meeks, L., P. Heit, and R. Page. 1995. *Drugs, alcohol, and tobacco: Teaching strategies*. Blacklick, OH: Meeks Heit.

Meeks, L., and P. Heit. 1996. *Totally awesome health*, Sixth grade manual. Blacklick, OH: Meeks Heit.

Olsen, L., R. St. Pierre, and J. Ozias. 1990. *Being healthy*, Teacher's Edition. Orlando, FL: Harcourt Brace Jovanovich.

Read, D. 1980. *Creative teaching in health*, 3rd ed. Prospect Heights, IL: Waveland Press.

Resources

Suggested Readings

Akers, R. L. 1992. *Drugs, alcohol, and society: social structure, process, and policy*. Belmont, CA: Wadsworth.

American Medical Association. 1990. *Healthy youth 2000*. Chicago: Author.

Appalachian Educational Laboratory. 1992. *R&D notes*, (Charleston,WV) 6(10).

Avis, H. 1996. *Drugs & life*, 3rd ed. Madison, WI: Brown & Benchmark.

Benard, B. 1993, Spring. Characteristics of effective prevention programs. *CenterPage*, Southeast Regional Center for Drug-Free Schools and Communities. Louisville, KY, 2(1).

Carroll, C. R. 1996. *Drugs in modern society*, 4th ed. Madison, WI: Brown & Benchmark.

Centers for Disease Control and Prevention. 1993. Youth risk behavior survey. *Journal of the American Medical Association*, 269(11).

Centers for Disease Control. 1990, April 27. *Current trends: Cigarette advertising—United States, 1988*, 39(16).

Fishbein, D. H., and S. E. Pease. 1996. *The dynamics of drug abuse*. Boston: Allyn and Bacon.

Hahn, D. B., and W. A. Payne. 1997. *Focus on health*. St. Louis: Mosby.

Hanson, G., and P. J. Venturelli. 1995. *Drugs and society*, 4th ed. Boston: Jones & Bartlett.

Hunton, H. T. 1991, November. Is your child using drugs? *Alternatives*, p. 1.

Langton, P. A. 1996. *The social world of drugs*. Minneapolis/St. Paul: West.

Levinthal, C. F. 1996. *Drugs, behavior, and modern society*. Boston: Allyn and Bacon.

Mintz, M. 1991, May 6. The nicotine pushers: Marketing tobacco to children. *The nation*.

National Commission on Drug-Free School. 1990, September. *Toward a drug-free generation: A nation's responsibility*. Washington, DC: Author.

Ray, O., and C. Ksir. 1996. *Drugs, society, and human behavior*, 7th ed. St. Louis: Mosby.

Schlaadt, R., and P. Shannon. 1990. *Drugs*, 3rd ed. Englewood Cliffs, NJ: Prentice Hall.

Sullivan, L. W. 1990, May 24. *Statement before the committee on finance*. U. S. Senate, Washington, DC.

Witters, W., P. Venturelli, and G. Hanson. 1992. *Drugs and society*, 3rd ed. Boston: Jones & Bartlett.

Videos

The following videos are available from Schoolhouse Videos & CDs, 4205 Grove Ridge Drive, Durham, NC 27703:

Prescription for health—alcohol addition
Why do people drink? People begin and continue to abuse alcohol for a number of reasons. Most frequently, alcohol fills a need in their lives. Learn the common reasons why most people abuse alcohol. (Item 8970)

High on life, not on drugs
An educational and entertaining program used by the FBI National Academy, and by thousands of teenagers, enforcement officers, teachers, clergy, and parents. An outstanding drug prevention program. (Item 5142)

Your family's health: Vol. 1: Talk to your doctor, Over-the-counter medicine
Six steps to well-being: Provides tips for finding the right physician and communicating the patient's needs. (53 minutes, Item 11682)

The following videos are available from Sunburst Communications, 101 Castleton Street, P.O. Box 40, Pleasantville, NY 10570:

Addiction: The problems, the solutions
Using a series of interviews with young people, a medical expert, and a clinical psychologist, explores what addiction is, who is vulnerable, and what can be done.

Drugs, your friends, and you: Handling peer pressure
Peer pressure can be a powerful influence on the decision to use drugs or alcohol, and young people don't always realize they can continue to respect their own best interests and say no. Program makes students aware they do have choices, then teaches specific techniques for dealing assertively with drug/alcohol pressures. (26-minute video, teacher's guide)

The truth about inhalants
Interweaving real-life vignettes and graphics on inhalants' dangers with tips on their safe use, offers a powerful indictment of inhalant abuse.

Tobacco and you
Interweaves a TV talk show on tobacco's health dangers with interviews with young teen smokers to show that

smoking is neither "cool," sexy, nor grown-up, but is instead a nonglamorous and socially offensive habit that is very hard to break.

The truth about alcohol
Alerts students to the facts they need to know about alcohol—what it is, how it acts on the body, and why young people are so vulnerable to its dangers. Encourages viewers to reexamine their thinking about alcohol, and helps them understand the problems caused by other people's alcohol abuse. (20-minute video, teacher's guide)

Why I won't do drugs
Designed for earliest drug education, helps young viewers make the connection between understanding and respecting your body and how drug use can harm it. Presents a positive, no-use message in terms students can easily relate to.

Professional Education Videos

A selection of videos for health professionals is provided. Evaluations are included for items that have been evaluated. The videos are available from the ARF (Addiction Research Foundation) Library for loan in Ontario. Call (416) 595-6987. Outside Ontario, contact the distributor.

Alcohol withdrawal syndrome (Video No. 2002, 1986; 48 minutes, $250)
Rating: none given (6-point scale)
Audience: health professionals
Producer: Addiction Research Foundation, 33 Russell Street, Toronto, ON M5S
2S1 1 (800) 661-1111/(416) 595-6059
Distributor: same

Synopsis: This program provides step-by-step training in an effective method of assessment and management of alcohol withdrawal syndrome. The method, developed in the Clinical Institute of the Addiction Research Foundation, helps ensure adequate and prompt treatment of the alcoholic patient and prevent serious complications of the alcohol withdrawal syndrome. The program includes three modules: (1) *Introduction*: The alcohol withdrawal syndrome is defined, causes and clinical manifestations are examined, and characteristics of withdrawal reactions are summarized. (2) *Assessment*: In order to determine the most effective treatment procedure, severity of withdrawal must be assessed. This module demonstrates the actual process of assessment, using simulations of a patient in minor and major withdrawal. (3) *Treatment*: Recommendations based on information recorded on the CIWA-A form are made for the management of minor and major withdrawal reactions. A variety of treatment approaches, both with and without drug therapy, are demonstrated.

Behavioral management of intoxicated and disruptive patients (Video No. 2006, 1980; not available for purchase)

Rating: none given (6-point scale)
Audience: health professionals
Producer: ARF, 33 Russell Street, Toronto, ON M5S 2S1
1 (800) 661-1111/(416) 595-6059
Distributor: same

Synopsis: This program illustrates a number of situations that admitting staff may have to deal with in the course of the day: a client who is overly aggressive; an older woman suffering from loneliness; an intoxicated man with an injury brought in by his friend; a woman with a minor injury (possibly self-inflicted). The various scenarios demonstrate safe ways of dealing with incidents ranging from the annoying to the potentially dangerous, both with and without drug therapy, are demonstrated.

Codependency: The what and why... (Video No. 1075, 1990; 23 minutes, $772)
Rating: 4.0 (6-point scale)
Audience: professionals whose work requires an understanding of codependency
Producer: Concept Media, 1419 Dubridge Ave., Irvine, CA 92714 (800) 223-7078
Distributor: RK Media Consultants, 107 Berkley Rd., Cambridge, ON N1S 3G8 (519) 622-5285

Synopsis: "Codependent" is a term originally used to describe people who "enable" the substance abuse of a partner or family member, for example, by ignoring the problem. The term has since been applied to people in relationships with compulsive gamblers, compulsive eaters, and others. In this video, the theories of leading writers in the codependency field (Melody Beattie, Claudia Black, John Bradshaw, Pia Mellody) are presented. In addition, actors mime some of the behaviors that lead to codependency, such as boundary violations, low self-esteem, and poor communication.

Evaluation: Good. Codependency is a somewhat controversial concept, since, as the definition has expanded, a large proportion of the population could now, in theory, be labelled codependent. For those who want to know more about the subject, this video would be a good primer. The narrative contains a lot of jargon, however, and is therefore best suited for professionals. The video seems aimed more at women than men; the early vignettes, for example, use the pronoun "she" exclusively.

Communication skills: A demonstration tape (Video No. 2011, 1984; 15 minutes, $65)
Rating: none given (6-point scale)
Audience: health professionals
Producer: Addiction Research Foundation, 33 Russell Street, Toronto, ON M5R
2S1 1 (800) 661-1111/(416) 595-6059
Distributor: Same

Synopsis: This interactive training tape is ideal for in-service use by addiction counselors. This course has been designed to assist counselors-in-training to learn techniques of listening and understanding with empathy, as well as clarifying, validating, and directing the flow of communication. The package includes user's notes and response-recording forms. The videotape is divided into two parts: (1) *reflective skills*, attending, paraphrasing, reflection of feeling, summarizing; (2) *directive skills*, probing, interpretation, confrontation.

Comprehensive drinker profile (Video No. 2104, 1989; 89 minutes, $30)
Rating: none given (6-point scale)
Audience: health professionals
Producer: University of New Mexico, CASAA, Albuquerque, NM 87131-1161 (505) 277-2805
Distributor: CASAA, Department of Psychology, University of New Mexico, Albuquerque, NM 87131-1161/(505) 277-2805

Synopsis: "Comprehensive" is the word for William Miller's step-by-step structured client interview. This is a pretreatment assessment of the client seen in the video *Motivational interviewing*. All details about drinking patterns, problems associated with drinking, kinds of drinks, self-image, personal habits, others' perceptions are surveyed in this intense assessment procedure.

The Door To Recovery: Community drug abuse treatment (Video No. 2135, 1989, 25 minutes, $8.50)
Rating: none given (6-point scale)
Audience: Health professionals
Producer: National Clearinghouse, Videotape Resource Prog., P.O. Box 2345, Rockville, MD 20847, 1 (800) 729-6686/(301) 468-2600

Synopsis: This video presents arguments and models for community-based treatment. Realizing that criminal justice is not the answer and that treatment is cheaper than jail, the producers present a number of U.S. programs. At Turning Point, clients are given duties and responsibilities and learn social skills and values. In another experimental program a client self-administers methadone at home in much the same way that a diabetic person uses insulin. In a client-run house in San Diego members are learning that just being off drugs is not enough, as one says, "I had to relearn my life." A counselor states that the community also has to learn that addiction is not just the concern of those in treatment, but is a social problem of concern to everyone.

Double trouble I: Mood and anxiety disorders (Video No. 1005, 1992, 30 minutes, US $295)
Rating: 4.0 (6-point scale)
Audience: health professionals; EAP; addiction specialists
Producer: Gerald T. Rogers, 5215 Old Orchard Rd. Suite #990, Skokie, IL 60077 (312) 967-8080
Distributor: Kinetic Communications Inc. 408 Dundas St. E. Toronto, ON M5A 2A5 (416) 963- 5979

Synopsis: Leo, a recovering alcoholic, feels paralyzed by depression. Neither his wife nor his boss can find a way to lift his spirits. Mary suffers from panic attacks and uses alcohol and tranquilizers to quell her symptoms, while her worried family tries to cope. The video dramatizes their symptoms and follows both through diagnosis and treatment. Leo is prescribed antidepressants (which don't violate his sobriety, his psychiatrist says), and psychotherapy helps him resolve long-standing feelings of grief and anger toward his father. Following detoxification, Mary follows a comprehensive program of therapy, relaxation, and other coping skills.

Evaluation: Good. The subject of dual disorders is emerging as a key issue in the health field. Professionals in the mental health field need to know more about drug use and its effects, and addictions professionals must learn more about some of the mood and personality disorders that may coexist with—or even prompt—alcohol or drug abuse. This video covers some of the basics, but seems geared more to the mental health professional than the addictions specialist. Viewers may find the attitudes of Mary's husband and therapist rather paternalistic.

Group therapy: The stages of group growth (Video No. 2019, 1988, 80 minutes, $250)
Rating: none given (6-point scale)
Audience: health professionals
Producer: Addiction Research Foundation, 33 Russell Street, Toronto, ON M5R 2S1 (416) 595- 6056/1-800-661-6111
Distributor: Same

Synopsis: This two-part program follows an open-ended counseling group through a four-month period. It depicts a group of drug- and alcohol-dependent individuals (a pressman, a nurse, a school teacher, a manager, an unemployed man, a school dropout). They learn to deal with their pain, conflicts, disappointments and their growth as individuals and as a group. They struggle with relapse, sexuality, inadequacy, loneliness, peer pressure, abstinence, and their relationship with the group leader.

In pain and out of luck (Video No. 1012, 1991, 29 minutes, $19.95)
Rating: 4.4 (6-point scale)
Audience: health professionals; general
Producer: Drug Policy Foundation, 4801 Massachusetts Ave. N.W., #400 Washington DC 20016, (202) 895-1634
Distributor: Same

Synopsis: Strict laws against the use of narcotic drugs may help stem drug abuse. But they may also impede physicians who wish to prescribe such drugs for patients in chronic pain. Physicians who "overprescribe" narcotic drugs risk investigation or suspension, but there are no real operating definitions of "overprescription"—just "community standards."

Multidisciplinary pain clinics may offer alternatives to narcotic pain killers, but not every patient can afford such care. This video examines the case of Dr. Harvey Rose, a California physician, who spent five years (and $140,000) fighting charges of overprescribing; then it features Dr.

Rose in a debate with a law professor and two doctors who are also members of state regulatory boards.

Evaluation: Good. The participants present an informed discussion of an important topic. Among the issues debated are whether patients should have to endure a life of chronic pain simply to prevent the possibility of dependence. There is also a discussion of the terms *addiction* and *dependence* and the difference between them.

The inebriated patient (Video No. 2089, $250)
Rating: none given (6-point scale)
Audience: medical and other health professionals
Producer: Canadian Learning Co, 95 Vansittart Ave., Woodstock, Ontario, Canada N4S 6E3/1 (800) 267-2977

Synopsis: This program outlines how medical emergency staff in a hospital might respond when presented with an intoxicated patient. In the example shown here a man, found collapsed, is brought into the hospital emergency room where staff attempt to treat and assess his injuries and condition. Ways are outlined to deal with a confused client while protecting the safety of the staff.

Motivation and change (Video No. 2036, 1989, 126 minutes, $250)
Rating: none given (6-point scale)
Audience: health professionals
Producer: Addiction Research Foundation, 33 Russell Street, Toronto, ON M5R
2S1 (416) 595-6059/1 (800) 661-6111
Distributor: Same

Synopsis: Program 1 explains motivation as an interactional process that is influenced by the characteristics of the client and the therapist, as well as by environmental factors. It covers the stages people go through as they change and the primary therapeutic strategies that help them move from one stage to the next. Program 2 demonstrates some methods that the helping professional can use in dealing effectively with resistance represented by the substance abuser. Resistance is defined as any client or counselor behavior that blocks the attainment of therapeutic goals. It is viewed as a natural part of the change process, because the prospect of change typically elicits anxiety and fear. This program also demonstrates the major components of the therapeutic process applicable to clients with addiction problems. Through the use of counseling skills, the interviewer assists the client in moving from stage to stage.

Motivational interviewing (Video No. 2103, 1989, 63 minutes, $30)
Rating: 4.4 (6-point scale)
Audience: health professionals
Producer: Project Coordinator, CASAA Research Division, Department of Psychology, University of New Mexico, Albuquerque, NM 87131-1161

Synopsis: William Miller discusses and illustrates the practice of "gentle confrontation" through empathy and reflection to elicit the client's cooperation in the assembly of a program to suit their particular needs. This video is in two sections. Part One (26 minutes) demonstrates an initial interview with a client, Peter, at risk for health and family problems resulting from excess drinking. Part Two (37 minutes) represents a third session with the same client after a thorough assessment, where results of tests are reviewed, and the client "contracts" to modify behavior.

Evaluation: Good. A realistic portrayal of the sometimes tedious, but often rewarding, process of motivating a person to address a substance abuse problem. The film would make a good training tool for addictions counselors. Unfortunately, a bland production makes the counseling process seem even more tedious than it really is. As well, the film could have benefited from showing a broader range of clients, including those with less severe problems.

Planning for success—preventing relapse (Kit No. 2043K, 1987, $99)
Rating: none given (6-point scale)
Audience: counselors and trainers, treatment professionals, and those in treatment
Producer: AADA Production and Distribution, 2000-10909 Jasper Ave., Edmonton, AB T5J 3M9 (403) 427-7319

Synopsis: Prepared by the Alberta Alcohol and Drug Abuse Commission, this kit provides counselors with a strategy for helping clients maintain abstinence. It uses education and skill development to prepare clients to: handle high-risk situations, reduce stress and develop a balanced lifestyle. The contents of this kit should be incorporated into the treatment process currently being used. Included in the kit is information for counselor reference and training, a pamphlet, overhead material, and client lectures.

Relapse prevention (Video No. 2025, 1992, 55 minutes, US $295.00
Rating: none given (6-point scale)
Audience: health professionals
Producer: Gerald T. Rogers, 5215 Old Orchard Rd., Suite 990, Skokie, IL 60077

Synopsis: Designed for the use of professional counselors dealing with clients who have relapsed. The what and why of relapse is explored: Interview demonstrations show how to help the client reduce the likelihood of relapse, identify warning signs, anticipate risk factors, achieve lifestyle balance, and to interrupt relapse when it occurs. Clients are encouraged to take action, change attitudes, develop structure, set goals, and participate in normal activities. Throughout the video, main points are highlighted, and the relapse process is reviewed at the conclusion.

Youth and drugs (Kit No. 2063K, $175.00
Rating: none given (6-point scale)
Audience: health, education and social service practitioners, police and corrections officers, youth workers, and anyone in routine contact with youth who may be or are beginning to experiment with drugs.
Producer: Addiction Research Foundation, 33 Russell Street, Toronto, ON M5R 2S1 (416) 595-6059/ 1 (800) 661-6111
Distributor: Same

Synopsis: The response to drug use has generally been in two areas: primary drug education and prevention programs, and tertiary treatment programs for those seriously involved with drugs. A third avenue of response, secondary prevention, has been largely neglected. This kit proposes to fill this gap by providing an in-depth course of professional development in secondary prevention. It will enable users of this kit to respond more effectively to young people who are developing problems in which drugs or alcohol play a part. The kit consists of a learner's manual in five units; six cases studies (on VHS); and a background book of reading. Prepared by Health and Welfare Canada and the ARF.

Web Sites

General Health

Resources for School Health Educators
http://www.indiana.edu/~aphs/hlthk-12..html

CDC Prevention Guidelines Database
http://wonder.cdc.gov/wonder/prevguid/prevguid.htm

Developing Educational Standards
http://putwest.boces.org/standards.html

Adolescent Health On-line
http://www.ama-assn.org/adolhlth/adolhlth.htm

See particularly the Adolescent Health Links at

<*http://www.ama-assn.org/adolhlth/gapslink/gapslnk2.htm#ADOL*>

PE Central
http://infoserver.etl.vt.edu/~/PE.Central/PEC2.html

Kathy Schrock's Guide for Educators
http://www.capecod.net/Wixon/health/fitness.htm

Health Education Forum
http://libertynet.org/~lion/forum-health.html

Education World—Subjects: Physical Education
http://www.education-world.com/db/phys-gen.shtml

The Life Education Network
http://www.lec.org/

American Cancer Society
http://www.cancer.org

Physical Activity and Health: A Report of the Surgeon General
http://www.cdc.gov/nccdphp/sgr/sgr.htm

American Social Health Association
http://sunsite.unc.edu/ASHA/

Adolescence Directory On Line (ADOL)
http://education.indiana.edu/cas/adol/adol.html

AIDS NOW! For Teens
http://www.itec.sfsu.edu/aids/aids.html

National Health & Education Consortium (NHEC)
http://www.nhec.org/

About Health
http://www.abouthealth.com/

National Parent Information Network
http://ericps.ed.uiuc.edu/npin/npinhome.html

Healthy People 2000
http://odphp.osophs.dhhs.gov/pubs/hp2000/default.htm

Drugs/Drug Addiction

National Clearinghouse for Alcohol and Drug Information
http://www.health.org/

Drug Education Page
http://www.magic.mb.ca/~lampi/new_drugs.html

Food and Drug Administration
http://www.fda.gov

Indiana Prevention Resource Center
http://www.drugs.indiana.edu/

National Institute on Drug Abuse
http://www.nida.nih.gov

Web of Addictions
http://www.well.com/user/woa

Join Together Online
www.jointogether.org

Mothers Against Drunk Driving
www.gran-net.com/madd/madd.htm

National Families in Action
www.niaaa.nih.gov/

Substance Abuse and Mental Health Services Administration
www.samhsa.gov

Tobacco/Smoking Cessation

American Lung Association
http://www.lungusa.org/

Master Anti-Smoking Page
http://www.autonomy.com/smoke.htm

Smoking and Health: A Physician Responsibility
http://www.chestnut.org/smoking.html

Tobacco BBS
http://www.tobacco.org/

Agency for Health Care Policy and Research
www.ahcpr.gov

American Dental Association Online
www.ada.org

American Cancer Society
www.cancer.org

American Heart Association
www.amhrt.org

CDC Office on Smoking and Health,
Tobacco Information & Prevention Sourcepage
www.cdc.gov/nccdphp/osh/tobacco.htm

Food and Drug Administration
www.fda.gov

Robert Wood Johnson Foundation
www.rwjf.org/

SAMHSA National Clearinghouse for
Alcohol and Drug Information
www.health.org

Substance Abuse and Mental Health Services
Administration
www.samhsa.gov

Food and Drug Safety

American Academy of Family Physicians
www.aafp.org

Administration on Aging
www.aoa.dhhs.gov/

FDA Center for Drug Evaluation and Research
www.fda.gov/cder/

FDA Center for Food Safety and Applied Nutrition
vm.cfsan.fda.gov/list.html

Food and Drug Administration
www.fda.gov

Institute of Medicine, Food and Nutrition Board
www2.nas.edu/Fnb/2102.html

NIH National Institute on Aging
www.nih.gov/nia/

USDA Food Safety and Inspection Service
www.usda.gov/agency/fsis/homepage.htm

Surveillance and Data Systems

Agency for Health Care Policy and Research Data and
Methods
www.ahcpr.gov:80/data

CDC National Center for Health Statistics
www.cdc.gov/nchswww/nchshome.htm

CDC Scientific, Surveillance, and Health Statistics, and
Laboratory Information
www.cdc.gov/scientific.htm

CDC WONDER
wonder.cdc.gov

Health Care Financing Administration,
1996 Statistics at a Glance
www.hcfa.gov/stats/stathili.htm

General Sites

American Medical Association
http://www.ama-assn.org

MedicineNet
http://www.medicinenet.com

Medscape
http://www.medscape.com

Oncolink
http://www.oncolink.upenn.edu

ParentsPlace.com
http://www.parentsplace.com

Thrive@ pathfinder
http://pathfinder.com/thrive

Links Only

Hardin Meta Directory of Internet Health Sources
http://www.arcade.uiowa.edu/hardin-www/md.html

Medical Matrix
ttp://www.5lackinc.com/matrix

Chapter Fourteen

Infectious and Noninfectious Conditions

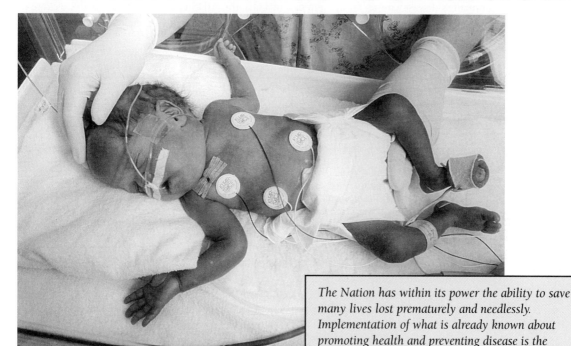

> The Nation has within its power the ability to save many lives lost prematurely and needlessly. Implementation of what is already known about promoting health and preventing disease is the central challenge.
>
> —Healthy People 2000

Valued Outcomes

After reading this chapter, you should be able to

- ○ describe the disease agents for infectious and noninfectious conditions
- ○ describe the typical stages through which a disease progresses
- ○ describe how the body is protected from disease
- ○ discuss the major childhood communicable diseases
- ○ discuss the human immunodeficiency virus (HIV)
- ○ discuss the types of cardiovascular disease and cancer
- ○ identify the risk factors associated with the major noninfectious diseases
- ○ discuss the recent trends in the diagnosis and treatment of diseases

Many conditions affect the quality of life. Over the past centuries, the types of diseases that have killed and debilitated humanity have changed. At one time, the infectious diseases were the big killers, but now the chronic diseases are the leading causes of death. Some say that the infectious diseases will again become our biggest enemy, in the form of the AIDS epidemic.

Communicable Diseases

At various times throughout history, such communicable diseases as the plague, smallpox, syphilis, and polio have been common throughout the world. Occasionally a disease such as the Legionnaire's disease causes an epidemic. Currently the AIDS epidemic threatens the welfare of our citizens. The common cold and influenza, and the persistence of the many childhood diseases, also are constant problems. (See Table 14.1.)

Table 14.1
The Pathogens

Type	Characteristics	Examples of Disease Caused
Viruses	The smallest pathogens. Composed of nucleic acid and protein. Made up of DNA or RNA but not both. Known as *obligate intracellular parasites* because they must live on living host. Penetrate cells and use cells' nucleic acid to replicate viruses. May burst out of cell, destroying it, or the cell degenerates and viruses are released as cell dies.	Warts; hepatitis A, B, C, D, E; measles; polio; mumps; oral and genital herpes
Bacteria	Single-cell micro-organisms, abundant in our environment, but very few are pathogenic to humans. Three common forms: rod-shaped or bacilli, round or cocci, and spiral or spirilla. Cause harm by releasing toxins (poisins), and need not invade cells to cause disease.	Tuberculosis, strep throat, tetanus, gonorrhea, Legionnaire's disease
Rickettsias	Now considered to be small bacteria. Resemble both viruses and bacteria. Like viruses, they are intracellular parasites. Transported by insects and other arthropod vectors.	Rocky Mountain spotted fever, typhus, Q fever
Fungi	Single-celled or multicelled plantlike organisms. Release enzymes that digest cells. Seek a favorable climate for reproduction on food or anywhere there is high humidity, warmth, and oxygen supply.	Candidiasis, ringworm
Protozoa	Single-celled microscopic parasitic animals. Release toxin and ezymes that destroy cells or interface with their functions.	Trichomoniasis, malaria, Amebic dysentery, African sleeping sickness
Metazoa	Multicellular parasitic animals. Vary in size from relatively small (pinworms) to a length of several feet, may lodge in various parts of the body and block the digestive tract, blood, and lymph vessels.	Pinworms, tapeworms, trichinosis

The Stages of Diseases

When a pathogen invades a human host, the reaction to this invasion proceeds through several broad phases. Figure 14.1 illustrates these typical stages. They include the incubation, prodromal, clinical, convalescence, and recovery stages. The **incubation stage** is the time between initial infection and the appearance of symptoms. The incubation period can be as short as a few hours (for the common cold) to years (as in the case of AIDS). The **prodromal stage** is the short period of time in which the body begins to react to the pathogens. Fever, headache, nasal discharge, and irritability are common. The actual characteristics of the disease are not yet apparent, and diagnosis may be difficult. The disease is usually highly communicable during this period. The **clinical stage** is the time when the disease is at its worst. The characteristics of the disease are readily identified. The **recovery stage** is the time in which recovery begins. The disease may still be communicable. The host may relapse, recover with immunity to the disease, recover but not have immunity, or recover from the disease but be a source (carrier) for the disease.

Figure 14.1
Typical Periods of Illness

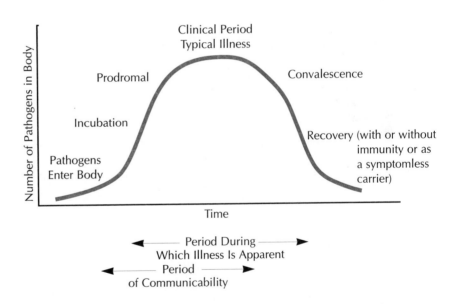

Protection against Diseases

For an infectious disease to invade a human host, some change must take place in either the host or the environment. The mere presence of a pathogen does not necessarily lead to infection; the host must be susceptible to the disease. Factors such as age, sex, stress, nutrition, and genetic makeup influence susceptibility. For a pathogen to gain entry to a human host, it must overcome several very effective barriers. These barriers are diagrammed in Figure 14.2.

Figure 14.2

The Body's Defenses against Disease

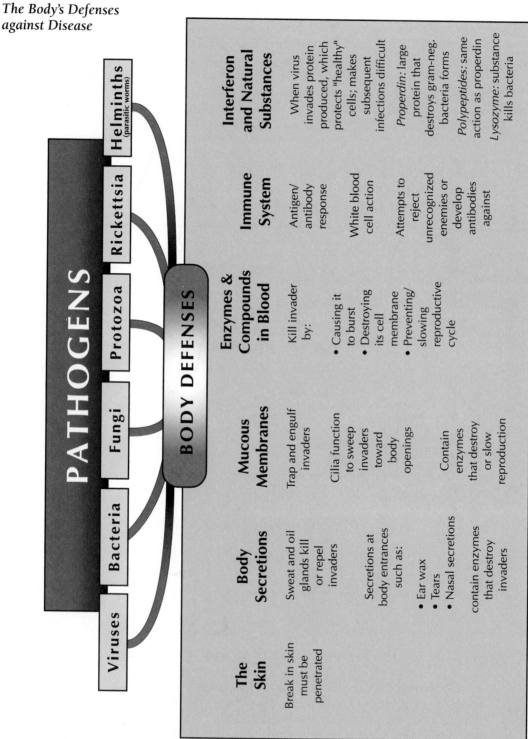

PATHOGENS

Viruses | Bacteria | Fungi | Protozoa | Rickettsia | Helminths (parasitic worms)

BODY DEFENSES

The Skin

Break in skin must be penetrated

Body Secretions

Sweat and oil glands kill or repel invaders

Secretions at body entrances such as:
- Ear wax
- Tears
- Nasal secretions

contain enzymes that destroy invaders

Mucous Membranes

Trap and engulf invaders

Cilia function to sweep invaders toward body openings

Contain enzymes that destroy or slow reproduction

Enzymes & Compounds in Blood

Kill invader by:
- Causing it to burst
- Destroying its cell membrane
- Preventing/ slowing reproductive cycle

Immune System

Antigen/ antibody response

White blood cell action

Attempts to reject unrecognized enemies or develop antibodies against

Interferon and Natural Substances

When virus invades protein produced, which protects "healthy" cells; makes subsequent infections difficult

Properdin: large protein that destroys gram-neg. bacteria forms

Polypeptides: same action as properdin

Lysozyme: substance kills bacteria

The Immune System

If the defenses listed in Figure 14.2 do not prevent development of a disease, the host body turns to another powerful line of defense. *Immunity* is the state of being protected against diseases or through the activities of the immune system. When the host is invaded by a pathogen, the immune system swings into action to destroy the infectious agent. Anything that invades the body and causes the immune system to react is called an *antigen* (foreign body). The body develops *antibodies* that destroy or lessen the effects of the invading antigen. Each type of antibody is specific for each type of antigen. For example, antibodies for measles have no effect on the common cold antigen.

The immune system works in several ways to protect against diseases and infections. The first is through the action of *phagocytosis*, which is the ingestion and destruction of pathogens by several different types of white blood cells (Thibodeau and Patton 1993). *Humoral immunity* is the protection provided by antibodies derived from B-lymphocytes. In *cellular immunity* T-lymphocytes are activated and attack microbes or abnormal cells such as viral or tumor cells. Figure 14.3 illustrates these three mechanisms.

Figure 14.3

Actions and Responses of the Immune System

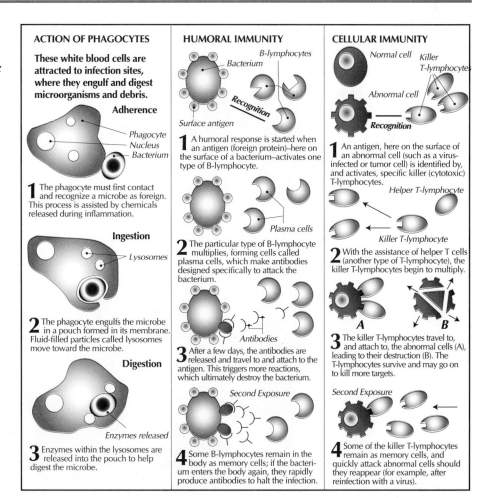

Lymphocytes are the type of white blood cells most responsible for the preceding actions. Two forms of lymphocytes are **T-lymphocytes** and **B-lymphocytes.** T-lymphocytes circulate through lymphatic tissue and the bloodstream, neutralizing antigens. **T-helpers** or **T-suppressor** cells either increase or release the response of other lymphocytes. B-lymphocytes produce antibodies. When stimulated by an antigen, these cells produce antibodies that destroy the antigens.

Immunity can be developed through having a disease **(natural immunity)** or through **artificial immunity.** Artificial immunity is acquired by vaccination with killed, attenuated (weakened) organisms, or **toxins** (poisons). Antibodies for a particular antigen can be injected that will provide short-term protection against a disease.

Selected Infectious Diseases

Diseases commonly found in the school include the common cold, influenza, strep throat, and the childhood diseases of chicken pox, mumps, and rubella (German measles). To a lesser extent,

Artificial immunity is acquired by vaccination.

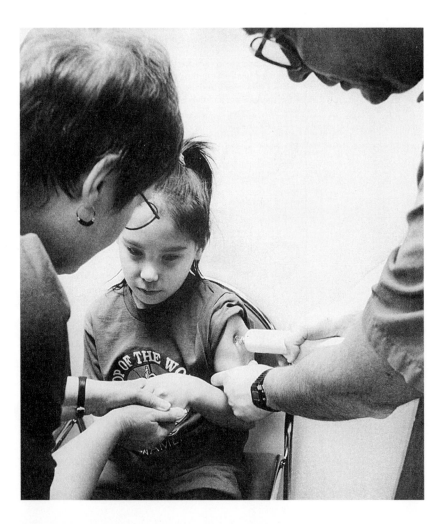

Health Highlight

Recommended Childhood Immunization Schedule—1995

Vaccine	Birth	2 Month	4	6	12	15 Months	18 Months	4-6 Years	11-12 Years	14-16 Years
Hepatitis B	HB - 1									
		HB - 2		HB - 3						
Diphtheria Tetanus & pertussis (DTP)		DTP	DTP	DTP		DTP		DTP	DT	
Haemophilus influezae type b (Hb)		Hb	Hb	Hb		Hb				
Poliovirus Oral Polio Vaccine (OPV)		OPV	OPV			OPV		OPV		
Measles, Mumps, Rubella (MMR)						MMR			MMR	

Source: Benenson, A. S. ed. *Control of communicable disease manual.* 1995. 16th ed. Washington, DC: American Public Health Association.

diseases such as infectious mononucleosis, hepatitis, and HIV are now affecting the classroom. In the school situation, childhood diseases constitute the greatest problem. Children face more days of restricted activity and school absenteeism because of these diseases. (See Table 14.1.)

Common Childhood Diseases

chicken pox

diptheria

German measles (rubella)

influenza

measles (rubeola)

meningitis

mumps (parotitis)

polio

rheumatic fever

scarlet fever

smallpox (variola)

strep throat

tuberculosis

whooping cough (pertussis)

The Common Cold

The cold is the most common of all the infectious diseases found in the school situation. A cold alone is not considered serious, but secondary infections resulting from improper care can be a problem.

There are more than 110 different viruses or rhinoviruses that can cause the common cold. Symptoms usually develop within twenty-four hours after exposure and include teary eyes, obstructed breathing, and a runny nose. When a fever is present, it indicates a secondary infection. Once a cold develops, it will run its course in seven to fourteen days.

There is no cure for a cold; antibiotics are of no benefit. Once a cold has developed, bed rest, good nutrition, and plenty of fluids are the best medicines. Over-the-counter drugs may mask symptoms, but they will not cure a cold. A cold is most contagious in the first twenty-four hours.

Strep Throat

Strep throat is commonly found in the school setting. The causative agent is the streptococcus bacterium. The infection is passed primarily through sneezing, coughing, or the use of soiled objects, such as handkerchiefs, that reach the mouth. Incubation time for strep throat is three to five days. Symptoms may include sore throat, fever, nausea, and vomiting. In some cases, people may develop a rash on the neck and chest area. Treatment is through the use of antibiotics. Students should be excluded from school until the fever and sore throat are gone for twenty-four to forty-eight hours.

Influenza

Influenza, or "flu," is a commonly experienced virus. Three forms of the virus are currently isolated, with a multitude of strains within each variety. Forms of the virus include "A" (the most pathenogenic), strain "B," and then "C." Short-term immunity may be acquired from any particular form, but this does not transfer to a different variety. Fortunately, the flu is not extremely hazardous to normally healthy people. However, death does result more frequently in adults over sixty-five, children under five, and people experiencing chronic diseases.

The symptoms of influenza include aches and pains, nausea, diarrhea, fever, and coldlike ailments. The best treatment for flu is ample bed rest, ingesting plenty of fluids, eating nutritious foods, and taking medicine, if prescribed. Although obvious symptoms last only a few days, a feeling of weakness may persist for some time, so extra rest may be needed. It is important to take extra care following the flu, so that complications do not develop. Because influenza is caused by a virus, Reyes syndrome can develop as a secondary disease. Children should not be given aspirin to relieve discomfort.

Infectious Mononucleosis

Infectious mononucleosis is thought to be initiated by the Epstein-Barr virus and is transmitted through saliva, hence its more common name, the "kissing disease." In reality, mononucleosis does not seem to be highly contagious. Initial symptoms may include moderate fever, discomfort, lack of appetite, fatigue, headache, and sore throat. Lymph nodes usually become enlarged, as does the spleen about one-third of the time. Occasionally mild liver damage may occur, leading to jaundice for a few days. Diagnosis is made using a blood test. A positive test indicates extremely high levels of white blood cells, as well as mononuclear cells. Treatment consists of possibly

Health Highlight

The Hepatitis B Occupational Risk Worksheet

Howard L. Taras

The U.S. Department of Labor's Occupational Safety and Health Administration (OSHA) protects workers from the dangers of blood-borne pathogens by mandating infection control guidelines in the workplace. In addition to educational responsibilities, school districts must make hepatitis B vaccinations available at no cost to all employees who have occupational exposure to blood and other secretions. In some school districts, employee job titles belie the fact that their work environment may place them at risk for Hepatitis B. Teachers and secretaries who regularly perform first aid, and building custodians who handle potentially infectious sharp objects are examples. Providing individualized counseling to each employee with increased risk for hepatitis B creates an administrative burden for school districts. The San Diego (California) Unified School District

designed a worksheet to assist employees with their own risk assessment (Figure 1). The worksheet does not replace comprehensive education on the communicability of blood-borne pathogens and its prevention. Employees should receive the worksheet after education has been received. The worksheet should not prevent individual employees from discussing their worksite exposure with a health professional. Qualitative terms such as "rarely" and "a few times" were used deliberately to encourage employees to speak to health professionals if they are uncertain about their relative risk.

Using the worksheet, the SDUSD employees assessed themselves into one of three broad categories of risk. Concomitantly, this practice relieved school health staff from answering the same questions from individual employees whose indications for the vaccine are either clearly present or absent.

worksheet on following page

prolonged bed rest, sound nutrition, and medicine for secondary problems, as indicated. For two to three months after recovery, the person may feel depressed, lack energy, and feel sleepy during the day. Symptoms may exist up to a year after infection.

Hepatitis

Five types of hepatitis have currently been isolated. Hepatitis A is often the result of poor sanitary conditions. Hepatitis A is a common infection in the United States, with almost half the adult population carrying antibodies against the virus. A gamma globulin provides protection against the virus if administered within ten days of exposure (Crowley 1992). Hepatitis B is currently transmitted primarily by addicts sharing contaminated needles, and through body secretions such as sweat, breast milk, and semen. Hepatitis B is more serious than hepatitis A, with a higher potential for liver damage. Hepatitis C resembles both A and B but is classified as neither. The majority of hepatitis occuring after blood transfusion is hepatitis C. There is a growing concern about sexual transmission of hepatitis C. Hepatitis D can only be contracted by a person suffering from hepatitis B. The C virus seems to intersect with hepatitis B to create a more severe form of the disease. It is most often spread among intravenous drug users. Hepatitis E also has been identified and is transmitted from feces contamination.

Health Highlight

Hepatitis B Occupational Risk Worksheet:
Guidelines for School Employees

At my worksite, I . . .

(Circle Frequency)

1. . . .am bitten by a student	Practically never	It occurs, but rarely	A few times a year	Regularly: more than 6–12 times a year
2. . . .am scratched by a student, drawing blood	Practically never	It occurs, but rarely	A few times a year	Regularly: more than 6–12 times a year
3. . . .clean up student's blood or body fluids containing blood (nose bloods, soiled tampons, saliva with blood, etc.)	Practically never	It occurs, but rarely	A few times a year	Regularly: more than 6–12 times a year
4. . . .clean and dress oozing or bloody wounds	Practically never	It occurs, but rarely	A few times a year	Regularly: more than 6–12 times a year
5. . . .perform medical procedures (such as draw blood, directly contact insertion sites of tracheal and gastric tubes)	Practically never	It occurs, but rarely	A few times a year	Regularly: more than 6–12 times a year
6. . . .handle sharp objects that are blood contaminated (includes maintenance workers exposed to such objects through torn garbage bags)	Practically never	It occurs, but rarely	A few times a year	Regularly: more than 6–12 times a year

Dr. Taras's Recommendations:
If exposure to blood occurs rarely, at most, your occupation is likely not placing you at increased risk. Reach a health professional after each exposure incident.

Dr. Taras's Recommendations:
If all exposure incidents together occur no more frequently than this, you are not at a significantly increased risk for Hepatitis B. Vaccine should be considered most seriously by those who circled more than three of these, by those with dry, cracked hands, and those who frequently have open cuts. Discuss your situation with a health professional.

Dr. Taras's Recommendations:
If you circled one or more on this column, you should strongly consider receiving the hepatitis B vaccine series. Discuss your eligibility with a health professional.

Source: Taras, H. L. 1994, March. The hepatitis B occupational risk worksheet. *Journal of school health* 64(3). Used with permission.

Treatment of any form of hepatitis is somewhat limited, and relapses may occur. Bed rest and inactivity may be necessary for months. Vaccinations are available against hepatitis A and B.

Human Immunodeficiency Virus (HIV)
and Acquired Immunodeficiency Syndrome (AIDS)

The human immunodeficiency virus (HIV) can lead to a complex array of diseases resulting in acquired immunodeficiency syndrome (AIDS). The Centers for Disease Control (CDC) list twenty-seven clinical conditions to be used in diagnosing AIDS, along with an HIV-positive seroconversion and a T-cell count of below 200 (CDC 1993). Table 14.2 provides the conditions used in diagnosing AIDS.

Although there is still no confirmed cure for HIV, several promising studies have produced results that may key the ultimate cure. A drug called AZT remains the benchmark of drugs used in treatment. However, researchers now have available a series of drugs that provide a powerful "cocktail" of antiviral drugs. This combination consists of drugs called *protease inhibitors*, AZT—the original antiviral drug used in treatment, and another powerful drug called 3TC, which is a chemical cousin of AZT. In a number of cases, this combination of drugs seemed to have forced the disease into remission. Questions exist concerning the possible long-term toxic effects, but for the present this antiviral cocktail is prolonging the lives of thousands of desperately ill people for several months and may continue to do so for years. Studies are now being conducted on HIV-positive individuals who are in the early stages of their infection, to determine if the disease can be eradicated (Cray and Park 1996, 65).

AIDS remains a devastating disease. It took 8 1/2 years for the first 100,000 cases of AIDS to be reported. In only 2 1/2 years the second 100,000 cases were reported. More than 50 percent of those cases reported since 1981 have since died. A study reported in 1995 AIDS cases have increased more rapidly among younger individuals who were born in 1960 or later, than among older Americans. In 1993 AIDS became the leading cause of death for Americans between the ages of twenty-five and forty-four. From 1993 to 1994, AIDS deaths among ages twenty-five to forty-four increased from 28,100 to 30,300 (CDC 1996). The best protection young people have is education, and practicing safer sex if they become sexually active. Figure 14.4 provides information on preventing the spread of HIV. Figure 14.5 provides sources of information for the nature of HIV, treatment, and prevention.

Individuals infected with HIV may experience a variety of symptoms or may appear to be quite healthy. However, even people with no obvious symptoms can transmit HIV to others. The indicators of possible HIV infection include conditions such as persistent diarrhea, dry cough, and shortness of breath; fatigue; skin rash; swollen lymph glands (neck, armpits, groin); candidiasis, unexplained fever or chills; night sweats (over several weeks); and unexplained weight loss of 10 percent of body weight in less than two months. Women may experience the same symptoms as well as abnormal Pap smears, persistent vaginal candidiasis, and abdominal cramping as a result of pelvic inflammatory disease (PID). These infections are a result of HIV infection and are caused by immunodeficiency, but they are not yet considered AIDS.

It was previously thought that HIV did little in the body immediately after infection and simply stayed within a few immune system T-cells for seven to ten years. It is now known that the real battle starts immediately within the lymph nodes, where day after day, year after year the body is in mortal combat battling the virus to a standstill before finally exhausting its immune response reserves (Cray and Park 1996, 64).

Table 14.2

Conditions Used in Diagnosing AIDS

1. **Opportunistic Infections (Infections that take advantage of a weakened immune system)**
   - *Pneumocystis carinii pneumonia* (PCP)—a type of lung disease caused by a protozoan fungus, which is usually not harmful to humans.
   - Tuberculosis—either *Mycobacterium aviumintracellulare* (MAI) or *Mycobacterium tuberculosis* (TB); MAI is most common among AIDS patients
   - Bacterial pneumonia—caused by several common bacteria
   - Toxoplasmosis—disease of the brain and central nervous system

2. **Cancers**
   - Kaposi's sarcoma—a cancer that causes red or purple blotches on the skin
   - Lymphomas—cancers of the lymphatic system
   - Invasive cervical cancer—more common in women who are HIV positive

3. **Other Conditions**
   - Wasting syndrome—involves persistent diarrhea, severe weight loss, and weakness
   - AIDS dementia—impairment of mental functions, mood changes, impaired movement as a result of HIV infection of the brain

4. **Other Infections**
   - Candidiasis (also called *thrush*)—a fungal infection that affects the vagina, mouth, throat, and lungs
   - Herpes—a common viral STD described later in this chapter
   - Cytomegalovirus—a virus that, in AIDS patients, can lead to brain infection, infection of the retina, pneumonia, or hepatitis

---

Currently ten subtypes of HIV are found around the world (Cray and Park 1996, 66) with the possibility of new subtypes mutating. HIV-1 is the type found in the vast majority of infected individuals in the United States. Two tests are currently being used to detect HIV. The ELISA is the antibody test initially used. If the ELISA results indicate that the patient has HIV, another test—the Western blot technique—is administered for confirmation. Since the ELISA is an antibodies test and it may take two to thirty-six months for antibodies to develop there is a possibility of a false negative test for HIV antibodies. Usually the Western blot shows clearly either HIV positive or negative. If there is an inconclusive Western blot test, a person should be retested in six months. Anyone who tests positive for HIV can transmit the virus. In addition to the above-mentioned test, a home-testing kit for HIV is now available. However, any results of home testing should be confirmed by a proper medical authority.

Primary transmission of HIV is through sexual contact. Secondary transmission occurs among intravenous drug users. Screening techniques have reduced the chances of receiving the HIV virus in blood transfusions to approximately one in one million. What has become a significant problem is the heterosexual transmission of the HIV virus. The World Health Organization has predicted that by the year 2000 heterosexual transmission will be the primary means of infection (Mann 1989). In fact, the AIDS epidemic that is possible through heterosexual transmission of HIV is staggering. Estimates are that a million Americans are already infected with HIV; thus, every sex partner in this group is at risk. Considering that the incubation period can be as long as ten years and that the HIV-infected person is unaware of the disease, transmission will grow

Figure 14.4

Preventing the Spread
of AIDS

Recommendations to reduce the possibility of becoming infected Include the following:

○ Practice abstinence or mutual monogamy.

○ Always use protection (that is, latex condoms and spermicide, such as nonoxynol-9) if having sex with multiple partners or with persons who have multiple partners.

○ Do not have unprotected sex with individuals with AIDS, those who engage in high-risk behavior, or those who have had a positive test for the AIDS virus.

○ Avold sexual activities that might cut or tear the rectum, vagina, or penis, such as anal intercourse.

○ Do not have sex with prostitutes.

○ Do not use IV drugs or share needles. Refrain from sex with IV drug users.

Figure 14.5

Information on AIDS
and HIV

CDC National AIDS Hotline
(800) 342-2437
Information on HIV and AIDS, free information available in several languages.

CDC National AIDS Clearinghouse
(800) 458-5231
Information on services and education services. Copies of Public Health Service publications available.

Lina National de SIDA (Spanish)
(800) 344-7432
24-hour hotline that provides information and referrals for HIV and AIDS. Local heath departments also have valuable information concerning HIV and AIDS.

geometrically. Another estimate that indicates the magnitude of the problem is that up to 70 percent of all HIV infections will result from heterosexual intercourse by the year 2000 (Jackson 1992, 40).

HIV infection is not contracted through contact with food, eating utensils, clothing, furniture, swimming pools, or insects. Such contact as shaking hands, coughing, sneezing or even living with an HIV-positive person will not transmit the disease. HIV has been found in tears, saliva, and urine, but transmission through contact with these substances has not been found to be directly implicated (Peterman 1986).

Chronic and Noninfectious Disease

Americans are commonly afflicted by chronic and noninfectious diseases. Diseases of this type are not "caught" but are developed over time, often are progressive in effect, and may be due to

Health Highlight

Natural History of Congenital HIV Infection

One major misperception regarding HIV infection and AIDS in children suggests these children are doomed to brief lives of nothing but pain, suffering, and early death. What actually happens to children born infected with the AIDS virus? How long do they survive? What is the nature of that survival?

The course of the disease is extraordinarily variable, as illustrated by two examples of real children followed in the pediatric AIDS Program. An infant girl, born to a mother with known HIV disease, never reached a development level beyond that of a two- to three-month-old infant. She could smile responsively, react to noises, and lift her head up, but never much more than that. Her head stopped growing, and she had to be fed with a gastrostomy tube. After two episodes of pneumonia, she developed heart failure and kidney failure and died at age fifteen months. A twelve-year-old boy was admitted to the hospital with abdominal pain and enlarged lymph nodes. His adoptive parents reported both parents had died of AIDS. His hospital record indicated that during his early years he had recurrent serious bacterial infections, successfully treated—a clinical syndrome now recognized as classic for pediatric HIV disease—and immune abnormalities that are now acknowledged as common and specific for HIV infection in children. But that was before 1980, and AIDS had not yet been described in anyone. At age twelve he was found to have HIV infection. At age fifteen he is now normally grown, a good student on the high school basketball team. He is sexually mature and sexually active. His situation is unusual, but hardly unique, and there will be many more like him.

The extremes include children with severe, early onset, rapidly lethal HIV disease, as well as those infected at birth who survive into elementary and high school years and possibly beyond. What is the "average experience," if such an experience exists? Large cohort studies, which follow a group of infected children from birth and document their survival and experience, can begin to provide an answer. Relatively few such studies exist, but those that do can offer some insight. The first study by Scott et al. reported on 172 children followed in their program at Jackson Memorial Hospital, Miami, FL, born through the beginning of 1988. The survival curve from that report showed an initial death rate the first two years of 25,910, after which occurred a relatively constant and lower death rate. Statistically, these data suggest that median survival in this cohort would be about six and one-half years. One-half the children would die before six and one-half years and one-half the children would survive beyond six and one-half years.

The largest cohort reported to date involved a study from Italy, where a national register collects data on HIV infection in children, reported in *Lancet* in May 1992. These are data from 573 children infected at birth. About 75 percent of these children showed some signs of HIV infection by the first birthday, and 90 percent by age two: not necessarily severe disease, but some sign of disease. Ten percent of two-year-olds had no clinical evidence of HIV infection, although they were infected. Mortality in the first year of life in the cohort was 9 percent. After that, the mortality rate held relatively constant at 3.5 percent per year to age seven. Seventy percent of the group is still alive at age six, and one-half the children statistically are expected to live beyond age eight.

The experience at Boston City Hospital includes current data on 56 infected children in the program. Their survival resembles that of other studies.

Most of the survival data presented in these other studies were collected without specific treatment being administered, as most preceded the use of antiretroviral drugs in children. We do not know to what extent the treatment being used today and planned for tomorrow actually will affect survival of children. Are we prolonging life with our treat-

Health Highlight–cont'd

ment? We assume some success, but data do not yet demonstrate that success.

All these data share a common problem. Because the cohorts form at different ages, most children cluster somewhere in the middle age ranges. A steep dropoff occurs at first, representing severe early disease, which we have not been very successful in treating. Most of the other children fall in a middle group. Some have severe disease but are still making it and are still alive, with that information hidden in the curve. A second mode of the bimodal distribution includes children in our program without severe early disease who are scattered across a wide range. As yet, no deaths have occurred in children who made it to three years, but we expect a death will occur. Most children will survive into the school years, and many are in school now.

What clinical syndromes and symptoms are experienced by children who make it to the school years? One relatively small study reported on school-age children in Africa, from ages five to twelve.

The chronic lung disease of pediatric AIDS—lymphoid interstitial pneumonitis—is seen in about 25 percent of the children. This disorder can be mildly symptomatic, or it can be more severe. It can resemble asthma and may respond to medications used to treat asthma. Enlargement of liver and spleen is seen in about 25 percent. Some children had pulmonary tuberculosis, as seen in many adults with HIV infection, more in New York City than in Boston. Retinal or eye dis-

ease occurs in a minority. Chronic ear infections and herpes zoster also are seen, as they are among the children we follow.

Pulmonary tuberculosis is the one complicating infection of concern for children in classrooms. Most infections that children with HIV disease contract tend to fall into two categories. The first category includes infections with common pathogens, which are disease-causing microorganisms that could produce disease in any child, such as *pneumococcus* or *Hemophilus influenza*. These organisms exist in the environment. If children have an ear infection, they may well be harboring one of these microbes in the ear. The child with HIV disease who has such an infection is no more a threat to other children in school than would be any other child with an ear infection. The second category is opportunistic infections, those microbes we all walk around with. Most of us have had, and may now be harboring, *Pneumocystis carinii* in our throats, yet we will not pass them to a healthy person with a normal immune system and make them ill. An opportunistic infection only has an adverse impact on individuals with compromised immunity.

In conclusion, none of these disorders represent a threat to children without HIV infection in the classroom—with the exception of pulmonary tuberculosis, which should be carefully monitored. Some communities face a problem with it, but as a rule it is less of a problem in children with HIV disease than it is in adults with HIV disease

References

G. B., Scott, C. Hutto, R. W. Makuch et al. 1989. Survival in children with perinatally acquired human immunodeficiency virus type I infection. *New England Journal of Medicine* 321: 1791.

P.A. Touo, M. Martino, C. Gabiano, et al. 1992. Prognostic factors and survival in children with perinatal HIV-1 infection. *Lancet* 336:221.

Source: A. Meyers. 1994. Natural history of congenital HIV infection. *Journal of school health* 64(1): 9–10. Used with permission.

Health Highlight

Support for Children with HIV Infection in School: Best Practices Guidelines

I. Preparation of the School Setting

1. An **advisory committee on HIV-related issues** shall be established for the school district and commissioned by the Superintendent. Membership shall be comprised of health professionals (community physicians, school nurses, and other child and adolescent health workers), parents, teachers, students, persons with HIV infection, attorneys, advocates, and persons representing diversity in the community. At regular meetings, matters shall be discussed concerning HIV that relate to administrative practices, legal and policy questions, educational programs, universal infection control standards, and student welfare. Consultants shall be used as appropriate.

2. The school district shall adopt **policy statements of relevance to students with HIV infection,** in collaboration with the advisory committee. These shall conform with state and federal laws and regulations, and draw on state-of-the-art medical and scientific information from appropriate government sources, documents from national organizations, research studies, and expert consultation. It may be helpful to use public hearings to gain input into these matters. The policy statements shall then be disseminated to all administrative levels, made available to staff, students, parents, and community leaders, and included in student and parent handbooks. They shall be reviewed at yearly intervals.

3. Staff education and inservice training concerning the issues of HIV infection, including transmission, prevention, civil rights, mental health, and death and bereavement, shall be carried out at least annually for all school personnel, including the school board. The program content shall be determined by a multidisciplinary team of appropriate individuals that shall include families of children with HIV infection and also persons with HIV infection. It shall aim to affect staff members' knowledge, feelings, attitudes, behavior, and acceptance of people who are HIV positive. For new employees, this education shall be built into the orientation program, and offered within three months of hire. Teachers responsible for instruction of students regarding HIV infection shall receive specific in-service training.

4. Universal precautions relating to bloodborne infections, as adapted for schools, shall be in effect. School clinics and nursing offices shall follow OSHA guidelines for health care facilities. It is the responsibility of the school district to ensure adequate gloves, bleach, sinks, and disposal containers. There shall be systems of quality assurance or monitoring to document compliance with universal precautions in all school settings. These matters shall be featured in the staff education program.

5. The school district shall provide **education relating to the prevention of HIV infection for students in grades K–12,** within the context of a quality comprehensive school health program. Delivered by trained teachers, health educators, and nurses, it shall be developmentally, culturally, and linguistically appropriate. It shall actively promote abstinence as the best protection, and shall also offer explicit information about the use and availability of condoms. Acknowledgment shall be given to the special needs of adolescents regarding emerging sexual orientation. An additional effect of this effort should be to enhance understanding of the needs of students, staff, and others who are infected with HIV.

II. The Enrollment Process

6. The parent, guardian, or student shall decide **whether or not to inform the school system** about HIV status or other health conditions. They may support the transfer of this information by another professional or person, including a personal physician or a case manager, but only in the context of strict informed consent procedures. It shall be recognized that disclosure of HIV status often involves revealing related facts, such as medication, parent condition, transmission, and other matters. Under no circumstances shall parents, guardians, or students be required by school personnel to obtain HIV testing or to release information about HIV test results on the student or other family members.

7. Few, if any, personnel in the school or school district shall **receive information about the HIV status** of a student. Determination of those who are to be informed is the prerogative of the parents, guardian, or student, and shall be made in the setting of consideration about special health care or social services that are needed while the student is in school. The terms "need to know" and "right to know" are usually not applicable for school staff, and are best eliminated. Specific release of information by the family as they wish it is obviously acceptable, but such material should then be treated confidentially regarding further dissemination.

8. **Information about a student's HIV status** shall not be included in the educational record, usual school health records, or any other records, that are accessible to school staff beyond those the parents, guardian, or student has determined should know. Documentation about specific health care

given by school nurses, counselors, clinicians, or other personnel to students with HIV infection shall be put in special health records kept in locked files. If the child changes schools, a plan for the transfer of these records shall be developed with the family and student.

III. Assurance of Appropriate Services

9. The **design of an individual student's program** shall be based on educational needs and not the status regarding HIV infection. The curriculum and other activities of a student with HIV shall be modified only as required per developmental and/or personal health needs. Exclusion or segregation of students solely on the basis of HIV infection is never appropriate.

10. **In-school health services** shall be provided as needed, including special regimens required because of HIV infection, but the origin of these programs shall not be identified at the classroom level. Specific "health care plans" may be formulated by school health personnel for students with symptomatic HIV infection. Notification for families about the presence of other communicable diseases at school (e.g., chicken pox) that place students at risk shall be forwarded universally.

Particular notification will be given to families who have informed key school personnel about HIV infection. School nurses, and others with appropriate training, shall participate in counseling for students regarding HIV matters, including the availability of testing. They shall establish quality linkages with youthserving HIV programs in the community that can provide culturally sensitive, age-appropriate medical, mental health, social, and drug treatment services.

IV. Other Elements

11. School administrators shall provide culturally sensitive information, technical

Health Highlight–cont'd

assistance/consultation, and access to resources on HIV issues to the **school's parents and families** through PTAs and other parent organizations. Appropriate issues for discussion include prevention, confidentiality, classroom educational services and related supports, and community resources.

12. Relevant to existing federal and state statutes, teachers, school health professionals, and other qualified employees shall have the **right to employment and confidentiality** regardless of their own HIV status or other health conditions. If they choose to disclose their HIV status to students or other staff this shall not have ramifications regarding employment.

Source: A. C. Crocker, et al. 1994. Support for children with HIV infection in school: Best practices guidelines. *Journal of school health* 64(1): 33–34. Used with permission.

genetic predisposition. Under normal circumstances, these conditions do not usually lead to death, but they are uncomfortable and, in more severe cases, can cause suffering. Although medicine is used in treatment, development of a wellness lifestyle may decrease both the incidence and the effects of these diseases.

The Cardiovascular System

Chronic diseases affecting the cardiovascular system are now among the leading causes of death. The cardiovascular system is complex and is subject to a range of diseases.

Anatomy and Physiology

The heart is composed of specialized muscle tissue, called *cardiac muscle*. This muscle is extremely thick and strong and has amazing endurance capacity. Although the heart is only the size of a fist and weighs a mere 8 to 10 ounces, it contracts an average seventy to eighty times per minute, 100,000 times per day, nearly a billion times in an average life of seventy years, and pumps 30 to 40 million gallons of blood.

On leaving the heart, blood travels throughout the body as part of the circulatory system. Blood containing oxygen and nutrients travels away from the heart, first in arteries, then arterioles, and then capillaries. It is through the very thin walls of the capillaries that oxygen, carbon dioxide, nutrients, and waste products are exchanged. Even the heart receives its nourishment in this manner. The waste products and carbon dioxide that are picked up by the blood are then returned to the heart in its deoxygenated state through venules (small veins) and then veins, before re-entering the vena cavae to the right atrium.

The heart has its own system for controlling its rhythmical pace. This mechanism begins with a group of specialized cells called the *sinoatrial node* or *pacemaker*. The sinoatrial node emits electrical impulses that travel toward the atrialventricular node (AV node) where there is a momentary pause before the electrical impulse is distributed through the bundle of HIS or AV bundle and then throughout the *Purkinje fibers*. Normally the heartbeat begins with the SA node. The SA node

Inactivity at any age contributes to heart disease.

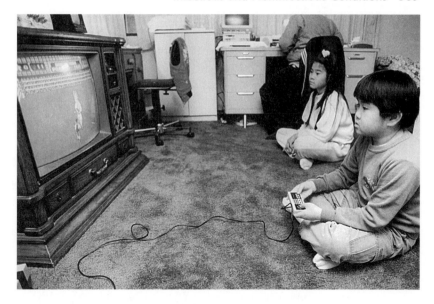

causes both atria to contract. As the electrical charge spreads to the AV nodes through the bundle of HIS (a band of fibers through which cardiac impulse is passed) and Purkinje fibers, the ventricles contract. This conduction of electrical charge occurs slightly later in the ventricles and accounts for the characteristic "lub-dub" heart sound through a stethoscope (Thibodeau and Patton 1995).

Types of Cardiovascular Disease

The most common cardiovascular diseases do not originate in the heart, but in the arteries. *Arteriosclerosis* is the generic term for a collection of diseases characterized by hardening of the arteries. The most common form of arteriosclerosis is known as *atherosclerosis*. Atherosclerosis is a degenerative disease that begins early in life, perhaps as early as two years of age. Atherosclerosis is the result of a buildup of plaque, fat, and other materials that aggregate at sites of damaged cells inside arterial walls. The earliest formations are composed of fatty streaks in the inner lining of the arteries. As atherosclerosis progresses, the arteries harden and thicken. With this hardening, the arteries begin to lose their ability to dilate and constrict, an ability needed to meet all the body's requirements for oxygen in the various parts. (See Figure 14.7.)

Over time, more and more plaque accumulates, gradually narrowing the flow of blood through the arteries. This narrowing can result in *ischemia,* diminished blood flow. Also, as channels narrow, the chances for developing a *thrombus,* or stationary blood clot, increase. If the channels become sufficiently narrow, a free-floating clot, or *embolus,* can become stuck and block blood flow, resulting in a heart attack, or *myocardial infarction.* A myocardial infarction may be severe enough to result in death or may be sufficiently mild so that heart function can return to normal. In either event, a certain amount of heart tissue dies, and heart tissue does not regenerate. In time, scar tissue can form, and if it is located in strategic areas, full recovery from a heart attack may not be possible. If atherosclerosis affects arteries going to the brain (the carotid and cerebral arteries), a stroke (shortage of blood to the brain) may result.

Figure 14.6
Diagram of the Heart

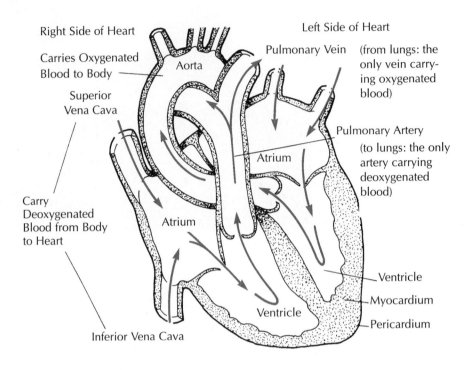

Right Side of Heart

Carries Oxygenated
Blood to Body

Superior
Vena Cava

Aorta

Left Side of Heart

Pulmonary Vein

(from lungs: the
only vein carry-
ing oxygenated
blood)

Pulmonary Artery

(to lungs: the only
artery carrying
deoxygenated
blood)

Atrium

Carry
Deoxygenated
Blood from Body
to Heart

Atrium

Ventricle

Ventricle

Myocardium

Pericardium

Inferior Vena Cava

Figure 14.7
*Progress of
Atherosclerosis*

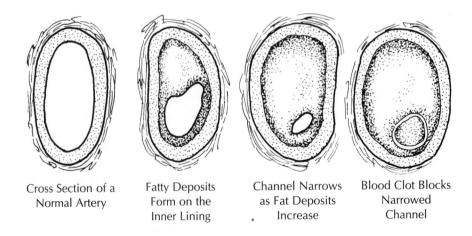

Cross Section of a
Normal Artery

Fatty Deposits
Form on the
Inner Lining

Channel Narrows
as Fat Deposits
Increase

Blood Clot Blocks
Narrowed
Channel

Coronary heart disease (disease of the coronary vessels, rather than of the heart itself) is the leading cause of death in the United States today. Coronary atherosclerosis is the leading form of coronary heart disease. Current research has indicated that some heart attacks may be caused by spasms (cramping) in the coronary arteries. The origin of these spasms is unknown at this time, although there is the possibility of a relationship between stress, tension, and heart spasms. Other experts believe that spasms are due to overabundance of calcium in cells that are being deprived of oxygen, or that the release of chemical substances at diseased sites causes the artery to close down. When these spasms occur in cases where sufficient atherosclerosis is present, the chances of having a heart attack increase. An aneurysm, a ballooning in an artery or vein due to weakened or damaged arterial walls, is another source of coronary heart disease. An aneurysm in arteries in the brain is another cause of stroke that occurs as a result of the hemorrhaging.

Other forms of heart disease include **congenital heart defects** that originate during the development of the fetus. These difficulties usually affect the septum or valves of the heart so that they do not function properly. In congestive heart failure, the heart has lost strength and cannot pump all the blood out of the chambers. Circulation is negatively affected. The number one reason for congestive heart failure is high blood pressure or *hypertension* that is uncontrolled, although it may also be due to a previous heart attack, atherosclerosis, or birth defect. Hypertension usually has no symptoms and may affect people of all ages, including children. Men are more susceptible than women to high blood pressure, and blacks are more susceptible than whites.

The common childhood illness of strep throat is the source of an infection that can cause **rheumatic heart disease.** Undiagnosed strep can result in rheumatic fever. In a portion of these cases, rheumatic heart disease results, causing damage to one or more of the heart's valves. Commonly known as a heart murmur, the valves in the heart either cannot fully open (stenosis) or do not close properly (insufficiency).

Figure 14.8

Results of Atherosclerosis on Arteries

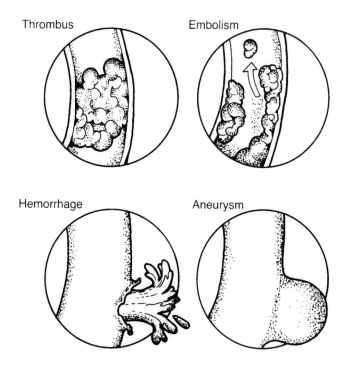

Thrombus

Embolism

Hemorrhage

Aneurysm

Table 14.3
Risk Factors for
Heart Disease

Major Risk Factors That Cannot Be Changed

1. Age   55% of all heart attacks attacks occur in people over 65. This age group accounts for more than 80% of the fatal attacks (American Heart Association, 1995).

2. Gender   Women have less heart disease than men, particularly before menopause. After menopause the heart attack rate among women increases significantly until the mid-60s, when women's risk is equal to that of men the same age.

3. Heredity   Father, grandfather, and brothers who dies of coronary heart disease before the age of 55 or female relatives (mother, grandmother, and sisters) who died of coronary heart disease before the age of 65 indicates a strong familial tendency.

Major Risk Factors That Can Be Changed

4. Cholesterol   There are several types of cholesterol. VLDL and LDL cholesterol have been referred to as the "bad" cholesterol or type that enhances the depositing of plaque in the lining of the arteries. HDL cholesterol in contrast "picks up" fat from the cells and linings of the arteries and delivers it to the liver, where it is degraded and eliminated or used to form other tissue.

5. Cigarette smoking   Tars, carbon monoxide, and nicotine adversely affect the body. The effects of these products increase heart rate, raise blood pressure, increase arterial spasms, reduce the ability of the blood to carry oxygen, and elevate cholesterol levels. Smoke destroys the alveoli in the lungs and paralyzes the cilia.

6. Hypertension   Systolic blood pressure is the force exerted against the arteries when the heart is contracting. Diastolic pressure is the force against the arteries when the heart is relaxed. These pressures are measured in millimeters of mercury (mmHg). As a result of hypertension, the heart receives inadequate rest between beats that produces muscle fibers which are overstretched and lose the ability to contract. This increases pressure, damages the kidneys, arteries, and accelerates atherosclerosis.

7. Inactivity   Research has shown that physical inactivity and heart disease was similar in magnitude to that of cigarette smoking, high serum cholesterol levels, and hypertension. Seventy-eight percent of Americans exercise too infrequently. In addition, exercise has a modifying effect on many of the risks for cardiovascular disease.

8. Obesity   There is a strong positive association between obesity and abnormal cholesterol and triglycerides, hypertension, and excessive production of insulin. These factors lead to increased likelihood of coronary artery disease and Type II diabetes.

9. Diabetes mellitus   Long-range complications that lead to degenerative disorders of the blood vessels and nerves. Diabetics often are victims of cardiovascular lesions and accelerated atherosclerosis. The incidence of heart attacks and strokes is higher among diabetics than nondiabetics. Diabetes increases the risk of coronary artery disease by two to three times the normal rate in men and three to seven times in women.

10. Stress   Experts agree that chronic stress produces a complex array of physiological changes in the body. Some of these physiological responses can constrict the arteries and increase the workload of the heart.

Angina pectoris is defined as chest pains. Angina is not a heart attack, nor is it a disease. It is a frequent symptom of coronary heart disease, however. An angina attack usually lasts less than five minutes, often after unaccustomed exercise or stress. A primary symptom is a squeezing sensation in the chest, as if a "weight" had been placed there. For some, it is pain somewhere else in the upper body, frequently the left arm, or feels similar to indigestion or heartburn. Angina usually subsides with rest and medication. The positive aspect of angina is that it is an early sign of progressive heart disease. For one-third of all victims, the actual heart attack is the first symptom. Recognized and properly treated, angina can lead to prevention of more serious heart disease or even a heart attack. The risk factors for cardiovascular disease are shown in Table 14.3.

Table 14.4

Blood Cholesterol and LDL-Cholesterol Levels for Children Ages Two to Nineteen

Cholesterol type	Cholesterol Levels (in mg per deciliter)		
	Normal	Moderately High	High
Total cholesterol	Below 170	170–185	Above 185
LDL cholesterol	Below 110	110–125	Above 125

Source: A. B. Elster and N. J. Kuznets. 1994. AMA guidelines for adolescent preventive services. Baltimore: Williams & Wilkins, p.102.

Table 14.5

Hypertension in Children

Age Group	Normal	Hypertension	
		Significant	Severe
1 mo–2 years	105/69	112/74	118/72
3–5	107/69	116/76	124/84
6–9	114/72	122/78	130/86
10–12	120/76	126/82	134/90
13–15	126/79	136/86	144/92
16–18	126/79	142/92	150/98

Source: Task Force on Blood Pressure Control in Children. 1987. *Pediatrics* 79 (1):1–25.

Cancer

The term *cancer* does not refer to one disease, but rather to a large group of diseases. Cancer is characterized by uncontrolled growth and spread of abnormal cells or *neoplasms*. These neoplasms often form a mass of tissue called a *tumor*. These masses or tumors can be *malignant* (cancerous) or **benign.** Benign tumors usually cause no harm. However, if they are located in an area where they obstruct or crowd out normal tissues or organs, benign tumors can be life threatening. For example, a benign tumor in the brain could restrict the flow of blood. Benign tumors are enclosed in a fibrous capsule that prevents their spreading to other areas of the body. To determine if a tumor is malignant or benign, a *biopsy* (microscopic examination of tissue) must be done.

Types of Cancer

There are four major categories of tumors: *carcinoma, sarcoma, lymphoma,* and *leukemia.* Carcinoma is the most common form of cancer. Cancers of the skin, breast, uterus, prostate, lung, stomach, colon, and rectum are examples of carcinoma. Sarcomas are cancers of the connective tissue. Muscle, bone, and cartilage cancers are examples of sarcomas. These cancers occur less often than the carcinoma, but usually spread more quickly. Lymphomas are cancers that affect the lymph nodes. Leukemia is cancer of the blood-forming cells, causing an overproduction of immature white blood cells. Data on the incidence of cancer appear in Figure 14.9.

Health Highlight

Cancer Terms to Know

Here are some terms commonly used in the language of cancer treatment:

antibody: a substance made by specialized cells in the body that defends you from infections due to viruses, bacteria, and other foreign substances

benign: a noncancerous growth

biopsy: removal and microscopic examination of tissue from a living body for diagnosis

cancer: a general term for more than a hundred diseases involving abnormal and uncontrolled growth of cells

grading: a method physicians use to identify the severity of cancer

malignant: a growth of cancerous cells

metastasis: the spread of cancer from part of the body to another; cells in the new site are like those in the original growth

remission: a lessening or stopping of symptoms of a disease when the disease is under control

staging: a numerical method indicating the extent to which the cancer has spread; helps determine best form of treatment and prognosis

tumor: a palpable mass; may be malignant or benign

How Cancer Spreads

Malignant tumors are not contained in a fibrous capsule. Consequently, the malignant cells can spread from one part of the body to another. This process of spreading is known as *metastasis*. Cancers metastasize by invading adjacent tissues or dislodging and moving through the blood and lymphatic vessels to other parts of the body. Early diagnosis is vital for any type of cancer. If the cancer metastasizes, treatment becomes much more difficult. As the malignant cells spread, they begin to disrupt the chemical functioning of the normal cells in the area they invade. The cancerous cells disrupt the RNA and DNA within the normal cells. When this disruption occurs, *mutant* cells that differ in form, quality, and function are developed.

Causes of Cancer

Even though the process of how malignant cells spread is understood, why this process occurs is not fully understood. Researchers have suggested that the DNA alters the cell in such a fashion as to allow the growth of cancer cells. These *oncogenes* (cancer-causing genes) are present in chromosomes, and

Figure 14.9
Leading Sites of New Cancer Cases & Deaths –1995 Estimates

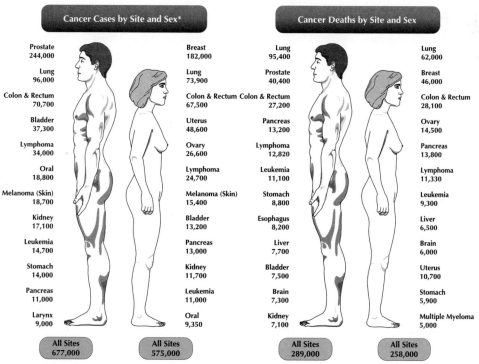

Cancer Cases by Site and Sex*				Cancer Deaths by Site and Sex			
Prostate 244,000		Breast 182,000	Lung 95,400			Lung 62,000	
Lung 96,000		Lung 73,900	Prostate 40,400			Breast 46,000	
Colon & Rectum 70,700		Colon & Rectum 67,500	Colon & Rectum 27,200			Colon & Rectum 28,100	
Bladder 37,300		Uterus 48,600	Pancreas 13,200			Ovary 14,500	
Lymphoma 34,000		Ovary 26,600	Lymphoma 12,820			Pancreas 13,800	
Oral 18,800		Lymphoma 24,700	Leukemia 11,100			Lymphoma 11,330	
Melanoma (Skin) 18,700		Melanoma (Skin) 15,400	Stomach 8,800			Leukemia 9,300	
Kidney 17,100		Bladder 13,200	Esophagus 8,200			Liver 6,500	
Leukemia 14,700		Pancreas 13,000	Liver 7,700			Brain 6,000	
Stomach 14,000		Kidney 11,700	Bladder 7,500			Uterus 10,700	
Pancreas 11,000		Leukemia 11,000	Brain 7,300			Stomach 5,900	
Larynx 9,000		Oral 9,350	Kidney 7,100			Multiple Myeloma 5,000	
All Sites 677,000		All Sites 575,000	All Sites 289,000			All Sites 258,000	

* Excluding basal and squamous cell skin cancer and carcinoma in situ (cancer that has not metastasized).

scientists theorize that stress, viruses, radiation, or some other *carcinogenic* (cancer-causing) agent activates these oncogenes. Other genes called *tumor-suppressor genes* slow it down. Whether these genes are present through genetics or develop because of exposure to some carcinogen is not known. A range of other factors may cause cancer.

Genetic Factors. Most cancers are not linked to genes. Whether there is an inherited tendency toward a cancer-prone immune system remains controversial. Because of the complexity of environment and lifestyle factors, it is unlikely a single cause will be discovered. Certain cancers, such as breast, stomach, colon, prostate, lung, and uterus, appear to run in families. Again, whether this is genetic or environmental remains a question.

Viral Cause. Although the evidence is still under investigation, there are indications that viruses enhance the probability for the development of cancer. There is evidence that the herpes viruses may contribute to the development of some forms of leukemia, Burkitt's lymphoma, Hodgkin's disease, cervical cancer, and some forms of leukemia (Donatelle, Davis, and Hoover 1991).

Diet. Although useful as preservatives, many food chemical additives and preservatives have been linked with cancer. For example, the cyclamate saccharin and the nitrosamines have been linked to cancer. It has been estimated that 40 to 50 percent of cancers derive from environmental chemicals such as pesticides, herbicides, preservatives, and other chemicals. The FDA has developed a list of over 14,000 chemicals suspected of causing cancer. Instead of concerning itself with all the ill effects of these chemicals, the American Cancer Society has developed the following nutritional guidelines for preventing cancer:

1. Eat a variety of foods. No one food provides all the nutrients. Eat a variety of foods such as fruit and vegetables, whole cereals, lean meats, fish, poultry without skin, beans, and low-fat dairy products.

2. Maintain desirable weight. Obesity increases the risks for colon, breast, gallbladder, and uterine cancer.

3. Avoid too much fat, saturated fat, and cholesterol. A low-fat diet may reduce the risks for cancers of the breast, prostate, colon, and rectum. A low-fat diet will help control weight and reduce the risk of heart disease.

4. Eat foods with adequate starch and fiber. Starch and fiber can be increased by eating more fruit, vegetables, potatoes, and whole-grain breads and cereals. A high-fiber diet helps reduce the risk of colon and rectal cancer.

5. Include foods high in vitamins A and C. Foods such as carrots, spinach, oranges, strawberries, and green peppers are high in vitamin C. Vitamin A can be found in dark green and deep yellow fresh vegetables. These foods may help reduce the risk for cancers of the larynx, esophagus, and lungs.

6. Include cruciferous vegetables. Foods such as cabbage, broccoli, brussel sprouts, and cauliflower may help prevent cancer. These are high in fiber.

7. Eat moderately of salt-cured, smoked, and nitrate-cured foods. Consuming these foods in large amounts is associated with higher incidence of cancer of esophagus and stomach.

8. If you drink alcohol, do so in moderation. Heavy drinking is associated with cancer of the mouth, throat, esophagus, and liver.

Warning Signals of Cancer

The American Cancer Society states that the following warning signs should be carefully monitored. The chances of survival are significantly better if early detection and diagnosis take place. None of the risk factors are sure indicators of cancer, but they should be checked by a physician. The warning signs are as follows:

1. change in bowel or bladder habits
2. a sore that does not heal
3. unusual bleeding or discharge
4. thickening or lump in the breasts or elsewhere
5. indigestion or difficulty in swallowing
6. obvious change in a wart or mole
7. nagging cough or hoarseness

Trends in Diagnosis, Treatment, and Research

The American Cancer Society states that anyone surviving cancer five years after diagnosis is considered to be cured. Continued emphasis is on the importance of early detection and treatment. Often the types of therapies will be a combination of several. The following is a partial list of the direction current methods used in treatment and research is proceeding (American Cancer Society 1993, 2–3; Kennedy 1992, 3).

1. A genetic fusing of cancer cells with normal cells can produce disease-fighting "monoclonal antibodies," specific antibodies tailored to seek out chosen targets on cancer cells. Their potential in the diagnosis and treatment of cancer is under study.

2. New approaches to drug therapy use combination chemotherapy and chemotherapy with surgery or radiation. New classes of agents are being tested for their effectiveness in treating patients who are resistant to drug therapies now in use.

3. New high-technology diagnostic imaging techniques have replaced exploratory surgery for some cancer patients. Magnetic resonance imaging (MRI) is one example of such technology under study. It uses a huge electromagnet to detect tumors by sensing the vibrations of the different atoms in the body. Computerized tomography (CT scanning) uses X rays to examine the brain and other parts of the body. Cross section pictures are constructed that show a tumor's shape and location more accurately than is possible with conventional X-ray techniques. For patients undergoing radiation therapy, CT scanning may enable the therapist to pinpoint the tumor more precisely to provide more accurate radiation dosage while sparing normal tissue.

4. Immunotherapy holds the hope of enhancing the body's own disease-fighting systems to control cancer. Interferon, interleukin-2, and other biologic response modifiers are under study. Recently, interferon was made available as the treatment for hairy cell leukemia, a rare blood cancer of older Americans. Interleukin-2 is under very active research in the treatment of kidney cancer and melanoma. Also under investigation are colony-stimulating factors that encourage production of white blood cells. This enables the patient to tolerate higher doses of medication while decreasing the chance of infection.

Health Highlight

Preventing Cancer:
Guidelines from the American Cancer Society

Primary prevention **refers to steps that might be taken to avoid those factors that might lead to the development of cancer.**

Smoking Cigarette smoking is responsible for 85% of lung cancer cases among men and 75% among women—about 83% overall. Smoking accounts for about 30% of all cancer deaths. Those who smoke two or more packs of cigarettes a day have lung cancer mortality rates 15–25 times greater than nonsmokers.

Sunlight Almost all of the more than 500,000 cases of nonmelanoma skin cancer developed each year in the U.S. are considered to be sun-related. Recent epidemiological evidence shows that sun exposure is a major factor in the development of melanoma and that the incidence increases for those living near the equator.

Alcohol Oral cancer and cancers of the larynx, throat, esophagus, and liver occur more frequently among heavy drinkers of alcohol.

Smokeless Tobacco Increased risk factor for cancers of the mouth, larynx, throat, and esophagus. Highly habit forming.

Estrogen For mature women, certain risks associated with estrogen treatment to control menopausal symptoms, including an increased risk of endometrial cancer. Use of estrogen by menopausal women needs careful discussion by the woman and her physician.

Radiation Excessive exposure to radiation can increase cancer risk. Most medical X rays are adjusted to deliver the lowest dose possible without sacrificing image quality. The ACS believes there is a potential problem of radon in the home. If levels are found to be too high, remedial actions should be taken.

Occupational Hazards Exposure to a number of industrial agents (nickel, chromate, asbestos, vinyl chloride, etc.) increases risk. Risk factor greatly increased when combined with smoking.

Nutrition Risk for colon, breast, and uterine cancers increases for obese people. High-fat diet may be a factor in the development of certain cancers

such as breast, colon, and prostate. High-fiber foods may help reduce risk of colon cancer, and can be a wholesome substitute for high-fat diets. Foods rich in vitamins A and C may help lower risk for cancers of larynx, esophagus, stomach, and lung. Eating cruciferous vegetables may help protect against certain cancers. Salt-cured, smoked, and nitrite-cured foods have been linked to esophageal and stomach cancer. The heavy use of alcohol, especially when accompanied by cigarette smoking or chewing tobacco, increases risk of cancers of the mouth, larynx, throat, esophagus, and liver.

Secondary prevention **refers to steps to be taken to diagnose a cancer or precursor as early as possible after it has developed.**

Colorectal Tests The ACS recommends three tests for the early detection of colon and rectum cancer in people without symptoms. The digital rectal examination, performed by a physician during an office visit, should be performed every year after the age of 40; the stool blood test is recommended every year after 50; and the proctosigmoidoscopy examination should be carried out every three to five after the age of 50, following two annual exams with negative results.

Pap Test For cervical cancer, women who are or have been sexually active, or have reached age 18 years, should have an annual Pap test and pelvic examination. After a woman has had three or more consecutive satisfactory normal annual examinations, the Pap test may be performed less frequently at the discretion of her physician.

Breast Cancer Detection The ACS recommends the monthly practice of breast self-examination (BSE) by women 20 years and older as a routine good health habit. Physical examination of the breast should be done every three years from age 20 to 40 and then every year. The ACS recommends a mammogram every year for asymptomatic women age 50 and over, and a baseline mammogram between ages 35 and 39. Women 40 should have mammography every 1–2 years depending on physical and mammogram findings.

Source: American Cancer Society (ACS). 1988. *Cancer facts and figures.* New York: ACS, p. 18.

5. Many cancers are caused by a two-stage process through exposure to substances known as *initiators* and *promoters*. Research scientists are exploring ways of interrupting these processes to prevent the development of cancer.

6. New technologies have made it possible to use bone marrow transplantation as an important treatment option in selected patients with aplastic anemia and leukemia. Bone marrow transplantation for other cancers is under study. The administration of larger doses of anticancer drugs or radiation therapy may be tolerated by some patients if their bone marrow is stored and later transplanted to restore marrow function (autologous bone marrow transplants).

7. Hyperthermia is a way to increase the heat or temperature of the entire body or a part of the body. It is known that heat can kill cancer cells. A cell temperature of 45 degrees C kills cancer cells. A temperature of 42–43 degrees makes the cell more susceptible to damage by ionizing radiation (X rays). Studies are under way to learn if hyperthermia can increase the effect of radiation or chemotherapy. The value of hyperthermia has yet to be established, and this technique, although appearing to be useful, is the cornerstone of many types of cancer quackery.

8. Improvements in cancer treatment have made possible more conservative management of some early cancers. In early cancer of the larynx, many patients have been able to retain their larynx and their voice; in colorectal cancer, fewer permanent colostomies are needed; and the surgery required in many cases of breast cancer is often more limited.

Respiratory Disorders

The term *allergy* can be used synonymously with the term *hypersensitivity*. In both cases, the reference is to an exaggerated response to an antibody-forming substance (antigen). Many people with the most common allergic disorders have an inherited tendency to develop this hypersensitivity. Although it may seem to those who suffer from allergies that the vast majority of people do experience hypersensitivity, each specific reaction is theoretically harmless to 80 percent of the population. Table 14.6 lists the more common respiratory disorders.

Asthma is most common in children. Because of their small airways, children are most prone to have problems with asthma. Childhood asthma tends to improve as the lung airways become larger. Older children tend to become relatively free of symptoms, yet may experience problems throughout their lives. If a child's asthma is more than mild, a proper treatment plan should be undertaken. This plan should be shared with the child's teachers so that he or she can fully participate in school activities.

Other Conditions

Diabetes Mellitus

Diabetes mellitus is a disease in which the inadequate production of insulin leads to failure of the body tissues to break down carbohydrates at a normal rate. It is a metabolic disorder referring to a complex hereditary and environmental interaction, resulting in abnormal secretions in insulin that, in turn, lead to metabolic and vascular manifestations. Diabetes can result from the secretion of too little insulin from the pancreas, insufficient numbers of insulin receptors on target cells, or

Table 14.6

Common Allergic or Sensitivity Reactions

Reaction	Causes	Symptoms	Relief
Hay fever	Pollen from trees, grasses, or weeds, molds; dust mites; furry animals	Stuffy nose; sneezing; runny nose, itching eyes and nose; watering eyes	Avoidance of allergens; medications
Eczema (atopic dermatitis)	Food allergies, contact with pollen, dust mites, furry animals, makeup, soaps, detergents	Patchy, dry, red itchy rash—often in creases of arms, legs, and neck	Avoidance; medication
Food allergies and/or sensitivities	Any food, but most common are eggs, peanuts, milk, fish, soy, wheat, peas, and shellfish	Vomiting, hives, diarrhea, or breathing/circulation problem	Avoidance of products
Asthma	Pollen, dust mites, cigarette smoke, furry animals, colds, changing weather, exercise, emotional stress	Coughing, wheezing, difficult breathing, chest tightness, coughing with exertion	Avoidance of what causes; medication; relaxation; breathing exercises

defective receptors that do not respond normally to insulin (Tate, Seeley, and Stephens 1994, 175). *Hyperglycemia* (high blood sugar) is the hallmark symptom of diabetes. Obesity is a contributing factor to lack of receptor sites in older people. Insufficient amounts of insulin are available to metabolize sugar, the primary source of fuel. When fat is metabolized without sugar, a residue called a *ketone body* develops, increasing acid in the bloodstream. Sufficient amounts of ketone bodies produce a diabetic coma and can cause death. The earliest symptom of characteristically elevated blood glucose levels is excessive urination.

There are two main types of diabetes mellitus. Type I (also called **juvenile diabetes** or insulin-dependent diabetes mellitus, IDDM) develops in young people and is usually caused by a lack of insulin secretion. Viral infection of the pancreatic islets or an immune response may be responsible for the development of the condition. This type of diabetes usually appears in people under the age of thirty-five, most commonly between the ages of ten and sixteen. **Type II diabetes** mellitus develops in older people and often does not result from a lack of insulin but from the reduced ability of the cells to respond to insulin. The onset is usually gradual and occurs mainly in people over forty. In some cases the combination of dietary measures, weight loss, and exercise can keep the condition under control without the injection of insulin. It is estimated that about 30,000 new cases of IDDM are diagnosed each year (Internet CDC Reducing the Burden of Diabetes 1996).

Insulin shock can develop when too much insulin is present. This occurs when a diabetic is either injected with too much insulin or has not eaten after an insulin injection. Disorientation, convulsions, and loss of consciousness may result.

Extra care with personal hygiene is part of treatment. Diabetics are very prone to infections, so it is important for them to maintain sterile conditions for shaving and to treat cuts and abrasions carefully. The feet and legs are particularly susceptible to infection. Long-term complications include heart disease, stroke, hypertension, blindness, kidney disease, nerve damage, dental disease, and amputations. Some new classes of drugs work in the small intestine to inhibit the absorption of carbohydrates (which raise blood sugar levels), while others stop the liver from producing excess amourts of sugar. A new type of insulin called Humalog supposedly is capable of acting more than twice as fast as other versions (Cray and Park 1996, 64).

Sickle Cell Anemia

Sickle cell anemia is an inherited blood disease that can cause pain, damage to vital organs, and, for some, early death. The effects of the disease vary greatly from person to person, but most people with the condition enjoy good health much of the time. Most cases of sickle cell occur among blacks and Hispanics of Caribbean ancestry. Approximately one in every 400 to 600 blacks and one in every 1,000 to 1,500 Hispanics inherits sickle cell. The physical growth of children with the disease is often slower than normal.

Normally, the red blood cells are round and flexible. However, the red blood cells of a person with sickle cell may change into a sickle shape within their blood vessels. The sickle cells tend to become trapped in the spleen and elsewhere and be destroyed. This results in a shortage of red blood cells, which causes the person to be pale, short of breath, easily tired, and prone to infections. Viral infection and vitamin deficiency can worsen the condition.

When the cells become stuck in the blood vessels, they lose oxygen. This loss of oxygen causes severe pain in the abdomen and chest. If the condition is long lasting, damage to the brain, lungs, or kidneys can even lead to death.

Sickle-cell anemia is not contagious, but it is inherited. Individuals may carry the disease (sickle-cell trait) but have no signs of the disease. When two persons who have the trait have a child, that child may inherit two sickle-cell genes and develop the disease. A test can identify people who either have the disease or carry the trait. Unfortunately there is no medication or therapy that will correct the effects of the disease-causing gene.

Epilepsy

The word *epilepsy* comes from the Greek word for seizures. Epilepsy is a disorder of the central nervous system characterized by sudden seizures, which usually last only a few minutes. Seizures are not always convulsive, and, even when they are, they are not as dangerous as they look. Epilepsy is not contagious, and, between seizures, epileptic children function normally. Seizures occur when there are excessive electrical discharges in some nerve cell of the brain. When this happens, the brain loses conscious control over certain body functions and consciousness may be lost or altered.

There are more than twenty different kinds of seizures. Only three will be described here

1. General tonic clonic seizures (grand mal) are the most disruptive in the classroom. The child becomes stiff and slumps to the floor unconscious. Rigid muscles give way to jerking, breathing is suspended, and saliva may escape from the lips. The seizure may last for several minutes, and the child will regain consciousness in a confused or drowsy state, but is otherwise unaffected.

Health Highlight

A Child with Sickle Cell Anemia in the Classroom

There may be a child in your class with the severe chronic disease sickle cell anemia. Your understanding of this handicap will help him (or her) on the road to learning.

Such a child is often thin and small for his age. When not experiencing physical discomfort, he is usually as active as any child in the class. Intelligence is not affected. As noted in earlier chapters, the majority of those affected are black, but the disease also occurs in people from Mediterranean countries, South and Central America, Caribbean countries, and southern India.

There are periods when the disease is more active (crises). These episodes often occur with colds and other infections and are more frequent in early childhood. At such times, the child becomes listless and complains of pain, usually in the back, extremities, or abdomen. The whites of his eyes may be slightly yellow. Most of these attacks will necessitate a week or two of absence from school. Sometimes, hospitalization and special procedures, such as blood transfusion, will be required.

The disease is due to a hereditary defect in the red blood cells, causing them to assume the crescent shape that gives the disease its name. The pains are due to aggregations of sickle cells causing a temporary blockage of the small blood vessels. These cells are subject to early destruction in the circulation, causing a chronic anemia.

Sickle cell anemia is inherited as a recessive trait affecting both males and females. Both parents, although apparently healthy, carry a recessive sickle cell gene. The affected child receives one such gene from each parent. When each parent has sickle cell trait, their offspring has a 25 percent chance of being normal, a 25 percent chance of having sickle cell anemia, or a 50 percent chance of having sickle cell trait. An examination of the blood by laboratory tests will show whether a person has sickle cell anemia or sickle cell trait. Individuals with the trait have a very small percentage of sickled cells in their circulation. They never develop sickle cell anemia per se, and as a rule, they are free of symptoms that could be attributed to the presence of an abnormal hemoglobin in their red blood cells.

Points for the Teacher to Keep in Mind

1. Sickle cell anemia is a chronic hereditary handicapping illness.
2. Crises cause frequent absence from school, especially in younger children.
3. Colds and other infections may precipitate crises.
4. Between crises, a child with sickle cell anemia may carry on the usual activity of his peer group, with the exception of strenuous sports.
5. The disease does not affect intelligence.
6. Education should be encouraged because this handicap will necessitate a sedentary occupation as an adult.
7. When long hospitalizations are required, children should be able to continue schoolwork in the hospital with the help of a visiting teacher.
8. Psychological problems may arise from adjustment to the handicap and the environment.
9. It is important that there be some activity in which the child can excel to gain acceptance with the peer group. This could be music, art, handicrafts, games, and so forth.
10. The disease tends to become milder as an individual grows into adulthood. Crises become less frequent and less severe after adolescence.

Source: Adapted from R. B. Scott and A. D. Kessler. 1988. *A child with sickle-cell anemia in your class (a guide for teachers).* Washington, DC: Center for Sickle Cell Disease, Howard University College of Medicine, pp. 1–4.

For tonic clonic seizures:

a. Keep calm. Ease the child to the floor and loosen his or her collar. You cannot stop the seizure. Let it run its course and do not try to revive the child.

b. Remove hard, sharp, or hot objects that may injure the child, but do not interfere with his or her movements.

c. Do not force anything between his or her teeth

d. Turn the child on one side to release saliva. Place something soft and flat under his or her head.

e. When the child regains consciousness, let him or her rest.

f. If the seizure lasts beyond a few minutes, or the child seems to pass from one seizure to another without gaining consciousness, call for medical assistance and notify his or her parents. This rarely happens but should be treated immediately

2. Generalized absence (petit mal) seizures, most common in children, usually last only for 5 to 20 seconds. They may be accompanied by staring or twitching of the eyelids and are frequently mistaken for "daydreaming," The child is seldom aware he or she has had a seizure, although he or she may be aware that his or her mind "has gone blank" for a few seconds.

3. Complex partial (psychomotor or temporal lobe) seizures have the most complex behavior pattern. They may include constant chewing or lip smacking, purposeless walking or repetitive hand and arm movements, confusion, and dizziness. The seizure may last from a minute to several hours.

≣ Summary

○ Micro-organisms (microbes) are living agents. Microbes that can harm humans are called *pathogens*.

○ There are six general types of pathogens—viruses, bacteria, rickettsiae, fungi, protozoa, and metazoa.

○ Every illness follows a pattern from the time the pathogen enters the body to the incubation period, prodromal period, typical illness, convalescence, and recovery.

○ The immune system protects against disease.

○ Body defenses include the skin, body secretions, mucous membranes, enzymes, blood compounds, and interferon.

○ Common diseases that can impact children include the common cold, streptococcal throat infection, influenza, infectious mononucleosis, and the various types of hepatitis.

○ HIV is the virus responsible for AIDS. It cannot be contracted through casual contact.

○ There are no cures for AIDS, but a combination of drug therapy seems promising.

○ Teachers must be aware of the emotional, social, and legal support an HIV-positive child needs.

○ The heart is a four-chambered organ, responsible for pumping blood to the body through a series of arteries, arterioles, capillaries, venules, and veins.

○ The risk factors for cardiovascular disease include heredity, sex, age, tobacco use, high cholesterol, hypertension, inactivity, obesity, diabetes, and stress.

○ Conditions of the heart and cardiovascular system include congenital heart defects, congestive heart failure, myocardial infarction, angina pectoris, hypertension, and rheumatic heart.

○ The term *cancer* is used to describe conditions characterized by uncontrolled cell growth.

○ Neoplasms (tumors) can be benign (noncancerous) or malignant (cancerous).

○ Types of cancer include carcinomas, sarcomas, lymphomas, and leukemia.

○ Cancer spreads through a process called *metastasis*.

○ Sickle cell anemia is an inherited blood disease that can cause extreme pain, damage to vital organs, and possible early death.

○ Epilepsy is a disorder of the central nervous system of which there are more than twenty types.

○ Three most common types of epilepsy are general tonic clonic (grand mal); generalized absence (petit mal); complex partial (psychomotor).

Discussion Questions

1. List and describe the pathogens.
2. Discuss immunity and the various protective mechanisms the body has to protect itself against disease.
3. Trace the stages through which a communicable disease typically progresses.
4. Describe the antigen–antibody response.
5. Select a communicable disease, and discuss its signs and symptoms.
6. Trace the possible physiological effects experienced by an HIV-positive person.
7. Trace the blood through the heart and circulatory system.
8. Describe the major risk factors for cardiovascular diseases.
9. What are the four types of cancer?
10. Describe how IDDM differs from NIDDM.
11. What considerations are necessary for a child with sickle cell anemia?

References

American Cancer Society. 1993. *Cancer facts and figures.* New York: Author.

American Heart Association. 1995. *Heart facts and stroke facts: 1995 statistical supplement.* Dallas, TX: Author.

American Medical Association. 1989. *Home medical encyclopedia.* New York: Random House.

Anspaugh, D. J., M. Hamrick, and F. Rosato. 1997. *Wellness concepts and applications.* St. Louis: Mosby.

Benenson, A. S., ed. 1985. *Control of communicative diseases in man.* 14th ed. Washington, DC: American Public Health Association.

Benenson, A. S., ed. *Control of communicable disease manual.* 1995. 16th ed. Washington, DC: American Public Health Association.

Berkow, R., ed. 1987. *The Merck manual of diagnosis and therapy.* 15th ed. Rahway, NJ: Merck.

Cray, D., and A. Park. 1996. The exorcists. *Time,* Special Issue 148(14): 64–68.

Crowley, L. V. 1992. *Introduction to human disease.* 2nd ed. Boston: Jones & Bartlett.

Donatelle, R. J. , L. G. Davis, and C. F. Hoover. 1991. *Access to health.* Englewood Cliffs, NJ: Prentice Hall.

Elster, A. B., and N. J. Kuznets. 1994. *AMA guidelines for adolescent prevention services (GAPS)*. Baltimore: Williams & Wilkins.

Engs, R., E. Barnes, and M. Wonty. 1975. *Health games people play*. Dubuque, IA: Kendal/Hart.

Green, L. W, and C. L. Henderson. 1986. *Community health*. 5th ed. St. Louis: Times Mirror/Mosby.

Hamann, B. 1994. *Diseases identification, prevention, and control*. St. Louis: Mosby.

Healthy people 2000—National health promotion and disease prevention objectives. 1990. Washington, DC: U. S. Department of Health and Human Services.

Jackson, J. K. 1992. *AIDS, STDs and other communicable diseases*. Guilford, CT: Dushkin.

Kennedy. C. C., ed. 1992. New methods to fight cancer. *Mayo Clinic health newsletter*. 10(2): 1-3.

National Cancer Institute Fact Book. 1987. Bethesda, MD: Office of Cancer Communications.

Ross, F. C. 1983. *Introduction to microbiology*. Columbus, OH: Merrill.

Scott, R., and A. D. Kessler. 1988. *A child with sickle cell anemia in your class*. Washington, DC: Center for Sickle Cell Disease, Howard University College of Medicine.

Silberner, J. 1990, January 29. Best ways to fight that cold. *U.S. News and World Report*.

Task Force on Blood Pressure Control in Children. 1987. Report of the second task force on blood pressure control in children. *Pediatrics* 79(l): 1–25.

Tate, P., R. R. Seeley, and T. D. Stephens. 1994. *Understanding the human body*. St. Louis: Mosby.

Thibodeau, G. A., and K. T. Patton. 1993. *Anatomy and physiology*. St. Louis: Mosby.

Thibodeau, G.A., and K. T. Patton. 1995. *The human body in health and disease*. St. Louis: Mosby.

Thomas, C. L., ed. 1984. *Taber's cyclopedic medical dictionary*. Philadelphia: Davis.

Chapter Fifteen
Strategies for Teaching about Infectious and Noninfectious Conditions

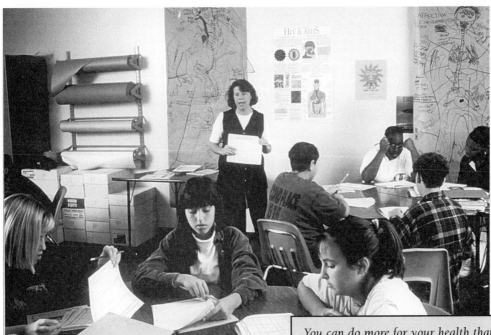

> *You can do more for your health than your doctor can.*
>
> —*Donald M. Vickery and James F. Fries*

Valued Outcomes

After doing the activities in this chapter, the student should be able to express and illustrate the following guidelines:

○ The diseases that are the leading causes of death in this century are the chronic diseases.

○ Infectious diseases originate from pathogens.

○ Protection against diseases is the work of the immune system.

○ The function of the heart is to pump oxygenated blood systematically and regularly through the body.

○ Noninfectious diseases often develop over time, are frequently progressive, and can be positively affected by a wellness lifestyle.

Many of the values that protect and direct us as we grow are fostered during the elementary years. Learning at an early age about pathogens, the stages through which disease progress, and lifestyles that are detrimental to high-level wellness can establish positive health values and habits. In addition, many chronic conditions detract from the quality of life for children. Awareness on the part of every teacher and child that children with chronic conditions can function effectively in the school setting improves the quality of life for the atypical child.

This chapter focuses on instructional strategies to help the elementary student learn about diseases.

Valued-Based Activities

How Did I Get It?

Valued Outcome: The students will be able to identify the risk factors associated with contracting an infectious disease.

Description of Strategy: Ask the students to think of someone who is extremely ill. Ask them to identify those factors that may have been associated with the sick person's illness. Write the responses on an overhead projector, butcher paper, or chalkboard. Make two lists and have the students identify which factors could have been better controlled if that person had followed a wellness lifestyle. After the activity the students can be assigned an Internet activity to discover information concerning some of the conditions identified and how they can be prevented.

Processing Questions:

1. How many of the illnesses/conditions are related to lifestyle?
2. What lifestyle factors put the individual at greater risk for developing the condition?
3. Are there factors that cannot be controlled? (Good place to point out that a wellness lifestyle can delay or prevent some of the genetic predispositions we have for certain diseases.)
4. Name some things you can do to prevent diseases.
5. What type of diseases/conditions would fall under the category of uncontrollable (hemophilia, for example)?

The Help I Get

Valued Outcome: The students will appreciate the many defenses the body uses to protect them from disease.

Description of Strategy: Provide the students with Figure 15.1. "The Help I Get," and ask them to identify each of the defenses on the handout. The various body defenses can be discussed in class or assigned as a group or individual activity for reporting findings back to the class.

Processing Questions:

1. What happens to our body defenses if we do not take care of our bodies?
2. Can you name all the body defense mechanisms?
3. How can we make sure our body defenses are operating at the highest level possible?
4. What are some lifestyle habits that inhibit our body defenses from operating at peak performance?

Health Highlight

A Most Preventable Situation

Chronic disease has replaced infectious or communicable disease as the leading cause of death in the United States. At the same time, however, some communicable diseases have been making a comeback. One such disease is measles, which has made a dramatic comeback. The major reason for this increase is the failure to immunize children at the recommended age intervals. This particular disease should be totally preventable if parents have accessibility to the health care system in the United States.

Figure 15.1
The Help I Get

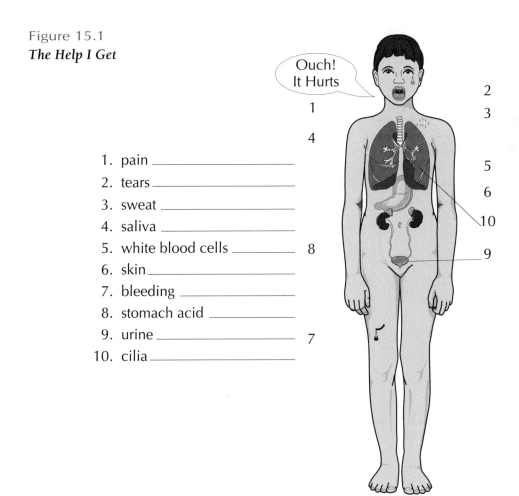

Ouch! It Hurts

1. pain _____
2. tears _____
3. sweat _____
4. saliva _____
5. white blood cells _____
6. skin _____
7. bleeding _____
8. stomach acid _____
9. urine _____
10. cilia _____

Values Statements

Valued Outcome: The students will examine issues and lifestyle factors associated with various conditions.

Description of Strategy: The following list contains several unfinished sentences that can help initiate discussion. The teacher can design her or his own questions to meet the individual needs of the children.

1. My heart is _____.
2. Smoking is _____.
3. Having someone sneeze on me _____.
4. I go to the doctor when _____.
5. A good diet _____.
6. People with diabetes should _____.
7. Cancer is _____.
8. If a friend had cancer, I _____.
9. Preventing heart disease _____.
10. AIDS is _____.
11. If I had a friend with AIDS, I _____.
12. Someone who is not feeling well should _____.

Facts and Myths

Valued Outcome: The students will determine what is true and false concerning various diseases and conditions.

Description of Strategy: The following are questions that students can be asked to vote on concerning heart disease, cancer, or infectious diseases. Other questions can be formulated for other topics. Have the children put their thumbs up if they agree and thumbs down if they disagree. Children can fold their hands if they have no opinion.

1. Do you think exercise is good for your heart?
2. Do you think your diet affects your heart?
3. Do you think exercise is good for your health?
4. How many think that there is no cure for cancer?
5. Can you get cancer from another person?
6. Can you get cancer from overexposure to the sun?
7. Can infectious diseases be spread by sneezing?
8. Do you think you should be around someone who is ill?
9. Does washing your hands help prevent disease?

Decision Stories

Your Heart's Eating Habits

Jenny's grandmother recently had a myocardial infarction, or heart attack. The grandmother was only fifty-four years of age. The heart attack was precipitated by the presence of atherosclerosis. Jenny's great-aunt, her grandmother's sister, died of heart disease when she was only sixty-one. Jenny's family eats a lot of food high in fat, and they all tend to be overweight. Jenny's mom and dad are concerned about the grandmother, and they are worried about Jenny's mom, who is thirty-four, and even Jenny, who is only eleven. The doctor has indicated that Jenny's family needs to change their eating habits, but they all really enjoy eating. Diets have never been successful in this family.

Focus Question: What are some options that Jenny and her family have in dealing with this problem?

Level: Fourth through sixth grades.

Moles Can Change

Andy's dad has a mole on his foot that has been changing in appearance. It is growing and is an unusual black color. The mole has been on his dad's foot for as long as he can remember, but it has only recently changed in looks. Andy's dad insists that it is only because of the way his shoes have been rubbing his foot. Andy's mom has expressed some concern due to the changes. Andy knows that an obvious change in a wart or mole is one of the warning signals of cancer.

Focus Question: What should Andy's dad do?

Level: Third through sixth grades.

Play Ball

Sam has allergies in the spring. This year he is ten years old and wants to try out for the school baseball team, but tryouts occur when his allergies bother him the most. His parents told him he should just stay inside during the spring and wait until his allergies clear up. Sam says that playing baseball is really important to him. All his friends play on teams, and they have a really great time. Besides, Sam doesn't have anyone to play with because all his friends are involved in sports.

Focus Question: Should Sam try out for the baseball team, or stay inside as his parents suggest?

Level: Second through fifth grades.

Dramatization

Two examples of dramatization are provided. These can be modified according to need and grade level.

Betty Bacteria

Valued Outcome: The students will be able to describe how communicable diseases are spread through lack of sanitary habits.

Description of Strategy: Younger students can act out a skit stressing the importance of cleansing wounds when they occur. Discussion can include topics such as the importance of washing all wounds, cuts, and scrapes, as well as preventive care, and washing hands at appropriate times. Ask the students to identify how germs are spread. Question the students on how they felt when they were becoming ill—list the systems on the board. Ask the children if they know how they "caught their disease." Introduce the skit by telling the children they are going to see one way diseases can be contracted. The characters for the skit include Betty Bacteria, Zach, the little boy, Mother, Narrator.

Materials Needed: The props for the skit include a medicine container, Band-Aid, piece of hose, and soap. A script should be provided for each child.

Script for Betty Bacteria

Narrator: It is Saturday afternoon. Mother is outside washing the car when Zach comes running up.

Zach: Mom! Mom! (Zach is crying). I hurt my leg and it's bleeding very badly! Mom, make it stop hurting! (Zach sits down and shows his mother his knee. Betty Bacteria is standing beside Zach's knee. She starts laughing.)

Betty: Now is my chance! I am going to get inside Zach's cut and make it all infected! I love to make people hurt! (Betty moves closer and closer to Zach's cut.)

Mom: I know just what to do, Zach. First, we are going to wash it so that no germs will get inside of it and make you sick. Wait here while I get the soap and some medicine and a bandage.

Betty: No! No! Don't use soap and water on me! I don't like soap and water! I can't live if soap and water are around and a cut is all clean. I better start making Zach's cut sick as quickly as I can. (Betty touches Zach's knee with her hand as Zach's mom returns.) (Mom picks up the hose and washes Zach's knee off. Betty jerks her hand back.)

Betty: Stop! Stop! I don't like water. Water will make me go away, and I want to hurt Zach! (Mom rubs the soap over Zach's knee and then rinses it off. Using a towel, she dries it and proceeds to rub an antibiotic on the cut. Betty is crying and starts to shrivel up and go away.)

Betty: This is no fun. I can't live with soap and water. Soap and water are the end of me. (Betty disappears off stage.)

Mom: Now your cut is nice and clean, and the medicine will keep any new germs from coming around and trying to hurt you. Do you feel better?

Zach: I feel much better now, Mom. Thanks for taking care of my cut.

Processing Questions:

1. What did you learn from today's lesson?

2. Can someone explain how disease germs are spread?

3. How can we prevent the spread of disease germs?

Role-playing—"Catching Cold"

Valued Outcome: The students will describe how sneezing can spread disease

Description of Strategy: Have the students role-play the following situation. Bill and Jay are eating lunch together. Bill has a cold. Bill sneezes and doesn't cover his nose and mouth while sitting beside Jay. Jay is wiping himself off when Aimee comes up and sits down beside them. She asks Jay why he is so upset.

Materials Needed: one spray bottle that can be used as the "sneeze"
Processing Questions:

1. Why do you think Jay is upset?

2. What should Bill have done when he had to sneeze?

3. Do you think Jay can catch a cold from Bill? Why?

4. Can Aimee catch the cold from Bill, since he just sneezed?

Discussion and Report Strategies

Disease Search

Valued Outcome: The students will be able to identify the most common diseases and discuss how they might have been prevented.
Description of Strategy: Have the students ask their parents which chronic and communicable diseases have been experienced within the immediate family (parents, grandparents, aunts, and uncles). These diseases would include heart disease, cancer, arthritis, allergies, measles, chicken pox, mumps, and so on. Students can then bring in lists of these diseases and turn them in to be placed on the board. Going down the list, have students raise their hands if someone in their family has had the disease. When finished, note the diseases that have been experienced the most, ranking from least to most common.
Materials Needed: responses can be placed either on the board or on butcher paper; marker to record responses
Processing Questions:

1. What seem to be the diseases experienced most by our group?

2. How many of the diseases listed have you personally had?

3. How could some of these diseases been avoided?

Name That Disease

Valued Outcome: Each student will be able to discuss the important signs and symptoms of various diseases.
Description of Strategy: Students working in groups can select a disease (infectious or chronic) and research the causes, signs or symptoms, and methods of treatment for the disease. The information should be placed on large sheets of paper and placed on the walls for each child to read. Oral reports may be given, using the large sheets as teaching aids.
Materials Needed: markers, butcher paper, and references for children to research the various diseases
Processing Questions:

1. What were some important points we learned about diseases in general?

2. For the diseases each of you read about, what were some facts that surprised you?

3. How are diseases treated?

What Should Be Done?

Valued Outcome: The children will be able to discuss what the school policy is concerning illness.
Description of Strategy: Allow the students to investigate the school policy on illness. Hold a discussion on appropriate actions to take when someone becomes ill. What should the teacher do? What should the students do? What is the responsibility of the school? How can the school nurse help (if one is available)? A variation of this strategy is to have the students write the policy and present it to the principal.
Materials Needed: copies of the school policy
Processing Questions:

1. Do you think the policies cover everything needed?
2. What would you do if a friend became ill?
3. What should be done if the school nurse is not at school when someone becomes ill?

Experiments and Demonstrations

Physical Fitness Test

Valued Outcome: After participating in the various fitness tests, the children will be able to discuss how being fit enhances their health.
Description of Strategy: Physical fitness can contribute significantly to the prevention of cardiovascular diseases. Several groups have developed fitness tests for school-age children. One of the newest is published by the American Alliance for Health, Physical Education, Recreation, and Dance (AAHPERD). Physical Best is a comprehensive fitness education and assessment program that has three components. They are (1) a health-related fitness assessment, (2) an education component, and (3) a set of awards to reinforce positive health changes and recognize personal achievement. The fitness assessment contains norms for girls and boys, ages five to eighteen years old. Further information can be obtained by contacting AAHPERD at 1900 Association Drive, Reston, VA 22091.
Materials Needed: The materials can be obtained from AAHPERD or other professional groups.
Processing Questions:

1. What did you learn about your physical fitness level?
2. How does being physically fit make you a more healthy person?
3. Does being physically fit protect you from diseases?

The Anatomy of the Heart

Valued Outcome: The children will be able to identify the various structures of the human heart and explain the function of each.
Description of Strategy: Ask the meat department at the local grocery to donate a beef heart for dissecting purposes. The class can observe as various structures of the heart are noted. The atria, ventricles, aortas, and various valves can be pointed out. The function of each structure also should be pointed out.
Materials Needed: rubber gloves, scalpel, paper towels, chart of the structures of the human heart

Processing Questions:

1. How many pumping stations does the heart have?
2. What functions does each part of the heart fulfill?
3. How does the blood get to the heart muscle?

Wash Those Hands

Valued Outcomes: The children will be able to discuss how germs are spread from person to person.

Description of Strategy: The purpose of this activity is to teach the students the importance of washing their hands. Stress that the hands must be washed before eating or touching food, before setting the table, and after using the restroom. Have the students spray water on a piece of dark colored paper. Explain that sneezes and coughs spray germs the same way water sprays on paper. Consequently the mouth must be covered each time a person sneezes or coughs, and the hands must be washed each time the person sneezes. Explain that the hands may look clean, but germs are still present. Demonstrate for the class the proper way to wash hands. Emphasize that germs hide on the front and back of their hands as well as between the fingers and under the nails.

Materials Needed: spray bottle of water, dark colored paper, soap, paper towels

Processing Questions:

1. Why is sneezing and coughing a good way to spread germs?
2. Why is it important to wash your hands?
3. How should we wash our hands?

Analyzing Cigarette Smoke

Valued Outcome: The children will be able to list the many harmful materials found in cigarettes.

Description of Strategy: This activity was developed by Dr. David White and Linda Rudisill. Due to the danger inherent in the chemicals involved, actual ingredients are not used. All ingredients represent by-products of cigarette use. The students are not informed as to what the ingredients represent. They are to guess, based on their knowledge. The entire script is provided for the activity.

Lesson Focus: How many of you have ever received products in the mail to sample, such as soap, shampoo, or toothpaste? The makers provide a small amount for us to try, and then we decide if we want to purchase the product. Suppose we could sample one of these products by breaking it down and trying the main ingredients, or analyzing it. (Teacher may want to discuss the meaning of *analyze*.) We might know much more about a product if we could analyze it, rather than simply trying a sample. The purpose of this lesson is to help you analyze a product that is used by millions of people in the United States. Its popularity, however, has been declining for several years. (Emphasize here that it is important not to comment on what the product is until instruction is complete. Have students write the name of the product on a sheet of paper when they think they have guessed correctly.)

Teacher Input: I will NOT ask you to sample these items as I describe them. When I have completed the discussion, you can then decide if you want to try them. Remember, if you do not want to try it, your grade will NOT be affected.

Point to balloons: The product that we are analyzing is associated with over 500 gases and several thousand chemicals. Since I would have to go to a lot of trouble to bring you over 500 gases, I just brought two of them in balloons. This balloon contains some *carbon monoxide*. Joe, after I describe the other chemicals, would you please inhale the gas in this balloon. This gas is odorless, colorless, and although this amount should not hurt you, this gas is deadly. When you use this product, your blood transports five to ten times more carbon monoxide than normal. This is because carbon monoxide binds to hemoglobin about 240 times more strongly than oxygen.

Now, Joe, I know what you are thinking. Why should only a guy try this? Sue, I would like you to choose a balloon and try it, too. Remember, if you use the average amount of this product daily, you will lose 6 to 8 percent of your body's oxygen-carrying capacity.

Point to other balloons: I have put another of the gases from this product in these balloons. This gas is *hydrogen cyanide*. Hydrogen cyanide is a gas that has been used in the gas chamber. When you use the product we are analyzing, the hydrogen cyanide paralyzes your cilia for 20 to 30 seconds. (Teacher may need to explain the functions of the cilia here.) Now, Carl, would you and Judy sample this ingredient by breathing the gas in these balloons? I'm fairly sure that the amount I have in here will not hurt you; however, remember that this gas paralyzes, or freezes, your cilia for 20 to 30 seconds each time you use this product.

Hold up the jar of flour (arsenic): In this jar I have a little arsenic. Kathy, would you sample this for us later? I have clean spoons for both you and Tom. Arsenic is a silvery-white, tasteless, poisonous chemical used in making insecticides. It looks like flour, and that is what it is mixed with in this jar. Arsenic is associated with the product we are analyzing.

Hold up a glass jar (about one cup) of chocolate syrup (tar): In this jar I have a brown sticky substance. If you use the average amount of the product we are analyzing, your body will collect about a cup of this brown, sticky substance a year. Tom, would you put your finger in this jar and then lick your finger?

Refer students to jar of clear syrup (nicotine): This substance is a poison. It can kill instantly in its pure form, but I have mixed it so that it will not kill you. It looks like clear syrup, so that is what it is mixed with. This poison is habit forming. It speeds the heart rate an extra 15 to 25 beats per minute, or as many as 10,000 extra beats a day. Also, it constricts the blood vessels and quickens breathing. George, would you sample this for us? Remember, a one-drop injection of this substance would cause death! Jean, you are so cooperative in class, would you mind doing this with George so he won't feel so uneasy? Also, when you use this product, this poison reaches your brain in only seven seconds. If it were not for this ingredient, people would probably not be interested in long-term use of the product we are analyzing.

Now, are you all ready to sample a few of the ingredients in this product? Before you answer, I want to give you some facts about this product. (Teacher can discuss or delete from this list, as is desirable.)

○ If you start using this product now and continue, you can expect to lose six and one-half years of your life.

○ If you use it a lot, your chances of dying between the ages of 26 and 65 are about twice as great as for those who do not use this product.

○ Over 100,000 physicians have quit using this product.

○ Before this day is over, approximately 4,500 young people will have tried or started using this product. By the time they graduate from high school, half the nation's teenagers will have used this product, 18 percent on a daily basis.

○ About 1.5 billion of these products are used by 54 million Americans for an average of about twenty-seven each day. The substances in this product are the primary cause of 360,000 known deaths a year, an average of 1,000 deaths a day.

○ Using this product is one of the largest self-inflicted risks a person can take. It is responsible for more premature deaths and disability than any other known agent.

○ More people die from using this product than seven times our annual death toll from highway accidents.

○ A pregnant woman who uses this product may be affecting the health of her unborn child. Comparing users with nonusers, users have a higher percentage of stillbirths, a greater number of spontaneous abortions and premature births, and more of the infants die a few weeks after birth. The child's long-term physical and intellectual development may be adversely affected.

○ This product will stain your teeth, and users often have bad breath.

You might say, "Surely a person can stop using this product whenever he or she wants to." My reply is "not necessarily." Remember the habit-forming substance we mentioned. Withdrawal symptoms for using this drug often include tension, irritability, restlessness, depression, anxiety, difficulty in concentrating, overeating, constipation, diarrhea, insomnia, and an intense craving for the product.

A few of the things I have not mentioned are:

○ If you use this product, you are 1,000 percent more likely to die from lung cancer than those who do not use it.

○ You are 500 percent more likely to die of chronic bronchitis and emphysema if you use it.

○ Average users of this product are 70 percent more likely to die of coronary artery disease. They also tend to suffer from more respiratory infections, such as colds, than nonusers.

○ Finally, this product is so dangerous that four rotating warning labels are required by law to be on the package.

If you were sent this product in the mail to sample, would you be likely to try it? If you received a box in the mail and, on the outside, these facts were printed, would you try it?
Have students name the product.
Lesson Closure
End the lesson with a statement about the importance of making wise decisions that influence your life in positive ways. For example, the teacher might say, "*You* have the power to influence your future in vital ways. The choice is up to you. No one can keep you from smoking, and it definitely will affect your entire life, however short or long it may be. Why start and get hooked? If you want to smoke, it is your life. But it is the only one you will ever get. The only safe cigarette is an unlit cigarette."
Materials Needed: four balloons (two representing carbon monoxide and two representing hydrogen cyanide), a small glass jar of flour (representing arsenic), one cup of chocolate syrup (tars), and a cup of clear syrup (nicotine)
Processing Questions:

1. Who is responsible for your using or not using cigarettes?

2. What are some of the bad things found in cigarettes?

3. What are some of the scariest things about cigarettes?

Source: D. M. White and L. Rudisill. 1987, August–September. Analyzing cigarette smoke. *Health education,* 50–51. Used with permission.

Minidocumentary for Cancer and Infectious Diseases

Valued Outcome: The students will be able to discuss cancer and many forms it can take.
Description of Strategy. Set the activity up like the "Sixty Minutes" or "20/20" TV programs. The concept is for each child to be a "star" of her own television show. Videotaping the show allows everyone to see the production again. The videotape would be good for showing at PTA functions.
How the Minidocumentary Works
Each student chooses a notecard on a particular area of cancer. On this card are several questions that she will research and discuss. They are also given a title for themselves and may choose their own names. As an example, a student chooses "cancerous tumors." Her card will read

Dr. _____, a leading oncologist from Harvard.

1. What are tumors?

2. What are two different types of tumors?

3. Are there any special tests to detect tumors?

4. Do tumors exhibit any special symptoms?

The rest is left up to the student. The student must find the correct answers and be able to report her findings on "TV." The following is a list that could be consulted for the remaining cancer topics.

1. physiology of cancer cells

2. cancerous tumors

3. most common causes of cancer

4. carcinogens

5. warning signals of cancer

6. tests for cancer

7. treatments for cancer

8. most common cancers in women

9. breast cancer

10. cancer of the uterus

11. most common cancers in males

12. lung cancer

13. cancer of the prostate gland

14. cancer of the testes

15. cancer of the larynx

16. oral cancer

17. skin cancer

18. cancer of the esophagus

19. cancer of the stomach

20. colorectal cancer

21. thyroid cancer

22. Hodgkin's disease

23. leukemia

24. cancer in children

25. the American Cancer Society

Two students must be chosen to fill the spots of commentator and interviewer. The commentator's job is to introduce the show and make some concluding statements at the end, whereas the interviewer is responsible for accepting the notecards from the specialists, introducing them, and asking the questions. (The students who have the most enthusiasm and originality seem to be best suited for these roles.) A small "set," consisting of chairs, a table, and a lamp could be constructed so that the camera operator can focus on both of the "stars" at once. To avoid confusion and allow continuity of the show while videotaping, a list should be posted so that everyone knows when her interview is coming up. The specialist takes her seat on the "set," gives her notecard to the interviewer, and when all is quiet, the camera operator gives a "ready . . . action!"

As soon as the interview is finished, the next specialist comes up and gets ready to go. The interviewee may also wear a lab coat and a stethoscope to add to the total effect. If each interview lasts one to two minutes, the whole show can be completed in a single class period. The students may be evaluated on their degree of research and their ability to answer the questions correctly. With a little enthusiasm, originality, and even humor, a fairly monotonous topic can be developed into an exciting and refreshing educational tool.

Even though cancer is a prime example of the topics that could be used, the minidocumentary does not need to be limited to cancer only. The same activity can be done using a variety of topics. The following is a list of possible topics for infectious diseases.

1. viruses

2. bacteria

3. fungi

4. protozoa

5. pathogens

6. incubation period

7. active immunity

8. passive immunity

9. diphtheria

10. whooping cough

11. tetanus

12. poliomyelitis

13. measles

14. German measles

15. mumps

16. chicken pox

17. common cold

18. influenza

19. tuberculosis

20. infectious mononucleosis

21. infectious hepatitis

Materials Needed: videotaping equipment, books and pamphlets for children to research the various topics, small set for videotaping (children can make)
Processing Questions:

1. What new information did you discover from the television program?

2. What do all the various conditions discussed seem to have in common?

3. What are some things we might do to protect ourselves against such diseases?

Source: This activity is reprinted with permission from *Health Education,* September–October 1983, 42–43. *Health Education* is a publication of the American Alliance for Health, Physical Education, Recreation and Dance, 1900 Association Drive, Reston VA 22091.

A microscope is an invaluable learning tool for students studying pathogens.

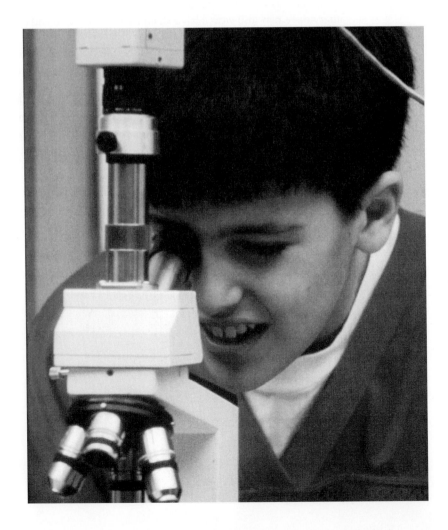

Draw a Bug

Valued Outcome: The students will be able to identify what pathogens cause various diseases.
Description of Strategy: Show pictures of the various pathogens (viruses, bacteria, fungi, and so on). Have the students draw and color one of the pathogens. On the board or overhead projector, list the names of various diseases. On their paper, have the students list the diseases caused by the pathogen they drew.
Materials Needed: pictures or drawing of the various pathogens and a list of diseases
Processing Questions:

1. How many diseases did the pathogen you drew cause?
2. Are some of them more serious than others?
3. How can a certain pathogen cause so many illnesses?

Things I Know, Things I'd Like to Know

Valued Outcome: The students will identify and answer areas of concern for various diseases.
Description of Strategy: Select several diseases or conditions for students to investigate. The students must write down what they think is true concerning each disease. Students can then list some questions (establish a minimum number) they have concerning each disease. During investigation, they can determine the accuracy of their ideas on their specific disease and learn the answers to the questions they have written.

Things I Know, Things I'd Like to Know

Disease or Condition

Things I know	T	F	Things I'd like to know	Answers
1. _____	___	___	1. _____	_____
2. _____	___	___	2. _____	_____
3. _____	___	___	3. _____	_____
4. _____	___	___	4. _____	_____
5. _____	___	___	5. _____	_____

Materials Needed: Charts on which the students can list what they know and what they want to know
Processing Questions:

1. Was any of the information you thought you knew incorrect?
2. What was one new thing you learned from the activity?

The "Bert Bird Knows" Mobile

Valued Outcome: The student will be able to list the risk factors associated with various diseases and conditions.

Description of Strategy: Have the students construct a mobile as shown in Figure 15.2. Each square would be a risk factor for cardiovascular disease or some other disease. The Bird can be reused as the children make cards for various other conditions or diseases.

Materials Needed: cardboard, paper, string, and lists of factors for whatever condition to be placed on the mobile

Processing Questions:

1. What can we do to protect ourselves against the factors listed on our Bert Bird?

2. Are any of the risk factors we have identified the same for other conditions?

3. Of the factors listed, what seems to be the most serious?

Figure 15.2
The Bert Bird Knows Mobile

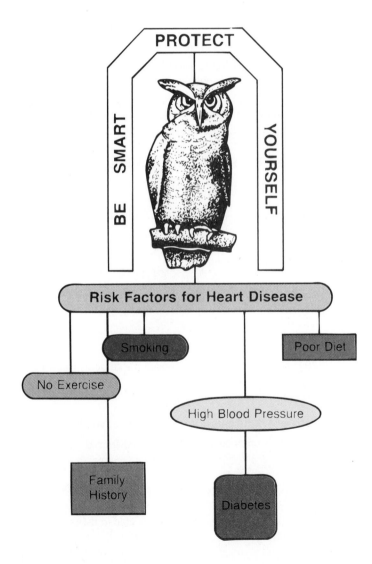

Puzzles and Games

Listed here are several suggestions for supplementing or building a lesson. Obviously the teacher must design and develop these activities to fit his or her students' abilities. They are great fun and provide excellent learning tools.

Word Search

Instruct students to find and circle the terms listed in the word search shown in Figure 15.3.

Figure 15.3
Heart Word Search

A	C	C	Q	E	J	D	W	S	D	M	F	Q	H	L	N	J	E	E
P	F	R	I	N	S	U	E	V	F	H	T	X	G	H	I	M	L	K
U	I	Y	R	S	Y	I	Y	V	N	Z	R	E	X	D	X	C	V	A
R	Z	V	W	H	R	V	O	S	W	Y	W	D	S	M	S	N	P	J
U	D	G	T	E	W	B	E	Z	Z	L	Z	O	K	U	V	S	H	A
W	G	P	T	O	N	N	R	I	T	Z	T	E	M	B	O	L	U	S
V	B	R	W	H	T	E	I	R	N	M	L	C	S	N	M	H	O	P
E	A	N	O	X	Y	H	M	G	K	S	A	Q	M	F	G	Z	V	Q
N	W	A	T	I	V	P	H	G	B	I	M	T	M	S	X	G	S	C
A	D	M	M	N	P	R	E	W	D	W	A	E	E	I	M	L	S	G
C	F	Z	C	Y	K	P	I	R	N	A	N	G	I	N	A	S	Y	W
A	U	R	X	W	O	A	A	N	T	D	O	A	P	A	S	Z	T	R
V	E	N	T	R	I	C	L	E	S	E	R	R	X	X	P	W	C	Q
A	S	T	R	O	K	E	A	P	T	G	N	X	T	W	J	F	B	N
K	R	T	A	H	U	M	V	R	S	V	W	S	A	A	B	S	H	A
C	F	S	S	Q	O	A	A	X	D	A	T	R	I	U	M	A	E	F
F	S	F	A	U	T	K	Y	G	V	I	D	X	S	O	O	I	B	N
I	O	L	S	F	I	E	O	N	R	O	U	W	R	J	N	Z	J	T
B	P	I	V	H	D	R	X	L	T	N	P	M	L	G	D	O	U	Y

Can you find these words?

CARDIACMUSCLE
VENTRICLES
VENACAVA
PLAQUE
VEINS
HYPERTENSION
PACEMAKER
EMBOLUS
ANGINA
AORTA
MYOCARDIUM
ARTERIES
ATRIUM
STROKE

Cancer Crossword Puzzle

Distribute copies of the crossword puzzle shown in Figure 15.4, and have each student complete one.

Infectious Diseases Word Search

For the word search in Figure 15.5, ask each student to find and circle the designated words.

Figure 15.4

Cancer Crossword Puzzle

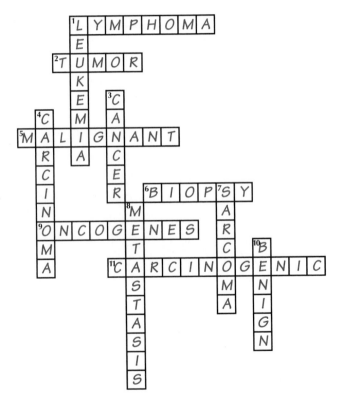

ACROSS
1. Cancer affecting the lymph nodes.
2. Abnormal growth.
5. A term used to indicate a cancerous growth.
6. Taking a small section of tissue to determine if it is cancerous is called a _____.
9. Genes thought to cause cancer.
11. Any substance that may cause cancer is a _____ agent.

DOWN
1. A type of cancer affecting the white blood cells.
3. Uncontrolled cell growth.
4. Cancer of the soft tissue.
7. Cancer of the connective tissue.
8. When cancer cells move from one location in the body to another location.
10. Noncancerous growth is a _____ tumor.

Figure 15.5
Infectious Diseases
Word Search

```
N E S Q Z S R E L L E G O L J D D L I T O
I M O M P G O T P I M I M M U N I T Y V N
T U B E R C U L O S I S T L U O P U A L C
E P G A O I N F L U E N Z A B U H B H E M
T F R S T I U X I T M Q M B R B T R S L E
A Z C L O I Q D O D N Y Y I B Q H B G I V
N U Q E Z S R M M U M P S P L B E I L D B
U D O S O Z Z A Y O F U N G I R R B H R F
S G B Y A N V Y E I N C U B A T I O N S O
E F J L D G B J L I N O G V A A W E Y X
G W J O V R A O I R A L N C S D E H I T G
H H I F M U C C T F C E O U I S J C R N H
F U K C H S T J J I W G N R H C Z D J Q N J
U N C A N K E S S O P I Y P E L G C U V N
M H B F H Y R I H T V L G T K W E H C Y N
R Y P I C L I T K F X Y F R I K O O I G M
J T W W R P A T G S H E P A T I T I S I S
V X M V R P D H K L T F N M T X L M I I O
W S O Y A B Q C P M Z N C Y L B K Z N I S
```

Can you find these words?

MONONUCLEOSIS

INCUBATION

DIPHTHERIA

PROTOZOA

TETANUS

VIRUS

POLIOMYELITIS

HEPATITIS

IMMUNITY

BACTERIA

MUMPS

TUBERCULOSIS

INFLUENZA

PATHOGEN

MEASLES

FUNGI

Word Scramble

Have your students unscramble the following words (correct order appears in parentheses after each word):

gahtposne (pathogens)

brmeisco (microbes)

suvries (viruses)

carebiat (bacteria)

stekracisit (rickettsias)

niguf (fungi)

orazotpo (protozoa)

nslehtmhi (helminths)

snxito (toxins)

trovesc (vectors)

tacinoibun gaste (incubation stage)

dalmroper tagse (prodromal stage)

yercover setag (recovery stage)

ityummin (immunity)

gatinen (antigen)

Hidden Message to Help Prevent Heart Disease

Have each student complete the following activity, and provide the following directions: Using the listed words, fill in the blanks in the sentences. Then place the answers in the spaces provided after all the sentences. The letters in the box reveal a hidden message.

pacemaker   veins

tobacco   embolus

aneurysm   stroke

hypertension   arteriosclerosis

cardiac

1. The heart is called the _____ muscle.
2. Cigarettes are made from _____.
3. Blood returns to the heart through the _____.
4. When a clot or vessel breakage occurs in the brain, that event is called a _____.
5. High blood pressure is known as _____.
6. A free-floating blood clot is called an _____.
7. _____ is the term for the collection of diseases characterized by hardening of the arteries.
8. The specialized group of cells called the *sinoatrial* node is also called the _____ of the heart.
9. Ballooning that occurs in weakened or damaged arterial walls is an _____.

Place your answers here for the secret message.

1.   c a r **d** i a c
2.   t **o** b a c c o
3.   v e i **n** s
4.   s **t** r o k e
5. h y p e r t e **n** s i o n
6.   e **m** b o l u s
7.   a r t e r i **o** s c l e r o s i s
8.   p a c e m a **k** e r
9.   a n **e** u r y s m

Resources

Books

Lammers, J. W. 1996. *I don't feel good—a guide to childhood complaints and diseases.* Santa Cruz, CA: ETR Associates. (Grades K–5)

Quackenbush, M., and Villarreal, S. 1995. *Does AIDS hurt? educating young children about AIDS.* Santa Cruz, CA: ETR Associates. (Grades K-3)

Scheer, J. K. 1995. *Teaching kids about how AIDS works.* Santa Cruz, CA: ETR Associates. (Grades K-6 curriculum guides)

_____ 1996. *Germ smart: Children's activities in disease prevention.* Santa Cruz, CA: ETR Associates. (Grades K-3)

Tillman, K.G., and Toner, P. R. 1990. *How to survive teaching health—games, activities, and worksheets for Grades 4–12.* West Nyak, NY: Parker.

Vickery, D. M., and J. F. Fries. *Take care of yourself: A consumer's guide to medical care.* 1993. Reading, MA: Addison-Wesley.

CD-ROMs/Computer Software

Mosby's medical encyclopedia for health consumers. A teacher resource that includes nearly 20,000 medical terms; audio pronunciations for over 4000 terms; more than 1200 full-color illustrations, video clips, and animations. (Teacher and grades 5 and up)

Pamphlets

HIV fast facts—The basics (Grades 6–9). Santa Cruz, CA: ETR Associates. Explains the difference between HIV and AIDS, how you get it, and prevention strategies.

HIV ABC's (Grades 6 and up). Santa Cruz, CA: ETR Associates. Comprehensive information on HIV.

Web Sites

American Heart Association (offers information on heart disease, prevention, nutrition, smoking cessation)
http://www.amhrt.org/

(Provides information on minority populations)
http://www.uvm.edu/~vdouglas/project.htm

(multimedia site on exploration of the heart)
http://www.fi.edu/biosci/heart.html

National Cancer Institute (wide range of cancer information)
http://www.nci.nih.gov/

(Offers an overview on skin cancer and a UV index)
http://www.maui.net/~southsky/introto.html

University of Pennsylvania Medical Center (OncoLink covers all aspects of cancer. Excellent source of information regarding cancer and cancer therapy)
http://www.cancer.med.upenn.edu/

American Lung Association (provides a list of programs and events that can be obtained from local area)
http://www.lungusa.org/

Joint Committee on Smoking and Health (fact sheet)
http://www.chestnet.org/smoking.html

Resource center focusing on tobacco and smoking issues
http://www.tobacco.org/

Center for AIDS Prevention Studies (presents a wide range of topics ranging from HIV testing to prevention)
http://www.caps.ucsf.edu/capsweb

Center for Disease Control (provides information on prevention of HIV, guidelines, and morbidity and mortality weekly reports)
http://www.cdc.gov/

(Links to AIDS-related information, information on other STDs)
http://www.niaid.hib.gov/

(Best starting place for cancer information; see the University of Pennsylvania Medical Center site listed earlier)
http://www.oncolink.edu

Videos

Come see what the Doctor sees (Grades 3–6). Students get to see and listen through doctor's instruments and learn various body functions. They also discover the "why" of blood and urine tests. Twenty-five-minute video available from Sunburst Communications, 101 Castleton Street, Pleasantville, NY 10570-0040.

Come see how we fight infections. (Grades 3–6). Describes how the immune system works and its various components. Viruses and bacteria are shown as well as how to keep the immune system strong and functioning properly. Twenty-five-minute video available from Sunburst Communications, 101 Castleton Street, Pleasantville, NY 10570-0040.

Coping with childhood cancer. (Grades 5–8). Program presents five open and honest interviews with family members of childhood cancer patients. Twenty-eight-minute video available from Films for the Humanities and Sciences, P. O. Box 2053, Princeton, NJ 08543-2053.

Kids and doctors. (Grades 1–6). Highlights the case of a ten-year-old boy with asthma and juvenile rheumatoid arthritis. Nineteen-minute video available from Films for the Humanities and Sciences, P. O. Box 2053, Princeton, NJ 08543-2053.

Zardip's search for healthy wellness. (Grades 1–5). A twenty-part series of animation, live action, and songs to promote an understanding of how the body works. Disease-oriented videos include *Germs, More Germs, The Doctor, Hospital Visit,* and *Laurie's Operation.* Fifteen-minute videos available from Films for the Humanities and Sciences, P. O. Box 2053, Princeton, NJ 08543-2053.

AIDS: The double connection. (Grades 5-8). Uses animated clay characters to explain how crack cocaine and other drugs can lead to unsafe sexual practices and to HIV infection. Explains how HIV is and is not transmitted. Eight-minute video available from The National Center for Elementary Drug and Violence Prevention, 117 Highway 815, P. O. Box 9, Calhoun, KY 42327-0009.

Chapter Sixteen

Nutrition

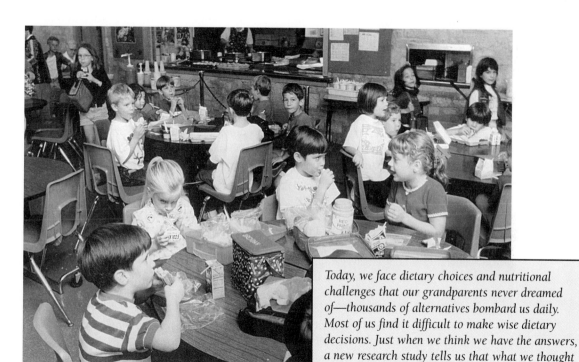

> Today, we face dietary choices and nutritional challenges that our grandparents never dreamed of—thousands of alternatives bombard us daily. Most of us find it difficult to make wise dietary decisions. Just when we think we have the answers, a new research study tells us that what we thought was true probably wasn't.
> —Donatelle and Davis (1996, 194)

Valued Outcomes

After reading this chapter, you should be able to

○ discuss the factors that determine food choices

○ describe cultural differences in eating patterns and preparation of foods

○ discuss the USDA's Food Guide Pyramid

○ list the basic function of the different categories of food

○ describe the Reference Daily Intakes

○ discuss the purpose of vitamins and minerals in the body

○ explain the benefits of antioxidants

○ list healthy ways to snack

○ describe the effect of hunger and malnutrition on a student's physical and intellectual development

❍ describe the characteristics of an anorexic and/or bulimic victim

❍ list several hints to help a student reduce or add weight

❍ determine the nutrient value of a food by reading the newly revised food label

Knowledge and Nutrition

Human beings must eat to survive. The well-nourished student is more apt to reach her full potential physically, mentally, and intellectually. Americans today have more health knowledge about nutrition than at any other time in history, yet this knowledge has not translated into proper nutritional and/or lifestyle behavior for all Americans. For years, the majority of Americans paid little attention to nutrition, other than to eat three meals a day, and perhaps, take a vitamin supplement, and fail to exercise. This lifestyle might have prevented major nutritional deficiencies, but medical evidence now links this American diet to a variety of chronic diseases, including obesity (Donatelle and Davis 1996, 194).

Americans live in a very food-affluent society, yet many Americans—not just the poor—are malnourished. An unwillingness to alter lifestyle to meet sound nutritional standards and concessions to convenience are often at the heart of it. In our fast-paced society, people opt to skip meals, especially breakfast, or to eat a poorly balanced meal at a fast-food restaurant. Many parents and teachers fail to provide good examples for their students concerning nutritional habits.

Nutrition education has been included as a priority by the U.S. Department of Health and Human Services in the Year 2000 Health Objectives for the Nation, as listed by the U.S. Surgeon General. The need for nutrition education is crucial. For example, American elementary school students have higher cholesterol levels than students from other countries. Studies indicate that sound school nutrition programs can produce positive outcomes (Miller, Telljohann, and Symons 1996, 13). Helping students develop sound nutritional habits should be one of teachers' major goals in elementary health instruction. To accomplish this, teachers must do more than simply provide information. They must counter the impact of television commercials and other sources. Also, they must help students recognize that although the food they eat is strongly influenced by their culture and their lifestyle, they can learn to control these influences. Teachers must also dispel misconceptions associated with food and nutrition, help students become informed consumers, and develop in them a sense of the importance of nutrition.

Food Habits and Customs

Every culture has its own food habits and customs. Approaches to nutrition are based in part on the food resources available. Food habits and customs in the United States reflect the multicultural nature of our society. At one time, there were significant regional differences in cooking and food preferences. Seafood was a major part of the diet on the East Coast. Wild game provided much of the meat eaten in the rural South. Mexican and Indian cultures influenced the cuisine of the Southwest. Today these regional differences have faded, largely as a result of refrigeration and modern transportation. It is now almost as easy to get fresh fish in Kansas as it is in Massachusetts. Cultural intermixing has also diminished regional differences, while at the same time expanding the range of dishes commonly eaten. Pasta, for instance, is no longer eaten only by Americans of Italian extraction. Chinese, French, German, Mexican, and Middle Eastern dishes have also become popular.

Economic, Personal, and Lifestyle Factors

As an affluent, multiethnic nation, we have a greater variety of foods and dishes to choose from than almost any other people on earth. This does not mean, however, that Americans can afford to eat anything they like. Inflation has influenced the eating habits of all Americans, rich and poor alike—but especially the poor. Those living near or below the poverty level often must subsist on cheap starchy foods, which are filling, if not particularly nutritious.

Although economics influences the American diet, as it does the diet of every nation, most Americans cannot blame lack of money for poor nutritional habits. Instead, we must look for the reasons in personal preferences and lifestyles. Personal preference for a food often is formed by reasons that have little or nothing to do with the nourishment that will be provided by that food. For example, parents typically pass their food preferences on to their children. People develop prejudices against foods because of bad experiences, such as when a food causes an allergic response or gastrointestinal upset. The most popular foods eaten by one's subculture and peer group also influence food choices. Finally, a food might be chosen because of the way it looks, smells, and tastes.

The national lifestyle also influences our nutritional habits. When the United States was mostly a rural, agrarian society, breakfast was a major meal. The main meal of the day was served at noon. These two meals provided the necessary energy for performing farm labor and chores. Evening dinner was typically a lighter meal. Today, the reverse is true. Most Americans eat a light breakfast, and some skip breakfast entirely. Lunch is also a light meal, often eaten in haste. The largest meal of the day is consumed in the evening, because there is more time to prepare and eat such a meal. Unfortunately, this meal is usually followed by general physical inactivity and then by sleep. This is one reason why so many Americans are overweight. Also, many overspice their foods, especially with salt and sugar. Others rush through their meals, which reduces the nourishment received from the foods.

There is not much that teachers and schools can do to change our hectic national lifestyle. However, many schools are recognizing the importance of providing nutrition to students—nearly two-thirds of all schoolchildren in the United States received about a third of their daily nutrients from the school food service program, including breakfast (Miller, Telljohann, and Symons 1996, 13). A good breakfast and lunch provides students with the energy they need for school and studying. In recent years, several studies have documented the benefits of breakfast consumption. Considerable research indicates that breakfast skipping impairs academic performance, whereas breakfast consumption has been associated with improved overall nutritional status. Breakfast skippers have been found to have significantly higher cholesterol levels, gain more weight, and have more body fat than breakfast consumers despite lower daily fat and cholesterol intake (Hales 1994, 139).

Teachers can also emphasize the value of a balanced, nutritional lunch and a reasonable evening meal. This is not to suggest that teachers should criticize the eating patterns of any student's family, and certainly not any religious dietary restrictions a family might have, but they can be a source of information about sound nutritional practices and encourage students to consider changes in their diet that could lead to sounder nutrition. Teachers can also stimulate students' curiosity about trying new dishes that could add needed variety to their diets.

Further, teachers should emphasize that snacking on junk food, such as candy, may spoil a student's appetite for a regular meal as well as contribute to tooth decay. Although children can benefit from snacking, they often fall into the habit of constantly eating the same foods. Snacks sometimes even substitute for, rather than supplement, children's regular meals, and these snacks may not provide the variety of nutrients these youngsters need. Thus, while snacking is regarded as

Health Highlight

Dietary Guidelines for Americans

The U. S. Department of Agriculture has established the following as Dietary Guidelines for Americans:

○ Eat a variety of foods.

○ Balance the food you eat with physical activity—maintain or improve your weight.

○ Choose a diet with plenty of grain products, vegetables, and fruits.

○ Choose a diet low in fat, saturated fat, and cholesterol.

○ Choose a diet moderate in sugars.

○ Choose a diet moderate in salt and sodium.

○ If you drink alcoholic beverages, do so in moderation.

Source: U.S. Department of Agriculture, U.S. Department of Health and Human Services. 1995. *Nutrition and your health: Dietary guidelines for Americans*, 4th ed. Washington, DC: U.S. Government Printing Office.

potential asset to the child's diet, it can become a liability if it results in more calories than are needed. Experts convened by the Center for Science in the Public Interest determined that foods marketed for children closely resemble junk foods. They determined that many of the kids' snacks have excessive amounts of fat, sodium, and sugar, which contribute to heart disease, cancer, and high blood pressure in later life (Bruess and Richardson 1994, 80).

Food is one of the delights of every civilization. In many cultures preparation of some dishes is an art. Eating a fine meal is an aesthetic experience, not just fulfillment of nutritional requirements, but even the simplest dish can provide great pleasure. Teachers can use this positive approach in presenting nutritional concepts. Too often nutrition is taught as a grim and dry subject, divorced from the human perspective. No wonder that students often emerge from health education with scorn for nutritional principles; they associate nutrition with the imagined somber atmosphere of a health food store!

Nutrients

Food's most basic function is to provide these nutrients to the body. Nutrients are the substances in food needed to support life functions. One vital way in which this is accomplished is by providing energy that the body needs. This energy, produced as a by-product of food consumption, is measured in calories. A calorie is defined as the amount of heat energy required to raise the temperature of 1 kilogram of water 1 degree Celsius. All foods have specific caloric values, and a given amount of food will produce a certain number of calories when broken down by the body.

The number of calories needed by the body daily depends on two factors: (1) the individual's basal metabolism and (2) the amount of energy expended in daily activities. Basal metabolism is the minimum amount of heat produced by the body when at rest. This heat, among other things, is necessary to maintain a normal body temperature. The amount of energy expended by an individual varies, depending on the activities of the individual. Thus, someone who engages in heavy physical labor each day needs more calories than someone who works in an office. Young students need fewer calories per day than active adults, because of the difference in body sizes.

According to the new standard called the Daily Reference Values (DRVs), most people should consume 2,000 calories daily. Young men, teenage boys, and all very active people need a greater number of calories daily (Mullen et al. 1996, 71–75). During periods of rapid growth, students also need more calories. For example, a ten-year-old boy requires an average daily intake of about 2,200 calories, with this amount rising to 2,900 calories by age thirteen. A ten-year-old girl requires an average daily intake of 2,200 calories, and 2,400 calories at age thirteen. Three categories of nutrients provide caloric energy: carbohydrates, fats, and proteins. Together, they make up most of the elements in the foods we eat.

Carbohydrates

Foods rich in carbohydrates form about half of the typical American diet. Carbohydrates are either simple sugars, derived from such foods as sugar and honey, or more complex compounds, derived from such foods as cereals and potatoes. For example, the sweet taste of corn and peas is due to the presence of carbohydrate compounds.

Carbohydrates are found in foods as monosaccharides, disaccharides, and polysaccharides. The monosaccharides are glucose (honey and fruits), galactose (human breast milk, fruits, and honey), and fructose (fruits and honey). The disaccharides are sucrose (a combination of glucose and fructose found in bananas, green peas, and sweet potatoes), lactose (a combination of glucose and galactose found in milk), and maltose (a combination of glucose and glucose used in candy flavor and brewing beer). Many adults, especially Asian Americans and African Americans, suffer from lactose intolerance. In other words, undigested lactose is not absorbed and remains in the gastrointestinal tract, resulting in bloating, a large amount of gas, and abdominal cramping. This malady can be treated through a diet that is high in protein, high in carbohydrate, low to moderate in fat, and high in calories. The polysaccharides are comprised of many glucose molecules and are the following: (1) glycogen (which is synthesized in the liver and muscles and serves as a reserve source of blood glucose, (2) cellulose (found in many vegetables), and (3) starch (found in plant seeds, cereal grains, and some vegetables).

Carbohydrates are broken down into glucose, and the metabolism of carbohydrates produces energy. Four calories are produced per gram of carbohydrates. If carbohydrates are not abundant in the diet, protein and fat have to be metabolized to produce needed energy. Carbohydrates must be constantly replenished in the blood, either by eating or by breaking down glycogen stored in the liver and muscles.

Carbohydrates are important in a student's diet and should comprise approximately 58 percent of total calorie intake. Foods rich in carbohydrates include rice, spaghetti, noodles, bread, breakfast cereals, and potatoes. Many vegetables, fruits, and fruit juices also contain some carbohydrates. Although candy and cookies are good sources of carbohydrates, the refined sugar they contain contributes to tooth decay and gum disease and does not provide additional nutrients. If foods such as milk, fruit, and vegetables (because they contain sugars) are eaten, the individual should brush and floss after the meal. If he cannot brush immediately after a meal, he should at least rinse out his mouth with water. Brushing and flossing before bedtime are especially important in reducing tooth decay. Fruits, vegetables, and juices make healthier snacks.

Proteins

Protein means "to come first." This suggests that proteins are essential nutrients. No organism can live, and almost no biological process can take place, without protein. A protein molecule is composed of smaller structures called *amino acids*. Some amino acids are termed *essential*, which means they must be provided by the diet, and some are termed *nonessential*, which means they are synthesized by the body. These amino acids are building blocks necessary for several body functions. Proteins are present in every cell, in enzymes, and in body secretions. Proteins provide calories but also serve other important and complex functions. They are important components of DNA and RNA molecules, which determine individuals' genetic makeup. Also, proteins help build new cells and tissues in growing students, maintain tissues that are already built, and play a role in the manufacture of blood, enzymes, hormones, and human milk. Furthermore, antibodies, which combat infection, are synthesized from proteins in response to infectious agents.

Proteins provide four calories per gram. Proteins should comprise about 12 percent of a student's total caloric intake. Most students require approximately 60 grams (g) of protein daily. Milk and meat products are excellent sources of protein. Poultry is another good source of this essential nutrient.

If a person eats a vegetarian diet, enough protein must be ingested to support normal growth and development, especially in students. This is called *complementary protein ingestion*, a dietary strategy that ensures that each food supplies some amino acids that the others lack. For example, peanut protein is combined with wheat, oats, corn, rice, or coconut, and soy protein is combined with corn, wheat, rye, or sesame. Nonmeat sources of protein include soybeans, dried beans, and nuts. Cereal grains, vegetables, and fruits contain vegetable protein, which must be augmented by other protein sources, as in tortillas and beans combined.

Fats

Fats, or lipids, are the most concentrated source of calories we ingest. Fats provide nine calories per gram, as compared with four for proteins and carbohydrates. There are two types of fatty acids: saturated and unsaturated. The dietary sources of saturated fatty acids are animal fat, beef, butter, chicken eggs, and whole milk. Unsaturated fats are found in vegetable oils, such as corn, olive, soybean, peanut, and safflower oils. The more saturated a fat is, the harder it is at room temperature. Although polyunsaturated fats were favored by nutritional researchers in the early 1980s, today many researchers believe that polyunsaturates may decrease beneficial HDL levels while reducing LDL levels. Monounsaturated fats seem to lower only LDL levels and thus are the "preferred" fats of the 1990s (Donatelle and Davis 1996, 208).

Fats are an important part of our diets. Their vital role is sometimes overlooked because of the association of fats with cardiovascular problems. However, fats serve several vital functions. The energy they provide spares protein for tissue synthesis. Fats also serve as carriers of the fat-soluble vitamins A, D, E, and K. As food, they provide satiety, because the rate at which a meal is emptied from the stomach is related to the fat content. The higher the fat content, the slower the food empties from the stomach.

Fats are an important part of all cells, membrane structures in the body, and tissues. In addition, fats provide protection in the adipose tissue just under the skin. This layer of adipose tissue also helps in maintaining the body temperature at a constant level despite changes in the environmental temperature. Similarly, fats provide a layer of protective shock-absorbing tissue between the kidneys, reproductive organs, and other organs. They also provide padding for the cheeks, palms of the hands, and balls of the feet. Finally, fats make foods more appetizing and flavorful.

Fats should comprise 30 percent of total caloric intake. These fats should be equally divided among polyunsaturated, saturated, and monounsaturated fats. The major food sources of fat are animal and vegetable fats, such as butter, cream, lard, and salad dressings. Olives and nuts also have a significant fat content.

Blood Cholesterol

An issue closely related to ingestion of fats, obesity, and health risks is blood cholesterol levels. Cholesterol is a vital part of the body, but too much of it can result in health risks. Cholesterol is a waxy, fatlike substance found mainly in the liver, kidneys, and brain. Most of the cholesterol is transported through the body as lipoproteins. There are different forms of lipoprotein, and they are classified by their density. The most important forms of lipoprotein are low-density lipoprotein cholesterol (LDL) and the high-density lipoprotein cholesterol (HDL). High levels of LDL indicate a cardiovascular risk. Many blood tests will provide only a total blood cholesterol reading, but a more important factor is the ratio of total cholesterol to HDL. The smaller the ratio, the less the cardiovascular risk.

Even though some foods might be labeled truthfully as containing no cholesterol, these foods might be high in saturated fats (such as coconut or palm oil), which will cause the body to produce more blood cholesterol. Although the body produces more cholesterol than is ingested through foods, the blood cholesterol level can be positively altered through a healthy diet. Generally, foods of animal origin, such as eggs and organ meats, should be reduced, whereas fruits, low-fat dairy products, vegetables, and whole grains should be increased. These foods will increase the amount of fiber in the diet, which will aid in digestion, increase intestinal motility, and possibly further lower cardiovascular risk. High-fiber diets are also beneficial in preventing constipation, obesity, hypoglycemia, heart disease, cancer, and diabetes (University of California at Berkeley 1992, 4).

Recent findings indicate the fish oils rich in unsaturated fats called omega-3 fatty acids actually change the chemistry of the blood to lower the cardiovascular risk. Specifically, these fatty acids lower blood triglycerides, highly saturated fats that contribute to blockage in the arteries. The oil in some seafood depresses LDL and raises HDL. Some seafoods high in omega-3 fatty acids are herring, mackerel, and salmon (U.S. Department of Health and Human Services 1992, 7).

In addition to the three major nutrients, water, minerals, and vitamins are vital to human nourishment.

Water

In considering nutrition, water is often overlooked, but it is second only to oxygen in importance to body functioning. A person can survive longer without food than water; there can be no life without water.

Water is an essential component of body structure. It also acts as a solvent for minerals and other physiologically important compounds. In the body, it transports nutrients to and waste products from the cells. Furthermore, water helps regulate the body temperature. Water comes from fluids and solids in the diet and is also produced by the metabolizing of energy nutrients within the tissues. The amount of activity and the climate are important factors influencing the amount of water a person needs. Because students usually participate in more physical activities, they perspire more and therefore need more water than many adults. Water is also lost through exhaled air. The recommended daily intake is the equivalent of six to eight glasses of water. Much of this is gained from solid foods.

Minerals

The body needs organic compounds, such as carbohydrates, fats, and proteins for proper nutrition, but it also needs inorganic materials, such as minerals. These inorganic elements are present in the body in small amounts, but they play a vital role in nutrition. The major minerals needed by the body are calcium, phosphorus, potassium, sulfur, sodium, chlorine, and magnesium. Food sources for these major minerals are:

calcium—milk, cheese, sardines, salmon, green vegetables

phosphorus—milk, cheese, lean meat

potassium—oranges, bananas, dried fruits

sulfur—eggs, poultry, fish

sodium—table salt, beef, eggs, cheese

chlorine—table salt, meat

magnesium—green vegetables, whole grains

Other mineral elements, known as *trace elements* and required in lesser amounts, are iron, zinc, selenium, magnesium, copper, iodine, fluorine, chromium, molybdenum, and cobalt.

Minerals function in the body in several ways. After the organic compounds have been oxidized, minerals remain to form actual body parts. For example, calcium, magnesium, and phosphorus are components of the bones and teeth. Minerals also act as regulators and are necessary to certain body functions. For example, minerals contribute to the water and electrolyte balance of the body and are important in the functioning of the transmission of nerve impulses. Minerals contribute to the osmotic pressure of body fluids and to the maintenance of neutrality—the acid–base balance of the blood and body tissues. Finally, they make possible the normal rhythm in the heartbeat.

Elevated amounts of some minerals may cause health problems. For example, elevated levels of sodium are associated with high blood pressure and cardiovascular disease. Restricting intake of salt, according to the American Heart Association, is safe, feasible, and probably useful in preventing hypertension in many Americans. Sodium can be restricted through the diet by reducing or eliminating salty foods, such as cured or processed meats; reducing or eliminating salt added to foods; experimenting with the flavor of other seasonings rather than using salt; reading labels and selecting low-sodium products; selecting fresh produce over frozen or canned; limiting the intake of processed foods; and considering sodium intake when selecting foods at fast-food restaurants (Bruess and Richardson 1994, 78).

A lack of essential minerals can cause malnutrition. For example, iron deficiency anemia is a major health problem in the United States and Canada and even more so in the rest of the world. Students deprived of iron will feel tired, and therefore may show a lack of motivation and less ability to work and play (Donatelle and Davis 1996, 216). This deficiency occurs most frequently in infants, adolescent males, and females during childbearing years.

Vitamins

No group of nutrients has captured the imagination of the public more than vitamins. Vitamins were discovered fairly recently, when physicians sought the cause of several diseases such as scurvy. They concluded that the chemical compounds called *vitamins* can make a great deal of difference to health. These vitamin-related discoveries have led people to equate good nutrition with vitamins, and some even thought vitamins contained the essential element for life.

The normal Recommended Daily Allowances (RDA) or Reference Daily Intakes (RDI) for vitamins are sufficient for optimal health. Few American suffer from true vitamin deficiencies if they eat a diet containing all the food groups at least part of the time. Nevertheless, Americans continue to purchase large quantities of vitamin supplements, which for the most part, are unnecessary and, in certain instances, may even be harmful. Overuse of vitamin supplements can lead to a toxic condition known as *hypervitaminosis* (Donatelle and Davis 1996, 211).

Vitamins are organic compounds required by every part of the body to maintain health and prevent disease. They must be provided by the diet because the body is not able to synthesize them in the required amounts. Vitamins foster growth, promote the ability to produce healthy offspring, maintain health, aid in the normal function of the appetite and digestive tract, and help the body's resistance to bacterial infections. Vitamins are classified as either fat soluble or water soluble.

Fat-Soluble Vitamins. Fat-soluble vitamins dissolve in fat and are found in the fatty parts of food and body tissues. They are stored in the body until needed, so it is not necessary to consume them every day. The fat-soluble vitamins transported by lipids through the body are A, D, E, and K. Vitamin A is important in promoting growth and health of body tissues as well as enhancing the function of the immune system. This vitamin also enhances vision by helping the retina function properly, permitting us to distinguish between light and shade and see various colors distinctly. A form of vitamin A is used by dermatologists to treat acne and other skin disorders. Overdoses of vitamin A may result in yellowish, dry, scaly skin and dry, irritated eyes.

Vitamin D is needed to prevent and cure rickets, a deficiency disease in which bones fail to harden. Vitamin E is an activator in certain enzyme reactions, and it protects vitamins A and C from being used up too quickly. Vitamin K is essential for the synthesis of prothrombin, a substance needed for normal blood coagulation.

Water-Soluble Vitamins. Water-soluble vitamins dissolve in water and are associated with the watery parts of food and body tissues. These vitamins are not stored by the body. Excess amounts are usually excreted in the urine and, therefore, should be provided in the diet on a regular basis. The water-soluble vitamins include the B vitamins and vitamin C, or ascorbic acid. The B vitamins are essential to daily human nutrition. Known as the B-complex group, they help body systems combat stress and maintain energy reserves. The B-complex group consists of vitamin B_1 (thiamine), vitamin B_2 (riboflavin), vitamin B_3 (niacin), vitamin B_5 (pantothenic acid), vitamin B_6 (pyridoxine), vitamin B_{12} (cobalamin), folic acid, and biotin.

Thiamine is necessary for carbohydrate metabolism. It aids in the release of energy from food. Riboflavin helps body cells use oxygen, promotes tissue repair, and helps the nervous system function properly. Niacin is essential to growth; without niacin, thiamine and riboflavin could not function properly in the body. Pantothenic acid helps increase vitality and influences glandular functions. Pyridoxine is necessary for healthy teeth and gums and helps maintain normal body cholesterol. Further, it aids in the production of antibodies. Cobalamin works in conjunction with folic acid and iron to build normal blood cells and prevent pernicious anemia. Folic acid aids in the proper growth and reproduction of blood cells and contributes to healthy skin. Biotin is necessary for the proper use of fats, carbohydrates, and protein. Biotin also helps produce antibodies.

Ascorbic acid is vital in preventing scurvy, in the formation and maintenance of collagen (the cementing material that holds cells together), in the normal metabolism of some amino acids, and in the function of the adrenal glands.

Vitamins sometimes serve as catalysts for important body functions. They are required only in small amounts and are vital to nourishment. They are unlike minerals, however, in that they do not become part of the body, as calcium does in the teeth and bones. Overdosing on vitamins can cause serious side effects: loss of coordination, nausea, rashes, diarrhea and fatigue. Excess amounts of the fat-soluble vitamins, stored in the body, can reach toxic levels. Even water-soluble vitamins, taken to extreme, can be dangerous. The key is moderation and a well-balanced diet featuring a range of healthy, vitamin-rich foods.

Food sources for some of the vitamins are:

A—liver, whole milk, butter, dark green leafy vegetables

C—citrus fruits, broccoli, tomatoes, potatoes

D—eggs, liver, fortified milk

E—margarine, salad dressing

K—egg yolk, liver, milk, cabbage

thiamin (B1)—pork, beef, liver, eggs, fish, whole grains, legumes

riboflavin (B2)—milk, green vegetables, cereals

pyridoxine (B6)—pork, milk, eggs, legumes

B12—seafood, meats, eggs, milk

niacin—milk, eggs, fish, poultry

folacin—spinach, asparagus, broccoli, kidney beans

biotin—milk, liver, mushrooms, legumes

Antioxidants

Certain vitamins, especially vitamins C, E, and beta-carotene (vitamin A) contain antioxidants. These antioxidants might play an important role in preventing heart disease, certain types of cancer and other chronic diseases. Antioxidants work by deactivating free radicals, activated oxygen molecules that are a natural by-product of the body metabolizing or burning oxygen. Free radicals can damage body cells, which leads to disease. Antioxidants are believed to prevent this cell damage. Vitamin E has been associated with a decreased risk of heart disease, oral cancer, and cataracts. Vitamin C has been associated with a decreased risk of high blood pressure and an increase in the levels of HDL. Vitamin C, beta-carotene, and vitamin E work together to decrease the risk for coronary artery disease. This information is very encouraging, but the American Heart Association and the American Cancer Society have cautioned us to wait for the results of more long-term studies on the effects of antioxidants (Mullen et al. 1996, 91–94).

Nutritional Needs

About fifty different nutrients are needed to maintain health. No food contains all the nutrients needed, not even milk, which is highly regarded in our society. Therefore, a variety of foods are required to satisfy nutritional needs. One way to assure this variety and to establish a balanced diet is to select foods each day from the types identified in the Food Guide Pyramid (Figure 16.1) by the U.S. Department of Agriculture. The Food Guide Pyramid emphasizes foods from five food groups shown in the three lower sections of the pyramid. None of the food groups is more or less important than the other—in order to be healthy, you need the appropriate number of servings as suggested from all the groups. The USDA Food Guide Pyramid was created as a food guide intended to provide practical information for eating a well-balanced diet (Hahn and Payne 1997, 107–8).

Characteristics of the Types of Food

Fruits are usually good sources of vitamin C, vitamin A, and fiber. Citrus fruits are especially good sources of vitamin C. Two to four servings daily (at least one of which provides vitamin C), each about equal in size to an orange, are recommended.

Vegetables are usually good sources of vitamin A, vitamin C, and fiber. Vegetables are low in calories if served without added fat. Deep green, leafy vegetables such as spinach, kale, collard

Figure 16.1
The USDA Food Guide Pyramid

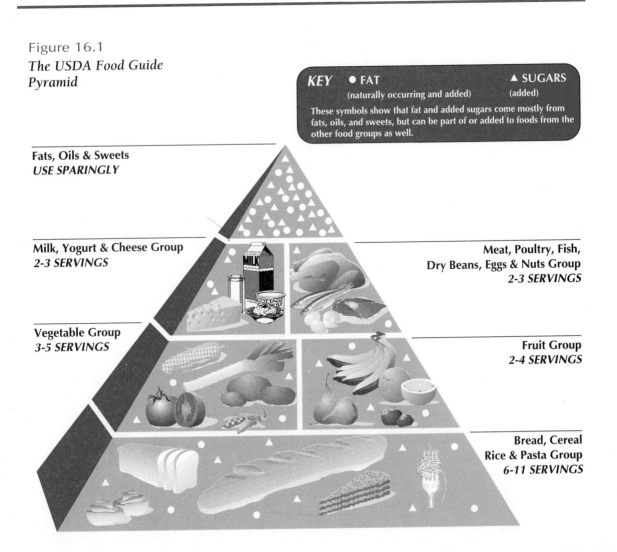

KEY   ● FAT   ▲ SUGARS
        (naturally occurring and added)   (added)
These symbols show that fat and added sugars come mostly from fats, oils, and sweets, but can be part of or added to foods from the other food groups as well.

Fats, Oils & Sweets
USE SPARINGLY

Milk, Yogurt & Cheese Group
2-3 SERVINGS

Meat, Poultry, Fish,
Dry Beans, Eggs & Nuts Group
2-3 SERVINGS

Vegetable Group
3-5 SERVINGS

Fruit Group
2-4 SERVINGS

Bread, Cereal
Rice & Pasta Group
6-11 SERVINGS

greens, mustard greens, and broccoli are high in vitamin A, vitamin C, and calcium. Orange vegetables such as carrots, sweet potatoes, and squash are also high in vitamin A. Three to five servings daily (at least one of which provides vitamin A), each about equal in size to a small potato, are recommended.

Bread, cereal, and pasta are high in iron, protein, and some B vitamins. Although the actual amount of protein is small in each serving, if many grain foods are eaten each day, part of the daily need for protein can be met. However, if these are the only sources of protein, they need to be combined with nuts and legumes to fulfill the needs for the required essential amino acids. Whole-grain products contain more fiber, vitamins, and minerals than refined products. Six to eleven servings daily, each about equal to the size of a slice of bread, are recommended.

Dried beans and peas are high in protein and iron. This food type also includes nuts, lentils, peanut butter, and tofu. These foods are usually low in cost and can be prepared a variety of ways. Nuts and peanut butter are high in fat and therefore high in calories. A combined total of two to three servings per day from this group and/or the meat, poultry, fish, and eggs group is recommended.

Meat, poultry, fish, and eggs are high in protein and iron. Lean meats, poultry without skin, and most fish are lower-calorie choices. A serving of this group is 3 ounces. A combined total of two to three servings per day from this group and/or the dried beans and peas group is recommended.

Milk and cheese are good sources of calcium and protein. Low-fat milk and cheese made from low-fat milk are lower-calorie choices. These low-fat products have the same amount of vitamins and minerals but a lower percentage of fat. Two to three servings are recommended daily for this food group.

Another group of food includes sweets and fats. These are added to other foods, thus increasing the number of calories. These "other" foods supply few nutrients for the calories they contain and are usually expensive. Beverages such as alcohol and soft drinks are included in this group. There is no recommendation for foods in this group; they should used sparingly.

Recommended Dietary Allowances

Another guide to proper nutrition are the Reference Daily Intakes (RDI), formerly known as the Recommended Dietary Allowances (RDAs). These are basic dietary guides for the population as a whole, and are designed to maintain good health. These recommendations have been set specifically as determined by the climate and general energy needs of the American population. Statistics were obtained from large groups of people living in the United States to establish the criteria for the recommended allowances. The Reference Daily Intakes are only estimates of the nutritional needs of Americans, but they are useful for dietary planning to ensure proper amounts of various nutrients.

Food Problems

Problems concerned with food have been a part of human life from the earliest times. In past ages, crop failures have led to famine and war. Even today, starvation kills hundreds of thousands of students and adults in very poor nations each year. Although there is also poverty in the United States, few students actually face the threat of starvation. Unfortunately, this does not mean that our nation does not have food problems. Many Americans are undernourished or malnourished. Overweight and obesity are also common.

Undernutrition

Typically, an undernourished person is also underweight, but this is by no means always the case. Undernutrition implies that the individual is not getting enough nutrients. This can occur even if the person is consuming more than enough calories. Thus, personal weight is not necessarily an indication of nutritive status. In the United States, malnutrition due to undernutrition is most likely to occur in infants, students, and adolescents, when nutritional requirements for tissue growth and development are high. When one is undernourished, the available proteins are depleted and the body begins to burn fat reserves. This process is known as *ketosis*. Undernutrition may cause blood sugar imbalances, lower basal metabolic rate, produce dehydration, provoke heart irregularity, inhibit growth, delay maturation, limit physical activity, and interfere with learning (Donatelle and Davis 1996, 254). The causes of undernutrition are many; poverty and lack of nutrition education are two major factors. In addition, many Americans are undernourished because they resist changing nutritionally deficient eating habits and patterns. Other practices dictated by cultural taboos, religious beliefs, and cultural patterns also sometimes lead to nutritional health problems. Occasionally the cause is physiological. A poorly functioning body might fail to use nutrients supplied to it. For example, a disease such as hyperthyroidism can affect growth regardless of the quality of diet.

Psychological factors can also lead to undernutrition. Hurried meals in haphazard settings may be harmful because of the type and amount of food as well as how the food is eaten. The noise and confusion that often accompany rushed meals can affect proper digestion.

An inaccurate perception of one's own nutritional state can bring on health problems such as anorexia nervosa, or nervous lack of appetite. This syndrome is characterized by loss of appetite, aversion to food, and weight loss. This condition should be considered a psychological disorder more than a simple eating disorder. It refers to a distinct psychological disorder in which a drive for thinness and a fear of fatness result in life-threatening emaciation and a host of other problems.

The central features of anorexia nervosa are difficult to specify because the disorder emerges over time as a complex mixture of the relentless drive for thinness, the effects of starvation, and commonly associated psychological disturbances (such as low self-worth and mistrust of others). A significant weight loss is one of the cardinal features of anorexia. The anorexic approaches weight loss with a fervor, convinced that her body is too large. Lost weight is viewed as "accomplishment . . . triumphant . . . powerful." The fact that slenderness is highly valued in our culture contributes to these attitudes held by anorexics. This drive for thinness is coupled with an extreme fear of becoming fat. This phobic fear of weight gain may express itself by the person weighing herself several times each day and becoming very anxious with any weight increase. An anorexic also has a distorted body image—unable to recognize her appearance as abnormal. She will insist that her emaciated figure is just right or even too fat (U. S. Department of Agriculture 1992, 19).

Anorexics are typically compulsive, perfectionistic, and very competitive. The anorexic sometimes suffers from a low self-image due to a feeling of incompetence, so he becomes consumed with losing weight to demonstrate to himself and others that he is in total control. Therefore, if a friend, parent, or teacher admonishes the anorexic for looking too thin, the anorexic may take this as a compliment, for it means others are aware of his disciplined approach to weight loss. Psychological counseling and family therapy are needed to correct some anorexic cases.

The long-term effects of anorexia include psychological problems such as obsessions, compulsions, paranoia, social withdrawal, and depression. They may become irritable, hostile, indecisive, depressed, defiant, and resistant to change. The arguments with parents and other authorities over eating habits become power struggles for control. The physical effects of anorexia nervosa are caused by overexercising, self-induced vomiting, and the use of laxatives and diuretics. Starvation can interrupt normal brain–body functions such as sleep, maintaining proper blood pressure, muscle weakness, immunity to disease, and sexual drive. Vomiting disrupts the potassium–sodium balance necessary for proper functioning of nerves and muscles (including the heart), and produces enamel erosion, tooth degeneration, and lesions in the esophagus.

The anorexic starts losing weight in order to become more popular, yet as the illness progresses, the anorexic becomes increasingly alienated from other people. Anorexia victims lose more than 25 percent of their total body weight. Girls are more affected than boys by anorexia nervosa, but the incidence among males is increasing (U. S. Department of Agriculture 1992, 19).

A related disorder is bulimia, in which a person eats large quantities of food during short periods of time and attempts to control weight by self-induced vomiting or laxative use. Bulimia is thought to result from a lack of self-esteem and a desire to become an "ideal" woman (Edlin and Golanty 1992, 145). This condition, like anorexia, can have serious health consequences, and medical help and counseling are essential.

The symptoms of undernutrition include fatigue, seizures, heart palpitations, thin bones, poor teeth, pale skin, dermatitis, inflamed eyes, sore tongue, fissures at the corners of the lips, muscular weakness, apathy, increased susceptibility to infections, shortness of breath, extreme nervousness, irritability, and sometimes weight loss (Mullen et al. 1996, 153–155).

A simple solution to the problem of undernutrition is to eat more of the proper nutrients, assuming these foods are available. If lack of knowledge is the only cause of the problem, then suggestions for proper food selection might remedy the situation. A balanced diet that includes a variety of foods, as well as moderation and balance, can be extremely beneficial to an undernourished student (U.S. Department of Agriculture 1992, 7).

Hunger and Learning

Hunger is a physiological and psychological state that occurs when food needs are not met satisfactorily. Research has shown that hunger definitely has an effect on learning behavior. Hunger increases nervousness, irritability, and disinterest in a learning situation. Students who are hungry will demonstrate a lack of interest in what is being taught and an inability to concentrate.

Hunger and malnutrition lead to weakness and illness. A variety of avitaminoses (vitamin deficiency disorders) can result from malnutrition. A student's development and brain function can be severely affected by hunger. Malnourished students are also more susceptible to infections, which can further lead to impaired growth.

Overweight and Obesity

Obesity is a prevalent condition among children and youth in the United States, and there is some evidence that the prevalence of obesity in children and youth may be increasing over the past two to three decades. Very little of this increase can be linked to heredity—lifestyle habits seem to play the primary role in the development of obesity. Because obesity has been shown to track from childhood into adulthood and because obesity is a risk factor for several chronic diseases, prevention and treatment of childhood obesity has become a recognized public health objective (Pate 1993, 1).

The health risks of obesity, such as degenerative diseases and shorter life span, may not be of immediate concern to elementary school students, but there are many other reasons for maintaining a correct weight. Obesity can be considered a physical handicap at any age because it affects physical activity. Also, overweight students face many emotional problems. In a society

Health Highlight

Obesity in Children and Youth Related to Inactivity

It has long been hypothesized that lack of physical activity could be a predisposing factor in childhood obesity. Over the past decade, two surveys of physical activity behavior in American children have been conducted. The national Children and Youth Fitness Study (mid-1980s) and the U.S. Centers for Disease Control and Prevention's Youth Risk Behavior Survey (YRBS) showed that a significant percentage of youth (20–30 percent) reported averaging less than one-half hour of physical activity per day. The YRBS results indicated that 50 percent of males and 75 percent of females fail to engage in moderate to vigorous activity on a frequent basis (three or more times per week). Girls tend to be less active than boys.

Physical inactivity is correlated with obesity. Those who exercise less have higher body fat. Also, it is possible that obesity may predispose youngsters to a less active lifestyle. Increased physical activity can decrease obesity in youth.

Source: R. Pate. 1993. Physical activity in children and youth: Relationship to obesity. *Contemporary nutrition* 18(2).

where "thinness" is emphasized, overweight students may be isolated and shunned, ridiculed, stared at, and rejected socially. As a result, overweight students may lose their sense of self-worth and withdraw from others. A complicating problem occurs when overweight students find satisfaction in nothing else except eating, which causes them to gain even more weight, further alienating them from peers.

Being overweight becomes a health problem when the person is 15 to 20 percent above normal. Of course, body build and an individual's lean-to-fat ratio also have to be taken into consideration. Different people gain weight in different places in the body. Those who typically gain weight in the lower portions of the body (usually females) do not have as many health risks posed as those who gain weight in the upper body (usually males). A person might have a stocky build and be over the desired weight for his height and age, but the percentage of body fat might be within the normal range. More often than not, however, obesity is self-evident.

Obesity is a problem influenced by the individual's physical, social, and emotional environment. Usually, the condition is due to a lack of exercise, overeating, improper food habits, or emotional problems. The increased popularity of video games and other sedentary activities has contributed to the lack of exercise in students. Some people simply enjoy food too much. Others overeat to reduce anxiety, using food as a tranquilizer. Still others eat because of anger or boredom. Family habits sometimes play a role in contributing to obesity. A family's pattern of lack of exercise, overeating, and improper snacking is easily incorporated into a student's lifestyle through imitation, thereby perpetuating obesity in the family.

Weight Control

Weight reduction demands self-discipline and commitment. An overweight individual must accept personal responsibility for the condition. If an emotional problem is the cause, that problem must be treated first to ensure long-lasting success at weight control, because the overweight condition is only a symptom of a deeper problem. Before any reducing plan is implemented, a physician should be consulted.

Obese persons must consume fewer calories than they expend daily, but this is easier said than done. Dieters should use a diet that is similar to the one to which they are accustomed so they do not feel as restricted and tempted to quit dieting.

Other techniques that have helped people lose weight are to

○ arrange to eat in one place only

○ remove all unnecessary fat when cooking and eating meat

○ avoid gravies, using herbs and spices for seasoning instead

○ start meals with filling, low-calorie dishes such soup or celery sticks

○ eat fresh fruit instead of canned

○ eat regular meals—missed meals may make you even more hungry during the day

○ use raw vegetables for snacks

○ eat baked, broiled, or boiled foods without adding fat

○ use a salad-sized plate rather than a dinner plate so the portions look larger

○ cut food into small bites and eat slowly

○ brush the teeth after each meal; sometimes the aftertaste of food can stimulate the appetite

○ exercise moderately and regularly

○ develop hobbies; sometimes people substitute food for friends and outside activities

Obesity is a preventable condition among children and youth in the U.S.

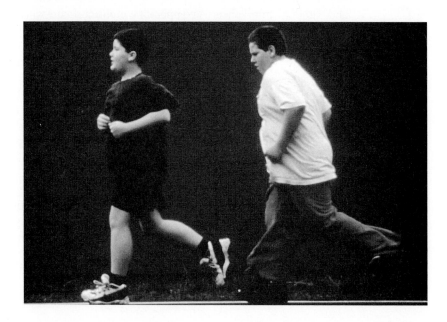

Care should be taken not to lose weight too rapidly. Rapid weight loss may result in exhaustion, kidney problems, dehydration, reduced cardiovascular output, decreased strength, decreased growth, and decreased endurance.

One point that should be kept in mind regarding a student's weight is ideal weight versus average weight. Some weight tables will provide data on "average" weight; but, as noted earlier, the average American student is overweight. Ideal weight tables should be used as the standard for evaluating weight.

Further, weight alone should not be the total issue. The student's body fat (or lean–fat ratio) is even more critical. If a student is "big boned," he may appear overweight, yet his body fat may be very acceptable. Conversely, a student with small bones may weigh in within an acceptable range but will actually have a body fat percentage that is unacceptable. Also, if a person couples a dieting program with an exercise program, that person may be losing fat and gaining muscle. Since muscles weigh more than fat, the result may not be lost pounds but rather lost fat—a healthy condition. However, since most dieters have been concerned only with how much they weigh, they may be disappointed that they are not losing weight. Again, the focus for a dieter should be on the lean–fat ratio, not weight alone.

Food label

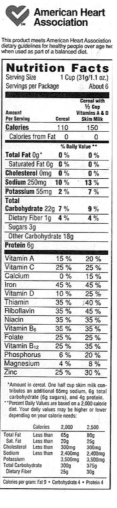

The Role of the Teacher

Teachers should provide accurate information concerning nutrition and teach students how to make wise decisions in order to help prevent undernourishment among students. They need to emphasize the importance of eating a good breakfast and lunch, as well as encourage sociability among students when they are eating. Teachers can help the students enjoy the taste, smell, color, and texture of food and thereby increase interest in it. In addition, teachers have an excellent chance to be exemplary role models by eating the right foods in the right way while at school.

Therapy and Counseling

Weight reduction is usually more successful when using a "buddy system" or peer support groups. Teachers can help by getting together several students who have a similar goal of weight reduction and having them eat together and share their concerns and problems. Teachers can also educate obese and overweight students about proper nutrition and encourage physical activity. To nurture the emotional health of the obese student, teachers need to offer security and acceptance without pitying or overprotecting the student. Being supportive will produce much better results than constant harassment or criticism. Trying to reduce the student's anxiety while helping build self-esteem and independence is also important.

Other Food Related Issues

Food Quackery

Obese individuals may understand the need to diet but may want to do so as painlessly as possible. Such individuals are vulnerable to fad diets advertised to help a person lose weight quickly. Some of these fad diets are restricted in variety, expensive, useless, and sometimes even detrimental to health. Most fad diets are directed at adults, rather than students, of course, but students are impressionable. It is important to put these diets into proper perspective. The fact is that most people who are overweight do not need to read a book on what to eat to lose weight. Simply eating somewhat less of everything will usually produce results, if the diet is followed conscientiously.

Food quackery is by no means confined to diet books or dieting clinics that employ dubious methods. The whole "natural and health foods" industry is considered quackery by many nutritional experts. Both of these areas prey on natural fears and uncertainties about foods and nutritional requirements. There is no accepted legal definition of what "natural foods" actually are and no way to keep entrepreneurs from selling granola, dried fruits, and so on at inflated prices, all the while hinting that these products are somewhat healthier for a person to eat. "Health foods," such as bee pollen and algae extracts, fall into the same category. Such foods are not harmful to health, but they are no better than foods obtained from ordinary sources. Advocates of "natural," "organic," and "health" foods claim that additives or pesticide residues in regular foods can cause disease or even lower the nutritional value of the food, but these claims are highly exaggerated. By and large, the Food and Drug Administration and other supervisory agencies do a good job in preventing possibly harmful or unsafe foods from reaching the market. Teachers can help students become informed consumers of food products and develop a good knowledge of nutritional principles. But nutrition should not become an obsession, as it is with many food faddists. Students should also be taught to recognize the difference between nutrition and food nostrums.

Food Labeling

A tremendous amount of nutritional information is available today, but many Americans are still misinformed and confused about the foods they buy and eat. Some FDA regulations have resulted in improved labeling designed to give a listing of nutrients in the product, and to make the information on food labels more meaningful to consumers (see Figure 16.2). For example, nutrients are listed on the label in order, beginning with the largest quantity. Typically, the label provides nutritional information based on one serving of the food product rather than on the entire can or package.

Manufacturers must use nutritional labeling when they add any nutrient to packaged food or when they make some nutritional claim for their products. Labeling is also meant to stop unsupported generalizations and fraudulent statements. Nutritional labeling of food products is being sought for nearly all foods. This would be difficult for some foods, such as fresh fruits, but labeling of all food products would be beneficial to the consumer.

The U.S. Food and Drug Administration (FDA) has proposed a major revision of the listing of nutrition information on labels. This proposal would change from RDA (now referred to Reference Daily Intakes—RDI) listing to "Daily Values" for the purpose of calculating the amount of nutrients that are in the food package. The FDA has established, in its Daily Values, age-adjusted average levels for vitamins, minerals, and protein recommended for various age/sex groups in the RDI, instead of the highest recommended values. Averaging for these nutrients was considered necessary by the FDA because it would be contrary to public health goals to base values for fat, for example, on the highest recommended intake. The new averaging approach for all nutrients would give consumers a more current, unified "measuring stick" to compare the content of all labeled nutrients among different foods. These Daily Values would include not only protein and several of the vitamins and minerals previously listed under the U.S. RDAs, but for the first time, fat, cholesterol, fiber, sodium, and other food components would be included (FDA 1992, 1–2). These changes would cause manufacturers to list certified color additives; label fruit and vegetable juices; display in grocery stores the nutrition information on the twenty most popular raw fruits, vegetables, and types of fish; require labels for virtually all packaged foods; define serving sizes; and define descriptors such as "light," "lean," and "low-fat" (Foulke 1992, 9).

Nutritional Education

In emphasizing sound nutrition to students, teachers need to make sure that the learning opportunities they provide are interesting and personalized. Students should be taught to help themselves make responsible food choices. Of course, the home and school have to work together to make the nutrition education of the student a success.

The School Lunch Program

School lunch programs began with the enactment of the National School Lunch Act in 1946. This federal legislation provided surplus agricultural commodities and federal funds to local school districts for the purpose of providing nutritious meals to children through a school lunch program. Federal government management of this program is the responsibility of the Department of Agriculture.

There have been a number of problems with these programs. For example, many schools do not meet the federal dietary guidelines for these programs, and a lot of food is wasted in the lunchrooms.

Figure 16.2
*FDA Revised Nutrition
Label*

Nutrition Facts

Serving Size: 1 cup (228g)
Servings Per Container 2

Amount Per Serving

Calories 260   Calories from Fat 120

	% Daily Value*
Total Fat 12g	20%
Saturated Fat 5g	25%
Cholesterol 30mg	10%
Sodium 660mg	28%
Total Carbohydrate 31g	10%
Dietary Fiber 0g	0%
Sugars 5g	
Protein 5g	

Vitamin A 4%	•	Vitamin C 2%	
Calcium 15%	•	Iron 4%	

* Percent Daily Values are based on a 2,000
calorie diet. Your daily values may be higher or
lower depending on your calorie needs:

	Calories:	2,000	2,500
Total Fat	Less than	65g	80g
Sat Fat	Less than	20g	25g
Cholesterol	Less than	300mg	300mg
Sodium	Less than	2,400mg	2,400mg
Total Carbohydrate		300g	375g
Dietary Fiber		25g	30g

Calories per gram:
Fat 9 • Carbohydrate 4 • Protein 4

Calories

Total calories are listed as well as calories from fat. So in a serving of this product, 120 of the 260 calories are from fat. To calculate percent calories from fat, divide the calories from fat (120) by the total calories (260) per serving and multiply by 100.
$120 \div 260 = .46$
$.46 \times 100 = 46\%$ of the calories are from fat.

Serving Size

Similar food products now list similar portion sizes which makes nutritional comparisons between products easier. Serving sizes are listed in common household (i.e. cups) and metric (i.e. grams) measures. The serving size listed now reflects amounts of food people typically eat.

% Daily Value

% Daily Value shows how a food fits into the overall daily diet based on a daily intake of 2,000 calories. Use these values as a guide to see if a food is high or low in a nutrient and to compare similar food products.

Daily Value Footnote

Some labels provide that daily values, the recommended intakes of the nutrients listed for both a 2,000 and 2,500 calorie intake. Your daily values may be higher or lower depending on your calorie intake.

Calorie Conversion Information

Some labels provide the number of calories in one gram of fat, carbohydrate, and protein.

The students criticize the school lunches for the quality of preparation and a dislike for the kinds and types of foods that are served—bland and lacking in nutrition (Miller, Telljohann, and Symons 1996, 13–15).

The goals of school lunches are to

○ provide one-third of the student's RDA

○ serve a minimum of five items with minimum portions

○ use resources provided by the government

○ appeal to students—if the school offers vending machines with other choices, however, the student will choose this instead of the school lunch

○ break even financially—a major problem, because most school systems operate on a limited budget

Even under these constraints, many school lunches provide varied and nutritious meals. A well-planned school lunch program provides excellent learning opportunities in nutrition. The federal school lunch program was established to provide nutritionally sound meals at low cost to students. These lunches can help students make good food choices while at school. This lunch consists of one-half pint of whole milk; 2 oz of lean meat, poultry, fish, or cheese; a three-fourths-cup serving of two or more vegetables or fruits or both; one slice of whole-grain or enriched bread or its equivalent; and one teaspoon of butter or fortified margarine. Some schools now offer alternative lunches of salads and/or sandwiches.

The educational impact of a lunch program can be important if it is used correctly. For students who bring their lunches from home, teachers need to provide several examples of nutritious sack lunches (for example, a sandwich including some type of lean meat and lettuce on whole-wheat bread, banana, raisins, and milk).

The cafeteria can be used as a place in which to help students learn table manners, sitting posture, and appropriate social behavior. The planning, preparation, and serving of meals by the cafeteria staff can also provide excellent learning opportunities for students.

▤ *Summary*

○ Although food is basic to human existence, food choices often have little to do with good nutrition.

○ Socioeconomic factors, personal preferences and habits, cultural customs, and religious beliefs are all determining factors in the food we select.

○ The eating habits of American students are often poor. This is due primarily to the habits of their parents, hurried lifestyles, and lack of nutrition education.

○ Snacking can be improved to help supplement an otherwise poor diet.

○ The development of positive lifetime eating habits in students is a critical issue.

○ Food's basic function is to provide nutrients to the body.

○ All foods have specific caloric values.

○ The USDA's Food Guide Pyramid and the Revised Recommended Dietary Allowance tables can be used to plan a healthy diet.

○ Food problems abound among students.

○ Hunger and malnutrition affect a student's growth and learning.

○ The number of overweight students is increasing.

○ Pressure from peers to be thin or to look good in order to be accepted by peers encourages anorexia and bulimia. These conditions are physical and emotional handicaps. Sometimes therapy and counseling are needed to correct these problems.

○ Food quackery preys on the fears and uncertainties people have regarding foods.

○ Students should be taught to distinguish between truth and misleading statements.

○ Food labels are provided on most foods to help determine the nutritional value of a food.

○ Students should be taught to make responsible choices about food.

○ Teachers and parents have to work together for nutrition education to be successful.

Discussion Questions

1. Describe why Americans' diets are typically insufficient even though we live in an affluent country.

2. What factors determine one's selection of foods?

3. Discuss the importance of complex carbohydrates in the diet.

4. Discuss some healthy ways to snack to enhance your diet.

5. List the food sources for proteins.

6. Differentiate between saturated and unsaturated fats.

7. Describe the importance of water to the body structure.

8. What beneficial roles do minerals play in body function?

9. Discuss the role of antioxidants in enhancing health.

10. Describe the use of the USDA's Food Guide Pyramid in selecting proper foods.

11. Discuss the typical characteristics of an anorexic victim.

12. Describe obesity as an emotional and physical handicap.

13. How can food labels be helpful to consumers?

14. Discuss the importance of the school lunch program.

References

Bruess, C., and G. Richardson. 1994. *Healthy decisions.* Madison, WI: Brown & Benchmark.

Donatelle, R., and L. Davis. 1996. *Access to health,* 4th ed. Boston: Allyn and Bacon.

Edlin, G., and E. Golanty. 1992. *Health and wellness: A holistic approach,* 4th ed. Boston: Jones & Bartlett.

Food and Drug Administration (FDA). 1992, February 12. *FDA backgrounder,* pp. 1–2.

Foulke, J. 1992, February. Wide-sweeping FDA proposals to improve food labeling. *FDA consumer,* pp. 9–13.

Hahn, D., and W. Payne. 1997. *Focus on health,* 3rd ed. St. Louis: Mosby.

Hales, D. 1994. *An invitation to health: The power of prevention,* 6th ed. Redwood City, CA: Benjamin/Cummings.

Miller, D., S. Telljohann, and C. Symons. 1996. *Health education in the elementary & middle-level school*, 2nd ed. Madison, WI: Brown & Benchmark.

Mullen, K., R. McDermott, R. Gold, and P. Belcastro. 1996. *Connections for health*, 4th ed. Madison, WI: Brown & Benchmark.

Pate, R. 1993. Physical activity in children and youth: relationship to obesity. *Contemporary nutrition* 18(2).

U.S. Department of Agriculture, U.S. Department of Health and Human Services. 1995. *Nutrition and your health: Dietary guidelines for Americans*, 4th ed. Washington, DC: U.S. Government Printing Office.

U.S. Department of Agriculture, Human nutrition information service. 1992, August. *Leaflet No. 572*. Rockville, MD: Author.

U.S. Department of Agriculture. 1992, December. *Dietary guidelines and your health*. Rockville, MD: Author.

U.S. Department of Health and Human Services. 1992, April. *Eating to lower your high blood cholesterol*. Washington, DC: Author.

University of California at Berkeley. 1992. Fast food: Decoding the menus. *University of California at Berkeley Wellness Letter* 8(9), 3.

Chapter Seventeen
Strategies for Teaching Nutrition

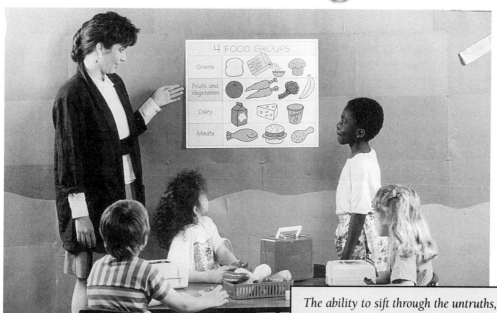

> The ability to sift through the untruths, half-truths, and scientific realities and select a nutrition plan designed to meet your individual needs is an essential health-promoting skill.
> —Donatelle and Davis (1996, 194)

Valued Outcomes

After doing the activities in this chapter, the student should be able to express and illustrate the following guidelines:

- ○ Nutrition plays a vital role in human development.
- ○ There is a close relationship between dietary practices and overall health.
- ○ The taste, sight, and smell of foods sometimes dictate food behavior.
- ○ One's nutritional status may affect one's self-image.
- ○ Food serves several functions in meeting body needs.
- ○ Food fads and fallacies can affect one's food behavior.
- ○ Caloric intake should be balanced with energy needs.
- ○ There are many individual and ethnic variations in food behavior.

○ Physical, psychological, and social factors affect personal food behavior.

○ There are healthy and unhealthy ways of losing weight.

○ A good breakfast is important for growing and learning.

○ Food is an important part of our lives.

○ Food nutrients can be classified as carbohydrates, fats, proteins, water, minerals, and vitamins.

○ Eating a variety of carefully selected foods is the best way to ensure that the body receives the proper amounts of the nutrients it needs.

○ The four basic food groups can serve as an aid in planning balanced, nutritious meals.

○ The lack of certain nutrients can lead to certain diseases.

○ Being underweight or overweight can lead to physical and emotional problems.

○ Maintaining a proper weight is an individual responsibility, but others can help if there is a weight problem.

○ Even if an individual does not have a weight problem, the person can be malnourished.

○ Simple foods can be nutritious and provide a well-balanced diet, if properly selected.

○ Trying new and different foods can be fun.

○ Junk foods, such as candy and soft drinks, can cause health problems if consumed too regularly.

○ Many people in the world do not have enough to eat.

○ Many people wrongly believe in food myths and food nostrums.

○ Food labels can provide useful nutritional information.

○ Money spent for food should be spent wisely.

A Flexible Approach to Nutrition

Teachers have the responsibility of helping students learn the basic principles of nutrition so that they will understand the important relationship between nutrition and health and will increase skill in solving food and nutrition-related problems. The concept of nutrition is quite abstract to younger elementary school children, often seen as somehow connected with but divorced from eating. Your job in teaching nutrition is to make that concept more concrete and real to your students by presenting learning opportunities that relate nutritional information to daily life. In other words, you must personalize the information so that students will internalize it and recognize its relevance to health.

Avoid a rigid, by-the-rules approach, and do not reduce nutrition education to a set of rules. Not only will a rule-based approach make nutrition seem grim, it will also cause children to reject sound principles as unrealistic. Help students to understand the motivations for choosing and eating certain foods, and that some of these motivations have little to do with the amount of nutrients to be attained from a certain food. For example, a person might be choosing a certain midafternoon snack because that snack was the one always offered by his or her parents, but that snack might not be as nutritious as another readily available snack.

Children and adults will change their habits only when they personally recognize the importance of doing so. Do not expect changes overnight. Encourage introspection, and foster positive decision-making skills. Act as a role model for changes you wish to bring about. Respect differences in tastes, likes, and dislikes. You will begin to see that your message is slowly getting through.

Value-Based Activities

The Food Guide Pyramid

Valued Outcome: Students will be able to rank their favorite food category in the Food Guide Pyramid.

Description of Strategy: Show the students copies of the Food Guide Pyramid, and review the six categories with them. Ask the students to observe the pyramid and to tell which food category is the most important one in our diet. Take a vote to see how many students think each category is the most important. Chart their responses on how they rank each category on poster board for future reference. Of course, the largest block on the pyramid, the grains, is the group from which we should eat the most. The grains make up the foundation of the pyramid, just as they should make up the foundation of our diet. Discuss the concept of foundations with the students. Instruct the students to write the names of at least five foods for each category. Then ask them to share their responses with the class. Make a large food pyramid using poster board and markers. Have students record the varied responses on the large food pyramid.

Materials Needed: copy of the Food Guide Pyramid, pencils, two poster boards, markers

Processing Questions:

1. What are the six food categories of the Food Guide Pyramid?

2. Which food category is the most important one in our diet?

Source: K. L. Siepak. 1994. *Keeping healthy*, Step-by-Step Science Series, Grades 4–6. Greensboro NC: Carson-Dellosa, pp. 28–30.

What's Healthy?

Valued Outcome: The students will be able to decide which breakfast foods are healthy and which are not healthy.

Description of Strategy: Divide the students up in groups of four to six students. Have the students get out two sheets of paper for the group. On one sheet of paper, write "Nutritious"; on the other sheet of paper, write "Not nutritious." Have the group decide what a nutritious breakfast is and write it down. Label the foods by their food groups. Then have them make up a breakfast that is not nutritious. Have a group discussion about their answers. After the discussion, do the same concept for lunch and dinner.

Materials Needed: paper and pencils for all students

Processing Question: Why is it important to eat a nutritious breakfast?

Nutrition Beliefs Survey

Valued Outcome: The students will be able to examine their values to determine if they agree or disagree with statements about nutrition.

Description of Strategy: Tell the students to check the appropriate column after each statement to indicate whether they agree or disagree with the idea:

	Agree	Disagree
1. An individual can avoid a cold by taking large amounts of Vitamin C.		x
2. Being overweight can be dangerous.	x	
3. Everyone should take vitamin supplements.		x
4. Before participating in a sports event, athletes should eat more protein foods than they usually eat.		
5. Honey and sugar are natural sweeteners with little difference in nutritive value.	x	
6. If a person wants to lose weight, the first things to eliminate from the diet are bread and potatoes.	x	

Materials Needed: handouts with the preceding statements, pencils for all students
Processing Question: What social and emotional factors help determine my beliefs about nutrition?

Source: Tennessee Department of Education. 1984. *Tennessee educates for nutrition now*. Nashville: Author.

Healthy Food Voting

Valued Outcome: The students will be able to determine if their favorite foods are healthy or unhealthy.
Description of Strategy: Start by asking students what their favorite foods are. Make a list of these on the chalkboard. After making these lists, make two separate columns with the following headlines: *Healthy* and *Unhealthy*. Then call out the list of favorite foods, and have the students vote whether each of the foods should go in the *Healthy* or the *Unhealthy* column.
Materials Needed: none
Processing Question: How can I change my diet if most of my favorite foods are unhealthy?

Nutrition Sentence Completion

Valued Outcome: The students will be able to complete nutrition-related statements with their own feelings and beliefs.
Description of Strategy: Have students complete the following statements with phrases that come to mind immediately on hearing the key phrase beginning the statement:

○ The most important meal of the day for me is . . .

○ Eating a good breakfast is . . .

○ My favorite foods are . . .

○ Eating right means . . .

○ I think that my present diet is . . .

○ Between-meal snacks should be . . .

○ One problem about nutrition for me is . . .

Materials Needed: handouts with the preceding statements printed on them, pencils for all students

Processing Question: Who can help you determine what is included in a good breakfast and/or snack?

Rank-Ordering Favorite Foods

Valued Outcome: The students will be able to clarify their values regarding their favorite foods.
Description of Strategy: Have each student prepare a list of three or four favorite foods or dishes from each section of the Food Guide Pyramid. Then tell the students to rank-order each food or dish, with the most favorite being labeled "1." Now have the students compare their lists. What class preferences seem to emerge? What are some individual preferences? Follow with a discussion of personal likes and dislikes.
Materials Needed: paper and pencils for all students
Processing Questions:

1. Do several of the students have the same favorite foods as you?

2. If they do not, why do you think that is true?

Values Continuum

Valued Outcome: The students will be able to explain how different eating lifestyles can affect one's nutrition.
Description of Strategy: Pass out continuum sheets. One end of the continuum represents a lifestyle where every meal is eaten at home under relaxed conditions. The other end of the continuum represents a lifestyle where every meal is eaten outside the home under hurried or hectic conditions. Have each student place an X on the continuum representing his or her assessment of eating lifestyle. Follow with a general discussion of how eating lifestyle may affect growth and development as well as emotional state.
Materials Needed: sheets with lines drawn to represent a continuum, pencils for all students
Processing Question: How does a hurried or relaxed eating lifestyle affect the digestion of the food we eat?

My Favorite Meal Is . . .

Valued Outcome: The students will be able to describe their favorite meals.
Description of Strategy: Have the students write about their favorite breakfast. Then have them write about their favorite lunch and supper. Have a group discussion about what they wrote. Ask them why this is their favorite meal. If it is not nutritious, ask them how they can make it nutritious. Have the students rank their meals from 1 to 10, from most nutritious to least nutritious. Discuss the results.
Materials Needed: paper, pencils
Processing Questions:

1. Why do you think you like the foods that you do?

2. Are the foods you like generally healthy?

What's for Lunch?

Valued Outcome: The students will be able to analyze the nutritious quality of their school lunches.

Description of Strategy: Have the students write down and analyze the school lunches for three days. After three days, have the students share what they thought about the school lunches. Discuss which food groups were poorly represented and which food groups were well represented. Have the students give their own opinions about the school lunches. As an instructor, make sure good things are said as well as bad.

Materials Needed: none

Processing Questions:

1. Did you enjoy these lunches?

2. Were you able to eat the types of foods you enjoy?

3. Did your analysis determine that your lunches were healthy? Unhealthy?

Decision Stories

Follow the procedures outlined in Chapter 5 for presenting decision stories such as the following.

What to Drink?

Al has just come inside from playing a game of football with his friends and is very thirsty. He opens the refrigerator and finds water, pop, and fruit juice.

Focus Question: Which drink would be best for Al to drink? Why?

Ken's Problem

Ken was cut when he tried out for the gymnastics team because he had limited energy and was not muscular enough. His problems were not related to an illness, but a physician suggested Ken's diet might be the problem. Ken decided he needed to eat more, so he began to snack on high-calorie foods such as doughnuts, cakes, and candy. At regular mealtimes he was not very hungry, so he ate less than usual. He gained weight, but lost endurance.

Focus Question: How should Ken change his eating habits to increase his endurance?

Source: Tennessee Department of Education. 1984. *Tennessee educates for nutrition now.* Nashville: Author.

Jane's Diet

Ten-year-old Jane decided that she needed to lose weight, because her jeans were too tight. Jane's best friend also tried a new diet recently where she could eat as much tomato juice or pineapple as she wanted, but no other foods were allowed. Her friend claimed that the diet was wonderful. Jane decided to try her friend's diet, but after three days, she was bored with only two foods, and she lacked energy. Jane quit the diet and decided that she is doomed to be fat.

Focus Question: What kind of diet could you propose for Jane to help her lose weight yet retain energy?

Source: Tennessee Department of Education. 1984. *Tennessee educates for nutrition now.* Nashville: Author.

Snacktime

John came home from school hungry. His mother told him that dinner would be late, so he could have a snack. She told him to go to the kitchen and get a piece of fruit to eat. But John remembered a candy bar that he had in his lunch box and thought of having that instead, even though he knew that the fruit would be better for him.

Focus Question: What should John do?

Fast Food

Tim doesn't like the food they serve in the school cafeteria. Some of his friends go to a fast-food restaurant near the school instead. He would like to go with them, but he knows that his parents want him to eat in the cafeteria.

Focus Question: What should Tim do?

Dramatizations

Eating for Special Needs

Valued Outcome: The students will be able to plan meals for people with special needs.

Description of Strategy: Have a couple of students in the class role-play patients in the hospital. Example: patient 1 is a sixty-seven-year-old man who has no teeth and an ulcer. Have each student think of a breakfast, lunch, and dinner that will fit his needs. Patient 2 is a seven-year-old girl who has had her tonsils removed and has a sore throat. Patient 3 is a forty-five-year-old man who is overweight and has a serious heart ailment. Make or plan a breakfast, lunch, and dinner for all the patients and then discuss the results.

Materials Needed: none

Processing Questions:

1. Why do some people need to avoid or have certain foods in their diets?

2. What would happen to these patients if they ate or avoided certain foods?

Star Search

Valued Outcome: The students will be able to describe various nutrition problems.

Description of Strategy: Divide the students in groups of four to six students. Have the students make up a song, poem, dance, or skit about a nutritional problem, such as eating too much junk food, or not eating foods from the four food groups. Have the students try to guess what the problem is and then discuss it. At the end of the class, reward everyone with star stickers, cookies, or whatever.

Materials Needed: none

Processing Questions:

1. Why do so many people in our country have nutritional problems when we have such a plentiful supply of food?

2. How can such nutritional problems affect our overall health?

Selling a Product

Valued Outcome: The students will be able to simulate nutritional advertisements.
Description of Strategy: Have the students divide up in groups of three to five students. Give each group a product. Have the group work together to think of a way to sell the product. Have each group come up in front of the class and try to sell their products. Have nutritious foods and nonnutritious foods as products. Discuss the product and the food group it belongs to.
Materials Needed: boxes, bags, and so forth, of different kinds of food
Processing Questions:

1. Why do companies use advertisements to sell their products?

2. How should we evaluate such advertisements to make sure we make wise nutritional decisions?

Foods That Keep the Body Healthy

Valued Outcome: The students will be able to identify certain foods that help keep the body healthy.

Description of Strategy: Draw an outline of three types of bodies: heavy, average, thin. Have students attach pictures to each body type that might result from a diet of these foods. Discuss with the students why an excess of certain foods can have a negative effect on the body.

To show the positive effect foods have on the body, have children role-play a race. Let two children who are going to "run in a race" role-play different ways of eating in preparation for the event. For example, one eats very nutritious, light meals, whereas the other eats high-calorie junk food. Let the two students enact what they would feel like while "running in the race."
Materials Needed: drawing of the body types, pictures of body types
Processing Questions:

1. What effect does food have on our body build?

2. What effect does food have on our energy level?

Role-Playing Nutrients

Valued Outcomes: The students will be able to describe the significance of nutrients, vitamins, and minerals through role-playing.
Description of Strategy: The students will assemble in cooperative groups. The teacher will assign each group a category—either nutrient, vitamin, or mineral. The group will then research their category and dramatize characteristics of their category. The nutrient-category students may use food representations to dramatize characteristics. Each group will present its dramatization to the class, and explain why they chose to dramatize the way they did. They will explain the significance of their nutrient, vitamin, or mineral and its relationship to a healthy diet.
Materials Needed: none
Processing Question: What are the important characteristics of each category of nutrients?

Sanitary Habits

Valued Outcome: The students will be able to identify sanitary and unsanitary work habits with regard to meal preparation.

Description of Strategy: Have students dramatize sanitary and unsanitary work habits while preparing, serving, and eating a meal. Have the remainder of the class observe the dramatizations and identify the errors.

Materials Needed: none

Processing Questions:

1. Why is it important to practice sanitary habits when preparing and eating a meal?

2. What habits can you change to become more sanitary when preparing and eating a meal?

Source: Tennessee Department of Education. 1984. *Tennessee educates for nutrition now.* Nashville: Author.

Meal Planning

Valued Outcome: The students will be able to plan numerous menus for various dietary situations.

Description of Strategy: Divide the students into groups, and provide each with one of the following situations to enact:

○ planning food to serve at a party for friends

○ planning breakfast menus for mornings when time for food preparation is limited

○ planning a dinner for a friend who is on a weight reduction diet

○ planning menus for an overnight camping trip

○ planning a dinner menu for a family gathering

○ selecting different foods from a buffet or cafeteria line

Materials Needed: none

Processing Question: How can planning menus enhance your nutrition?

Source: Tennessee Department of Education. 1984. *Tennessee educates for nutrition now.* Nashville: Author.

Proper Manners

Valued Outcome: The students will be able to identify appropriate and inappropriate eating behaviors in various settings.

Description of Strategy: Assign groups of students the task of role-playing eating in various settings (such as pizza parlor, family restaurant, picnic, school cafeteria). For each setting, have some students exhibit behaviors that would be appropriate, and have different students exhibit inappropriate behaviors.

Materials Needed: none

Processing Question: What are appropriate behaviors when eating in public places?

Source: Tennessee Department of Education. 1984. *Tennessee educates for nutrition now.* Nashville: Author.

Choosing from a Menu

Valued Outcome: The students will be able to select foods from a restaurant menu.
Description of Strategy: Bring several actual menus from area restaurants, or let students make menus. Let several students enact a situation in which they are seated in a restaurant and make choices from the menu. Have others play the role of waiter/waitress to help guide the diner's choices.
Materials Needed: pen and paper
Processing Question: Why is it important to know how to order from a menu in a restaurant?

Food and Energy

Valued Outcome: The students will be able to role-play eating various foods in preparation for a race.
Description of Strategy: Let two children that are going to "run in a race" role-play different ways of eating in preparation for the event; for example, one eats very nutritious and light while the other eats high-calorie junk food. Let the two students enact what they would feel like while "running the race."
Materials Needed: none
Processing Questions:

1. What foods should you eat to prepare for a race or other endurance activity?

2. What effect would poor food choices have on one's endurance?

Which Nutrient Am I?

Valued Outcome: The students will be able to identify characteristics of various nutrients, vitamins, and minerals.
Description of Strategy: Assign various nutrients, vitamins, and minerals to individual students. Let them research the nutrient, then dramatize characteristics of the nutrient to the class. For example, for a fruit, the student could simulate planting, growing, harvesting, shipping, buying, eating, and digesting the food. Let the observers guess from the dramatization which nutrient is being enacted.
Materials Needed: none
Processing Questions:

1. What are the characteristics of the individual nutrients, vitamins, and minerals?

2. Why is it important to know these characteristics?

Garden Puppet Show

Valued Outcome: The students will be able to demonstrate different foods that are grown in the garden, and be able to tell the benefit of each food for the body.
Description of Strategy: Let students make puppets of different foods that are grown in the garden. Let them enact a scene in a garden in which the various foods tell what they will do for the body when they are eaten.
Materials Needed: paper lunch bag or cloth for puppets, markers
Processing Question: How do various garden-grown foods help our bodies function better?

Dieting Puppets

Valued Outcome: The students will be able to demonstrate the problems some individuals have in gaining weight and losing weight.
Description of Strategy: Prepare several puppets, some to represent thin people trying to gain weight and others, overweight persons trying to lose weight, and still others, anorexic or bulimic people. Have the puppets sitting at a table during a meal discussing why they are eating (or not eating) various foods.
Materials Needed: paper lunch bags or cloth for making a puppet, telephone
Processing Questions:

1. Why do some thin people try to lose more weight?
2. How can such behavior affect that person's health?

Nutrients on Trial

Valued Outcome: The students will be able to determine essential functions of the nutrients of the body.
Description of Strategy: Have the students conduct a mock court having nutrients on trial. Give the students situations in which the nutrients on trial are accused of not being useful to the body. The nutrients' defendants must defend their essential function in the body.
Materials Needed: none
Processing Question: What are the useful functions provided by each food?

Cafeteria Selection

Valued Outcome: The students will be able to select a meal by choosing foods from each level of the food pyramid.
Description of Strategy: Using food pictures, set up a "cafeteria line" from which students will choose a meal to place on a tray. Have students take turns being the cashiers—checking to see that choices include food from each level of the Food Guide Pyramid.
Materials Needed: food pictures from magazines, scissors, glue, paper
Processing Question: Why do we need foods from each level of the pyramid?

Food Puppets

Valued Outcome: The students will be able to select foods that provide a balanced diet.
Description of Strategy: After discussing the Food Guide Pyramid and the nutrients they provide, have the class make puppets representing the various foods within the pyramid. Prepare a skit that explains how the foods work together to provide a balanced diet containing all essential nutrients, including water.
Materials Needed: lunch bag or cloth for making a puppet
Processing Question: How can combinations of foods help enhance our health?

Stranger in a Strange Land

Valued Outcome: The students will be able to discuss typical foods eaten in different countries.
Description of Strategy: Divide the class into small groups. Have each research the foods and

dishes eaten in a different nation, such as Mexico, India, Malaysia, Germany, Japan, and Greece. Then have the students in each group prepare models or drawings of different typical dishes served in their assigned nation. You act the part of a traveler, just arrived in the country and very hungry. Ask about each dish the children have to offer. What is it made of? How does it taste? How does one actually eat it? Follow with a general discussion of different ethnic foods.

Materials Needed: paper, markers

Processing Questions:

1. How do other countries' eating habits differ from ours?

2. Why should we know about other cultures' dietary habits?

Discussion and Report Techniques

Eat for Fitness

Valued Outcome: Students will identify why the body needs a variety of foods.

Description of Strategy: Show students the growing figure (made of paper) and gradually unfold it so that it grows. Engage students in a discussion of what helps bodies grow (exercise, rest and sleep, and food; heredity also plays a part in how much we grow). Talk about the role of food in helping the body grow and how different foods help build up different parts of the body.

Brainstorm with the class other reasons for needing a variety of food. Include the following:

○ to give us energy (our fuel to keep our engine running, the more active we are the more energy, or calories, we use)

○ to keep us healthy (keeps bones and teeth strong)

○ to prevent sickness (helps body fight off germs)

Make a chart for the classroom of the reasons for a healthy, balanced diet. Students may want to make this chart themselves in small groups and then come together to combine their reasons onto one big class chart.

As an activity, have the students color, cut out, and assemble the growing figure. Use tape or fasteners to join the pieces. Show the class how to fold on the dotted lines and then gradually unfold the paper doll to make it grow.

Summarize the lesson by allowing each student to read what is written on their figure, and then allow some time or questions and discussion.

Materials Needed: student activity sheet (one per person), a sample student activity figure to use as a lesson visual, chart paper, crayons (optional)

Processing Questions:

1. What if you loved watermelon and ate only watermelon for breakfast, lunch, dinner, and snacks, everyday? Would that be the best way to help your body grow? Why or why not?

2. What kinds of foods are best for our bodies? (Sweets are not "best.")

Source: G. Ezell. 1992. *Healthy living 2: Healthy and growing.* Grand Rapids, MI: Christian Schools International, p. 135.

Building a Pyramid

Valued Outcome: The students will be able to construct a model of the Food Guide Pyramid with an understanding of the Dietary Guidelines for Americans.

Description of Strategy: Discuss the Dietary Guidelines for Americans and the Food Guide Pyramid and their meanings. Explain that the model they will create will be three-dimensional. To help with the construction of the pyramid, draw an outline of one on the chalkboard. On one side, have the students write in the food groups where they belong on the pyramid. On another side, ask the students to write in the recommended number of daily servings for each group. And on the third side, have them write in a type of food for each food category. On the last open side of the triangle (the bottom), ask the students to write their favorite food. Discussion may include other foods that fall into the various food groups, what food group their favorite food is a part of, or how many servings they have had from each food group on that particular day.

Materials Needed: poster board, scissors, pencil/crayons

Processing Questions:

1. What effect does eating a variety of foods have on our bodies?

2. By following the Dietary Guidelines for Americans, what diseases may we reduce our chance of getting?

Source: L. Meeks and P. Heit. *Totally awesome health*, Fourth grade manual. Blacklick, OH: Meeks Heit.

Keeping in Balance

Valued Outcome: Students will apply knowledge of food groups and daily minimum requirements to plan a balanced daily menu.

Description of Strategy: The major issue in nutrition for most students is not scarcity of foods from each of the four food groups, but making the right choices from among the wide range of food available to them. Although at this age most students are dependent on the choices of their adult caregivers, this lesson may help them to choose whether or not to eat the food the adults provide, and the knowledge to make good snack choices.

Write the numbers 3-2-4-4 on the board, and have students recall what they stand for—the amount or number of servings needed daily (minimum) of each of the food groups. Write the names of the food groups over the numbers.

Have each student plan a day's menu. Follow these steps: Direct students to write down the names of food groups at the top of a sheet of paper. Then list an appropriate number of choices under each grouping. (For example, vegetables, fruit: orange juice, banana, carrot sticks, lettuce.) On a second sheet of paper have them write the headings *Breakfast, Lunch, Dinner, Snack.* Then direct them to write under each heading what they would choose to eat for each meal. They must plan a balanced day's diet with sufficient servings from each of the groups. They can refer to the listings of food group names and choices for help. Extras can be included, but they must be in the moderate amounts. Have pairs of students share their work and check on whether their partner's choices add up to a balanced menu.

As an activity, give students opportunity to "produce" one of the meals on their menu. They can draw, color, and cut out the food items (from magazines and so on) and paste them on a paper plate. If time permits, have students share their meals. In closing, tell the students that today they have used what they know about the four basic food groups to plan healthy meals. This knowledge has now given them the power to make healthy choices in their diet. We can all be smart eaters.

Materials Needed: paper plates, magazines, markets, scissors, crayons, and various art supplies

Processing Questions:

1. After the students have created their menus, ask them what other foods should or could be added to make up the day's quotas?

2. How different are the menus they have made in class to the meals they eat everyday?

3. What changes if any should they make in their diets? in what areas?

Source: G. Ezell. 1992. *Healthy living 2: Healthy and growing*. Grand Rapids, MI: Christian Schools International, p. 135.

"Gregory, the Terrible Eater"

Valued Outcome: The students will present their understanding of the four basic food groups by creating a menu.

Description of Strategy: The purpose of this activity is for the students to review and present their understanding of the need for balanced meals and an understanding of the food sources for proteins, carbohydrates, fats, minerals, and vitamins. *Note:* Have the students save food ads from local papers for a month before the assignment. Begin the lesson by reading the book *Gregory, The Terrible Eater*, by Mitchell Sharmat, and then discuss with the class if Gregory had received any good advice for his eating habits. Ask the students if their parents have ever tried this approach to entice them to eat foods that they dislike. Next, review the Food Guide Pyramid and sources of proteins, carbohydrates, fats, vitamins and minerals. Then divide the class into groups of three and four students each. Assign the groups the projects of planning a three-meal-a-day menu for five days. Use the newspaper food ads to figure the cost of their menus. Stress that economy is important. Each group presents its menu to the class and must be able to defend its selections. Record the total coats of each menu, and then have a group construct a bar or line graph to show the differences in the menu costs.

Materials Needed: newspaper food advertisements; graph paper; children's book *Gregory, The Terrible Eater*, by Mitchell Sharmat; markers

Processing Questions:

1. What are the categories in the Food Guide Pyramid?

2. What are some examples from each category?

This Is What We're Looking For!

Valued Outcome: Students will know which foods belong to which category in the Food Guide Pyramid.

Description of Strategy: Display a poster for each of the categories in the Food Guide Pyramid. Have students bring in clippings from magazines, newspapers, and so forth of different foods. Have students glue pictures to the designated poster (one for each of the food categories in the pyramid) in a certain area of the classroom.

Materials Needed: Poster board, glue, food advertisements

Processing Question: Why are specific foods placed in a particular category?

Planning a Healthy Menu Using the Food Guide Pyramid

Valued Outcome: The students will use their knowledge of the Food Guide Pyramid to plan a healthy meal.

Description of Strategy: When starting this activity, the teacher must review the categories within the Food Guide Pyramid. After reviewing the food categories, explain to the class that they are going to design a menu for one meal, that includes something from each food group. The teacher will then pass out a sample menu and discuss it with the class. The teacher will encourage creativity in this project. When the students are done with their menu for a meal, have them share with the class and discuss whether or not it meets the requirements. Have the students take their menu home and with the help of their parents write the recipes of their meal. Then have all the students turn in a final copy to you. The teacher will then take all the recipes and make a classroom cookbook.

Materials Needed: copies of a sample menu, writing paper, writing utensils, binder in which to keep the recipes included in the cookbook

Processing Questions: How is it helpful to our diet to plan a menu?

Calories In, Calories Out

Valued Outcomes: Students will

1. learn how calories are stored to keep the body functioning and to get energy for physical activities

2. learn how the calories we eat are related to the calories used for activity

Description of Strategy: Hand out a sheet that shows on the left side the amount of calories for servings of particular foods. On the right side of the page are activities. Listed by each activity are the number of calories that would be used per minute of performing that activity. On the bottom of the page are problems (described as follows) for each student to solve using the information at the top. Tell the class that the problems will be solved through class discussion. Read each of the problems to the class. After sufficient time to work the problem independently, have the class discuss the problem together. Use this worksheet as a springboard for further discussion.

Sample problems:

1. Ray ate enough pizza to bike for 153 minutes. What happens if Ray ate more pizza but still biked for only 153 minutes? (He will get more energy from pizza than he needed, so the body will store the extra energy.)

2. What do you suppose will happen to Ray if he eats the same amount of pizza and bikes for longer than 153 minutes? Do you suppose he will run out of energy and stop pedaling? (No.) Why do you think that? (Accept any reasonable response.)

Materials Needed: teacher-made "Calories In, Calories Out" worksheet

Processing Questions:

1. True or false: your body needs calories for energy?

2. True or false, calories come from eating foods?

3. True or false, different activities done for the same period of time use up different amounts of calories?

Source: National Dairy Council. 1987. *Nutritional health guide*, Fifth Grade. Rosemont, IL: U.S. Department of Education, p. 13.

Foods I Eat

Valued Outcome: The students will be able to keep a diary and determine family eating habits.
Description of Strategy: Have students keep a diary of what they eat, where they eat, when they eat, why they eat, and how much they eat over a three-day period. Have them record their family's eating habits to see if those habits are similar or different from the student's eating habits.

Sample Chart:

Time	Foods	Servings	Place	With Whom

Materials Needed: chart for each student
Processing Question: Why do we eat sometimes even when we are not hungry?

Do You Want to Eat this Food?

Valued Outcome: The students will be able to read and interpret food labels for various products.
Description of Strategy: Have students compare the nutrition labels from various foods, such as waffles, potato chips, soup, yogurt, and ice cream. Have the students determine which they would rather eat according to the nutrition labels.
Materials Needed: food labels from various products
Processing Question: Why is it important to be able to understand food labels?

Reporting on the Food Guide Pyramid's Categories

Valued Outcome: Students will become familiar with different foods in the pyramid categories and their nutritional value.
Description of Strategy: Divide the class into six groups and assign each one to a specific food category. The groups will study their category, discovering what foods are in the category, what nutrients are found in them, how many servings we should eat daily, and what benefits and potential problems result from eating these foods. The groups will create a presentation for the class, including oral reports, visual aids, and possibly some samples of foods in their category. If the class does an exceptional job, you can arrange for them to make the presentation to other classes.
Materials Needed: supplies for visual aids, samples of foods (pictures)
Processing Questions:

1. What nutrients are found in the foods in each category?

2. How many servings should we eat daily of each category?

Source: K. L. Siepak. 1994. *Keeping healthy*, Step-by-Step Science Series, Grades 4–6. Greensboro, NC: Carson-Dellosa, p. 31.

Nutrition I.Q.

Valued Outcome: The students will be able to test their nutrition knowledge by answering the questions.

Description of Strategy: The teacher will hand out to each student a sheet containing the following questions. The teacher then can have the students turn in their independent work or discuss the questions as a class.

True or False

1. You'll get proper nourishment if you just eat a variety of foods.

2. People who don't eat meat, poultry, or fish can still stay healthy.

3. Food eaten between meals can be just as good for your health as food eaten at regular meals.

4. Fresh vegetables cooked at home are always more nutritious than canned or frozen vegetables.

5. A high-protein, low-carbohydrate diet is ideal for losing weight.

6. When dieting, avoid starchy foods, such as bread and potatoes.

7. If you weigh what you should, you're getting proper nourishment.

8. Milk contains all the essential elements of a good diet.

9. Give a child all the foods he wants, and he will never suffer from malnutrition.

10. Dark bread has the same caloric value as white bread.

11. Once a person stops exercising, muscle fibers change to fat.

12. Women in their childbearing years need more iron than men do.

Materials Needed: test sheets and pencils for all students

Processing Question: Why is it important to our health to have a good nutrition IQ?

Being Healthy!

Valued Outcome: The students will be able to explain the effects of a proper diet on their physical and mental health.

Description of Strategy: Have the students write down four to six sentences on how they feel when they eat nutritious foods. Have them write how they feel mentally, physically, and emotionally. Then, have them do the same thing on how they feel when they eat nonnutritious food. Write the three aspects of health on the board, and discuss the answers.

Materials Needed: pencil and paper for all students

Processing Question: How can food affect your ability to learn?

Grocery Shopping

Valued Outcome: The students will be able to purchase foods efficiently from a "grocery store."

Description of Strategy: Give each student $20 in play money. Have a variety of food labels set up on a table with their prices. Make note cards for fruits and other products that you don't have labels for. Tell the students that they need to purchase food for two people for three days. Have them shop for the food they'll eat by writing down the food item and its cost. Discuss the results by asking a variety of questions. Who here has bought enough food for three meals a day? Who has bought something from each category of the Food Guide Pyramid?

A field trip to the grocery store is an excellent nutrition strategy.

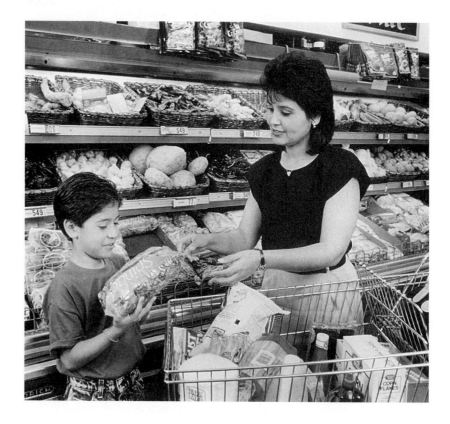

Materials Needed: food labels, note cards
Processing Questions:

1. Why is it important to plan a budget for buying food?
2. What can you learn about a food from reading the label?

Healthy Breakfasts

Valued Outcomes:

1. The students will be able to explain why we need a good breakfast.
2. The students will be able to choose healthy breakfast foods.

Description of Strategy: The teacher will give each child a magazine that he or she can cut pictures from. The students will cut out enough pictures to create a balanced breakfast. They will glue these pictures onto a sheet of construction paper labeled "A Healthful Breakfast."
Materials Needed: magazines, glue, scissors, construction paper, markers or crayons
Processing Questions:

1. Why is breakfast called the most important meal of the day?
2. What types of foods are good to eat at breakfast?

Eating for Healthy Teeth

Valued Outcome: The students will be able to identify foods that are good for the teeth.

Description of Strategy: The teacher will write: "Healthy" and "Unhealthy" on the board. Write one or two words under each category as an example. Then divide the class into groups of three or four. Say, "Please work as a group. Copy the chart and words off the board. As a group, complete the chart by listing healthy foods for teeth under the 'healthy' side and the unhealthy foods under the 'unhealthy' side." Walk around the room to monitor for understanding. Allow time for them to complete the assignment. When all groups have finished, have the class help you complete the chart on the board. Have them explain why they put certain foods under certain categories.

Have students bring in at least ten pictures—drawn or cut out of magazines—of healthy and unhealthy foods for our teeth. Pictures cut out of magazines must be glued or taped on paper. Label pictures "healthy" or "unhealthy."

Materials Needed: magazines, glue or tape, paper

Processing Questions:

1 What are the healthiest foods to eat for our teeth?

2. What are the foods to avoid hurting our teeth?

Healthy Weight

Valued Outcome: The students will be able to explain the benefits of being at a healthful weight.

Description of Strategy: The teacher will write the following menus on the chalkboard.

Menu 1: skim milk, bran muffin, fruit salad, broiled chicken, whole-grain rice, beans

Menu 2: chocolate milkshake, cheeseburger, french fries, and chocolate chip cookies

Ask the students which lunch is healthier.

The teacher will list the seven diet goals on the chalkboard:

1. Eat a variety of foods.

2. Be at a healthful weight.

3. Eat few fatty foods.

4. Eat more fiber.

5. Eat less sugar.

6. Use less salt.

7. Do not drink alcohol.

The teacher will have students write the diet goals on a 3- x 5-inch file card. They should keep the file card with them and refer to it at mealtimes until they have memorized the goals. This will help them become accustomed to considering the diet goals when selecting foods. The teacher will discuss each diet goal. For example:

1. *Eat a variety of foods.* The teacher will ask students to identify the food groups and give the number of servings from each group that should be eaten daily.

2. *Be at a healthful weight.* The teacher will explain how your body works best when you are at the weight that is right for you. Let the students know that the doctor can tell them if they are at a healthful weight. The teacher will explain to the students that they can make wise choices to help them be at a healthful weight and how important it is to exercise.

Materials Needed: 3- x 5- file cards
Processing Questions:

1. Why should you follow the seven diet goals?

2. What are some ways nutrients help your body?

3. Why is it important to be at a healthful weight?

Classifying Healthy and Unhealthy Snacks

Valued Outcome: After completing the week's activity centers, the students will be able to categorize healthy and unhealthy snacks.

Description of Strategy: The teacher will introduce each center as follows: "Today, class, we are starting a new week, and the topic is nutrition. All our centers this week will be related to nutrition."

○ "First we have the Book Center. There are many books to read and look at. There will also be a couple of books you can listen to."

○ "Next we have the Block Center. In here I encourage you to use your imagination and relate something you build to healthy and unhealthy snacks."

○ "Next we have the Writing Center. Here you can make your own nutrition journal by tying some decorative paper together. Today's topic is to draw or tell about the snacks that you like to eat."

○ "Next we have the Cooking Center, where you can mix your own healthy snack. After you mix together the appropriate ingredients, you can take your mix to the eating area and enjoy it. You will be mixing things like Chex cereal, pretzels, peanuts, raisins, and popcorn in a little bag and shake it all together. Then it is ready to eat."

○ "Next we have the Art Center. In art today we are going to make a collage of healthy and unhealthy snacks. Look through the magazines and find pictures of either healthy snacks or unhealthy snacks. Then glue them on your piece of paper. Try choosing only healthy and unhealthy snacks for your collage. You can also make caterpillars out of the styrofoam pieces and the toothpicks."

○ "In the Math Center, you will sort the snacks into two piles of healthy and unhealthy snacks. There will be a checklist on the back of the title card."

○ "In the Language Arts Center, there is a worksheet and on the worksheet there are both healthy and unhealthy snacks. Color the healthy snacks."

○ "In the Science Center, you will taste healthy and unhealthy snacks, and chart how well you liked each snack. Then as a class we will look at the results to see who liked what the best."

○ "In the Game Center there will be several games to play, such as X's and O's from Cheerios, Hangman using the Alphabet cereal, and the usual games that are there."

Materials Needed: paper, nutrition books, building blocks, decorative paper, healthy and unhealthy snacks, sandwich bags, magazines, title cards

Processing Question: What types of food provide the healthiest snacks?

Healthy Snacks

Valued Outcomes:

1. The students will be able to describe the function and role of snacking in relation to their eating habits.
2. The students will be able to identify healthy snacks.

Description of Strategy: Have students compare their eating habits with those needed for good nutrition by writing down their favorite snack foods. Ask students if these foods belong to the Food Guide Pyramid categories. Compare favorite snack foods to nutritious snack foods. If favorite foods do not belong to basic food groups, what nutritious foods can be eaten instead? Eat a smart snack with the class. Have the students plan the snack time based on their regularly scheduled lunch time. Have a simple snack of popcorn or cheese and crackers, or if students brought various items from home, have a tasting party. Challenge students to use their knowledge of good snacking to think of five smart snacks that would sell in a "snack store." Consider setting prices on items and having students work out some math problems on the bottom or back of the worksheet.
Materials Needed: healthy snack foods
Processing Questions:

1. Is it a good idea to include snacks as part of your diet?
2. If you snack, are there healthy snacks that will enhance your health?

Learning about the Food Guide Pyramid

Valued Outcomes:

1. The students will identify the levels in the Food Guide Pyramid
2. The students will demonstrate the ability to select foods in each category.

Description of Strategy: Pass out some magazines and have students cut out pictures of different foods. As you cut out these pictures, think about the Food Guide Pyramid. Try to find a picture to represent each food category. If they find a picture of a food that represents more than one food category, have them try to identify the different groups represented by that food.

After students appear to have each category well represented, list each food group on the board. For foods that have ingredients from different categories, list the food as a whole, and then the ingredient in that category. Continue the list until it is sufficient to indicate students have a clear understanding of what foods belong in what categories.

Using the food pictures, set up a "cafeteria line" from which students will choose a meal to place on a tray. Have students take turns being the cashiers—checking to see that choices include food from each food group.
Materials Needed: magazines with food pictures, scissors, trays borrowed from cafeteria
Processing Questions:

1. What categories are in the Food Guide Pyramid?
2. What foods are in each category of the pyramid?

School Cafeteria Menus

Valued Outcome: The students will be able to write sample menus incorporating a variety of foods from the school lunch program.
Description of Strategy: Have the school dietitian bring various cafeteria menus to class and show how variety is incorporated into them. Have students write sample menus incorporating a variety of food characteristics for the school lunch program.
Materials Needed: pen and paper
Processing Question: Does your school lunch menu have foods from each category of the Food Guide Pyramid?

Food Advertisements

Valued Outcome: The students will be able to identify merchandising methods used in making foods more appealing.
Description of Strategy: Assign students to observe food advertisements on television and in magazines and newspapers. Have them notice merchandising methods used to make foods more appealing and interesting. Have students report their observations to the class.
Materials Needed: magazines and newspapers
Processing Questions:

1. How are food advertisements produced to make you want to buy and eat that particular type of food?

2. Do you think food advertisements have enticed you to buy a food that you did not actually need?

Food Safety

Valued Outcome: The student will be able to identify food safety legislation.
Description of Strategy: Have students conduct library research to determine federal and state legislation that helps ensure food safety for the public. Have them present this information in written or oral reports.
Materials Needed: none
Processing Questions:

1. What organizations protect our health by ensuring that the foods we eat are safe?

2. What kinds of laws are in effect to make foods safer?

Weight Management Programs

Valued Outcome: The students will be able to learn healthy weight reduction methods.
Description of Strategy: Invite a leader of a weight reduction group that stresses balanced nutrition in its program to discuss the effect and health implications of prolonged overeating and crash diets. Have students submit questions on cards in advance to be answered by the resource person.
Materials Needed: index cards
Processing Questions:

1. What are the dangers of dieting improperly?

2. Why are fad diets so popular?

"Candy Machines in the Schools" Debate

Valued Outcome: The students will be able to debate whether candy machines should or should not be installed in the school cafeteria.

Description of Strategy: Should candy machines be placed in the school cafeteria? Have two debate teams argue the issue. Act as moderator and keep the debate on track. Then follow with a general class discussion.

Materials Needed: none

Processing Questions:

1. Why are candy machines present in some schools?

2. Does the presence of some machines encourage poor eating habits on the part of some students?

Food Label Activity

Valued Outcome: The students will be able to identify and report on regulations concerning labeling food.

Description of Strategy: Have students research the regulations concerning labeling of packaged foods and present their reports either orally or in writing. Individualize the activity by having each student prepare a report on a specific food product. Then have the student discuss his or her findings in class, explaining what information is contained on the label of the package. Later, put all the packages on display so that students may examine them.

Materials Needed: various packaged foods

Processing Questions:

1. Why do packaged foods have labels?

2. How can such labels help us eat healthier?

Diet Modification

Valued Outcome: The students will be able to compare different diet modifications.

Description of Strategy: Give students a problem such as modifying diets for athletes or planning inexpensive party menus. Have them consult at least three different sources of information. Compare the conclusions that might be reached from the information derived from the three sources.

Materials Needed: none

Processing Questions:

1. How do professional nutritionists help us eat healthier?

2. Why is it important to plan the meals for such events?

Brainstorming about Nutrition

Valued Outcome: The students will be able to brainstorm concerns about the school food service program.

Description of Strategy: Organize students into several groups. Have them identify students' concerns about the school food service program and brainstorm about potential solutions to the

Hands-on activities enhance the learning of health concepts.

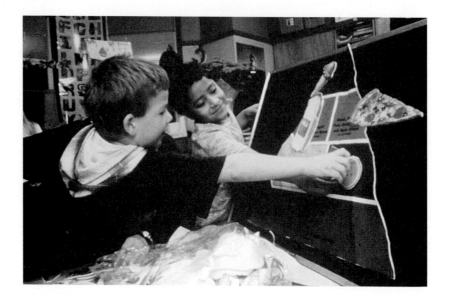

problems they have identified. Have them summarize their ideas and present them to the school dietitian.

Materials Needed: none

Processing Questions:

1. How would you rate your school food service program?

2. What barriers to effectiveness do most school food serve programs face?

Food Patterns over the Years

Valued Outcome: The students will be able to list the changes over the years concerning food patterns.

Description of Strategy: Have students interview grandparents or others of that age to see how food patterns have changed over the years. Have them report on how and why the patterns have changed.

Materials Needed: none

Processing Questions:

1. How have eating patterns changed since your grandparents' day?

2. Do you eat healthier now as a child than your grandparents did when they were your age?

Pyramid Essay

Valued Outcome: The students will be able to identify foods from the Food Guide Pyramid that he or she likes the least and the best.

Description of Strategy: After a discussion of the Food Guide Pyramid, have the students write a short essay about the food group they like the best and the least, along with their favorite and least favorite foods in the groups.

Materials Needed: a poster of the Food Guide Pyramid
Processing Questions:

1. What is the purpose of the Food Guide Pyramid?

2. Which levels do you like the most? the least?

Experiments and Demonstrations ——————————

Vitamins for Nutrition

Valued Outcome: Students will be able to determine the vitamin content of several different beverages.
Description of Strategy: The students will list several different vitamins found in foods and beverages. Vitamin C will be chosen by the teacher, and then the students will discuss the reason we need vitamin C. They will then discuss what beverages they think vitamin C is found in. Then they will conduct an experiment for testing the content of the beverages. A test solution will be made. This is done by combining 3 mL cornstarch to 50 mL of water in a pan. This will be boiled until the cornstarch dissolves. After cooling, 5 mL of this solution will be added to 125 mL of cold water. One drop of iodine will be added, which will make the solution blue. Ten mL of the blue solution will be placed in a test tube. The test tube will be labeled with the name of the beverage being tested. Then 25 drops of the beverage being tested will be added. The students will then record the results. Vitamin C will turn the blue solution clear. The clearer the solution, the more vitamin C in the beverage. The students will record the color of the solution before and after the beverage is added. One test tube will only contain the test solution for comparison. The students will then line up the test tubes in order from the least amount of vitamin C to the most. If needed for comparison purposes, a white sheet of paper may be placed behind the test tubes. Once the students have determined the liquid with the most vitamin C, they will look at the nutritional labels and compare the least amount and the most amount of vitamin C.
Materials Needed: cornstarch, water, pan, hot plate or stove, spoon, tincture of iodine, beverages to test (orange juice, soft drinks, water, apple juice, lemonade, tea, and milk), test tubes, eyedropper
Processing Questions:

1. Why do we need vitamin C?

2. If we don't get enough vitamin C in our diets, what will happen to our bodies?

3. What other vitamins are needed for a healthy body?

Source: D. Vaszily and P. Perdue. 1994. *Bones, bodies, and bellies.* Glenview, IL: Scott Foresman, p. 60.

Fats: Hidden But Tasty

Valued Outcome: Students will be able to find fat in foods.
Description of Strategy: Give students pieces of brown paper (a little larger than notebook paper), and tell them to write their names on them. Let the students choose twelve foods to test, or let them test everything you brought. Instruct them to take a piece of the food and rub it in one spot on their papers. If they are testing something like seeds or chips, they should break the pieces of food to

ensure that whatever is inside the food will be tested. Tell the students to rub only one piece of food at a time, and once they have rubbed that food to circle the rubbed spot and label the circle with the food's name. This way they will know what they have tested. Set the papers in a warm location to dry. When the papers have dried, tell the students to find theirs and observe them. Can they tell where fat is? Fats will be absorbed into the paper, making it appear translucent. Are they surprised to see fat residue from some of the foods? Instruct the class to make graphs indicating the foods that had fat in them. Discuss the importance of considering the fat content in foods before eating. If we are to have low-fat diets, we must consider the amount of fat naturally in some foods, such as peanut butter or mayonnaise. Often people mistakenly assume that we are supposed to eat some extra fats and oils because they have a block on the Food Guide Pyramid. Fats are found in so many foods already that we don't need to add them to anything to get enough in our diets.

Materials Needed: brown paper bags, pencils, variety of foods to test, including corn chips, potato chips, bologna, hot dogs, glazed doughnuts, mayonnaise, peanut butter, cheese, sunflower seeds, pecans or other nuts, apples, bananas, lettuce, cooked rice, cooked noodles, potatoes, butter, margarine, popcorn, chocolate chips, carrots, cooked or canned pinto beans, celery, coconut, and oranges

Processing Questions:

1. What is the importance of considering the fat content in foods before eating?

2. Of the foods tested, are the majority of the fatty ones in any one particular food category?

Source: K. Siepak 1994. *Keeping healthy*, Step-by-Step Science Series, Grades 4–6, Greensboro, NC: Carson-Dellosa, p. 34–35.

Is It Healthy Or Not?

Valued Outcome: The students will be able to determine if a group of foods comprises a healthy meal.

Description of Strategy: Set up a couple meals on a table. Have a real nutritious meal, a nonnutritious meal, somewhat nutritious, etc. Split the class up in groups. Have the groups go to each meal and look at them. Have them guess if the meal is nutritious or not. Give them five to seven minutes at each station. Tell them that they are not allowed to talk to anyone. Have them write whatever comments they want to about the meal. Then have the groups get together and discuss what they wrote. Have a group discussion about every meal. Let the groups explain what they wrote and why.

Materials Needed: food, plates, glasses, utensils

Processing Question: What criteria did you use to decide if a meal was nutritious or not?

Fats and the Heart

Valued Outcome: The students will be able to describe the effects of a poor diet on the heart.

Description of Strategy: Have a picture of the heart on the wall. Point out the different valves. Explain how the blood enters and leaves the heart. Ask a variety of questions about the heart. Show the fact that if you eat too much junk food that contains fat that you can block one of the valves. When a valve is blocked it can cause the heart to beat abnormally. If the heart doesn't beat normally, then it can stop and this can cause a heart attack. Also, bring in pieces of fat. Try to get a pound of fat so they can see what it looks like when you gain a pound of fat.

Materials Needed: picture of the heart

Processing Questions:

1. How do healthy foods help the heart function better?
2. How do unhealthy foods harm the functioning of the heart?

Complete Proteins

Valued Outcome: The students will be able to describe complete proteins.

Description of Strategy: Explain how complete proteins are ones that contain just the right amounts of all nine essential amino acids. Animal sources of protein (meat, fish, eggs, milk, and milk products) contain complete proteins. Plant sources of protein (dried beans, peas, nuts, breads, and cereals) contain incomplete proteins. These are low in one or more essential amino acids. Have cards made that have the names of foods that provide incomplete proteins written on them ("Beans," "Rice," "Grains"). Take two blank cards and put them together. Label this "Complete protein." Then take one incomplete protein card and add another incomplete protein card to show how to make a complete protein, such as "Beans and Rice." Explain the fact that this is what most vegetarians do, because they don't eat meat.

Materials Needed: note cards

Processing Questions:

1. What role does protein play in our diet?
2. What would happen to the body if we did not eat enough of the right kind of proteins?

Using Disclosing Tablets

Valued Outcome: The students will be able to determine how well they brush their teeth after a meal.

Description of Strategy: Give each student a disclosing tablet—a chewable tablet that will color the plaque and calculus, acid, bacteria, and food buildup on our teeth that we cannot see. Instruct the students chew up the disclosing tablet. After the students have chewed the tablet, have them look in a mirror to see what their teeth look like. Pass out toothbrushes and toothpaste (these can be supplied by the local dental society), have them brush their teeth and check them again in the mirror. Allow them to continue brushing their teeth until less of the disclosing color is on the teeth.

Materials Needed: disclosing tablets, toothbrushes, toothpaste, mirrors (if there isn't one in the room)

Processing Questions:

1. Why is it important to brush and floss after eating?
2. How do disclosing tablets help us determine if we are brushing correctly?

Eating Fewer Fatty Foods

Valued Outcomes:

1. The students will be able to identify fatty foods and follow a plan to eat fewer fatty foods.
2. The students will be able to identify sources of fiber by reading cereal box labels and follow a plan to eat more fiber.
3. The students will be able to identify different kinds of sugars and follow a plan to eat less sugar.

4. The students will be able to determine salt content and follow a plan to eat less salt.

Description of Strategy: The teacher will use bacon and an apple for demonstration. The teacher will place the two foods on a section of a grocery bag. Demonstrate how the bacon will leave a grease spot on the bag. The teacher will explain to the students that this same material can collect on artery walls.

The teacher will use empty cereal boxes and have the students read the cereal labels to determine which cereals contain sources of fiber. The teacher will instruct the students to create a name for a cereal that tells the consumer that the cereal contains fiber.

The teacher will write the following words on the chalkboard: *sucrose, maltose, fructose, lactose,* and *corn syrup.* Explain that these are words for different kinds of sugar. The teacher will add the word *sodium* and explain that this word is used for salt. Have the students pretend they are sugar and salt detectives. They are to read labels at home to find what kinds of foods contain sugars and salt. The students should make a list of five foods that contain sugars and five foods that contain salt.
Materials Needed: slices of bacon, an apple, empty cereal boxes
Processing Questions:

1. Why should we eat more fiber? How does that make us healthier?

2. Why should you keep your arteries clear of fat?

3. Why is it important to eat foods with fiber?

4. Why should you eat less sugar?

5. Why should you use less salt?

6. Why is it important to read food labels?

Differences in Milk

Valued Outcome: The students will be able to compare the taste of various milk products.
Description of Strategy: Display a collection of milk products: whole, skim, evaporated, condensed, powdered, chocolate, buttermilk, etc. Compare the various milk products as to taste, smell, feel, consistency, and appearance.
Materials Needed: varieties of milk products
Processing Questions:

1. What purposes do milk serve in our diet?

2. Which type of milk is healthiest?

3. Which type of milk do you prefer?

Make Egg Nog

Valued Outcome: The students will be able to make egg nog.
Description of Strategy: During the winter holiday season, have children make egg nog from a recipe. Have the students beat 4 eggs with a beater, add 1/4 cup sugar, 1/4 teaspoon salt, 1/2 teaspoon vanilla, 1 quart milk, and a dash of nutmeg. Beat until thoroughly mixed, then serve.
Materials Needed: 4 eggs, a beater, 1/4 cup sugar, 1/4 teaspoon salt, 1/2 teaspoon vanilla, 1 quart milk, and a dash of nutmeg.
Processing Questions:

1. How do food traditions begin for special events such as holidays?

2. Does your family have any such traditions centered around food?

Food Diary

Valued Outcome: The students will be able to record foods eaten for two or three days and determine the status of the food in the Food Guide Pyramid.

Description of Strategy: Have the students keep a food diary for themselves for two or three days. Have them list foods they eat, being as specific as possible, such as fried or baked, amount eaten. Have them look up each food in the food pyramid. Have them record the total of foods eaten in each of the food groups after the three days.

Materials Needed: Food Guide Pyramid, chart, food log

Processing Questions: How can keeping a food diary enhance your nutrition decisions?

Food Labels

Valued Outcome: The students will be able to identify the nutritional content from various food labels.

Description of Strategy: Distribute different food labels, and have students answer the following questions about their food: name, net weight, largest ingredient, additives, serving size, calories per serving, percentage of RDA for the vitamins and minerals.

Materials Needed: food labels

Processing Questions:

1. Why do foods have labels?
2. What important information can be found on food labels?

Preparing Cafeteria Food

Valued Outcome: The students will observe the cafeteria personnel preparing food.

Description of Strategy: Take the class to the cafeteria to observe a food being prepared, such as bread. To make the experience more interesting and informative, have the school dietitian explain each step in the process.

Materials Needed: none

Processing Questions:

1. What did you learn from the preparation of the food in the cafeteria?
2. What sanitary activities did you observe in the food preparation?

Foods Eaten in the Cafeteria

Valued Outcome: The students will observe various foods eaten by students in the school cafeteria.

Description of Strategy: Have students observe (using an observation form) the kinds and amounts of foods eaten by students in the school cafeteria. Record the kinds and amounts of foods eaten by students at each grade level, if possible.

Materials Needed: observation form

Processing Questions:

1. Do most students in your school eat healthy lunches in the cafeteria?
2. Does your school lunch program offer various alternatives for eating?

Food Waste

Valued Outcome: The students will identify foods that are wasted by the students in the school cafeteria.

Description of Strategy: The previous experiment could be followed up with a food waste survey to determine which foods are not eaten from each food group. Have students make a graph of the information and present arguments to increase selection of the food groups that are not chosen or eaten often.

Materials Needed: food waste survey, graph paper

Processing Questions:

1. Do you think a lot of foods are wasted in your cafeteria?

2. What types of food are wasted the most?

3. What environmentally healthy can be done with the wasted food?

Food Preparation

Valued Outcome: The students will be able to prepare a food in a variety of ways.

Description of Strategy: Have students conduct a laboratory experiment in which they prepare one specific food in several different ways. Have them evaluate their perceptions of the food prepared in each way.

Materials Needed: a quantity of a specific type of food

Processing Question: Why is it important to know different ways to prepare the same type of food?

Food Cleanliness

Valued Outcome: The students will be able to prepare and observe agar plates of certain contaminating bacteria.

Description of Strategy: Prepare agar plates to show the growth of bacteria resulting from lack of personal cleanliness. For each plate, have a student contaminate by coughing, sneezing, touching with dirty hands, touching with washed hands, or placing a hair in it. Have students view the plates the day prepared and several days later to determine how personal cleanliness affects the growth of bacteria.

Materials Needed: agar plates

Processing Questions:

1. How can germs be spread through unsanitary behavior around food?

2. How can we prevent our food from being contaminated?

Source: Tennessee Department of Education. 1984. *Tennessee educates for nutrition now*. Nashville: Author.

Microbe Growth

Valued Outcome: The students will be able to observe how heat inhibits the growth of microbes.

Description of Strategy: Have students do an experiment that illustrates how hot a food must be to keep microbes from growing. Heat water to 150° Fahrenheit. Use a meat thermometer to determine temperature. Have students take a few sips with plastic spoons to see how hot the water feels to the lips and tongue. Then cool it to 140°F, the point at which microbial growth of organisms begins, and have them taste again. Ask students to give examples of hot foods that frequently are allowed to cool to 140°F, and discuss the problems associated with this practice. Also, discuss measures that can be taken to prevent them.

Materials Needed: meat thermometer, water, hot plate

Processing Questions:

1. Why is it important to heat foods prior to serving?

2. How does the heating process enhance the quality of the foods?

Source: Tennessee Department of Education. 1984. *Tennessee educates for nutrition now.* Nashville: Author.

Food and the Five Senses

Valued Outcome: The students will be able to utilize food to demonstrate the five senses.

Description of Strategy: Use a food, such as an apple, to teach about the senses. Cut the apple, and ask the students how the apple looks different on the outside and inside (using sight). Give everyone a chance to smell an apple that has been cut and one that is whole. Which has more of an odor (smell)? Have the students determine if the apple is warm or cool, soft or firm, light or heavy (touch). Have students bite into an apple and describe the sound (hearing). Have the students describe whether the taste was sweet, bitter, or salty (taste).

Materials Needed: apple

Processing Question: How do the various senses work together to enhance our enjoyment of foods?

Puzzles and Games

Food Dominoes

Valued Outcome: Students will identify and match foods from the same food categories

Description of Strategy: Divide students into groups of four. A copy of the set of "Food Dominoes" should be given to each group to cut out. (May be laminated for greater durability.) Each domino has two parts, each part representing a separate food category in the Food Guide Pyramid. Five dominoes are doubles in which foods of the same food category appear on both sides. The double multifood domino is always put aside as the starter for the game. The remaining dominoes are shuffled or mixed and turned face down. Each player picks out five and turns them face up in front of him or her. After the double multifood domino has been placed in the center of the playing area, the first player may place one of his or her dominoes to one end of the double domino if the picture matches. The second player may try to match the double domino or the food end on the other end of the second domino played. The play continues with the third and fourth players. Only one domino may be played at each turn. Dominoes are played lengthwise instead of at right angles. The only exception to this rule is in the case of doubles (both ends represent the same food category), where right angles are permitted. A double is always played crosswise to the end it matches. This creates two new directions in which the dominoes may be played. If a player cannot make a match, he or she must draw from the remaining, face-down dominoes until he or she is able to play. If he or she draws the last remaining domino and is still unable to play, he or she must "pass" and try again on his or her next turn. The first player to use all of his or her dominoes wins. Or, if no further plays can be made, the player with the least number of dominoes left wins the game. A copy of the Food Guide Pyramid may need to be made available for reference.

Materials Needed: copies of "Food Dominoes" sheets for each group of students, scissors, a copy of the Food Guide Pyramid

Processing Question: What foods are in the different food categories of the Food Guide Pyramid?

Source: M. W. Fischer. 1996. *Health & safety curriculum*, Primary manual. Grand Rapids, MI: Instructional Fair/TS Denison, pp. 15–17.

Nutrient Game

Valued Outcome: The students will be able to display knowledge of the nutrients by grouping them properly.

Description of Strategy: Make up six big poster board cards that have one of the six nutrients on it. Then make up smaller cards that have different foods written on it. Give each student a card. Six students will have the poster boards while the rest of the students will have the note cards. In this game, the students will walk around and try to group themselves to the nutrient they belong in. However, no one is allowed to speak in this game. The students should try to work together as fast as they can. The group who gathers first wins. However, everyone in their group must belong to that nutrient or they are disqualified.

Materials Needed: poster board, note cards

Processing Question: Why is it important to include a variety of nutrients in our diet?

Alphabet Game

Valued Outcome: The students will be able to spell the names of foods and nutrients correctly.

Description of Strategy: Divide the students up in three groups. Each group will have construction paper with one letter of the alphabet written on each piece of paper. Some letters will be written twice. The instructor will ask the students a question. The group must work together to think of an answer and then spell the word correctly. Each student should only have one letter in his or her hand. They should be standing in a straight line with the word spelled correctly. The group who can do this first wins. *Example:* "This nutrient is responsible for building new cells and tissues in growing children." *Answer:* "protein."

Materials Needed: cards with a letter of the alphabet on each one

Processing Question: What is the function of each nutrient?

Learning the Food Guide Pyramid

Valued Outcome: The students will be able to describe the Food Guide Pyramid.

Description of Strategy: Assign four to five students to each group. On each table there should be some magazines, paper bags, poster boards, scissors, and glue. Each student should have his or her own paper bag. Have the students cut out different foods from the magazines and place them in their bags. Then have the students exchange bags with each other. Tell the students to remove the different foods from the bag and paste it on the correct poster board according to the category in the Food Guide Pyramid it belongs to. Once the students finish, have each group show their poster boards. At the end of class, hang the posters around the classroom.

Materials Needed: magazines, paper bags, scissors, glue, poster boards
Processing Questions:

1. What are the categories in the Food Guide Pyramid?
2. Why is it important to know the various categories in the Food Guide Pyramid?

What Kind of Food Am I?

Valued Outcome: The students will be able to guess types of food from clues.
Description of Strategy: Say "Now we are going to play the 'What kind of food am I?' game." Tape the name of a food on each student's back. "No one is allowed to tell you what your food is, and you are not to tell them the name of their food." Once everyone has become a food, start the game. Call them up to the board one at a time. Have them turn around so their classmates can see the food. The classmates will start describing (one at a time) the food—which food group the student belongs to, the shape, color, or size, or even other foods it might taste good with or be found in. After each hint, the student may guess which food she or he is. After they guess their food, write it on the board under the correct category. Allow students to keep their food tags.
Materials Needed: tape, paper for food tags
Processing Question: What types of clues (characteristics) about foods will help identify those foods?

Label Scavenger Hunt

Valued Outcome: The students will be able to identify certain foods just by reading the food labels.
Description of Strategy: Give several food labels (that have been removed from the products) to groups of students. Have them try to determine what food each of the ingredient labels are describing. Points can be awarded to the groups on the basis of guessing the correct food from the labels.
Materials Needed: food labels
Processing Question: How can the information from food labels help us to identify foods?

Food Scavenger Hunt

Valued Outcome: The students will be able to participate in a scavenger hunt using costs as the criteria.
Description of Strategy: A variation on the preceding game is the following: Ask parents to help students conduct a scavenger hunt in local groceries or kitchens at home. Have them look for the following: a food that costs more than $5 per pound, the least expensive form of milk per liquid ounce, the most expensive form of potatoes per pound, and the least expensive form of peaches per pound. After the hunt, compare results and discuss the factors involved in the cost of various foods.
Materials Needed: pen and paper
Processing Questions:

1. Why are some foods more expensive than others?

2. If a food is more expensive, does that always mean that it is more nutritious?

Source: Tennessee Department of Education. 1984. *Tennessee educates for nutrition now*. Nashville: Author.

Brown Bag Contest

Valued Outcome: The students will be able to prepare and share a brown bag lunch where no refrigeration is available.
Description of Strategy: Have a contest to plan the most interesting and nutritious brown bag lunch for a situation where refrigeration is not available. Have the students prepare, display, and eat the lunches.
Materials Needed: lunch prepared by students
Processing Questions:

1. Can a brown bag lunch be as nutritious as a school cafeteria-prepared meal?

2. What are some healthy choices that can be included in a brown bag lunch?

Source: Tennessee Department of Education. 1984. *Tennessee educates for nutrition now*. Nashville: Author.

Food Alphabet

Valued Outcome: The students will be able to list the names of foods for each letter of the alphabet.
Description of Strategy: Divide the students into teams, and assign each team a number of letters of the alphabet. For example, one team can be assigned letters *A* through *E*, the next team letters *F* through *J*, and so on. Challenge each team to write down at least one food for each letter assigned to the team.
Materials Needed: pen and paper
Processing Question: What are the names of foods that start with each letter of the alphabet?

Cultural Foods Game

Valued Outcome: The students will be able to make food cards representing different cultures' foods.
Description of Strategy: To make cards, paste or draw pictures of food in the center of the card. Write name of food at the top of the card. The player must recognize the country when he sees name of food. Suggested number of cards is 30 for two to four players, more for larger groups.
How to Play:

1. Shuffle the deck well.

2. Deal five cards to each player face down.

3. The player on the dealer's left draws one card from the deck. He may either keep the card, or discard it right side up next to the pile. If he keeps the card, he must discard another (at all times the player must have five cards in his hand).

4. The opponent (s) may either take the card that is right side up or draw from the pile. He discards.

5. The game continues until a player has five different cultures of food represented by his cards.

6. The player lays down his hand for his opponent(s) to see and check. If correct, he is then declared the winner.

Variation:

Players can decide to play for one culture of food. In which case six cards should be made for each of five cultures. When a player sees the first five cards he is dealt, he can decide which country he has more food representing. This will determine which country he plays for, and he will try to get a "set" of cards for that country. The first player to get a set is the winner.

Materials Needed:

1. One package 3- x 5-inch index cards.

2. Pictures of foods from countries studied. These pictures can either be cut out of magazines, from food boxes, or drawn. Foods from Mexico, France, China, Germany, Italy, and Hawaii are especially interesting to study.

Processing Questions:

1. What are some foods from other countries that are different from ours?

2. Why is it important to know about other cultures' foods?

Food Guide Pyramid Bingo

Valued Outcome: The student will be able to participate in bingo using food lists instead of numbers or letters.

Description of Strategy: Distribute bingo cards to the students. The cards will have several columns across, with each one labeled to represent a different category of the Food Guide Pyramid. The spaces below each column will have the name of a food within that food category. Draw cards with the names of various foods on them, and read them aloud to the students. The students will place tokens over the names of the foods on their cards, and the first person to match four words across is the winner.

Materials Needed: bingo cards

Processing Questions:

1. What are the different categories of foods within the Food Guide Pyramid?

2. Why is it important to know foods within each category?

Wheel of Food

Valued Outcome: The student will be able to participate in a game identifying certain foods from the Food Guide Pyramid.

Description of Strategy: This game is set up like "Wheel of Fortune." The spinner spins the wheel indicating from which food category the secret word will be chosen. Students serving as card holders will be given the correct cards for a food name. The blank sides of these cards will be held toward the class until the letter turner is instructed by his or her assistant to turn the card. Remind the children that the food they will be trying to spell out will come from the food category chosen.

This first team, or student, chooses a letter, and if correct, they continue. If the first team/student is incorrect, the second team/student get a turn and so on. The team to turn or guess all letters and spell the name of the food is the winner.

Materials Needed: wheel, cards, Food Guide Pyramid chart

Processing Questions:

1. What are the different categories of foods within the Food Guide Pyramid?

2. Why is it important to know the foods within each category?

Other Ideas

Food Guide Pyramid Posters

Valued Outcome: The students will be able to work as a group to make a bulletin board made of posters including the various categories of the Food Guide Pyramid.

Description of Strategy: Assign four to five students to each group. On each table there should be some magazines, paper bags, poster boards, scissors, and glue. Each student should have a paper bag. Have the students cut out different foods from the magazines and place them in their bags. Then have the students exchange bags with each other. Tell the students to remove the different foods from the bag and paste them on the correct poster board according to the food category it belongs to. If a student has a question about a specific food, the group can help the student out. Once the students finish, have each group show their poster boards. Have the students share with the instructor which foods they had problems placing and discuss it. At the end of class, hang the posters around the classroom.

Materials Needed: magazines, paper bags, scissors, glue, poster boards

Processing Question: Which foods did you have trouble placing in the proper category? Why?

Nutrition Self-Portraits

Valued Outcome: The students will be able to draw a picture that describes how the foods they eat help them become healthy.

Description of Strategy: Have the student draw a picture of him- or herself in the center of a piece of paper. Then have the students draw around their pictures all kinds of nutritious foods that they like to eat. Display the self-portraits around the room.

Materials Needed: paper, crayons or markers

Processing Question:

1. Why is it important to eat nutritious foods?

2. How do nutritious foods enhance our health?

Diet and Athletic Performance

Valued Outcome: The students will be able to research and report on the relationship between proper diet and improved athletic performance.

Description of Strategy: Have the students research the relationship between proper diet and improved athletic performance. One suggestion would be to have them interview a local high school athlete or coach for his or her own eating behaviors.

Materials Needed: none
Processing Questions:

1. What effect does a healthy diet have on athletic performance?

2. What effect does a poor diet have on athletic performance?

3. What types of foods should be eaten to enhance athletic performance?

Field Trips

Valued Outcome: The students will be able to participate in a field trip relating to food or dairy products.

Description of Strategy: Arrange to take the class on a field trip to a dairy, bakery, food processing plant, or other nutrition-related operation. Be sure to prepare your class thoroughly for the trip before they go. Discuss the nature of the operation that they will see. Explain the processes they will observe, and have the students prepare a list of questions they will want to ask.

Materials Needed: none
Processing Questions:

1. How do the processes of food preparation vary in the different nutrition-related operations?

2. What sanitary practices did you observe in the processing of foods?

Poster Contest

Valued Outcome: The students will be able to construct a poster using topics concerning all aspects of food.

Description of Strategy: Each week assign a theme for individual posters, using such topics as the Food Guide Pyramid, table manners, essential nutrients, and so on. Post the completed art in the classroom or in the school cafeteria.

Materials Needed: poster board
Processing Questions:

1. How do such signs serve as reminders for good food-related behavior?

2. What are some essential messages that should be related through such signs?

References

Donatelle, R. J., and L. G. Davis. 1996. *Access to health,* 4th ed. Boston: Allyn and Bacon.

Ezell, G. 1992. *Healthy living 2: Healthy and growing.* Grand Rapids, MI: Christian Schools International.

Fischer, M. W. 1996. *Health & safety curriculum,* Primary Manual. Grand Rapids, MI: Instructional Fair/TS Denison.

Meeks, L., and P. Heit. 1996. *Totally awesome health,* Fourth grade manual. Blacklick, OH: Meeks Heit.

National Dairy Council. 1987. *Nutritional health guide,* Fifth grade. Rosemont, IL, National Dairy Council.

Siepak, K. L. 1994. *Keeping healthy,* Step-by-Step Science Series, Grades 4–6. Greensboro, NC: Carson-Dellosa.

Smolin, L., and M. Grosvenor. 1994. *Nutrition: Science and applications.* Fort Worth, TX: Saunders.

Tennessee Department of Education. 1984. *Tennessee educates for nutrition now.* Nashville: Tennessee Department of Education.

Vaszily, D., and P. Perdue. 1994. *Bones, bodies, and bellies.* Glenview, IL: Scott, Foresman.

Suggested Readings

Bruess, C., and G. Richardson. 1994. *Healthy decisions.* Madison, WI: Brown & Benchmark.

Donatelle, R., and L. Davis. 1996. *Access to health,* 4th ed. Boston: Allyn and Bacon.

Edlin, G., and E. Golanty. 1992. *Health and wellness: A holistic approach,* 4th ed. Boston: Jones & Bartlett.

FDA. 1992, February 12. *FDA backgrounder,* pp. 1–2.

Foulke, J. 1992, February. Wide-sweeping FDA proposals to improve food labeling. *FDA consumer,* pp. 9–13.

Hahn, D., & W. Payne. 1997. *Focus on health,* 3rd ed. St. Louis: Mosby.

Hales, D. 1994. *An invitation to health: The power of prevention,* 6th ed. Redwood City, CA: Benjamin/Cummings.

Miller, D., S. Telljohann, and C. Symons. *Health education in the elementary & middle-level school,* 2nd ed. Madison, WI: Brown & Benchmark.

Mullen, K., R. McDermott, R. Gold, and P. Belcastro. 1996. *Connections for health,* 4th ed. Madison, WI: Brown & Benchmark.

Pate, R. 1993. "Physical Activity in Children and Youth: Relationship to Obesity." *Contemporary nutrition* 18(2).

U.S. Department of Agriculture, Human Nutrition Information Service. 1992, August. Leaflet No. 572. Rockville, MD: Author.

U.S. Department of Agriculture. 1992, December. *Dietary guidelines and your health.* Rockville, MD: Author.

U. S. Department of Health and Human Services. 1992, April. *Eating to lower your high blood cholesterol.* Washington, DC: Author.

U.S. Department of Agriculture, U.S. Department of Health and Human Services. 1995. *Nutrition and your health: Dietary guidelines for Americans,* 4th ed. Washington, DC: U.S. Government Printing Office.

University of California at Berkeley. 1992. Fast food: Decoding the menus. *University of California at Berkeley Wellness Letter* 8(9): 3.

Yarian, R., ed. 1996. *Health 95/96.* 13th ed. Guilford, CT: Dushkin.

Videos

The following videos are available from Schoolhouse Videos & CDs, 4205 Grove Ridge Drive, Durham, NC 27703.

Teen health series: Nutrition and diet. An interesting look at diet, loaded with tips, do's and don'ts and experts' advice on proper nutrition. (Grades 5–9, 30 minutes, Item 6736)

Teen health series: Eating disorders. Moving interviews with several young people who have suffered from anorexia nervosa and bulimia, plus therapists discussing these potentially fatal disorders. (Grades 7–12, 30 minutes, Item 6732)

The following videos are available from Sunburst Communications, 101 Castleton Street, P.O. Box 40, Pleasantville, NY 10570.

Real people: Coping with eating disorders. Gives viewers revealing insights into eating disorders by documenting the stories of three young people—an anorexic, a bulimic, and a compulsive overeater. Interweaving their stories, a specialist discusses the pattern, symptoms, and treatment of eating disorders.

Come see about nutrition and exercise. Presents details about food groups, fiber, vitamins, cholesterol, weight control, disease prevention, exercise, and energy metabolism. Helps students understand the Food Guide Pyramid.

Web Sites

General Health

Resources for School Health Educators
http://www.indiana.edu/~aphs/hlthk-12..html

CDC Prevention Guidelines Database
http://wonder.cdc.gov/wonder/prevguid/prevguid.htm

Developing Educational Standards
http://putwest.boces.org/standards.html

Adolescent Health On-line
http://www.ama-assn.org/adolhlth/adolhlth.htm

See particularly the Adolescent Health Links at
<*http://www.ama-assn.org/adolhlth/gapslink/gapslnk2.htm#ADOL*>

PE Central
http://infoserver.etl.vt.edu/~/PE.Central/PEC2.html

Kathy Schrock's Guide for Educators
http://www.capecod.net/Wixon/health/fitness.htm

Health Education Forum
http://libertynet.org/~lion/forum-health.html

Education World—Subjects: Physical Education
http://www.education-world.com/db/phys-gen.shtml

The Life Education Network
http://www.lec.org/

American Cancer Society
http://www.cancer.org

Physical Activity and Health: A Report of the Surgeon General
http://www.cdc.gov/nccdphp/sgr/sgr.htm

American Social Health Association
http://sunsite.unc.edu/ASHA/

Adolescence Directory On Line (ADOL)
http://education.indiana.edu/cas/adol/adol.html

AIDS NOW! For Teens
http://www.itec.sfsu.edu/aids/aids.html

National Health & Education Consortium (NHEC)
http://www.nhec.org/

About Health
http://www.abouthealth.com/

National Parent Information Network
http://ericps.ed.uiuc.edu/npin/npinhome.html

Healthy People 2000
http://odphp.osophs.dhhs.gov/pubs/hp2000/default.htm

Nutrition

American Cancer Society Guidelines
www.cancer.org/todguide.html

American Dietetic Association
ww.eatright.org

American Heart Association
www.amhrt.org

Food and Drug Administration
www.fda.gov

International Food Information Council
ificinfo.health.org

NIH National Cancer Institute 5 a Day Program
www.dcpc.nci.nih.gov/5aday

Office of Disease Prevention and Health Promotion
odphp.osophs.dhhs.gov

U.S. Department of Agriculture
www.usda.gov

Eating Disorders

Alliance to Fight Eating Disorders
http://www.fsci.umn.edu/~AFED/

Eating Disorders: Anorexia Nervosa and Bulimia
http://www.pb.net/usrwww/w_fishy/ed.htm

Eating Disorder Support Page
http://www.geocities.com/SunsetStrip/3761/

Eating Disorders in Males
http://www.mhsource.com/edu/psytimes/p950942.html

National Institutes of Mental Health
http://www.psych.med.umich.edu/web/psychRef/disorder/eating.htm

Food and Drug Safety

American Academy of Family Physicians
www.aafp.org

Administration on Aging
www.aoa.dhhs.gov/

FDA Center for Drug Evaluation and Research
www.fda.gov/cder/

FDA Center for Food Safety and Applied Nutrition
vm.cfsan.fda.gov/list.html

Food and Drug Administration
www.fda.gov

Institute of Medicine, Food and Nutrition Board
www2.nas.edu/Fnb/2102.html

NIH National Institute on Aging
www.nih.gov/nia/

USDA Food Safety and Inspection Service
www.usda.gov/agency/fsis/homepage.htm

Surveillance and Data Systems

Agency for Health Care Policy and Research Data and Methods
www.ahcpr.gov:80/data

CDC National Center for Health Statistics
www.cdc.gov/nchswww/nchshome.htm

CDC Scientific, Surveillance, and Health Statistics, and Laboratory Information
www.cdc.gov/scientific.htm

CDC WONDER
wonder.cdc.gov

Health Care Financing Administration,
1996 Statistics at a Glance
www.hcfa.gov/stats/stathili.htm

General Sites

American Medical Association
http://www.ama-assn.org

MedicineNet
http://www.medicinenet.com

Medscape
http://www.medscape.com

Oncolink
http://www.oncolink.upenn.edu

ParentsPlace.com
http://www.parentsplace.com

Thrive@ pathfinder
http://pathfinder.com/thrive

Links Only

Hardin Meta Directory of Internet Health Sources
http://www.arcade.uiowa.edu/hardin-www/md.html

Medical Matrix
http://www.5lackinc.com/matrix

Chapter Eighteen

Intentional and Unintentional Injuries
(Accident and Violence Prevention)

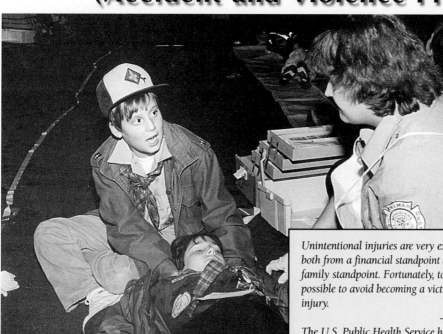

Unintentional injuries are very expensive for our society, both from a financial standpoint and from a personal and family standpoint. Fortunately, to a large extent it is possible to avoid becoming a victim of an unintentional injury.

—*Hahn and Payne (1997)*

The U.S. Public Health Service has identified violence as a leading public health problem that contributes to significant death and disability rates among Americans.

—*Donatelle and Davis (1996)*

Valued Outcomes

After reading this chapter, you should be able to

○ discuss the difference in intentional and unintentional injuries

○ discuss the major human and environmental causes of accidents

○ describe the characteristics of an accident-prone person

○ discuss young people's attitudes toward violence

○ list the ways for a child to protect him- or herself against violence

○ list the ways for a child to protect him- or herself against adult and stranger abuse

○ describe why risk taking is a necessary evil

○ discuss the major parts of a school safety program.

◯ contrast a positive approach to safety education with a negative approach

◯ discuss the growing violence problem in U.S. society

Children and Accidents

Unintentional accidents (accidents that no one intended to occur) are the leading cause of death among elementary school children (Mullen et al. 1993, 257 pp. 253–260). The reasons for this are many: First, children are extremely active. They are constantly exploring and testing their environment. In addition, they are often ignorant or unaware of the consequences of the risks they take. And finally, they have simply not yet learned to be as cautious as they should be.

Also, children and others are the victims of intentional injuries (those in which someone intended to harm another). Violence on the part of adolescents and preadolescents has been growing (Botsis-Alexander et al. 1995, 253–260). Since at least 1985, nearly one million young people have been victims of violent crimes each year. Among urban children ages ten to fourteen, homicides are up 150 percent, robberies are up 192 percent, and assaults are up 290 percent (Donatelle and Davis 1996, 568).

The Need for Safety Education

Fortunately, most accidents that happen to children are not serious or fatal. Unfortunately, accidents occur enough to make safety an extremely important part of elementary health instruction. As a teacher, your involvement in safety education is imperative because of the number of accidents that occur while the child is at school. Your efforts, combined with those of the school administration, can make a difference. It is very important for teachers to periodically review and comply with school district policies concerning safety and first-aid procedures to be followed.

The number of accidents among children is unnecessarily high. Although accidents will always occur, given the characteristics of children, accidents don't "just happen." In most instances, they are caused by human error or carelessness, and these factors can be positively influenced by safety education. Children do not have to learn safe behavior through trial and error; they do not have to continue having accidents in order to recognize the importance of safety. They can be taught the elements of safety in a positive way that will result in fewer accidents of all types, both at school and away from school. As a teacher of health education, this should be one of your major goals. The elements of safety education are

◯ *knowledge about accident prevention*—which creates an awareness of accident potential and problem areas;

◯ *promoting positive attitudes*—which enable a person to judge the potential value of making a behavioral change;

◯ *behavioral practices*—which allow the individual to consistently and safely perform an action (Miller, Telljohann, and Symons 1996, pp. 182–183).

This chapter presents an overview of the elements of safety education and violence prevention. Topics include risk taking and safety procedures, positive characteristics of safety, accident prevention, violence and violence prevention, types of accidents, and the school safety program.

Safety and Risk Taking

We take risks in almost any of our activities, from going to school or work in the morning, to cooking or eating a meal, to engaging in daily tasks and recreational activities. If safety were our only concern, logically many of these efforts would have to be curtailed: One could be hit by a truck while crossing the street, choke on a piece of food, or suffer a fatal injury while at work or at play. What is an "acceptable" degree of risk depends on the needs and desires of the individual and the activity. Some adults, for instance, make their living by engaging in highly risky activities—race drivers, deep sea divers, law enforcement officers, and so forth. Such individuals are often held in high esteem by the rest of the population, demonstrating that risk taking is viewed positively in our society.

Fostering Safety Behavior

Children develop an unrealistic view of risk taking, and this attitude may tempt them to enter into situations that are potentially very hazardous. This, combined with their natural curiosity and energy, can greatly increase the chance of serious accidents. Part of your job in teaching safety education is to make children aware that unnecessary risk taking is not socially endorsed behavior, and that it is important to safely prepare for necessary activities in which there are some risks involved. This cannot be accomplished, however, by simply providing your students with a list of safety "don'ts." Children, especially younger children, should be emphatically warned of dangers in the environment. However, the "don't" approach to safety education is a negative one, and one that is not likely to influence behavior.

A Positive Approach to Safety

You are more likely to influence children's behavior toward safer personal practices when you take a positive approach. Emphasize that safety is largely a matter of individual choice and responsibility. Although an acceptance of risk is a part of living, embracing risk without recognizing and accepting the possible consequences is not wise. In considering role models, point out that even adults who make their living in the most hazardous of ways do all they can to minimize the risk involved.

As in all areas of health education, stress the importance of personal decision-making skills. Accidents happen not because of chance or fate, but because of the inherent risk involved in the activity combined with the possibility of human error. When children understand and internalize this concept, they will be in a better position to enhance their own personal safety. By recognizing their own choices and responsibility, they will begin to be better able to assess the risk involved in a given activity and to take steps to minimize the possibility of making errors when engaged in that activity.

To become mindful of safety, a person must become analytical. What are the risks involved in the activity contemplated? What can be done to lessen those risks? After determining the probable answers to these questions, the individual can then act accordingly. The process of becoming analytical about decision making begins in childhood. You can do much to help children develop analytical decision-making skills by providing a variety of learning opportunities that require them to think before they act.

Of course, you cannot expect a child to have the analytical skills of a competent adult, and therefore you must also supervise children's activities to prevent needless accidents. This supervision should take place in the classroom, gymnasium, cafeteria, hallways, and playground. As much as possible, however, relate your supervision to individual decision-making skills. Always keep a positive approach to safety.

The Accident-Susceptible Individual

Everyone has heard the terms "accident prone" or "accident susceptible," and among your students there will be a few who could be so characterized. It is important to recognize that being accident susceptible is usually not synonymous with being unlucky.

Children and adults who have more than the typical number of accidents are often psychologically disposed to self-harmful behavior (Pruitt and Stein 1994, 276). Some of the emotional factors related to accident susceptibility are subconscious guilt, for which the accidents serve as punishment, and the desire to escape from problems.

Accident-susceptible individuals are often impulsive, unable to form close relationships, or hostile to authority. For such individuals, simply providing information about safety procedures and encouraging the development of decision-making skills may not be enough. Special attention and counseling are often necessary to help the person understand the root of the real problem. Personality characteristics of children are often good indicators of their proneness to accidents. Special attention should be given to children who are daydreamers, tend to be absent-minded, are easily frustrated and tend to lose their tempers quickly, and try to gain attention by showing off. All such individuals may have a higher accident rate than average for their age group.

Accidents

Causes of Accidents

Before the solution to a problem or the cure for a disease can be found, the source of the problem or cause for the disease must be examined. About 85 percent of all accidents are attributable to human error. The implication is that appropriate safety education aimed at changing human behavior could reduce accidents. Many of these accidents are due to risk-taking behaviors, poor attitudes toward safety, environmental hazards, and some physiological factors (Pruitt and Stein 1994, 275–276). Some physiological factors that could contribute to accidents are sensory impairments (such as faulty vision), fatigue, and medical disorders (such as epilepsy).

Types of Accidents

Accidents involving schoolchildren can be classified into five categories: school, traffic, recreational, home, personal, or disaster. Disaster situations include floods, hurricanes, tornadoes, and earthquakes. As these are general emergencies involving a large segment of the population, they will not be detailed here.

School Accidents. Most school accidents occur in physical education classes, during playground activities, and in sports contests. These activities expose the students to greater levels of risk.

Plan carefully to ensure maximum safety. First of all, the teacher in charge should make sure that sports and playground equipment are in good condition and suitable for the activity. Work closely with school administrators, other faculty members, and the school custodians. Equipment that is not in use should be stored so that it does not interfere with the ongoing activity. Swings and other play equipment should be inspected regularly. The playground should also be routinely inspected for hazards, including broken glass, and damaged fencing before children are allowed to play.

Next, be sure that all physical activities are properly supervised by an adequate number of faculty members. Some schools now require teachers supervising playground activities during school to stand and watch children carefully rather than completing paperwork or other distracting activities. Teachers should confine all activities to designated areas, and make sure that the activity of one group of children does not interfere with that of another group. Keep any activity you are supervising well ordered, and watch for signs of fatigue. When a child becomes tired, the chances for an accident increase. Finally, when your students have finished the activity, make sure that equipment is properly stored. Lock all equipment cabinets to prevent unauthorized, unsupervised use.

Safety in the hallways, stairways, cafeteria, and other parts of the school outside the actual classroom should be maximized by teacher supervision. Stress the importance of polite, considerate behavior, rather than simply demanding that students follow rules. Hall monitors should not be allowed to function as prison guards. Work with school administrators and custodians to keep the school environment free of potential hazards. Stairways should have banisters and adequate lighting. Water fountains should have the appropriate amount of water pressure—not too low to cause children to bump their teeth and not too much to cause water to spill on the floor. Spills of any sort should be wiped up promptly, and litter should be removed. Doors to maintenance areas should be locked.

In the classroom itself, make sure that you also maintain a safe environment. Keep equipment and supplies stored until they are needed. Supervise all activities closely. If you prepare any experiment or classroom demonstration that could be hazardous, do not take unnecessary risks. For example, if a demonstration involves the use of a sharp object or a chemical, do not have students help you. Also, be especially careful with any electrical apparatus.

A safety concern that has received considerable attention in the schools is the danger of asbestos. Asbestos has been widely used as an insulating material in schools for many years and other commonly occurring items, such as brake linings in cars. Asbestos is considered a danger to health only if the insulation is disturbed regularly through contact. If this happens, fibers that can block breathing passages will be released into the air. Problems such as chronic lung conditions and cancer may result from long-term exposure to damaged asbestos insulation (Mullen et al. 1993, 290). Many school systems are replacing asbestos with safer types of insulation.

Traffic Accidents. Going to and from school accounts for few school accidents. This is surprising when one considers the potential dangers that children face as pedestrians, bicyclists, and bus and auto passengers. The low accident rate speaks well for school safety patrols and pedestrian and bicycle safety programs. Nonetheless, traffic accidents do occur, and they are often serious. Help your children recognize the importance of following established safety procedures when they are pedestrians, bicyclists, and vehicle passengers.

As pedestrians, children should understand how to interact with motor vehicles. Traffic laws are designed not only for operators of motor vehicles but also for pedestrians. Each has an obligation to the other, a point you should stress. Help younger children learn the meaning of traffic signs and signals, and explain the reasons behind traffic regulations. Youngsters usually do not appreciate the physical principles involved in the operation of a motor vehicle and do not

Being safe in and around the school bus is an important part of a student's life.

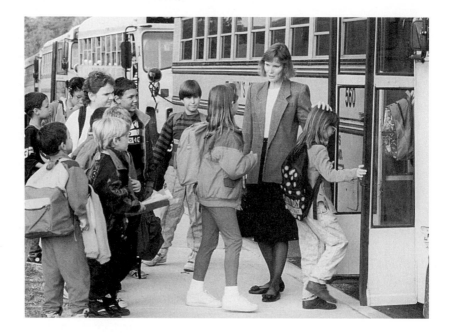

understand that a car cannot stop on a dime or that the child can see the car much better than the driver can see him or her. Further, children often become so engrossed in their own activities that they simply do not consider the vehicular traffic around them. They may dart into the street after a ball without thinking.

Bicycle safety should also be emphasized. Children often assume that traffic laws and regulations apply only to motor vehicles. They see themselves not as operators of vehicles—which they are—but rather as mounted pedestrians. To some degree, this is a values-related issue and must be approached as such. That is, children do not see themselves as being irresponsible when they fail to heed traffic regulations because they place themselves in another category when they ride their bikes.

Most children are regular passengers on school buses and in family vehicles. Because of the large numbers of children being transported to and from schools in buses and cars, children need to become aware of proper safety practices in buses and cars.

Drivers of school buses are responsible for supervising students during their ride. Cooperate with drivers in establishing firm guidelines for safe student behavior while loading, riding, and unloading the buses. Unruly students can easily distract a driver so that an accident results. Make clear the possible consequences of unruly behavior, and point out that the well-being of many people can be affected by poor behavior. Also provide instructions for safe behavior. Children should enter the bus in an orderly manner and move to their seats swiftly but with care. They should remain seated during the ride. Books, lunch boxes, and other objects should be kept out of the aisles. Windows should remain closed unless the driver opens them. If windows are opened, children should not stick their arms out or throw trash from them. Finally, students should remain well clear of the bus when it is approaching the bus stop and after they have departed.

As automobile passengers, children should also be aided in developing safety practices. Emphasize that even though it may look easy, driving a car requires the full attention of the operator. Children should not distract the driver and should not lean out of windows. Stress the importance of wearing safety belts, even if the parents of some children do not regularly use them.

Many states in America are now requiring the use of safety belts by some passengers. Many other states are considering such legislation. Not wearing a safety belt is essentially irrational behavior. Reasons given for not using belts are many. Some drivers find them constricting or uncomfortable. Others say that they are not needed for short trips. A few claim to fear being trapped inside the vehicle in case of an accident. None of these reasons hold up. The truth is that people refuse to wear safety belts either because of simple laziness or because of a belief that somehow preparing for an accident by wearing a belt will actually allow an accident to take place! Not wearing a belt is a psychological device called *denial*.

Recreational Accidents. A large portion of recreational accidents happen to children in and around water. Thus water safety should be an important component of the instruction that you provide. All children should be taught to swim at an early age. This is something that you can encourage by getting parents and children involved in organized recreational programs. Even if children know how to swim, however, the danger of accidental drowning always exists. Most drownings happen to people who are not dressed for swimming, which implies that they were not planning to be in the water. Victims usually fall into the water, whether in a home pool, from a boat, or by a river or lake. Emphasize to your children that any body of water should be treated with respect and caution, including a flooded drainage ditch. In your discussion of water safety, include the rules for boating safety, such as always wearing a life preserver.

Camping and hiking activities contribute to many recreational accidents. Falls from cliffs and other high places result in hundreds of fatalities and injuries each year. Stress the importance of being cautious in unfamiliar terrain. Skateboards also cause many recreational accidents among children. The popularity of skateboards is currently on the wane, but use is still high, as is the number of resulting accidents. Emphasize the need for proper protective equipment. Also note that skateboards should not be used on streets. A collision between a car and a child on a skateboard can be fatal for the child.

Teach about forms of recreation popular in your area, such as snowmobiling, hunting, and fishing.

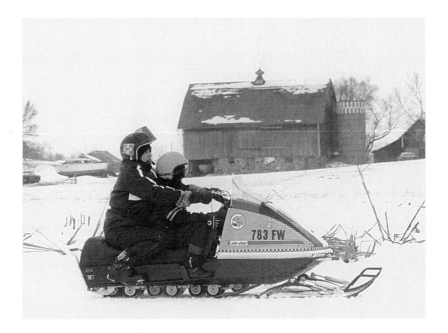

Your treatment of recreational safety should also include any forms of recreation popular in your area, such as snowmobiling, iceskating, hunting, and fishing. The following suggestions (Ibrahim and Cordes 1993, 326) increase safety in winter sports:

1. Participants may choose to carry a pack with high-energy food, water, or juice, and a thermos of tea or hot chocolate.

2. Study a map and monitor the weather before undertaking a trip.

3. Observe and mark checkpoints.

4. If lost, avoid the temptation to move on—backtrack following your own tracks.

5. Understand the hazards of frostbite and hypothermia—for example, wear apparel that provides adequate protection from the cold without preventing freedom of movement.

Home Accidents. "There's no place like home" implies that home is a pleasant place to be. Unfortunately, there's no place like home for accidents, either. More accidents happen in the home than in any other place, partly because most people spend a great deal of time at home. The leading cause of death in the home is fire. Most home fires occur in the kitchen and bedroom. For the latter, smoking in bed is often the cause. Home safety, including fire safety, is primarily a parental responsibility, but you can help by making your students aware of possible hazards. Work with parents and children to ensure that every family has a fire safety and fire evacuation plan.

For younger children, emphasize the danger of playing with matches or with the kitchen stove. Encourage parents to install smoke detectors. Teach children what to do if a fire breaks out in the home, especially at night. Too often, frightened children seek shelter in a closet or other enclosed area rather than fleeing. Follow each fire drill in school with a discussion of home fire drills. Every member of the family should know the evacuation route and an alternative route if the primary one is blocked by smoke or flames.

Poisonings are another common home accident, especially among younger children. Explain the dangers of ingesting any substance, such as medicines, food that may have gone bad, and household chemicals. Make sure that parents understand the dangers of accidental poisonings from such substances as aspirin, and encourage them to keep a list of emergency procedures on hand. Also, inform parents and children of the telephone number of the local poison control center. Electrical appliances are a common source of home accidents. Make sure that your children understand the danger of playing with any electrical device. Also discuss how electrical overloads can lead to home fires.

Your instruction in home safety techniques should include specific recommendations, such as not leaving toys or other objects on stairs or sidewalks, having adequate ventilation when running internal combustion motors, and wearing protective eye equipment when using power tools or lawn equipment. Encourage parents to do all they can to keep the home a safe environment for themselves and their children. For example, you may wish to prepare a checklist for children to take home to their parents. Discussion of items on the checklist can provide a valuable learning experience for all involved.

Just as a family should have a home evacuation plan in case of fire, it should also have a general disaster plan. Encourage children and their parents to work out a plan for any disaster that might hit their community. Depending on the locale, disasters might include earthquakes, floods, tornadoes, or extreme blizzards. Each family member should know what to do in case a disaster strikes.

Children and Violence

According to the Healthy People 2000 Midcourse Review, which follows the progress of target goals in several health areas, the United States is only progressing on three of the eighteen objectives in the area of violence. For example, suicide among young men is escalating, the homicide rate is rising, and both firearm-related deaths and assault injuries are increasing (Hahn and Payne 1997, 402).

The United States leads the industrialized world in homicide rates, with handguns being involved in most of the homicides. In 1993 a total of 24,526 people were murdered in the United States; however, data indicate that the homicide rate is now actually dropping in the United States. Speculation about the reasons for this decline focuses on better community policing effort, the 1994 passage of the Federal Crime Act and state laws, such as provisions that mandate life sentences without parole for repeat violent offenders (Hahn and Payne 1997, 403).

Children are becoming involved in violence at ever younger ages, both as victims and as perpetrators. The threat of firearms is the greatest concern, but no single factor can be blamed as the cause of violence (Hechinger 1994). Poverty, unemployment, hopelessness, lack of education, inadequate housing, poor parental role models, cultural beliefs that objectify women and empower men to act as aggressors, lack of social support systems, discrimination, ignorance about people who are different, breakdowns in the criminal justice system, stress, economic uncertainty, and a host of other factors may precipitate violent acts (Donatelle and Davis 1996, 569).

Health Highlight

Young People's Attitudes toward Crime and Violence

A recent survey considered young people's attitudes toward crime and violence. These young people reported the following:

1. Many of these young people reported that they did not always feel safe.

2. More than one in three thought violence was a serious problem in their communities.

3. Three in four believe conditions were not changing or were growing worse.

4. Seven in ten either did not know or did not think they could do anything to help prevent crime in their neighborhoods.

Overall, this survey showed that awareness and fear of crime influence the behavior of many young people.

Source: National Crime Prevention Council, National Institute for Citizen Education in the Law, Department of Justice, Office of Juvenile Justice and Delinquency Prevention, Washington DC. 1995. *Between hope and fear: Teens speak out on crime and the community.* Survey conducted by Louis Harris & Associates, New York, New York, p. 232.

Violence is learned, and can be combatted through teaching alternatives. No single strategy, institution, or discipline can create the change needed to reduce violence in America. Preventing violence requires long-term commitments, a comprehensive set of strategies, and new partnerships focused on prevention of, not responses to, youth violence (Prothrow-Stith 1995, 95–101).

The teaching of prosocial behavior at home and in school must be accompanied by the provision of health and social services to children and families. Conflict resolution and mediation programs show promise in reducing violence. Violence prevention curricula are among the import-ant efforts schools can make. These efforts can be supported by community and youth organizations (Hechinger 1994, 17).

Also, younger students respond well and listen to older students. At the fourth through sixth grade level, peer-led activities are effective (Botsis-Alexander et al. 1995, 253–260).

Personal Safety

Becoming a victim of violent behavior or sustaining an unintentional injury can harm your health as much as any of your own unhealthy behavior. Intentional injuries reflect violence committed by one person acting against another person. Categories of intentional injuries include homicide, robbery, rape, suicide, assault, and abuse (Hahn and Payne 1997, 403).

Unfortunately, many children suffer from injuries inflicted on them by adults, sometimes parents or relatives of the children and sometimes by strangers. Children need to be taught to trust their feelings when they do not feel right about a person or a situation. For example, if they are being touched by an adult, and the touch feels uncomfortable, the child needs to know to inform another adult. Emphasize to children that they have a right and a responsibility to determine when and how they wish to be touched. Teach them to assert their own "personal space," or privacy. They need to be taught to keep their distance from people that make them feel most uncomfortable.

Each child should be taught to be more aware of his or her surroundings—that is, be aware if someone is following you. Walk in the middle of the sidewalk, and try to walk with someone else. Stay away from dark places when you are alone. Tell them it is all right to scream if they are approached by someone intending them harm.

The School Safety Program

Instruction in safety education should be only one part of your school safety program. The total program should consist of these components:

- providing instruction by and for faculty, staff, and students
- planning and implementing safety procedures
- providing safe transportation, including bus travel, walking, and bicycle safety
- establishing accident reporting and recordkeeping procedures
- making sure there is liability insurance protection for staff
- providing emergency health care for all people attending or employed by the school
- creating a safe environment

The school should define the responsibilities of each person involved in the safety program, and instruct each person regarding specific duties or responsibilities. Supervision should be pro-

Health Highlight

Home Alone!

An increasing number of children spend time at home alone while their parents are working. For this reason, certain rules should be followed to ensure the personal safety of these children:

1. Always keep the doors locked, and never permit a stranger to enter the house.

2. Become familiar with appropriate ways to respond on the telephone (for example, never say that you are home alone).

3. Know how to use the telephone to summon help (for example, parent's work numbers) in an emergency (for example, fire or a stranger at the door).

4. Know the emergency telephone numbers in the community (for example, police and fire department).

5. Have a trusted neighbor you can call or go to if you become scared or upset.

Source: D. Miller, S. Telljohann, and C. Symons. 1996. *Health education*. Madison, WI: Brown & Benchmark, p. 202.

vided for all school activities, including travel to and from school, physical education, playground time, and after-school gatherings.

Some schools have established school safety councils to develop rules, policies, and procedures for safe living within the school and for school activities. Safety councils provide excellent learning opportunities and allow for student involvement. For example, a school safety council could do a needs assessment or accident survey for the school. This procedure makes the students and others involved aware of the accident situations in their school environment, helping to prevent future accidents.

Generally, any accident that causes a student to miss school, go home from school, or that involves property damage should be reported. Some schools have specific forms for reporting any type of accident in or around the school. Accident reports can provide data for studying accident trends in the school environment. They are also valuable in the event of lawsuits filed against the school.

First-Aid Skills

First aid means just that—providing aid before more qualified medical help can be obtained. Adults and children alike should have some knowledge of first aid procedures so they can aid an accident victim in an emergency. Often such knowledge can make the difference between life and death in extreme cases. However, first aid should never be dispensed casually, and not at all if more qualified help can be obtained quickly. As a classroom teacher, you should learn basic first-aid procedures and instruct your students in them. Most often, first aid procedures are used in common, everyday incidents involving cuts, nosebleeds, sprains, and so on.

Children should have some knowledge of first aid procedures to be of help in emergency situations.

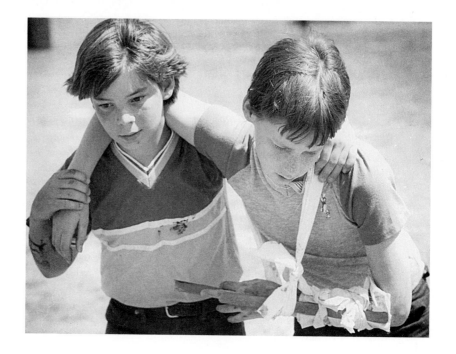

Begin your own preparation by checking with the school administration and medical personnel to determine established procedures for handling medical problems and emergencies. This is extremely important as far as liability is concerned and cannot be stressed too strongly. In most instances, you will probably be told not to offer any medical assistance except under clearly life-threatening circumstances or when there is no possibility of obtaining more qualified assistance. In some instances, however, administering first aid may be acceptable and provided for in the school safety program.

Keep in mind that first aid is not treatment; instead, it is protection of the victim until treatment can be given. The purpose of first aid is to offer emergency care, prevent further injury, lessen the victim's pain, and ward off unnecessary complications, such as shock. While this is being done, help should also be sought.

Emergency Situations

The best way to prepare yourself to handle an emergency medical or accident situation is to become qualified to handle emergencies. If you are not qualified, you should become qualified by taking a first-aid and CPR class through the American Red Cross, National Safety Council, and/or American Heart Association to become qualified. You will gain hands-on experience in dealing with a variety of situations and will have a chance to practice basic first-aid skills before you actually have to use them.

Appendix A details the first-aid procedures to follow in specific emergencies.

≣ *Summary*

○ Elementary school children are subject to many injuries, some intentional and some unintentional.

○ Accidental deaths are the leading cause of death for this age group, but deaths and injuries from violence are on the rise.

○ Children are becoming involved in violent behavior in increasing numbers, both as perpetrators and victims.

○ Safety education that covers both safety and violence prevention should be a vital part of health instruction.

○ Safety education will help students to increase their awareness of the accident problems and causes, provide them with factual knowledge about safety, help them adjust to new, unfamiliar environments, and heighten their potential for living full, productive lives.

○ Positive, safe behavior should be seen by the students as an important part of living.

○ The emphasis in safety education should be on positive attitudes and values.

○ Learning opportunities in safety should be designed to help students recognize potentially hazardous situations, develop a sense of responsibility for their own safety and others, and make wise decisions regarding their behavior.

○ Do not provide safety instruction that is limited to accident statistics, safety rules, or scare tactics. Instead, stress that living is much more enjoyable when a person is safe.

○ Teach the students how to prevent violence in their own lives, and how to respond if they are faced with violence.

○ As the teacher, you should set a good safety model for your students.

○ The classroom and other parts of the school environment should be examples of safe, efficient places to work and live.

○ Teachers should be aware of their responsibility regarding liability in various school situations.

○ Because so many accidents happen to children while they are attending school, teachers should learn basic first-aid skills to treat injuries resulting from accidents.

○ Students should also learn how they can be of help in emergency situations.

Discussion Questions

1. Describe the factors that lead to a disproportionate number of accidental deaths among children.

2. Discuss the reasons for some taking risks in our society.

3. How can we teach children to assume a positive approach to safety?

4. Describe the emotional makeup of an "accident-prone" individual.

5. Discuss the ways to make a playground safer for children.

6. Describe the proper behavior for a child while riding on a school bus.

7. Discuss the steps to take when confronted by someone who is threatening to attack you.

8. Enumerate the rules for children to follow to ensure their personal safety from strangers.

9. Discuss the first-aid procedures to follow in a breathing emergency.

10. Discuss the types of educational programs to prevent violent behavior.

References

American National Red Cross. 1993. *Community CPR workbook*. Washington, DC: American Red Cross.

Botsis-Alexander, J., et al. 1995, Summer. Parental loss and family violence as correlates of suicide and violence risk. *Suicide and life threatening behavior* 25(2): 253–260.

Donatelle, R., and L. Davis. 1996. *Access to health,* 4th ed. Needham Heights, MA: Allyn and Bacon.

Hahn, D., and W. Payne. 1997. *Focus on health*. St. Louis: Mosby-Year Book.

Hechinger, F. 1994, Winter. Saving youth from violence. *Carnegie quarterly* 39(1).

Ibrahim, H. and K. Cordes. 1993. *Outdoor recreation*. Madison, WI: Brown & Benchmark.

Miller, D., S. Telljohann, and C. Symons. 1996. *Health education*. Madison, WI: Brown & Benchmark.

Mullen, K., R. Gold, P. Belcastro, and R. McDermott. 1993. *Connections for health,* 3rd ed. Madison, WI: Brown & Benchmark.

National Crime Prevention Council, National Institute for Citizen Education in the Law, Department of Justice, Office of Juvenile Justice and Delinquency Prevention, Washington, DC. 1995. *Between hope and fear: Teens speak out on crime and the community*. Survey conducted by Louis Harris & Associates, New York, New York.

Prothrow-Stith, D. 1995. The epidemic of youth violence in America: Using public health prevention strategies to prevent violence. *Journal of health care for the poor and underserved* 6(2): 95–101.

Pruitt, B., and J. Stein. 1994. *Healthstyles: Decisions for living well*. Fort Worth, TX: Saunders College.

Chapter Nineteen
Strategies for Teaching Safety and First Aid

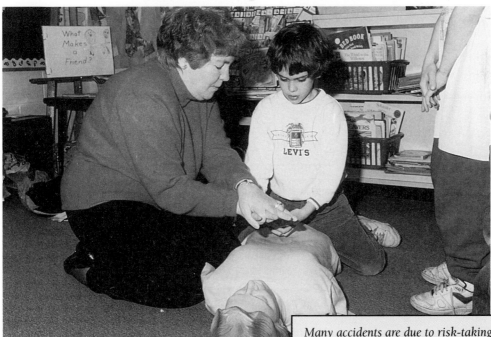

> Many accidents are due to risk-taking behaviors and poor attitudes toward safety.
> —Pruitt & Stern (1994, 275–276)

Valued Outcomes

After doing the activities in this chapter, the student should be able to express and illustrate the following guidelines:

○ Each person is to a large degree responsible for his or her own personal safety.

○ Peers exert a tremendous influence over safety practices.

○ Obedience to safety rules can enhance the quality of life.

○ Risk taking is a part of living, but unnecessary risk taking greatly increases the risk of harm to oneself and to others.

○ The degree of risk in any particular activity can often be determined by analytical thinking.

○ Some rules and procedures for safe behavior can help prevent accidents in the home, school, and community.

○ Hazardous conditions should be corrected when possible.

○ There are many people and community agencies who can help in the time of accidents.

○ Elementary school children have more fatal accidents than any other age group.

○ More than half of all accidents involving children happen at school.

○ Playground rules are important for safe activities.

○ Elementary students need to practice safe behavior in traffic.

○ Home and school fire escape routes should be practiced frequently.

○ Acting without thinking often results in an accident.

○ Individuals who are accident prone often have ulterior motives for such behavior.

○ Basic first-aid skills are important for everyone.

○ Improper first aid can do more harm than good.

○ Safety is not just a matter of "luck."

○ Safe behavior must be learned.

Fostering Safety Behavior

Progress has been made in virtually every area of health education in this century, including disease prevention, environmental sanitation, and nutritional habits. If there is one area of health education that has lagged behind, it is safety and accident prevention. Many laws have been passed, especially in the area of traffic safety. Some states are passing mandatory safety belt and stiffer drunk driving laws. These laws should help save more lives on the road; however, despite these and other legislative safety efforts, thousands of Americans die or are injured each year because of needless accidents. The situation will not change significantly until Americans reject an attitude of apathy toward safety, and adopt a lifestyle of safe behavior.

Value-Based Activities

Safety Habits Beliefs

Valued Outcome: The students will exhibit their beliefs about safety habits.
Description of Strategy: Before spending time discussing safety rules and habits, the students will complete a series of questions that show how they feel when it comes to safety. Then as a class, the students will begin to learn about safety rules and regulations. The questions are as follows:

1. I wear a helmet when I ride a bicycle because . . .

2. I can avoid falling by . . .

3. I think the most dangerous type of safety violation is . . .

4. The safest place to walk is . . .

5. I always swim with an adult present because . . .

6. The most important thing I can do when mowing the lawn is . . .

7. The best thing I can know when there is a fire is . . .

8. I need to take cover in a tornado because . . .

9. The best place for poisons to be kept is . . .

10. In case of an emergency, I need to know how to call the local emergency numbers because . . .

11. I always fasten my safety belt in the car because . . .

12. I think that most important thing that I can do to try to remain safe is . . .

Materials Needed: paper and pencils
Processing Questions:

1. Why do we need safety rules and regulations?

2. If we don't follow rules, what might happen?

3. Why did you select what you did for the most important thing you can do to try to remain safe?

Safety Voting

Valued Outcome: The students will be able to respond to safety-related statements based on their values.
Description of Strategy: Have your students raise their hands to agree or disagree with the following statements:

Some accidents are caused by people showing off.

All the medicines in my house are stored in a safe place.

Some medicines can be taken without parents' permission.

I know the number of the local poison control center.

I read labels on all medications before I take them.

It is important to wear a safety belt even on short trips.

Materials Needed: none
Processing Question: What variables help you determine your values about safety practices?

Safety Sentence Completion

Valued Outcome: The students will be able to complete sentences with their own values-related beliefs.
Description of Strategy: Have your students complete the following statements. Then, on a volunteer basis, discuss the values implicit in each statement:

Wearing a safety belt is . . .

Driving while drunk is . . .

All students should be required to participate in fire, tornado, or hurricane drills because . . .

To me, safety education means . . .

Accidents are the result of . . .

As a pedestrian, I should know . . .

People who drive should be aware of . . .

The costs of accidents are . . .

I would become personally involved if someone were hurt in an accident if . . .

Educating others about preventing accidents can be organized by . . .

Materials Needed: handouts with the preceding statements, pencils for all students
Processing Question: How can your attitude toward safety improve your safety?

Decision Stories

Valued Outcome: The students will be able to answer the focus question in each of the following decision stories.

Description of Strategy: The teacher and students will follow the procedures outlined in Chapter 5 for decision stories.

Fire!

Marilyn is alone in her house. She goes into the hallway on the second floor and sees flames coming from the room down the hall. The flames are between Marilyn and the only staircase to the downstairs part of the house.
Focus Question: What should Marilyn do?

Students need to be safe pedestrians.

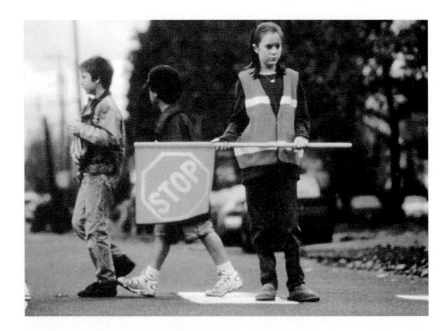

The Hill

George and Frank like to ride their bikes to school. There is a hill on the way to school. Near the top of the hill, there is a stop sign. If they stop, getting over the hill is difficult. George usually stops, but Frank never does. George has to get off his bike and start again. Frank kids him about this and calls him a chicken. George does not want to seem a coward to his friend but he knows that he should stop for traffic signs.
Focus Question: What should George do?

Safety Belts

Jack's friend, Warren, and Warren's parents came to Jack's house to take Jack and Warren to a party. When Jack got into Warren's parents' car, he noticed none of Warren's family were wearing their safety belts, and the one at his seat was hard to find. Jack had always been taught to wear his safety belt, but he was afraid he would embarrass Warren and his parents if he were the only one in the car to wear his safety belt.
Focus Question: What should Jack do?

The Raft

Jason and his friends are playing by a river near their home. Some of the boys decide to build a raft. They are going to use it to cross the river. They find some wood on the river bank and start making the raft. But it doesn't look too sturdy to Jason. When the time comes to put the raft in the water, Jason has his doubts. What if the raft falls apart while the boys are on it? Jason knows how to swim, but swimming might be difficult with his clothes on. Also he is not sure the others can swim.
Focus Question: What should Jason do?

The Stranger

Beth and her sister Harriet are walking home from school. Just then a car pulls up by the curb. The driver is a man Beth and her sister have never seen. He asks them their names, and they tell him. Then the man says that he is a good friend of their father. He says that their father has asked him to pick them up and take them for a ride. The stranger offers to buy the girls some ice cream, too.
Focus Question: What should Beth and her sister do?

The First Real Party

Tammy was a shy girl. She rarely got invited to parties. Sam, a friend at school, asked Tammy if she would like to come with him to a party this Friday night. Tammy accepted, thinking this would be her chance to get to know some more people. At the party, some of the kids are smoking and drinking. Sam wanted Tammy to smoke and drink too. He said this would help her come out of her shell.
Focus Question: Should Tammy smoke and drink at the party?

Medicine

Tina is getting over a cold. It is nothing serious, but she stayed home from school for two days. Now she is back. Her cold is almost gone, but she is still coughing. At lunch, Tina sits with her

friend Pam. Pam has been taking medicine for an infection that she has. "It's real good stuff," Pam says to Tina. "I'll bet it would make your cough go away just like that. Why don't you try some?"
Focus Question: What should Tina do?

Emergency Care

Mary came home from school and found her grandmother lying at the foot of the stairway unconscious. She could not lift her.
Focus Questions:

1. Who should Mary call?
2. What else should she do for her grandmother?

Dramatization

Emergency Skits

Valued Outcome: Students will evaluate what they can do as individuals to prevent accidents and what to do when an emergency arises.
Description of Strategy: Have a group of students pantomime a make-believe emergency. Ask them to include how the emergency happened, who needs help, and the best ways to give assistance to the injured people. Then have another group of students pantomime some safety behaviors. Ask other students to guess the behavior and explain how each helps prevent accidents.
Materials Needed: none
Processing Questions:

1. What is the proper sequence of events that should take place in the event that an emergency occurs? (Stay calm, quickly notify a teacher or the school office, use first aid to help the student until other help arrives.)
2. How can I contribute to the prevention of accidents?

Source: *Being healthy*, Teacher's Resource Book. 1990. Orlando, FL: Harcourt Brace Jovanovich, p. 115.

Medical Emergencies

Valued Outcome: Students will be able to demonstrate first-aid techniques for injuries that require immediate attention.
Description of Strategy: This activity is to be performed after an extensive study on first-aid techniques. Begin by asking students if anyone has ever been personally involved in an emergency situation. Ask students to share their experiences with the class. Then ask students to get in groups of three. Have each group choose a skit in which they can act out a medical emergency such as choking, bleeding, or drowning. Have the students demonstrate the proper first-aid techniques.
Materials Needed: none

Processing Questions:

1. Although first aid begins with action, what is stressed in first-aid training?

2. What are some accidents which could result in a need for first-aid treatment?

3. When should a person use CPR?

Source: Adapted from B. Getchell, R. Pippin, and J. Varnes. 1989. *Health*, Teachers edition. Boston: Houghton Mifflin, p. 539.

Using Assertiveness to Protect Personal Safety

Valued Outcome: Students will be able to demonstrate assertiveness and refusal skills.
Description of Strategy: After a discussion of what passive, aggressive, and assertive behaviors involve, have students volunteer to act out the following three situations. Follow each one with a discussion about the situation.

Skit 1

Mary: May I borrow five bucks? I'll pay you back later.

Susan: No. I need the money. I have to buy a few things.

Mary: If you let me borrow it, I can buy this new tape I've been wanting. You trust me to pay you back, don't you?

Susan: I trust you, but I need the money for myself right now.

Mary: I don't understand why you won't let me borrow the money. You know I always pay you back, right?

Susan: Yeah.

Mary: Do you trust me?

Susan: (somewhat depressed) Yeah, here's the money.

Discussion: What happened in this situation? Susan wasn't assertive enough in the beginning so Mary made her friend feel guilty by implying that Susan didn't trust her. The point isn't whether Susan trusts Mary but whether Susan wants to let Mary borrow the money. What forms of body language were involved?

Skit 2

Mary: May I borrow five bucks? I'll pay you back later.

Susan: I know you'll pay me back, but I don't want to lend any money right now. Sorry.

Mary: You sound like you don't trust me!

Susan: Oh, I trust you. I just don't want to let *anyone* borrow any money right now. I know I'll need the money later.

Mary: Yeah, you'll need it later, but I need it right now!

Susan: True, but I just can't let you have it. Sorry.

Discussion: What happened this time? Susan assertively refused to let Mary borrow the money. She didn't make excuses, she wasn't pushed into feeling guilty, and she didn't let the conversation turn into a dispute about trust.

Being assertive means being as strong or stronger than a person who is pressuring you. For most of us, the hardest pressure to handle comes from our peers. What works when friends gang up and really pour on the pressure? Watch Susan handle this situation:

Skit 3

Susan: What's up, guys?

Mike: We're waiting for you. We have a great plan.

Bill: The theater is having a special matinee of three sci-fi films. We're all going.

Susan: All right! When does it start?

Mike: Twenty minutes. We'd better get moving.

Susan: Twenty minutes? Are you skipping class? I can't skip class. I have chemistry and English this afternoon.

Source: American School Health Association. 1994, March. *Journal of school health* 64(3): 128–130.From *Education for self-responsibility II: Prevention of drug use*, produced with funds from the U.S. Department of Education, Drug-Free Schools and Communities Act, Joe Wiese, Program Director for Drug Use Prevention Education.

Avoiding Threatening Situations

Valued Outcome: Students will generate ways to avoid threatening situations.
Description of Strategy: Cut one of the large sides from a carton. Then draw an outline of a car in the shape of a convertible, and cut around the outline. You will need this shape because you will place a chair behind it so it appears that you are driving. You will also be able to reach out from the side of the car. Select a student to stand 10 feet away from the car. Tell this student to pretend (s)he is walking down the street and to do what you say. Pretend you have a photograph of a puppy, and say to the student, "Excuse me. I lost my puppy and I have a picture of her. Could you come over here so I can show you her picture? She is lost and I want to know if you saw her." As the student approaches the "car," reach out and grab him or her by the arm. Then tell the class that if you were a stranger who wanted to harm this person, you easily could have dragged him or her into the car.

With this example in mind, emphasize that you should never approach a car with a stranger inside. Reinforce the concept that most strangers are nice people; however, there are certain rules that need to be followed in situations involving strangers, and keeping away from strangers in automobiles is one of those rules. Discuss what the students should do in the event that they are approached by a stranger in a car. Explain that they should run in the direction *opposite* to the car's direction. They are to run in the opposite direction because if a person inside the car wanted to attack them, the car would have to travel backward or turn around and that would be difficult to do. If a person were to run away in the same direction as the car was traveling, it would be much easier for the stranger to catch this person. Explain to students that it is also important to remember as much as possible about the car and the stranger. For example, the student could remember the color of the car, what kind of car it is, and what the stranger is wearing. You can practice this aspect of the activity by drawing and attaching a license plate to the car. Do not tell the class what you have done.

Then have another student volunteer to be walking along the street. Pretend that you stopped your car and asked this student to come closer to see the photograph of your lost puppy. Tell the student to act in the correct way. (Run away in the opposite direction the car is traveling.)

Materials Needed: a cardboard carton from the grocery or appliance store, chair, scissors, pencil
Processing Questions:

1. Whom do I consider strangers?

2. When is it okay to talk to people I do not know?

Source: L. Meeks and P. Heit. 1996. *Totally awesome health*, Kindergarten manual. Blacklick, OH: Meeks Heit, pp. 384–385.

Emergency Call Role-Play

Valued Outcome: Students will identify what an emergency is and will know the procedure for getting help in an emergency.
Description of Strategy: Discuss what an emergency is and what to do when an emergency happens. Have students write the local emergency number and their telephone number, name, and address on a piece of paper. A class list of names, addresses, and telephone numbers should be available for reference. As students finish this activity, have them use this worksheet to practice emergency calling in role-play. Encourage them to take their assignment home and review facts and the calling procedures with their parents. (It is important for the students to practice calls on both rotary and touch-tone model phones.)
Materials Needed: pencils, paper, rotary telephones and touch-tone telephones
Processing Questions:

1. What is an emergency?

2. What should you do in an emergency?

3. How do you make an emergency call?

Source: G. Ezell. 1992. *Healthy living*, Grade 1. Grand Rapids, MI: Christian Schools International, pp. 147–148.

Disaster Drama

Valued Outcome: The students will be able to learn first-aid procedures during a disaster.
Description of Strategy: Have the students enact a "mock disaster." Set up the classroom as if a tornado or hurricane had hit the area, and the students are the only trained first aiders who can help. Assign some students to be "victims" with a variety of injuries, and the other students will play the parts of emergency care personnel who will perform first aid for the "victims."
Materials Needed: first-aid kits, bandages
Processing Questions:

1. How can you help during a disaster?

2. What first-aid skills would you need to know?

House Fire

Valued Outcome: The students will be able to enact a home fire drill.
Description of Strategy: Assign the role of parents and children to several students. Have them enact a situation in which a fire takes place in a "home" (set up in the classroom). Have some "family members" downstairs while some are upstairs, and others are blocked from any doorway exit.
Materials Needed: none
Processing Questions:

1. Why is it important to have a preplanned escape route from your home in case of a fire?

2. Do you have two escape routes planned?

School Bus Behavior

Valued Outcome: The students will be able to identify proper conduct on a bus.
Description of Strategy: Students are in groups. Each group is given a situation that has happened on the bus and the students must decide what should be done.

Case 1. Two students are fighting.

Case 2. Two students are sitting on the same seat; one student wants the window up, the other student wants the window down.

Case 3. A student is holding his arms and head out of the window.

Materials Needed: two chairs
Processing Question: Why is it important to behave well on the school bus?

Looking for Hazards

Valued Outcome: The students will be able to identify hazardous areas in the school setting.
Description of Strategy: Assign students to go to various rooms in the school and look for hazards: shop rooms, cooking and sewing classes, and gym classes. Students are to report the findings. In one week, the students return to the same classes and see if the hazard still exists.
Materials Needed: form with rooms in the school listed
Processing Questions:

1. What safety hazards are typically found in schools?

2. What can students do to help eliminate these hazards?

Phoning for Help

Valued Outcome: The students will be able to learn the proper technique for using the phone during an emergency situation.
Description of Strategy: In many emergency situations, assistance can be obtained by telephoning the proper authority or agency. Stress the importance of knowing whom to call and what to say on the telephone. Have the students prepare a list of emergency telephone numbers, including those of the fire department, the poison control center, and so on. Then have them role-play emergency situations. One student plays the part of the telephone operator or official. Another student then phones for help. Point out that information given over the telephone should be stat-

ed clearly and accurately. Let each student role-play the part of an emergency caller at least once. Follow the activity with general discussion of proper use of the telephone.
Materials Needed: telephone book, pen, and paper
Processing Questions:

1. Do you know the phone numbers of your local fire department, etc?

2. What information should you give over the phone in case of an emergency?

Accident Pantomime

Valued Outcome: The students will be able to enact various accidental situations.
Description of Strategy: Assign various accident situations to individual students. These could include careless improper use of tools or kitchen implements, and so forth. However, no props are used. Instead, each child must act out the behavior using mime techniques. The children should observe each performance, and note how human error leads up to the "accident" that finally occurs.
Materials Needed: none
Processing Questions:

1. What is meant by human error?

2. What types of human error lead to accidents with kitchen implements?

Safety Puppet Show

Valued Outcome: The students will be able to demonstrate their ability to react in emergency situations.
Description of Strategy: Have children make or use puppets (such as, "Safe Susan" and "Hazardous Harry") to perform safety-related skits. Topics could include disaster situations, handling medical emergencies, fire safety, recreational safety, and safety in the home.
Materials Needed: paper bag or cloth for making puppet, markers
Processing Questions:

1. Why is it important to plan ahead for disaster situations?

2. How can you help your family during a disaster?

Commercials for Safety

Valued Outcome: The students will be able to prepare a script on different safety hazards.
Description of Strategy: Discuss public service safety messages that children may have seen on television. Then have students prepare individual 30-second or one-minute scripts that offer safety advice on specific safety hazards. Some children may want to work in small groups to dramatize the situation under discussion. Others may want to use props, such as an electrical appliance, to demonstrate a safety concept. Encourage imagination.
Materials Needed: per the individual student
Processing Questions:

1. What safety messages have you seen on television?

2. How do they help prevent accidents?

School Safety

Valued Outcome: The students will be able to determine safe and unsafe behavior for the school environment.

Description of Strategy: Assign the roles of teacher, students and principal to several students. Have the "students" enact several school situations, such as, running in the hall, horse-playing around the water fountain, and so forth. Following these enactments, have the students make a list of "safe" and "unsafe" rules for the school environment.

Materials Needed: pen and paper

Processing Questions:

1. What dangerous activities by students at school cause accidents?

2. How can you help eliminate some of these dangerous activities?

Pedestrian/Driver Safety

Valued Outcome: The students will be able to understand the importance of road signs for traffic safety.

Description of Strategy: Set up various "road signs" around the classroom as in an intersection. Assign the roles of driver and pedestrian to several students. Have the "drivers" pretend they are driving on a busy street, while the "pedestrians" try to cross the street at a busy intersection. Also let them simulate this activity without signs to demonstrate what traffic would be like if they did not have signs and rules to guide them. (This simulation could also be done with the students playing the roles of bicycle rider and automobile driver.)

Materials Needed: materials to make road signs

Processing Questions:

1. What road signs do you have in your neighborhood?

2. How do road signs help prevent accidents?

Safety Attitudes

Valued Outcome: The students will be able to role-play positive and negative attitudes concerning safety.

Description of Strategy: Attitudes play a large part in safety behavior. Have students role-play people with positive and negative attitudes (such as, *positive:* consideration, maturity, courtesy, honesty; *negative:* selfishness, impatience, childishness, competitiveness, showing off, daydreaming, and risk taking) while participating in several activities (such as bicycling, playing various activities).

Materials Needed: none

Processing Questions:

1. How does one's attitude about safety cause or prevent an accident?

2. What are some examples of positive safety attitudes? of negative safety attitudes?

Discussion and Report Techniques————————————

Safety in the Home

Valued Outcomes: Students will become aware of

1. their responsibility to prevent accidents

2. the potential safety hazards at home

3. the poison prevention rules

Description of Strategy: Show students visuals of different areas in a house. Give students plenty of time to examine the pictures, and then present these safety rules: Don't drink, eat, or taste any unknown substances; don't use tools meant for adult use only. Review the symbols for poison and other hazardous materials. Display the symbols throughout this unit. Teach the following "alert" words: *warning, caution, danger, poison.* Identify places students may see these words.

    Direct students to think of ways they can improve safety in each room in their own home. Obtain stickers (Mr. Yuk or Officer Ugg) from a poison control center, and distribute them so students can label potentially dangerous substances found in their homes.

Materials Needed: teacher visuals of household danger areas; symbols for hazardous substances or labels with warning signs and symbols. *Optional:* Contact local poison control center for stickers to label poisonous substances in the home.

Processing Questions:

1. What are accidents, and why do many people have them?

2. What kinds of ways did you think of to improve safety in each room?

3. What are some choices we can make to prevent accidents both to ourselves and others?

Source: G. Ezell. 1992. *Healthy living 2: Healthy and growing.* Grand Rapids, MI: Christian Schools International, p. 157.

Emergency First Aid

Valued Outcome: Students will be able to identify priorities and make logical decisions in emergency situations.

Description of Strategy: Give one discussion sheet (including the following situations) to each student for completion. After students have finished, ask for volunteers to share their answers with the class. Ask the students to explain their answers. Lead the class in a group discussion on each emergency.

Materials Needed: discussion sheets for each student (see as follows)

Processing Questions:

1. Should anyone at the scene of an accident or emergency administer first aid? Why or why not?

2. Is incorrect first aid better than no first aid at all?

3. Explain the importance of acting quickly and calmly, but at the same time carefully thinking through each step of aid given.

Source: K. Bridge. 1989. *Health*, Student Activities. Boston: Houghton Mifflin, p. 130.

Emergency!

Valued Outcome: The students will be able to identify the correct action to take in emergency situations.

Description of Strategy: Each of the following items describes an emergency that was handled incorrectly. Read each item. Identify the incorrect action and tell why it was incorrect. Explain what you would do in the situation.

1. Leroy was hit in the head by a moving swing and was knocked unconscious. Since it was a very hot day, his friend Eddie moved him into the shade before going for help.

2. While Liz was baby-sitting for the Jacksons, two-year-old Timmy drank some liquid from an unlabeled bottle. When Liz found him, Timmy was pale and sweaty, with stains from whatever he drank around his mouth. Liz immediately gave him some syrup of ipecac to make him vomit. Then she called the poison control center.

3. While José and Ben were sledding, José was thrown from his sled, hitting his head on a rock. Although conscious, he felt nauseated and too dizzy to walk. Before going for help, Ben covered José with his coat and gave him some hot chocolate from their thermos to keep him warm.

4. Nancy and Kayla were in the park, eating hamburgers and talking. Kayla, who had been lying on her back while she ate, suddenly jumped up and made strange wheezing sounds as if she couldn't breathe or speak. Nancy saw that Kayla was probably choking and ran to get some water for her.

Materials Needed: none

Processing Question: Why is it important to know the correct action to take in emergency situations?

Safety Rules

Valued Outcome: Students will review safety rules covered at earlier levels.

Description of Strategy: The purpose of this lesson is to stimulate discussion on a review of basic safety rules. The students will also be assigned an activity where they will report information from articles based on safety rules. To begin the discussion and review on basic safety rules, write on the chalkboard names of accident categories (for example, falls, burns, poisonings, traffic accidents) or of broad safety categories (for example, fire safety, pedestrian safety, bike safety, swimming safety, boating safety, preventing electric shock, food safety). Divide the class into groups, and have each group develop a list of safety rules for one category. The rules should be short—if possible, no more than four to five words. Go over the lists with the full class. Add any important rules that were omitted. Promote class discussion by asking why safety in each of these categories is important. Make sure to touch on each category. After the discussion, assign the students to different groups. Have each group look for articles about accidents in one category covered in the lesson. Groups will report their findings back to the class and discuss the articles and identify the safety rules that apply to the situations described.

Materials Needed: chalkboard, magazines

Processing Questions:

1. Why is safety important?

2. Should we have only broad safety rules that cover every category or should we have specific safety precautions for each individual category? Why?

3. What are some safety precautions you follow in your favorite category?

Source: G. Ezell. 1993. *Healthy living*, Grade 6: *Health inside and out*. Grand Rapids, MI: Christian Schools International, pp. 257, 258.

Illegal Weapons

Valued Outcome: The students will identify safety tips to help them obtain assistance when confronted with dangerous situations.

Description of Strategy: Discuss violence and weapons. Explain that there has been an increase in violence in schools because of young people carrying weapons illegally. Discuss steps to take when they see a student carrying a weapon or if they see a weapon in the school building or anywhere else. Emphasize that they should stay away from the student carrying the weapon. They should tell a teacher or a counselor what they saw. These steps are responsible actions to take to protect themselves. To prepare for this teaching strategy, using a marker, make a shoe box look like a safe. You can do this by drawing a circular combination lock and a handle that can be used to open the safe at one end. Use scissors to cut a slit on the top of the box. After discussion about violence and weapons, instruct students to consider guidelines they can practice to be responsible and to protect themselves. Each student is to write a safety tip (s)he can practice if (s)he sees a weapon. After they each write a tip on a piece of paper, they are to fold the paper and slip it through the slit on the top of the safe (the shoe box). After the students have written their safety tips and placed them in the safe, explain that what is contained within the safe is the right combination of information that can be applied to the very serious job of being safe around weapons. Open the safe, and have each student select one of the safety tips. Make sure that a student does not get the tip that (s)he wrote. One at a time, have students read the safety tips to the class. Discuss each tip. Remind them that no matter where they see a weapon, they need to behave responsibly.

Materials Needed: shoe box, marker, scissors

Processing Questions:

1. What would I do if I saw someone carrying a weapon?

2. Who could I tell if I saw someone carrying a weapon?

Source: L. Meeks and P. Heit. 1996. *Totally awesome health*, Sixth-grade manual. Blacklick, OH: Meeks Heit, pp. 163–164.

Poison Poster

Valued Outcome: The students will be able to identify various poisonous substances.

Description of Strategy: Have students cut pictures out of magazines representing known poisonous substances, and glue them on construction paper. Underneath the pictures, have them write down a safety rule about the particular substance. The students could take turns reporting to the class about the poison in their picture.

Materials Needed: magazines, scissors, pen, paper, glue, construction paper

Processing Questions:

1. What poisonous substances are in your home?

2. What safety rules do you have in your family about those poisonous substances?

Disaster Demonstration

Valued Outcome: The students will be able to demonstrate proper behaviors during various disasters.

Description of Strategy: Assign groups of students to demonstrate the proper behaviors during various disasters, such as tornado, hurricane, earthquake. Have them give instructions to the other students, and actually carry out the drill.

Materials Needed: none

Processing Questions:

1. What types of disasters could occur in your area?

2. Does your family have a plan to follow if such a disaster occurs?

Alcohol/Drinking Report

Valued Outcome: The students will be able to relate activities of various organizations that deal with drinking and driving.

Description of Strategy: Assign several students the project of reporting on the activities of several groups, such as Students Against Drunk Drivers (SADD) and Mothers Against Drunk Drivers (MADD). Other related topics in these reports could include their state's drunk driving laws. A related activity could be to have the class establish a SADD chapter in the school.

Materials Needed: none

Processing Questions:

1. Is there a SADD or MADD chapter in your town?

2. How have these groups helped to reduce drunk driving in your state?

Safety Belt Debate

Valued Outcome: The students will be able to debate the topic "wearing safety belts" against "not wearing safety belts."

Description of Strategy: Choose two teams of students to research the use of safety belts in automobiles. One team should argue that wearing safety belts, even for short trips, can save lives and prevent needless injuries in case of an automobile accident. The other team should present reasons why many people don't bother or refuse to wear safety belts. Have the class decide which argument is more based on fact.

Materials Needed: none

Processing Question: Why is it important to wear a safety belt every time you ride in a car?

Presentation by Safety Officials

Valued Outcome: The students will be able to invite community service employees to speak to the class.

Description of Strategy: Students select five representatives from the community to visit the class. Students are in charge of asking the officials to come. Officials could be fire, police, emergency personnel, and so forth.

Materials Needed: none

Processing Question: What role in safety do firefighters play? Police? Emergency personnel?

Safety Diary

Valued Outcome: The students will be able to list hazards that occur during holidays.

Description of Strategy: Students should list major holidays. Students should make a list of accidents or safety hazards that occur more during that particular holiday. On another list, the students write ways in which those accidents could be reduced or prevented.

Materials Needed: pen and paper

Processing Questions:

1. How can the major disasters be prevented?

2. If such a disaster cannot be prevented, how can we plan in order to reduce the number and severity of accidents?

Nuclear Disaster Evacuation

Valued Outcome: The students will learn the specifics of a nuclear disaster evacuation.

Description of Strategy: Have a local safety official discuss the various reasons for an evacuation during a nuclear disaster. Also, have them detail exactly how evacuation routes were planned for their specific town.

Materials Needed: none

Processing Questions:

1. Do you have any nuclear power sources near your home?

2. Are you familiar with the evacuation routes in the event of a nuclear disaster?

Experiments and Demonstrations

Responding to Emergency Situations

Valued Outcome: The students will learn about emergency situations and how to respond.

Description of Strategy: The students will be divided into groups of four. Each group will be given an emergency situation. They are to research the proper way to respond to the situations. Then they will make a poster describing the techniques or steps in the process. Each group will take a turn and will demonstrate their response to the situation. Some possible situations are

1. The house catches on fire while you are asleep. You smell smoke and wake up. What should you do to get out of the house safely? Then what do you do?

2. You are waiting for your ride to pick you up at the mall. A car pulls up. A man offers you some candy. What do you do?

3. While you are at a restaurant eating, the man at the next table starts choking. No one is noticing. What do you do?

4. You are alone at home. You hear on the television that a tornado has been spotted in the area. You need to get to safety. Where do you go, and what do you do?

5. You are making a fried egg when the stovetop catches on fire. It is a small fire but you don't want it to spread. What do you do?

6. Your baby sister has fallen in the pool. You pulled her out, but she is not breathing. What do you do?

7. Your best friend has fallen, and her knee is bleeding. What is the best thing to do?

8. You get a nosebleed. What do you do?

9. Your brother was trying to light a fire, and he burnt his hand. How do you treat it?

10. Your sister falls, and she thinks her leg is broken. What should you do?

Materials Needed: first-aid kit, bandages, fire extinguisher
Processing Questions:

1. Why is it important to know first aid?

2. Should you be trained to do CPR or can you do it anytime on your own with no training?

Source: D. Vriesenga. 1991. *The human body*, Whole Language Theme Unit. Grand Rapids, MI: Instructional Fair, p. 3.

Basic Water Safety/Reaching Assists

Valued Outcome: The student will discuss safety rules and perform various reaching assists.
Description of Strategy: Water safety is very important for children to learn. This lesson shows children at a young age, basic safety rules for swimming pools or lakes and how to help out a distressed swimmer by the use of a reaching assist. Procedures are as follows:

1. Have the students give safety rules that they already know. As they give the rules, also explain why each is important and why it should be followed.

2. Go over any safety rules that were not previously mentioned and why each is important.

3. Explain what a distressed swimmer is and again emphasize safety rules.

4. Ask the students what they would do if they encountered a distressed swimmer. Emphasize getting help in that situation.

5. Explain reaching assists and give a demonstration using the shepherd's crook.

6. Ask the students what else could be used for a reaching assist. Demonstrate the use of arms and legs for reaching assists.

7. Demonstrate assists with any other equipment that is available.

8. Have the students practice reaching assists in pairs, starting with arms and legs.

9. Have the students try reaching assists with various equipment.

10. Go over reaching assists and safety rules and how they tie together. Finish with a summary of the safety rules.

Materials Needed: swimming pool, rescue tube, shepherd's crook, or reaching pole
Processing Questions:

1. Why is it necessary to demonstrate reaching assists?

2. What are some basic water safety rules?

3. How are these two components related?

First-Aid Demonstration

Valued Outcome: The students will be able to identify and become familiar with various first-aid procedures.
Description of Strategy: Take several classes to demonstrate the proper first-aid procedures used in various emergencies, then allow time for the students to master these procedures.
Materials Needed: first-aid kit
Processing Questions:

1. What first-aid procedures can you perform?

2. When do you think you would have to use such procedures?

Cafeteria Poisons

Valued Outcome: The students will be able to identify poisonous substances in the cafeteria.
Description of Strategy: Have students cooperate with school cafeteria personnel in an activity to make the cafeteria safer. Let the students walk through the cafeteria and determine which substances may be poisonous or harmful. Have the students make poison stickers to be placed on each container of a poisonous or harmful substance.
Materials Needed: stickers, pen
Processing Questions:

1. What poisonous substances are present in your school cafeteria?

2. How can poison stickers help prevent accidents with these poisons?

Tool Safety

Valued Outcome: The students will be able to become familiar with proper tool safety.
Description of Strategy: Bring a variety of tools, appliances, and common implements to class and discuss the safe use of each. Demonstrate items that are appropriate to your age group. These might include scissors, knives, hand tools, small electrical appliances, gardening equipment, and kitchen equipment.
Materials Needed: hand tools, small kitchen appliances, electrical appliances, scissors, knives
Processing Questions:

1. What tools, appliances and implements do your parents or guardians use around the house and/or yard?

2. What are the possible safety problems that might accompany the use or misuse of these tools?

Learning to be safe while riding a bicycle can prevent many accidents.

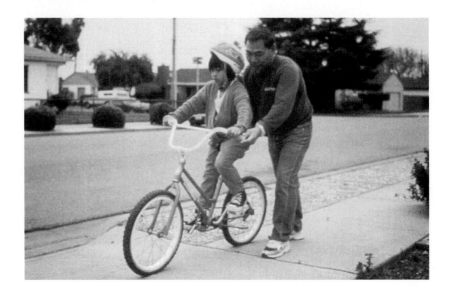

Bicycle Safety

Valued Outcome: The students will learn and be able to demonstrate proper bicycle safety.
Description of Strategy: Assign different tasks related to bicycle safety to several students. Have some students bring their bicycles to class to demonstrate the safety devices on the bicycle, such as reflectors on the pedals. Have other students demonstrate how to inspect their bike for possible safety problems and how to correct the problem. Let others actually ride their bicycles through a simulated traffic scene to demonstrate safe riding behaviors.
Materials Needed: bicycles
Processing Questions:

1. In what kind of traffic do you ride your bicycle?
2. Why is it important to have the proper safety devices on your bicycle?

Safety Belt/Restraining Devices

Valued Outcome: The students will be able to learn proper safety belt procedures.
Description of Strategy: Have a local safety official come to class to demonstrate the proper procedures for wearing safety belts for children and adults and restraining devices for infants. Let the students practice the correct way of placing an "infant" (doll) in several different types of restraining devices.
Materials Needed: dolls, car seat
Processing Questions:

1. Where do most accidents occur (near your home)?
2. Why is it important to wear safety belts *every time* you ride in a car?

The Hug of Life

Valued Outcome: The students will be able to demonstrate the Heimlich maneuver.

Description of Strategy: Have a trained representative from the American Heart Association demonstrate the proper use of the Heimlich maneuver if this knowledge is appropriate for your age group. Emphasize that this is only conducting a mock demonstration, and be careful not to apply too much pressure.
Materials Needed: none
Processing Questions:

1. How does the Heimlich maneuver work to help a person who is choking?

2. How does this procedure work differently for children and adults?

Resuscitation Annie

Valued Outcome: The students will learn mouth-to-mouth resuscitation.
Description of Strategy: If you have a CPR mannequin model available, demonstrate the proper technique for mouth-to-mouth resuscitation. Contact your local chapter of the American Heart Association for assistance in presenting this demonstration.
Materials Needed: CPR mannequin
Processing Questions:

1. How does resuscitation help a victim of a breathing problem?

2. Can you perform these procedures?

Fire Extinguishers

Valued Outcome: The students will be able to learn the proper techniques of using a fire extinguisher and be able to identify the various classes of extinguishers.
Description of Strategy: Show the students how to operate the extinguisher. Identify the difference classes of extinguishers.

Class A—used for wood, paper, or textile fires

Class B—used for oil, grease, or paint fires

Class C—used on electrical equipment

Materials Needed: fire extinguishers from each class
Processing Questions:

1. Does your family have a working fire extinguisher in your home?

2. Do you know how to use the extinguisher?

Puzzles and Games

Simon Says: Be Safe

Valued Outcomes:

1. Students will review pedestrian and car safety.

2. Students will be introduced to bike safety.

Description of Strategy: Show students pictures of traffic signs and ask them to identify the meaning of each sign. Review basic pedestrian rules with the class. Elicit the rules from the class, and write them on the board or on a chart. Add any rules the students miss. Include the following:

○ Walk on the sidewalk or grass away from the curb. Watch out for cars backing up in driveways.

○ Cross the street at the corner. Stay in the crosswalk if there is one.

○ Look all ways for cars before crossing. Listen for approaching cars. Watch for turning cars (and bicycles).

○ If there is a traffic or crossing light, obey the light.

○ Walk rather than run across the street.

Perhaps you can mark off an "intersection" on the classroom floor and have students practice watching for cars and crossing the street.

Take the classroom on an imaginary car ride. Ask students to think about how they can be safe while they're riding. Then tell them to pretend they are riding in a car. To add interest, add sound effects of getting in a car, closing door, and starting the car. You may ask, "What are ways to be safe in a car?" (Wear safety belts, sit quietly, don't distract the driver.) Have the class pretend to buckle up and stay buckled up until you say they have arrived at their destination.

Then have the class pretend to be riding bikes on a sidewalk. Again, add sound effects to simulate a bike ride. Ask, "What are ways to be safe while we're riding bikes on the sidewalk?" Include the following:

○ Dress properly. Tie shoelaces and avoid clothes that can catch in the bike chain.

○ Keep bikes in good repair.

○ Watch what's going on around you; watch out for cars backing out of driveways.

○ Keep both hands on the handlebars. Don't try to carry things.

○ Watch out for pedestrians on the sidewalk.

○ Avoid loose gravel or broken cement.

○ Wear bike helmets

Finally, arrive back home and park the bike in an appropriate place.

Play a Simon Says game to review the safety rules. Call it a Safe Simon Says game. If Simon says a safety rule, have students pantomime the rule. But if Simon suggest unsafe behavior, have students put their hands up in a stop gesture or sit down.

Materials Needed: pictures of traffic signs. *Optional:* chart paper; use masking tape to mark off an "intersection" in the classroom.

Processing Questions:

1. Which safety rule is the hardest for you to remember or to follow?

2. Why is knowing safety rules not enough? (We need to choose to follow them.)

3. How can following safety rules to help us to respect others and ourselves?

Source: G. Ezell. 1992. *Healthy living 2: Healthy and growing.* Grand Rapids, MI: Christian Schools International, p. 159.

Short Fuse/Long Fuse

Valued Outcome: Students will identify effective approaches to conflict resolution that exclude fighting.

Description of Strategy: Make a three-color ball of yarn. Cut three-foot strips of each color of yarn. Using the sequence of red, yellow, and green, tie the ends together, and make a new three-color ball of yarn. Have students sit in a circle. Show students a piece of red yarn. Explain that the red yarn represents a fuse—a short fuse. Show them a piece of yellow yarn as you tie it to the piece of red yarn. Explain that the yellow yarn represents ways to cool off. This gives you more time because the fuse is now longer and less likely to "blow." Next, show a piece of green yarn and tie it to the end of the yellow yarn. The green yarn has lengthened the fuse even more. The green yarn represents healthy ways to resolve conflict. Give the three-color ball of yarn to one student in the circle. Ask that student to wrap the yarn around his or her finger. Suppose it is yellow. Because yellow represents ways to cool off, the student mentions one way to cool off, such as going for a long walk.

Suppose his or her finger was wrapped in red yarn. Because red represents a short fuse, (s)he will mention a way of resolving conflict that would be harmful. If his or her finger was wrapped in green yarn, the student would mention a healthy way of dealing with conflict, since green represents healthy ways to resolve conflict. Students are to continue passing the ball of yarn around until everyone in the class has had an opportunity to wrap yarn around his or her finger, check the color, and respond by mentioning a way to resolve conflicts that is represented by the color of the yarn. After the web is complete, explain that students will experience many conflicts in their lifetime. They should notice that the people connected to them—friends, family, and so on—have different styles of resolving conflict. Stress that it is important to resolve conflicts in healthful ways and to stay away from people who have short fuses and choose to resolve conflicts in harmful ways.

Materials Needed: ball of red yarn, ball of yellow yarn, ball of green yarn, scissors

Processing Questions:

1. What conflicts have I experienced with different friends?

2. Did I resolve these conflicts in the most healthful way possible?

3. If not, what could I have done differently?

Source: L. Meeks and P. Heit. 1995. *Violence prevention, Totally awesome teaching strategies for safe and drug-free schools.* Blacklick, OH: Meeks Heit, pp. 360–361.

Safety with Lightning

Valued Outcome: Students will be able to interpret information and generalize.

Description of Strategy: Discuss with students the danger of swimming during a thunderstorm: If lightning strikes the water, it can give the swimmer an electric shock. Read the activity with the students. Be sure students understand that the puzzle is made up of four separate sentences. The answer to the puzzle is, Come out of the water. Lightning might strike the water. Then electricity could travel through the water. It could travel to you and give you a shock.

You may wish to have students make up other word puzzles using different water safety rules. Let students exchange puzzles with their classmates.

Materials Needed: copy of puzzle for each student

Processing Questions:

1. What are some general rules you should obey when in the water?

2. How can following the safety rule help save lives?

Source: Scott, Foresman. 1990. *Health for life*, Teachers edition. Glenview, IL: Scott, Foresman, p. 134.

Flashcard Safety Game

Valued Outcome: Students will be able to give recommendations applied to recreational safety.
Description of Strategy: Make flashcards with the following pictures on one side. On the other side, write a message to go along with the picture. Drill the students every day for a week to see if they will remember the "Rules for Recreation."

Picture	Message
car seat with safety belt	Be safe when riding in the car!
a red cross	Visit the Red Cross to learn how to cope with unexpected injuries.
champagne glasses	Alcohol use increases the likelihood that people will get hurt.
eyes with glasses	Protect your eyes from injury and sunlight.
child swimming in water	Learn to swim! Drowning occurs most frequently to people who never intended to be in the water.
a road sign	Obey the laws. Many laws are directly related to the safety of the participants.
a thermometer	Be aware of weather conditions. Always be prepared for bad weather. Sudden shifts in the weather can turn outdoor activities into tragedy.

Materials Needed: 4- x 6-inch flashcards; markers
Processing Questions:

1. Why is it important to take safety precautions anytime I go outdoors?

2. What are some outdoor activities that I enjoy?

3. How might I safeguard myself when doing these things?

Source: Adapted from W. Payne and D. Hahn. 1992. *Understanding your health*, 3rd ed. St. Louis, MO: Mosby-Year Book, p. A8.

Which Sign Am I?

Valued Outcome: The students will be able to identify various traffic signs
Description of Strategy: Have the class design a poster of several traffic signs. After a discussion of traffic signs, split the class into teams. Call out certain clues about a sign, and have a member of one team come to the front of the room and point to the sign on the poster, explain what the sign means, and where you might find it.
Materials Needed: poster board, markers, scissors

Processing Questions:

1. How can traffic signs help prevent accidents?

2. Where do you find the different types of traffic signs, and what do they mean?

Safe Route Home

Valued Outcome: The students will be able to determine the safest route home from school.
Description of Strategy: Have students map out a safe route to their home from their school. The students could have their parents provide input to help chart the safest route.
Materials Needed: pen and paper
Processing Questions:

1. How do you travel from school to home?

2. If you walk or ride your bicycle, do you have a safe route planned?

3. If you walk from the school bus stop to your home, do you have a safe route planned?

Other Ideas

Violence Prevention

Valued Outcome: Students will participate in a cultural awareness activity.
Description of Strategy: Combine classes of the same grade for one class period for a week-long cultural volunteer mentor-training workshop. Increase an awareness of the concerns and issues of various ethnic backgrounds that can be the basis of a mutual support network. Following this collaboration, set regular meeting times for those interested in continuing as cultural volunteer mentors. This may end up being a tremendous service to your school and will facilitate tolerance and provide a means to redefining diversity.
Materials Needed: resources with information regarding cultural diversity
Processing Questions:

1. Of what things about your culture are you most proud?

2. What are some things that you wish other people would see as positive attributes about your culture?

3. What are some ways your culture is different from other cultures?

4. Why do people of other cultures look down on certain things about cultures that are different from their own?

Source: Adapted from J. White. 1995, January–February. Violence prevention in schools. *Journal of health education* (AAHPERD, Reston, VA) 26(1): 52.

Fire Escape Plans

Valued Outcome: The students will be able to identify a safe evacuation of their homes in case of a fire.
Description of Strategy: Ask students to draw a basic plan showing the layout of their residences. Have the students discuss a fire evacuation route and an alternate route with their parents, and

then ask them to show these routes on their drawings, using different colored arrows for the two routes. Each student should be able to explain why the routes are the best ones to use in case of a home fire.

Materials Needed: construction paper, paper, pen, scissors

Processing Questions:

1. Do you have two escape routes planned from your bedroom?

2. Where will your family plan to meet outside in the case of a fire in your home?

Traffic Safety Obstacle Course

Valued Outcome: The students will learn the importance of traffic signs.

Description of Strategy: Set up a simulated "obstacle course" on the playground illustrating such traffic hazards as busy intersections, unmarked intersections, and so on. Mark each potentially hazardous part of the course with traffic safety signs, including speed limit signs, yield signs, and pedestrian signals. Have some children go through the course on their bicycles, while others play the part of pedestrians. Discuss the importance of following traffic safety signs, signals, and regulations.

Materials Needed: poster board, markers, scissors, construction paper

Processing Questions: Why is it important to practice negotiating traffic obstacles?

First-Aid Kits

Valued Outcome: The students will be able to identify the important contents of a first-aid kit.

Description of Strategy: Instruct the students on what items should be kept in a first-aid kit for the home, then have each student make his or her own first-aid kit. These kits could include strips of cloth for bandages and dressings, Band-Aids, tongue depressors (for a small splint), 1-inch and 2-inch roller gauze.

Materials Needed: first-aid kit, including strips of bandages, Band-Aids, tongue depressors, gauze

Processing Questions:

1. Do you have a first-aid kit in your home?

2. How can such a kit help reduce the severity of accidents in the home?

Field Trips

Valued Outcome: The students will be able to inspect a fire station and learn how it operates.

Description of Strategy: If feasible, take the class on a field trip to the local fire station or other safety agency outlet. Prepare the class thoroughly for what they will see, and have them write down a list of questions they wish to ask those in charge.

Materials Needed: pen and paper

Processing Questions:

1. What items are in the fire station (or on the truck) to help reduce the effects of a fire?

2. How does each safety agency help the public prevent accidents?

Safety Guest Speakers

Valued Outcome: Students will be able to identify safety procedures from various areas of safety and accident prevention.

Description of Strategy: For one week, have a guest speaker come to speak to your class each day. Include someone from the following backgrounds: a CPR/first-aid instructor, a water safety instructor; a firearms safety instructor; a professional from a poisoning, burn, or other trauma center; a fire safety representative; someone from the American Red Cross; or a highway safety instructor. At the end of the week, have each student report on the things he or she felt were the most important addressed by the guest speakers.

Materials Needed: paper and pencil

Processing Questions:

1. What is the importance of each of the roles of the guest speakers?

2. What can you do as a contributing member of your household and classroom to promote safety and accident prevention?

Source: Adapted from F. Sizer and E. Whitney. 1988. *Life choices: Health concepts and strategies.* St. Paul West, p. 455.

References

American School Health Association. 1994, March. *Journal of school health* 64(3). Kent, OH (From *Education for self-responsibility II: Prevention of drug use*, produced with funds from the U.S. Department of Education Drug-Free Schools and Communities Act, Joe Wiese, Program Director for Drug Use Prevention Education.): 128–130.

Being healthy, Teacher's Resource Book. 1990. Orlando, FL: Harcourt Brace Jovanovich.

Bridge, K. 1989. *Health, student activities.* Boston: Houghton Mifflin.

Ezell, G. 1992. *Healthy living, grade 1.* Grand Rapids, MI: Christian Schools International.

Getchell, B., R. Pippin, and J. Varnes. 1989. *Health*, Teachers edition. Boston: Houghton Mifflin.

Meeks, L., and P. Heit. 1996. *Totally awesome health.* Blacklick, OH: Meeks Heit, p. 163–164.

Meeks, L, P. Heit, and R. Page. 1995. *Violence prevention totally awesome teaching strategies for safe and drug-free schools.* Blacklick, OH: Meeks Heit.

Payne, W, and D. Hahn. 1992. *Understanding your health*, 3rd ed. St. Louis: Mosby Yearbook.

Richmond, J. B., E. T. Pounds, C. B. Corbin. 1990. *Health for life*, Teachers edition. Glenview, IL: Scott, Foresman.

Sizer, F., and E. Whitney. 1988. *Life choices: Health concepts and strategies*, St. Paul: West.

Vriesenga, D. 1991. *The human body*, Whole Language Theme Unit. Grand Rapids, MI: Instructional Fair.

White, J. 1995, January–February. Violence prevention in schools. *Journal of health education* (AAHPERD, Reston, VA) 26(1).

Resources

Books

American National Red Cross. 1996. *Community CPR workbook.* Washington, DC: American Red Cross.

Botsis-Alexander, J., and others. 1995. Summer. Parental loss and family violence as correlates of suicide and violence risk. *Suicide and life-threatening behavior* 25(2).

Donatelle, R., and L. Davis. 1996. *Access to health*, 4th ed. Boston: Allyn and Bacon.

Hahn, D., and W. Payne. 1997. *Focus on health.* St. Louis: Mosby-Yearbook.

Hechinger, F. 1994, Winter. Saving youth from violence. *Carnegie quarterly* 39(1).

Ibrahim, H., and K. Cordes. 1993. *Outdoor recreation.* Madison, WI: Brown & Benchmark.

Levy, M. R., M. Dignan, and J. H. Shirreffs. 1997. *Life & health*, 5th ed. New York: Random House.

Miller, D., S. Telljohann, and C. Symons. 1996. *Health education.* Madison, WI: Brown & Benchmark.

Mullen, K., R. Gold, P. Belcastro, and R. McDermott. 1993. *Connections for health*, 3rd ed. Madison, WI: Brown & Benchmark.

National Crime Prevention Council, National Institute for Citizen Education in the Law, Department of Justice, Office of Juvenile Justice and Delinquency Prevention. 1995. *Between hope and fear: Teens speak out on crime and the community*. Survey conducted by Louis Harris & Associates, New York, New York.

Prothrow-Stith, D. 1995. The epidemic of youth violence in America: Using public health prevention strategies to prevent violence. *Journal of health care for the poor and underserved* 6(2): 95–101.

Pruitt, B., and J. Stein. 1994. *Healthstyles: Decisions for living well*. Fort Worth, TX: Saunders College.

Videos

The following videos are available from Sunburst Communications, 101 Castleton Street, P. O. Box 40, Pleasantville, NY 10570.

Student workshop: Solving conflicts
Designed as a hands-on workshop in conflict resolution skills. Mini-dramas raise problems students will recognize as straight out of their own lives, giving them practical help with their school, peer, and home relationships. (26-minute video, 12 student worksheets, teacher's guide in three-ring binder)

Student workshop: What to do about anger
Designed as a hands-on workshop in anger management skills to help children get along better with friends, family, and authority figures. Program teaches students the difference between angry feelings and angry behavior, how to handle anger by controlling how they act, and how to deal with angry energy in safe, positive ways.

Getting better at getting along: Conflict resolution
Provides an introduction to conflict resolution by demonstrating essential techniques. Shows students that when they express themselves clearly and listen carefully, they improve their ability to solve problems, are able to take greater responsibility for themselves, and get better at getting along, in and out of school. (16-minute video, eight student worksheets, teacher's guide, plus . . . full-color poster, game, audiocassette of songs, English/Spanish, send-home pages and extra activity pages)

Come see what first aid can do
In this engaging and humorous program on first aid, viewers learn how to treat injuries and burns, watch a cut heal, and much more. Program details important first-aid facts, explains why certain treatments work, and shows how to use the Emergency Response System to get help.

First aid: New techniques: Series A
True-to-life first-aid emergencies draw the viewer into this lively program on practical first aid, safety precautions and rescue techniques.

Kids for safety
Combines catchy song lyrics with colorful graphics to teach students all about bicycle, fire, and personal safety. Advising viewers that "keeping safe is up to you," presents easy-to-learn rules for riding bicycles, preventing fires at home, and staying safe when home alone or in other potentially dangerous situations. Uses reviews and quizzes to reinforce the points made.

Real people: Violence in the family
Designed to offer understanding and real help to teens who live in the estimated one out of four families in which violence occurs. Interweaving first-person accounts by teens who grew up in violent homes, dramatic stories, and interviews with experts, program helps viewers distinguish between what is normal family life and what is not, and learn coping skills.

The following video is available from Schoolhouse Videos & CDs, 4205 Grove Ridge Drive, Durham, NC 27703.

Emergency Action
Learn step-by-step how to help someone during a medical emergency. The information included can save a life. (Item 4621)

CD-ROM

(Available from Sunburst Communications)

Safety monkey
Help Safety Monkey make his home, school, and neighborhood safe.

• Teaches safety in 16 various settings

• Hundreds of safety tips

• Colorful animation that kids love

• Easy navigation for young learners, ages 3–8

• Original songs teaching safety

This fun and engaging disc teaches important lessons about safety. Kids learn how to spot and correct unsafe situations and when to get a grown-up's help. In lively, 3-D animation, Safety Monkey and his friends make Swingland safe again.

Web Sites

General Health

Resources for School Health Educators
http://www.indiana.edu/~aphs/hlthk-12..html

CDC Prevention Guidelines Database
http://wonder.cdc.gov/wonder/prevguid/prevguid.htm

Developing Educational Standards
http://putwest.boces.org/standards.html

Adolescent Health On-line
http://www.ama-assn.org/adolhlth/adolhlth.htm

See particularly the Adolescent Health Links at <*http://www.ama-assn.org/adolhlth/gapslink/gapslnk2.htm#ADOL*>

PE Central
http://infoserver.etl.vt.edu/~/PE.Central/PEC2.html

Kathy Schrock's Guide for Educators
http://www.capecod.net/Wixon/health/fitness.htm

Health Education Forum
http://libertynet.org/~lion/forum-health.html

Education World—Subjects: Physical Education
http://www.education-world.com/db/phys-gen.shtml

The Life Education Network
http://www.lec.org/

American Cancer Society
http://www.cancer.org

Safety/Accident Prevention

American Automobile Association Foundation for Driver Safety
http://webfirst.com/aaa

Driver's Support
http://www.veta.se/

Not One More!
http://www.frisk.com/not/

Travelers' Safety
http://werple.mira.net.au/%7Ewreid/bali_p2h.html

American Academy of Orthopaedic Surgeons, Prevention of Injuries
www.aaos.org/wordhtml/press/prevent.htm

CDC National Center for Injury Prevention and Control
www.cdc.gov/ncipc/ncipchtm.htm

Consumer Product Safety Commission
www.cpsc.gov

HRSA Children's Safety Network
www.edc.org/HHD/csn

Indian Health Service
www.tucson.ihs.gov

National Fire Prevention Association
www.wpi.edu/fpe/nfpa.html

National Highway Transportation Safety Administration
www.nhtsa.dot.gov

National SAFE Kids Campaign
www.oclc.org/safekids

National Safety Council
www.nsc.org

University of Pittsburgh Injury Control Resource Information Network
www.pitt.edu/ icrin/index.htm

U.S. Fire Administration
www.usfa.fema.gov

Violent and Abusive Behavior

National Committee for the Prevention of Child Abuse
www.childabuse.org/new.html

Hawaii
www.hawaii.gov/health/index.html

Massachusetts
www.magnet.state.ma.us/dph/dphhome.htm

CDC National Center for the Injury Prevention and Control
www.cdc.gov/ncipc/ncipchm.htm

Pavnet Online
www.pavnet.org

Educational and Community-Based Programs

CDC National Center for Chronic Disease Prevention and Health Promotion
www.cdc.gov/nccdphp/nccdhome.htm

Health Resources and Services Administration
www.hrsa.dhhs.gov

Healthy Cities Online
www.healthycities.org

Office of Minority Health Resource Center
Washington State Department of Health
www.doh.wa.gov

Occupational Safety and Health

American Industrial Hygiene Association
www.aiha.org

CDC National Institute for Occupational Safety and Health
ww.cdc.gov/niosh/homepage.html

Department of Energy, Environment, Safety, and Health InfoCenter
nattie.eh.doe.gov/map.html

Department of Labor
www.dol.gov/

DOL Mine Safety and Health Administration
www.msha.gov

Occupational Safety and Health Administration
www.osha.gov/

CDC National Center for Health Statistics
www.cdc.gov/nchswww/nchshome.htm

CDC Scientific, Surveillance, and Health Statistics, and Laboratory Information
www.cdc.gov/scientific.htm

CDC WONDER
wonder.cdc.gov

Health Care Financing Administration
1996 Statistics at a Glance
www.hcfa.gov/stats/stathili.htm

General Sites

American Medical Association
http://www.ama-assn.org

MedicineNet
http://www.medicinenet.com

Medscape
http://www.medscape.com

Oncolink
http://www.oncolink.upenn.edu

ParentsPlace.com
http://www.parentsplace.com

Thrive@ pathfinder
http://pathfinder.com/thrive

Links Only

Hardin Meta Directory of Internet Health Sources
http://www.arcade.uiowa.edu/hardin-www/md.html

Medical Matrix
http://www.5lackinc.com/matrix

Chapter Twenty

Consumer Health

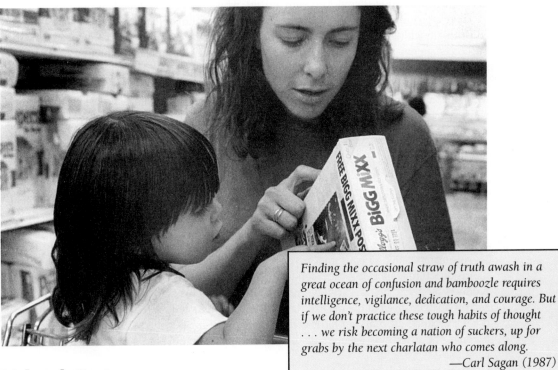

Finding the occasional straw of truth awash in a great ocean of confusion and bamboozle requires intelligence, vigilance, dedication, and courage. But if we don't practice these tough habits of thought . . . we risk becoming a nation of suckers, up for grabs by the next charlatan who comes along.
—Carl Sagan (1987)

Valued Outcomes

After reading this chapter, you should be able to

- ○ analyze the role of advertising in consumer purchases
- ○ list various advertising approaches
- ○ discuss how quackery affects health care
- ○ state criteria for selecting a health care professional
- ○ state criteria for selecting a health care facility
- ○ list the rights of the consumer
- ○ discuss private and governmental agencies that help protect the consumer

A Nation of Consumers

We are all consumers. A consumer is anyone who selects and uses products to fulfill personal needs and desires. Consumer products range from the clothes we wear to the foods we eat to the over-the-counter drugs we buy for self-medication. Consumer services include those provided by physicians, dentists, and other medical professionals. In this chapter, we examine the area of **consumer health**, which is defined as the intelligent purchase and use of products and services that will directly affect one's health. At first, this may seem only a small percentage of consumer goods and services, but in fact many more are health related than may be supposed. For example, buying a car may not seem to be a health-related matter, but it is, at least in part. One car might be a safer vehicle because it is equipped with airbags, while another automobile is not.

This chapter cannot discuss all aspects of consumer health, only the more directly health-related issues. In addition to products and services, we look at consumer psychology and how various forces attempt to manipulate consumer attitudes and behavior. In addition, we discuss consumer rights, consumer-oriented legislation, and government agencies, and the role of the teacher in consumer health education. Some of the information may seem to be very adult oriented, but if children are going to be wise consumers in their adult years, the process must begin in the elementary school years.

Advertising and Consumer Behavior

Everyone has consumer needs and desires. From childhood, we are barraged with advertising that attempts to foster these needs and desires so that one blurs into the other. A need becomes a desire, and a desire is perceived as a need. Our economic system is built on supply and demand, and producers do all that they can to nurture a growing demand.

This manipulation of consumer psychology and behavior begins in early childhood, often by means of Saturday morning television commercials aimed specifically at young children. Typical products promoted are toys, candy, and breakfast cereals. As students grow older, the messages and products change but the message is still one of persuasion. In fact, the methods used to advertise the products are quite sophisticated. By law, advertising of any kind may not be false or misleading. The advertising agencies do an excellent job of stimulating desire and creating a belief about need.

Businesses spend over $60 billion a year on advertising; more money is spent on advertising health products than any other category of items. Approximately 5 to 35 percent of the gross sales of drugs and health aids is spent on advertising (Cornacchia and Barret 1993). A great deal of psychological research goes into advertising so that the target group, whether children, teenagers, homemakers, young adults, or older adults, can be effectively reached and manipulated. The entire point of this endeavor is to get consumers to buy a particular product or engage in a specific activity. Advertising does not seek to inform, but to persuade.

There are dozens of different brands of products to choose from. In many ways, the U.S. consumer is fortunate to have so great a choice. Competition for the consumer dollar also stimulates the development of better and more efficient products and services. Consider the level of quality that would be available if only one brand of each type of product or service were offered. By providing us with so much choice, however, our economic system also makes it more difficult to make correct and informed decisions about purchases. Many of the products on the market are virtually indistinguishable from one another as far as quality and effectiveness are concerned. Price may be the only difference, and even that may not be much of a factor. For example, all brands of aspirin are basically the same in quality and effectiveness, regardless of advertising claims to the contrary.

Because the purpose of advertising is to persuade, most advertising contains little informational content. Even that which appears to be informational is carefully selected so that the product being advertised will appear to be uniquely better in some way. Certainly, no manufacturer could be expected to state, "Our product is no different from our competitors' products, but please buy ours anyway."

Advertising Approaches

Advertising is a sophisticated kind of manipulation. Advertising experts understand that, despite the lack of information conveyed about the actual merits of a product, consumers can be convinced that one particular brand should be sought out from among the dozens of very similar products on the market. The reason for this is that advertising seeks to appeal, not to the rational aspects of human psychology but instead to the irrational aspects. By making a particular product sound more appealing, *for any reason*, an advertiser can increase the market share of the product. This can be done in a variety of ways, almost all of them noninformational in nature. Here are typical approaches used to create appeal. It is important to remember that the same appeals are used on children as on adults. Table 20.1 contains some of the most common advertising techniques.

Many advertisers combine the approaches mentioned in Table 20.1 with visual and/or emotional imagery. Whether in a magazine ad or television commercial, the visual aspects of the advertisement are just as important as the written or spoken message. If the visual message of the commercial is pleasant, the reader or viewer will more likely associate positive thoughts with the product. Students should be made aware of the powerful stimuli provided by advertisements. Consumers must learn to recognize that there is a great deal of puffery in almost any commercial

Packages and advertisements can be powerful stimuli. Students should be made aware of this.

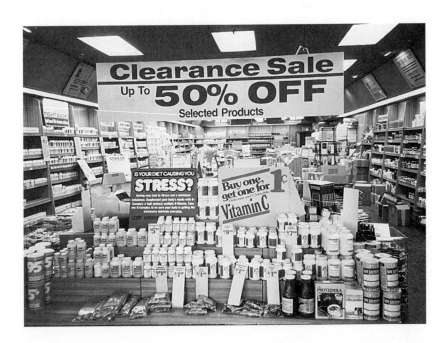

Table 20.1
Common Advertising Techniques

Techniques	Appeals	Questions to Ask
bandwagon	Typical phrases: "everyone uses, nation's leading, used by millions, preferred by most, used for more than twenty years"	Is it really true? Who says?
comedy appeal	use of humor to promote product "Morning Mouth"	Does the product really work?
costs	cost effective, less than competition	Is the cost really less? What is the quality?
effectiveness	most effective, relieves pain, itch, protects, easy to use	What is the evidence? How long is it effective? Does it really work?
endorsements/testimonials	use actors, athletes, dentist, physicians to promote	What are their qualifications to endorse the product?
scientific appeal	use of phrases such as "many doctors recommend," "hospital tested" if a person is usually an actor or actress	Is the information accurate? What evidence? Where did the information come from?
slogans/humor	humorous lyrics, cartoon characters, phrases	Do any actually apply to product?
snob appeal/superiority	famous person or use of phrases such as "people who know." Use of words *long-lasting, natural, extra strength.* Contains some ingredient from Europe, etc.	Does the person really know? What is the real implication of *the words used?* Does it work as claimed?
social	Makes you more attractive, smell better, more socially acceptable	Does the product really work?

or advertisement, regardless of the approach used to convey the message. Often there is little difference in effectiveness between one health product and another, and price is not a big factor either. We are all manipulated by advertising, and even if a person actually feels better about using one product over another, usually there is no difference in health consequences whether Brand X or Brand Y is selected. For children and adults, what is important to their consumer health is to develop an understanding of how advertising seeks to manipulate them, so that, when more serious health problems arise, they will not be deceived by advertising claims. Perhaps most important, the limited effectiveness of all OTC drugs and self-medication must be recognized.

Other Influences on Product and Service Choices

Consumer decisions are influenced not only by advertising but also by an individual's level of education, family beliefs, religion, socioeconomic status, community, and personal goals. A host of other factors may be involved, including one's physical and emotional needs, motives, and personality (Corry 1983). People may model their buying patterns and selections on those of family members, friends, or peers. The more status or importance that the person being modeled has, the greater the influence that person has.

With all these influences, it might seem that a person can hardly be blamed for sometimes making poor choices about consumer health products and services. But this denies personal responsibility. Not everything can be blamed on advertising or outside influences. People often make harmful health decisions quite independently of either. They may use advertising claims to shore up these decisions, for example, by relying on OTC products in an attempt to cure ill health when they actually know that they should be seeking more effective medical treatment. Such individuals are only too willing to create a false sense of security or relief by accepting advertising claims uncritically or by enlarging on such claims themselves in order to find easy answers where no such answers exist. In the final analysis, consumers can make informed choices if they want to do so. As with other aspects of wellness, each individual must accept self-responsibility. Consumers can then seek out information on products and services, analyze each on its own merits, and make better decisions accordingly.

Consumer Myths and Misconceptions

Some consumer health myths might be classified as folk beliefs. Although not based on any scientific facts, many of these myths are widely believed. In some instances, belief in certain of these myths can lead to unwise consumer health decisions. For example, a belief that "organic" or "natural" foods are somehow better than regular produce available in stores can lead to wasteful spending on overpriced specialty products. Some consumer health myths are believed because the person is desperate for relief. Sufferers of arthritis, which is an incurable condition at present, may wear a copper bracelet in the hope that perhaps the myth about the curative properties of copper really has some truth to it. They may also spend money on mud baths or other worthless forms of supposed therapy. As some of these treatments do provide relaxation, leading to a feeling of temporary relief, they are not entirely without value, but consumers who place their faith in them are deluding themselves as to long-term benefits.

Consumer misconceptions also lead to wasteful spending and, occasionally, to actual harm to health status. Perhaps the most common misconception is that producers manufacture only products that are needed; therefore, if a product is on the market, it must be fulfilling a need. In fact, many products are marketed to create a need that does not actually exist. For example, many mouthwashes, tonics, and other nostrums provide few health benefits. However, most consumers believe that any product that continues to be sold must be meeting a real need. Constant advertising reinforces this misconception. Even the better educated are often ignorant about consumer health information and hold many misconceptions. For example, when college students were surveyed concerning their knowledge of health care, only 49 percent responded correctly to a series of questions on the subject. Of this same group, 42 percent believed that health articles printed in popular magazines were always checked for scientific accuracy before publication.

Clearly, consumers must become better informed if they are to make wise consumer health decisions. They must recognize the negative impact that myths and misconceptions can have on personal health. They must also become more aware of how advertising seeks to manipulate consumer behavior and learn to reject appeals to the irrational in favor of facts and accurate information. Obtaining factual information about health products and services is not always easy. By law, advertisers must tell the truth about their products, prove the claims they make, be specific about any guarantee or warranty, and avoid making misleading statements. In addition, the advertising code subscribed to by most business advertisers puts forth similar guidelines. However, most products are still made to sound more effective than they really are. It is ultimately the consumer's responsibility to see through this puffery and make wise decisions accordingly. To accomplish this, children and adults must strive to become intelligent health consumers. Cornacchia and Barrett (1993, 10–11) offer six guidelines for intelligent consumers:

1. The intelligent consumer is well informed and knows how to make sound decisions.

2. The intelligent consumer seeks reliable sources of information.

3. The intelligent consumer is appropriately skeptical about health information and does not accept statements appearing in the news media or advertising at face value.

4. The intelligent consumer is wary of inept practitioners, pseudo practitioners, and pitchmen in the business and medical worlds and can identify quacks and quackery.

5. The intelligent consumer selects practitioners with great care and questions fees, diagnoses, treatments, and alternative treatments.

6. The intelligent consumer willingly "speaks out" by reporting frauds, quackery, and wrongdoing to appropriate agencies and law enforcement officials.

Quackery

There are many models of medical treatment. Some of them are valid and time tested; some are new and their advocates are working to gain acceptance. Others, however, do not seek scientific validation and, in fact, avoid scientific inquiry. The first category of medical models is comprised of conventional medicine practiced by physicians who are licensed and certified in their fields. The second category includes such approaches to health care as biofeedback and holistic health, which may be of value in treating certain health conditions. The third category is quackery, the use of worthless approaches that often promise miraculous results.

Quacks usually try very hard to appear scientific. Their offices may closely resemble conventional physicians' offices, even to the framed degrees (but often from diploma mills) on the walls. They may dress as physicians, in a white laboratory coat or with stethoscopes around their neck, employ scientific-looking gadgets, and use scientific-sounding mumbo jumbo to explain their supposed treatments. But it is all a sham, and a quack will always find an excuse for not permitting the form of quackery to be subject to independent scientific scrutiny. Although some quacks may sincerely believe in the efficacy of their treatments, most are simply out to victimize the consumer to make money.

Quackery flourishes in the United States for a variety of reasons. The primary reason is ignorance. Many Americans do not know the difference between legitimate and illegitimate medical practitioners. Anyone who claims to be a doctor or a healer is taken at face value. Another reason quackery exists is that quacks often promise cures or relief that legitimate medical practitioners cannot offer. For those suffering from incurable diseases, the false hope that quacks hold out may seem irresistible. As nothing else can help them, they turn to quacks in desperation. People also sometimes consult quacks because they hope to get around the high cost of legitimate medical attention; the quack promises a quick and inexpensive cure. In other instances, people turn to quacks because they wish to avoid surgery or other involved legitimate medical treatment. Some individuals may not realize the difference between scientifically proven methodologies and legitimately trained professionals versus those who are trained in treatments that are outside this body of knowledge. Still, of course, many people actually believe the flimflam claims made by quacks (Payne and Hahn 1991).

Quackery can involve deception in several areas, such as medicine, drugs, healing devices, and diets. Some of the warning signs of quacks include (Hamrick, Anspaugh, and Ezell 1986, 69) the following:

1. offers of a guaranteed, quick cure for an illness with a "miracle" drug or treatment
2. uses of fear strategies to convince the patient of his or her need for the cure
3. claims of victimization by other physicians or the American Medical Association
4. underrating traditional medical practice
5. no use of surgery
6. use of devices, gadgets, and secret formulas to convince patients that their illness is cured

If quacks cannot effect cures, why do so many people continue to have faith in them? In some instances, quacks do seem to provide relief or cures. In such cases, the patient may be a hypochondriac with no actual physical problem. If the person believes that help is being provided, the "problem" disappears. In cases where an actual problem does exist, the natural healing powers of the body may be responsible for a cure attributed to a quack. Finally, temporary relief or remission may be mistaken for a cure.

Not only is the consumer's pocketbook short-changed in quackery treatments, medications, and devices, but people's health can be undermined. Quackery delays proper treatment and increases the possibility of a more serious outcome. Using good sense and seeking information from physicians or some reputable agency is a good start to finding proper information (Greenberg and Dintiman 1992, 491). Some nonprofit agencies that may be able to help provide reliable information and referrals include the Consumer's Union, American Cancer Society, Arthritis Foundation, American Heart Association, American Lung Association, American Medical Association, American Dental Association, and the Better Business Bureau.

Health Care

The U.S. health care delivery system is beginning to evolve. Rising medical care costs, as well as the ever-increasing number of uninsured or underinsured, are significant factors contributing to many of the proposed changes. The reasons for increasing health care costs include current reimbursement practices, increasing technology, and rising physicians' fees and other health care salaries. Another factor in high health care costs, particularly in hospitals, is the costs of care for the poor, uninsured, and underinsured. The poor and the elderly are the ones who suffer most from the current health care delivery system. Government programs such as Medicare and Medicaid help, but for many individuals the portion of the bills not paid by these programs is still financially overwhelming.

Paying for Health Care

Health care cost in the United States is expensive and is continuing to increase in cost. For the year 1994 national health care expenditures were estimated to be $910 billion, with the projected expenditures to be over $1 trillion by the year 2000 (Vincenzino 1994). The vast majority of Americans cannot afford the costs of medical care without some form of health insurance. Health insurance is a contract between an insurance company and either an individual or group for the payment of medical costs. Health insurance usually entails the individual or group to pay a premium to the insurance company each month. The insurance company then pays for all or part of the health care costs, depending on the type of coverage provided.

Medical Insurance

As fees for medical and health care services continue to climb, it is more important than ever to have adequate medical insurance. Today, many workers are covered by a group plan at their place of employment. Typically, such plans pay 80 percent of medical costs, with the individual responsible for the remaining 20 percent. Premiums for this coverage are paid for by employer contributions and employee pay deductions. Group insurance plans typically have a deductible that the insured is responsible for paying before costs are covered by the insurance company. Most of these plans provide good coverage, but one problem is that the insurance coverage ceases if the employee leaves the company.

A variation of the third-party reimbursement method of medical insurance as described in the previous paragraph includes the use of preferred providers (PPOs). Under the PPO system, a plan is provided by an employer to minimize insurance claim filing and costs. The employer contracts with an insurance company and specific health care providers. The employee agrees to use only the health care professionals and institutions under contract. The employer and employee pay lower insurance premiums, the insurance companies save on paperwork and claim filing, and physicians increase their patient load.

Many people pay for their own medical insurance. Self-employed people, of course, have no other choice. Taking out personal and family medical insurance has certain advantages—the type and amount of coverage can be tailored to individual needs. However, the more extensive the coverage desired, the more expensive the premiums will be. Nonetheless, every individual should try to have some sort of medical insurance.

Where the role of medical insurance will change and if it will exist under the present structure is not known, because the Clinton administration has yet to restructure the health care system. It does seem that the present system will be changed or at least modified over the next few years.

Health Maintenance Organizations

As the debate about national health insurance continues, other attempts to provide better, more economical health care have been made. One promising approach is the health maintenance organization (HMO). These private health care centers provide prepaid group programs that offer a full range of medical services. Good HMOs emphasize preventive medicine. They are trying to keep their patients well, rather than using the crisis-oriented approach of most physicians. The philosophy behind the HMO approach is that it is cheaper to keep people well than to treat them after they become ill. Several advantages and disadvantages are characteristic of this form of care, as in all forms of medical care. Many HMOs have suffered from poor financial management, and this approach to health care still needs refinement.

Government Health Insurance

Two examples of government insurance plans are Medicare and Medicaid. Medicare is financed by Social Security taxes and is designed to provide health insurance for people sixty-five years and older, the blind, severely disabled, and those requiring specialized treatments such as kidney dialysis. Medicaid is underwritten by federal and state taxes. It provides limited health benefits for people who are eligible for assistance from two programs: Aid to Families with Dependent Children (AFDC) and Supplementary Security Income (SSI).

When to Seek Health Care

Sometimes it is difficult to determine when to seek health care attention. Some people tend to wait too long before seeking health care, while others may seek help unnecessarily. For many, the ability to tolerate discomfort determines whether they seek help or not. Health care decisions are largely personal and based on the perceived severity of the symptoms. Being in tune with one's body and having knowledge of the signs and symptoms of illness can help someone make the decision to seek or wait to get medical attention.

Several symptoms indicate the need for medical attention. Blood present in urine, feces, vomit, or sputum, or other body orifice all indicate need for medical advice. Pain in the abdomen, especially when accompanied by nausea, may indicate a wide range of conditions, ranging from appendicitis to pelvic inflammatory disease—all of which need a physician's attention. A stiff neck accompanied by fever may indicate meningitis. And obviously, any disabling injury requires prompt medical assistance (Anspaugh, Hamrick, and Rosato 1994, 272).

Presence of fever is another area of concern when someone is deciding to seek medical care. A fever is an indication that the immune system is working to fight an infection. If left untreated, a fever may damage various body organs and structures. Self-treatment in the form of aspirin, acetaminophen, or ibuprofen usually lowers temperature. However, if there is no improvement in 24–36 hours or a low-grade temperature continues over a period of time, a physician should be consulted. Fever in children should always be discussed with a physician.

Selecting a Health Care Professional

Nearly everyone should have a primary-care physician. If a medical emergency arises, a person can seek help immediately from a trusted health care professional who knows the patient's history. Just as important, by having a personal physician or other health care professional, a person can better maintain good health by means of regular checkups or consultations with the provider about health concerns. A health care professional should be selected carefully. Some suggestions are listed here (Hamrick, Anspaugh, and Ezell 1986, 39, 40, 53):

1. Choose your physician while you are in good health. If you wait until a medical crisis arises, you will have to rely on whomever you can find. Having a physician you trust and feel comfortable with *before* a crisis will lessen anxiety in a crisis.

2. To locate physicians who are accepting new patients, telephone the local county medical society. You can find the number in the telephone book yellow pages. If you are not sure what kind of physician you need, such as a specialist or a general practitioner, the medical society can also offer some initial advice. Generally you will be given the names of two or three physicians you can call. A local hospital can also be a good source of information about physicians who are accepting new patients.

3. Select a board-certified family practitioner for a family physician, a pediatrician for children, and a gynecologist for females (see the Health Highlight for other types of specialists).

4. Check the credentials of physicians you are considering. Don't be afraid to ask questions about how the person is keeping current in the field.

5. Get details about office hours, emergency care, whether house calls will be made, and so forth. Also try to determine how long a patient usually has to wait before seeing the doctor.

6. Determine the fee schedule for checkups and different types of treatment. Doctors often base their fees on recommended prices recorded in a fee schedule book produced by the American Medical Association. The fees are recommended ranges, not fixed prices, and a physician may charge on the high or low end. Keep in mind that the most expensive physician is not necessarily the best.

7. Choose a physician who is able to communicate with you in terms you can understand. You have a right to know what is going on during any treatment, and the doctor has an obligation to keep you informed. Regardless of their medical skills, however, some physicians are better communicators than others.

8. Choose a physician you feel comfortable with. The doctor's age, sex, and personal manner may all be factors that make you more comfortable or less comfortable. Set up an appointment to talk with the professional to see whether he or she is willing to communicate openly and honestly.

9. Choose a physician you can have confidence in. Even if the person is highly qualified and well thought of in the profession, you may be put off by some personal quality.

10. Don't be afraid to change physicians if you are not satisfied with the way you are being treated. Find a doctor with whom you feel comfortable.

Ask questions! The more questions, the fewer mistakes and the more power patients have in the doctor–patient relationship (Devita 1995).

Choosing a Health Care Facility

If given a choice, few people would select the use of a health facility such as an emergency room or hospital. Unfortunately, most people will need the services of these facilities at times throughout their life. Consequently, knowing what to consider when choosing a health care facility should be weighed long before it is needed.

Emergency rooms should be used only in an absolute emergency. Most ERs are understaffed, overcrowded, and harried. In addition, if the personnel view a particular situation as less serious, long waits can be usual. Tests that may be needed are more difficult to arrange, and the cost for ER care is higher than those of a visit to a physician's office.

When there is time to select a hospital, it is wise to discuss with your physician the options that are available. Many times, physicians hold admitting privileges at more than one hospital. Every attempt should be made to find out as much as possible about the hospital. Some possible questions to consider include

1. Why does your physician use this hospital?

2. What is the patient-to-nurse ratio?

3. What are the room rates?

4. What are the costs of laboratory services, X rays, and so on?

Health Highlight

Health Care Specialists

Name of Specialist	Field of Specialty
Medical Specialists	
Allergist	Allergic conditions
Anesthesiologist	Administration of anesthesia (for example, surgery)
Cardiologist	Coronary artery disease; heart disease
Dermatologist	Skin conditions
Endocrinologist	Diseases of the endocrine system
Epidemiologist	Investigates the cause and source of disease outbreaks
Family practice physician	General care physician
Gastroenterologist	Stomach, intestines, digestive system
Geriatrician	Diseases and conditions of the aged
Gynecologist	Female reproductive system
Hematologist	Study of blood
Immunologist	Diseases of the immune system
Internist	Treatment of diseases in adults
Neonatologist	Newborn infants
Nephrologist	Kidney disease
Neurologist	Nervous system
Neurosurgeon	Surgery of the brain and nervous system
Obstetrician	Pregnancy, labor, childbirth
Oncologist	Cancer, tumors
Ophthalmologist	Eyes
Orthopedist	Skeletal system
Otolaryngologist	Head, neck, ears, nose, throat
Otologist	Ears
Pathologist	Study of tissues and the essential nature of disease
Pediatrician	Childhood diseases and conditions
Plastic surgeon	Use of material to rebuild tissues
Primary-care physician	General health and medical care
Proctologist	Disorders of the rectum and anus
Psychiatrist	Mental illnesses
Radiologist	Use of X rays
Rheumatologist	Diseases of connective tissues, joints, muscles, tendons, and so on
Rhinologist	Nose
Surgeon	Treats diseases by surgery
Urologist	Urinary tract of males and females and reproductive organs of males

Health Highlight-cont'd

Dental Specialists

Dentist	General care of teeth and oral cavity
Endodontist	Diseases of tooth below gum line (performs root canal therapy)
Orthodontist	Teeth alignment, malocclusion
Pedodontist	Dental care of children
Periodontist	Diseases of supporting structures
Prosthodontist	Construction of artificial appliances for the mouth

Other Specialists

Chiropractor	Emphasizes the use of manipulation and adjustment of body structures to treat disease
Naturopathic physician	Emphasizes lifestyle and dietary therapies in the prevention and treatment of disease
Optometrist	Examines and tests eyes for visual defects
Osteopath	Emphasis on structural integrity of the body; uses manipulation along with medical therapies
Podiatrist	Care and treatment of the foot
Psychologist	Study of human behavior

5. How frequently does the hospital perform the procedure you require?
6. Have there been or are there now any malpractice charges against the hospital?
7. Can you tour the hospital?
8. Be familiar with your rights as a patient (See Health Highlight "Your Medical Rights").

Choosing a hospital is serious business. Don't be afraid to ask questions, your life may depend on it.

Health-Related Products

Americans spend billions of dollars each year on health care products ranging from over-the-counter drugs to cosmetics. Many of these products are used to help relieve symptoms, aid in curing illnesses, and provide cosmetic effects. Unfortunately many products are not needed, don't provide the advertised effect, and may have the potential to harm health.

Over-the-Counter (OTC) Drugs

There are more than half a million OTC health care products. These vary widely from mouthwashes to pain relievers. In fact, some of the most beneficial OTC drugs can also create problems. For example, pain relievers such as aspirin and ibuprofen (a nonsteroid anti-inflammatory drug) can damage the lining of the stomach, which can lead to ulcers, among other problems. Large

Health Highlight

Your Medical Rights

As a patient in the health care system, you have the right

1. As a parent, to stay with your children during tests and treatments, provided you don't interfere with medical treatment or are not suspected of child abuse.

2. To request that a relative or friend accompany you during a test or treatment or hospitalization, unless you are in a semiprivate room.

3. To see your medical records and to copy certain parts of your record. Not all states currently allow the patient to do this. Check the laws of your individual state.

4. To emergency care, whether you have insurance or not.

5. To refuse to sign any form. The health care provider can also refuse to provide treatment without your authorization.

6. To a second opinion—but your doctor can also stop treating you for challenging him or her.

7. To leave the hospital at any time, even against medical advice or without paying the bill.

8. To refuse or stop any treatment, whether or not it's experimental.

9. To an itemized, detailed bill for all medical services.

10. To know the results of all tests unless the doctor has reason to believe that the information will be harmful (for example, a depressed patient might become suicidal on hearing the information).

dosages have been associated with kidney damage. Another pain reliever, acetaminophen, also relieves pain and reduces fever. This is the drug of choice for relieving pain in children. However with heavy doses the drug can cause bleeding and liver damage. All the above-mentioned pain relievers should be taken with a full glass of water to reduce irritation to the lining of the stomach.

Two other frequently used OTC products also provide good examples of potentially hazardous use. Nasal sprays relieve congestion by shrinking the blood vessels in the nose. If used for too long, more and more spray is required to maintain effectiveness and the vessels begin to swell, actually making the congestion worse. This is called the rebound effect. Furthermore, prolonged use can result in bleeding and partial or complete loss of the sense of smell. Another product that holds potential misuse problems is laxatives. Many people, especially the elderly, consider a daily bowel movement necessary. Chronic use of laxatives destroys much of the flora in the intestinal tract, making constipation even worse. Bulk laxatives are better, but exercise and a high-fiber diet are much safer alternatives for promoting normal defecation.

Cosmetic Products

Many health care products are intended to be used externally. Some of these have little effect but, due to massive advertising campaigns and misconceptions about their effectiveness, are extensively used. These products include the following:

Skin Products. Some products are designed to prevent or cure acne, rejuvenate skin, prevent body odor, or protect against excessive sunlight. Acne products, in conjunction with washing the face with a mild soap, may help control the condition. Over-the-counter skin rejuvenators have never been shown to be effective at actually changing skin properties, regardless of the claims that are made! A moisturizer can help with the dry skin associated with aging, although it does not actually change the skin. Retin A, a prescription drug, does seem to help delay skin deterioration and restore a more youthful appearance for those individuals who can use it. Retin A irritates the skin and may result in peeling, blotching, or other undesirable side effects. Deodorants and antiperspirants can help control body odor but no product can prevent sweating in extremely hot weather or during exercise (nor is this desirable because sweating is the body's primary means of cooling itself). Regular washing is essential if the bacteria and other odor-causing substances are to be removed.

Hair Products. Hair products run the gamut from removing hair to restoring, cleaning, and coloring the hair. There are several products designed to remove hair. Shaving can be used in almost all circumstances and is a safe method of hair removal except for the risk of cutting oneself. Tweezers can be used to pluck unwanted hair but present some danger of infection because the adjacent skin may not be clean. Chemicals can be used to soften and remove hair at the root; wax can be warmed and used to tear hair from the roots as it hardens on the skin; and a fine pumice stone can be used to prevent hair from growing above the skin. Although these products are usually safe, if sometimes painful, there is always the possibility of skin reactions, irritations, and infections. A dermatologist should be consulted if any symptoms appear.

Most hair-restoring products do not work. Most products advertised in the media have not been proven to be effective. A drug invented by the Upjohn Company called Minoxidil (Rogaine) does seem to grow limited amounts of hair in some people. Rogaine can now be purchased over-the-counter, however, it has never been shown to totally restore hair (Folkenberg 1989, 11). Surgery can replace hair loss but it is extremely expensive, painful, and may take a year or two to complete. Certainly before considering surgery, the person should gather multiple medical opinions.

Products used to clean the hair are generally safe. There are a wide variety available, and personal preference is usually the primary criteria for selecting a particular product. Some people may have allergic reactions to hair products, but this tends to be atypical. Most people consider dandruff a hair problem, but it is actually a scalp problem. The scalp tends to slough off dead skin cells, or dandruff. If hair is washed daily, dandruff is not usually a problem, so it is unnecessary to purchase a special hair product to help fight dandruff—any hair-cleaning product will serve to remove the flakes. People with a severe problem may wish to use an antidandruff shampoo, however. The FDA considers antidandruff shampoos to be a drug. These products can help control dandruff but they cannot cure it. Dandruff may represent a social or psychological problem but usually poses no medical or health threat unless it is a symptom of psoriasis, seborrhea, or dermatitis, which require a physician's attention.

Hair-coloring products should be used with caution since many of these products can cause skin irritation or harm the eyes with direct contact. These products are used for cosmetic reasons only. Consequently, care should be used by testing the product on a small area of the hair prior to covering all the hair with the product.

Mouth Products. Mouth products include toothpaste, mouthwashes, and gargles. There are many toothpaste products that, when used with dental flossing, serve to protect against tooth decay. Living in an area where the water supply contains fluoride also helps prevent dental cavi-

OTC products must be checked carefully.

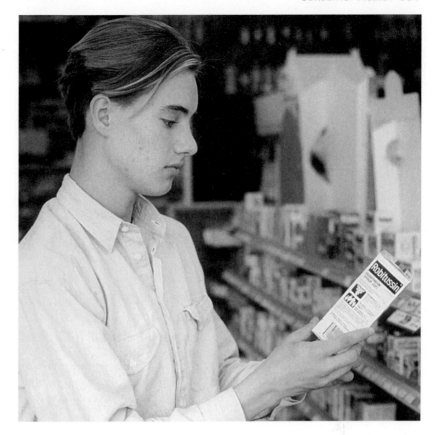

ties. A toothpaste with fluoride should be used. It is unwise to purchase a toothpaste with whiteners since they contain abrasives that damage the teeth.

Mouth washes and gargles do little to eliminate unpleasant odors or treat a sore throat. Since unpleasant odors do not develop in the mouth but are carried from the intestines to the lungs and expired, these products can only mask smells. Bad breath also may be a symptom of other conditions such as infections, tumors, or diabetes (Cornacchia and Barrett 1993). Mouthwash can only mask these odors. In fact, excessive use can actually dry the mucous membranes, making a sore throat even more irritated.

Consumer Rights and Protection

One of the basic premises of wellness or high-level health is that individuals should be responsible for their own health behavior. This is certainly true for consumer health. With so much competition for every dollar spent, and with so much available to buy, consumers need to guard against wasteful spending on products and services of dubious value. For the most part, consumers do not protect themselves properly through informed consumer health behavior. Fortunately, government agencies and private organizations have stepped in to establish consumer rights and offer some protection. On 15 March 1962, President John Kennedy sent to Congress his "Special Message on Protecting the Consumer Interest" (Cornacchia and Barrett 1993). The message stated that additional legislative and administrative actions were required to assist consumers in the exercise of their rights. Kennedy outlined these rights:

○ *right to safety:* to be protected against the marketing of goods that are hazardous to health or life

○ *right to be informed:* to be protected against fraudulent, deceitful, or misleading information or advertising

○ *right to choose:* to be assured that consumer interests will receive full and sympathetic consideration in the formulation of government policy on consumer matters

In 1970 and 1971, Mary Gardiner Jones of the Federal Trade Commission and consumer activist Ralph Nader further extended the definitions of consumer rights to include these rights:

○ the right to expect quality of design, workmanship, and ingredients in products and services

○ the right to be charged fair prices

○ the right to receive courteous and respectful treatment from firms

○ the right to expect consumer products and services whose use by the consuming public is consistent with the values of a humane society

○ the right to redress of legitimate grievances related to purchased products and services

These consumer rights, of course, are meaningless unless they are backed up with the power of legislation. Over the years, hundreds of federal, state, and local laws have been passed to ensure the rights of consumers and to protect consumers from fraudulent or harmful products and services.

Consumer Protection Agencies

Many federal agencies work to protect the consumer. One of the most active of these agencies is the Food and Drug Administration (FDA). Responsibilities of the FDA include periodic inspection of foods, drugs, devices, and cosmetics. The agency demands proof of the safety and effectiveness of any new drug before it is marketed and has the power to recall possibly unsafe drugs or other substances from the market. The FDA also enforces the law against illegal sales of prescription drugs, investigates therapeutic devices for safety and truthfulness of labeling claims, and checks importation of foods, drugs, devices, and cosmetics to ensure that they comply with U.S. laws.

Another government agency, the Federal Trade Commission (FTC), is responsible for eliminating unfair or deceptive practices in commerce that curtail competition. In other words, this agency prevents the free enterprise system from being suppressed by a company creating a monopoly on a product or service, or by fraudulent trade techniques. The FTC has the authority to stop the dissemination of advertisements of foods, drugs, devices, or cosmetics when such action is in the best interest of the consumer. Also, if a label on a product is misleading, the FTC can order the withdrawal of that product from the shelves.

The Consumer Product Safety Commission, established by the federal government in 1973, protects the public against unreasonable risks of injury from products. This commission oversees the enforcement of the Flammable Fabrics Act, the Federal Hazardous Substances Act, and the

Poison Prevention Packaging Act, among many others. Under these acts, the Consumer Product Safety Commission is responsible for regulating the manufacture for sale of all highly flammable wearing apparel and fabrics. This is especially helpful for the consumer, because the majority of fabrics used in today's clothing burn quite easily.

In January 1964, President Lyndon Johnson established the President's Committee on Consumer Interests. This committee was replaced by the Office of Consumer Affairs in 1971. The main purpose of this office is to act as a consumer voice in the presidential administration. This organization also coordinates all governmental activities in the field of consumerism; conducts investigations on consumer problems; handles consumer complaints; facilitates communication on consumer affairs between the government, business, and the consumer; and helps disseminate helpful information to the consumer.

Various department-level organizations within the federal government also aid the consumer. The U.S. Department of Commerce encourages industry to avoid packaging proliferation that can lead to consumer confusion in shopping. This department can request mandatory packaging standards. The organization also provides statistics on population, gross national product, corporate profits, personal income, retail sales, balance of payments, manufacturing, and housing—all of which help the government and consumer understand the present status of the nation's economy. The Department of Labor provides the consumer price index (CPI), the measure of changes in the nation's economy and currency. This agency also surveys employment trends and studies prices of various commodities. The Department of Agriculture (USDA) inspects meat and food animals before slaughter to prevent any diseased meat from reaching the stores. The USDA establishes grades to meat to help the consumer in identifying the different levels of quality. The U.S. Postal Service investigates any incidence of mail fraud and regulates attempts to sell worthless or harmful merchandise or medicines through the mails.

Private Agencies

Many private agencies also assist the consumer by providing accurate, unbiased information about products or by attempting to eliminate fraud and deception by businesses. For example, Consumer's Union publishes *Consumer Reports*, a magazine that provides impartial information about products. This publication informs the consumer about the best buys and the most reliable products. *Consumer Reports* also helps the consumer by interpreting advertising on many products.

Better Business Bureaus are private, nonprofit, business-supported groups that help the consumer mediate misunderstandings between customers and businesses. These groups provide information about a company, help resolve complaints against companies, foster ethical advertising and selling practices, alert consumers to bad business practices, and provide the media with informational materials on consumer subjects. Better Business Bureaus have no legal powers, but they can arbitrate between consumer and business. When illegal practices are discovered and a business refuses to cooperate, the matter is turned over to the appropriate law enforcement agency. These bureaus are one of the more important sources of help to which consumers may turn when they need assistance, especially in regard to health products and devices (Cornacchia and Barrett 1993).

Many cities have chambers of commerce that are supported by businesses in that community. These organizations publish a business consumer relations code of ethics. Their work is quite similar to a Better Business Bureau in that they act as liaisons between the consumer and business. They also protect the consumer by attempting to eliminate fraudulent business practices.

Health Highlight

Newsletters: Reliable Health-Related Information

Newsletter	Address
Consumer Reports Health Letter	Consumers Union 256 Washington Street Mount Vernon, NY 10533
Environmental Nutrition	52 Riverside Drive New York, NY 10024-6599
Harvard Health Letter	P. O. Box 420333 Palm Coast, FL 32142-0300
Mayo Clinic Health Letter	P. O. Box 53889 Boulder, CO 80322-0300
Nutrition Action Healthletter	Center for Science in the Public Interest Suite 300 1875 Connecticut Avenue NW Washington DC 20009-5728
Tufts University Diet and Nutrition Letter	P. O. Box 57857 Boulder, CO 80322-7857
University of California, Berkeley Wellness Letter	Health Letter Associates P. O. Box 412 Prince Street Station New York, NY 10012-0007

Even with all these government and private agencies working to protect the consumer, however, it remains the individual's responsibility to be informed about products and services in order to increase the probability of satisfaction when purchasing a product.

Teaching Consumer Health Education

Consumer health education teaches consumers (children) to learn to make wise decisions about buying and using products and services, especially in health-related areas (Corry and Galli 1985). Children need to become knowledgeable about consumer rights and consumer responsibilities. They (like their adult counterparts) have rights as outlined earlier in the chapter, but rights are balanced with responsibilities. These responsibilities include seeking out accurate information about products and services, being skeptical of advertising claims, recognizing the differences between needs and desires, and making wise consumer choices. This process must begin early in life and be fostered throughout the elementary school years. Even though the information presented in this chapter may seem more appropriate for adults the concepts that lead to becoming an effective consumer as an adult are instilled in each child early in life.

The most effective way that all consumers, regardless of age, can protect themselves in the area of consumer health is through preventive health care. By learning about proper nutrition, exercise, and health care, students can avoid the need for many consumer health products such as tonics, diet products, or some other worthless health product or service.

The importance of critical thinking cannot be overemphasized when it comes to teaching consumer health education. Children must recognize that just because a product is advertised on television or in a newspaper it is not necessarily worthwhile or useful. They should learn to see how wants can be fostered artificially. In addition, they should learn not to accept advertising claims or promises without thinking. Children need to conceptualize that much of what is said in a commercial is meaningless. For example, a product may be touted as "new" or "improved." Is "new" necessarily better? "Improved" in what way? If a product is advertised as being "25 percent more effective," students should ask, "More effective than what?" Generally, no answer to these questions can be found.

The intent of consumer education is not to teach children what to buy, but rather how to buy. Students should be encouraged to get the facts, comparison-shop, consider the consequences of all purchases, and budget their money the same as any wise adult would do. By learning the importance of wise consumer behavior, children can incorporate the concepts taught into their own value system. Finally, children should be informed of their rights as consumers and what recourse they have if they are victimized in the marketplace. All consumers have legal rights. Exercising these rights can help put an end to shoddy and deceitful health care practices and services as well as worthless health care products.

▤ *Summary*

○ A consumer is anyone who selects and uses goods and services.

○ Consumer health education is concerned with those products that directly or indirectly affect personal health.

○ Consumers become aware of available products primarily through advertising.

○ Advertising seeks to manipulate consumer psychology and behavior by confusing wants with needs and by fostering desires.

○ Many advertisements for health products seek to give the impression that the products are more effective than they actually are.

○ Consumers are persuaded to buy a product because of a variety of appeals.

○ Quackery is widespread in the United States despite legal measures designed to prevent it.

○ Resorting to a quack can prevent a person from getting proper or even life-saving treatment.

○ Many people today either are not insured or are underinsured.

○ Private insurance companies, HMOs, and governmental plans help meet needs and reduce costs, but do not fill the needs of all citizens.

○ A physician and health care facility must be selected with care.

○ Private and government agencies help protect consumer rights, evaluate the quality and effectiveness of health-related products, and police business practices.

○ The primary responsibility of each consumer is to become knowledgeable when making health-related consumer decisions.

❍ Helping children to learn to become informed, wise consumers is a vital part of teaching consumer education.

Discussion Questions

1. How does advertising manipulate consumer psychology and behavior?

2. Discuss the most typical advertising approaches.

3. Describe the influences, other than advertising, that affect consumer behavior.

4. List and discuss some common health-related consumer myths.

5. Discuss the teacher's role in combatting consumer misconceptions.

6. Discuss the role of Better Business Bureaus in protecting consumers' rights.

7. What are some considerations that should be made when selecting a physician?

8. What are some of the agencies that help protect the health consumer?

References

Anspaugh, D. J., M. Hamrick, and F. D. Rosato. 1994. *Concepts and applications of wellness*. St. Louis: Times Mirror/Mosby.

Cornacchia, H., and S. Barrett. 1993. *Consumer health: A guide to intelligent decisions*, 5th ed. St. Louis: Mosby-Yearbook.

Corry, J. 1983. *Consumer health: Facts, skills, and decisions*. Belmont, CA: Wadsworth.

Corry, J., and N. Galli. 1985. The role of the school in consumer health education. *Journal of school health* 55:4.

Devita, E. 1995. The decline of the doctor–patient relationship. *American health* 13(7): 63–65, 105.

Folkenberg, J. 1989. Hair apparent? For some, a new solution to baldness. *FDA consumer* 22:10.

Greenberg, J. S., and G. B. Dintiman. 1992. *Exploring health—Expanding the boundaries of wellness*. Englewood Cliffs, NJ: Prentice Hall.

Hamilton, P. 1982. *Health care consumerism*. St. Louis: Mosby.

Hamrick, M., D. Anspaugh, and G. Ezell. 1986. *Health*. Columbus, OH: Merrill.

Olsen, L., K. Redican, and C. Baffi. 1986. *Health today*, 2nd ed. New York: Macmillan.

Payne, W. A., and D. B. Hahn. 1991. *Understanding your health*, 2nd ed. St. Louis: Times Mirror/Mosby.

Price, J., N. Galli, and S. Slenker. 1985. *Consumer health: Contemporary issues and choices*. Dubuque, IA: Brown.

Quackery: A brief manual. 1984, October. *Harvard Medical School health letter* 9:12, 1–2.

Sagan, C. 1987, February 1. The fine art of baloney detection. *Parade magazine*, pp. 12–13.

Vincenzino, J. V. 1994. Developments in health care costs—an update. *Statistical bulletin* 75(1): 30–35.

Chapter Twenty-One
Strategies for Teaching Consumer Health

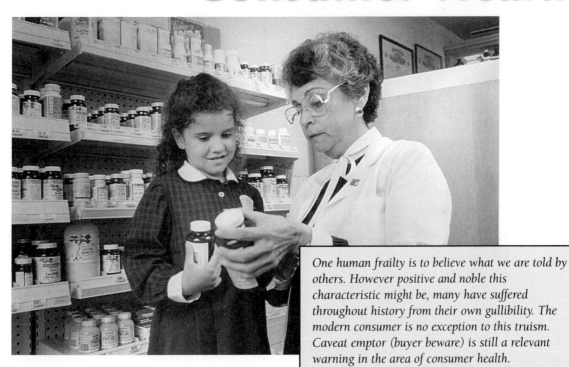

One human frailty is to believe what we are told by others. However positive and noble this characteristic might be, many have suffered throughout history from their own gullibility. The modern consumer is no exception to this truism. Caveat emptor (buyer beware) is still a relevant warning in the area of consumer health.
—*Warren E. Schaller and Charles R. Carroll, 1976*

Valued Outcomes

After having done the following activities, the student should be able to explain and illustrate the following statements:

○ Health products and services should be used only when needed.

○ It is important to obtain accurate information concerning health care products and services.

○ Not all products and services are worthwhile or necessary.

○ Advertising seeks to persuade rather than to inform.

○ Many advertising claims are inflated or misleading.

○ One's family, friends, and peers influence choice of products and services.

○ Labels on all health care products should be read carefully, and the directions should be followed closely.

○ The existence of widespread quackery in health products and services must be recognized.

○ There are many ways to spot quack products and services.

○ Quack products and services are useless or dangerous.

○ Medical attention should be obtained only from qualified and recognized professionals.

○ Many government and private agencies work to protect the consumer.

○ Federal, state, and local laws enforce the rights of the consumer.

○ The best way to make wise consumer decisions is to become informed about the facts concerning products and services. Making wise consumer decisions is ultimately a personal responsibility.

Establishing Consumer Behavior Patterns

The patterns established in childhood of appraising, selecting, and using consumer products and services can influence an individual's physical, psychological, and social well-being for a lifetime. To choose wisely requires accumulating knowledge and formulating attitudes about different kinds of products and services. Children must learn that products and services differ in quality, worth, and intrinsic value. They must also recognize how advertising and social forces influence ideas about needs and desires. Above all, they must understand that the responsibility for making wise consumer decisions ultimately is a personal one.

Consumer health pertains to products and services that either directly or indirectly relate to personal health. Broadly speaking, almost any product or service purchased can in some way be health related. For example, choice of foods has a bearing on nutrition. Choice of clothing relates not only to physical needs but also to psychological expression of personality. Choice of discretionary purchases, ranging from toys to jewelry to stereo equipment, affects income available for necessities.

Health Highlight

A Thought on Generic Drugs

Substantial savings to consumers can be obtained through the use of generic drugs. Generic drug sales have increased dramatically since 1984 when Congress passed the Drug Price Competition and Patent Term Restoration Act. The Food and Drug Administration issues guidelines to ensure that generic drugs retain the same quality and potency as brand-name drugs. Almost 80 percent of generic drugs are produced by brand-name firms in their manufacturing plants. The FDA's Office of Generic Drugs conducts reviews and approves generic drugs for marketing.

What does this suggest to you concerning generic drug use?

Most directly health-related products and services include OTC drugs, cosmetics, and medical and dental treatment.

In this chapter, both the rights and the responsibilities of the consumer are emphasized. A variety of suggestions for learning activities will assist you in helping children establish responsible consumer behavior patterns.

Value-Based Activities

Valued-based activities are designed to assist children in developing their critical thinking skills, personalize information, and establish those concepts that are conducive to high-quality wellness. Teachers can design a variety of activities that are value based, depending on the content being discussed. Some suggestions follow.

Why Do I Buy?

Valued Outcome: The students will be able to identify reasons they purchase various products.
Description of Strategy: Have each student think of a product that he or she buys from time to time. It can be any sort of product, not necessarily a health-related one. Ask the students the following questions. Have the students explain and discuss the answers they give. How do they relate their decisions to their values?

1. How does advertising convince consumers to buy a product?
2. If your friends use a certain product, would you use it also?
3. Does cost affect what you buy?
4. If you didn't like a product, but it was the only kind available, would you buy it?
5. If you had your choice of two products, one in a bright colorful box and one in a plain box, which would you buy?
6. Would you buy a product because your family likes it?
7. Does the quality of a product matter?
8. Would you try several brands to find one you like?
9. Do you tell other people about products you like/buy?
10. What kind of products would you buy because of an associated name; in other words, because of who wears them or whom they represent?

Assessing Attitudes

Valued Outcome: The students will be able to analyze why they purchase products.
Description of Strategy: Copy and pass out the following list of statements, and have students assess their own attitudes about each one. By doing so, the children will become more aware of why they make choices.

	Agree	Disagree	Not Sure
1. Most television commercials give accurate information about the product advertised.	____	____	____

	Agree	Disagree	Not Sure
2. If my friends have a certain product, I usually want to buy that product, too.	_____	_____	_____
3. I only buy products that I need.	_____	_____	_____
4. Advertisers must tell the truth.	_____	_____	_____
5. Only products and services that are useful are sold.	_____	_____	_____
6. I sometimes buy things that I don't need.	_____	_____	_____
7. There is not much point to saving money.	_____	_____	_____
8. Sometimes I buy things without knowing very much about how good they are.	_____	_____	_____
9. Health care products are always safe to use.	_____	_____	_____
10. The products I buy for myself can affect my health.	_____	_____	_____

Processing Questions:

1. What seems to be most important in determining why you buy a product?
2. Are there products you buy that perhaps you could do without?
3. Are any of the products you buy potentially harmful to you?
4. Do all the products you buy seem to be as good as you had thought they would be?

Budget Diary

Valued Outcome: The students will develop insight into the reasons they purchase products. *Description of Strategy:* Have each student keep a notebook diary of all purchases made for a week or longer. Every purchase made should be recorded in the diary, along with the reasons for that purchase. Money spent on food, snacks, toys, video games, school supplies, transportation, books and magazines, pet supplies, hobbies, and health care products should all be recorded. Explain to the class that the amount of money each student spends is not as relevant as how the money is spent. After the diaries have been completed for the assigned time period, have each student analyze his or her purchases and answer these questions:
Processing Questions:

1. What items did you buy that brought you a great amount of pleasure?
2. What items did you buy that disappointed you?
3. Do you think that you spent any money unwisely? Why?
4. Does this diary suggest ways that you could budget your spending money better? How?
5. What does this diary tell you about your consumer habits? Are there patterns in the way you spend your money?

Answers to these questions should be written out so that students can clarify their thoughts better and come to personal conclusions about their patterns of consumer behavior. On a volunteer basis, have students explain to the class what they learned from this activity. Follow with a general discussion.

I'm a Wise Consumer Because . . .

Valued Outcome: The students will be able to identify their positive purchasing habits.
Description of Strategy: Ask each student to complete the statement "I'm a wise consumer because . . ." in twenty-five words or less. Each written answer should be based on actual behavior or attitudes. Discuss each student's response in a general class discussion. Ask students to explain what values their statements are based on.
Processing Questions:

1. Were you able to identify reasons why you are a good consumer?
2. What makes you a wise consumer?
3. What do you consider before buying a product?

Health Fact or Fiction

Valued Outcome: The students will be able to identify factual health related information.
Description of Strategy: Give each student a set of the following questions, and ask him or her place a checkmark in the blank under the appropriate answer.

	Agree	Disagree	Not Sure
1. Raw eggs are more nutritious than cooked eggs.	____	____	____
2. Eating an egg a day is harmful.	____	____	____
3. Fish and celery are brain foods.	____	____	____
4. Frozen orange juice is less nutritious than fresh.	____	____	____
5. All fruits and vegetables should be eaten raw.	____	____	____
6. It is dangerous to leave food in a can that has been opened.	____	____	____
7. Drinking too much water will make you retain fluid.	____	____	____
8. Drinking ice water causes heart trouble.	____	____	____
9. If one vitamin pill a day is good, two are better.	____	____	____
10. Meat is fattening.	____	____	____
11. Toast has fewer calories than bread.	____	____	____
12. Special diets help people with arthritis.	____	____	____
13. Acupuncture is a reliable method of treating illness.	____	____	____
14. Cooking with an iron skillet increases the amount of iron in the food cooked.	____	____	____
15. Cooking with aluminum pots and pans may increase the likelihood of getting Alzheimer's disease.	____	____	____

Processing Questions:

1. What are some additional statements you have heard concerning health fact/fiction?
2. Why does misinformation begin concerning health?

Decision Stories

Follow the procedures outlined in Chapter 4 for presenting decision stories such as these.

Broken Promises

Ricardo saw a model car advertised on television. It looked like a fun toy. He saved up his money and bought the model. But when he opened the package, the car didn't look as well made as it did on television. He started playing with it and the car broke. He was angry and disappointed. He felt like throwing the car away, but it had cost a lot of money.
Focus Question: Was it Ricardo's fault that the car broke?

Vitamins for Vera?

In her health class, Vera has been learning about the importance of vitamins for good health and growth. She wonders if she is getting enough vitamins, because sometimes she feels tired and worn out. One day, Vera's mother asks her to go to the grocery store to buy some milk. While at the store, Vera sees a shelf with many different kinds of vitamin pills on it. She has some money of her own with her. Maybe she should buy some vitamins. Then she might feel in better health.
Focus Question: What should Vera do?

Munch or Lunch

Mike likes to play video games. He spends a lot of his money playing Munchman, his favorite video game. He is getting better and better at it, but playing Munchman often leaves him without any money for other things. His parents give him lunch money every day. Up to now, he hasn't spent this money on anything except lunch. But maybe he could cut a few corners. Maybe he could buy less for lunch and use the rest of the money to play video games.
Focus Question: What should Mike do?

Music, Music, Music

Marsha likes music. She spends a lot of her money buying records and tapes. One day, Marsha sees an advertisement for a tape club in a magazine. For only $10 she can buy any three of her favorite albums on tape through the mail. Marsha sends off a money order, and in a few weeks her three selections arrive. She is very pleased. The tapes are great, and for $10 they are a real bargain. However, the next month three more tapes arrive in the mail, but Marsha didn't order them. Still, there is a bill along with the tapes. The bill is for $25.
Focus Questions:

1. Does Marsha have to pay for the new tapes?

2. How can she find out about her consumer rights in this matter?

Shampoo of the Stars

Valerie's friends have been telling her about a new shampoo called Hairdoyoudo. They say that it makes their hair feel soft and pretty. Valerie has also seen the product advertised on television. A famous young model says that she uses it. The model has beautiful hair. Valerie would like to use

Wise consumers read labels carefully and compare various brands before making purchases.

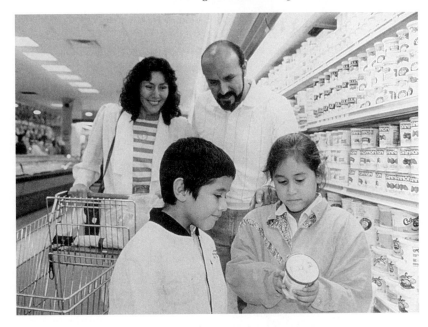

Hairdoyoudo, too, but her mother buys another brand of shampoo. It costs much less than Hairdoyoudo and seems to work fine. Valerie asks her mother to buy Hairdoyoudo, but she refuses. She says it is overpriced. Valerie is very put out. She wants her hair to look as nice as her friends' hair. But how can that be if she has to use another shampoo?
Focus Question: What should Valerie do?

Spots and Shaun

Shaun has acne. He is very embarrassed about his spots and blemishes. One day he sees an advertisement for a new acne medication in a magazine. The advertisement promises a "miracle cure." It says that the product will cure acne in thirty days. The product has a money-back guarantee, but it can only be purchased by mail. The advertisement also says that the product has a secret ingredient that no other product has. It sounds like just what Shaun has been looking for, even if the product does cost $12.95 a tube.
Focus Question: Should Shaun send off for the product?

Other Teaching Strategies

The Home Medicine Cabinet

Valued Outcome: The students will be able to discuss the types of medicines and drugs they have in their homes and the purposes of each.
Description of Strategy: Assign the students the task of investigating their own medicine cabinets. A list can be made of all medicines, their cost, their purpose, and the effectiveness as

ascertained by the user. Also to be listed and then discarded are medicines that have expired. These lists can be compared in class to learn the average number and kinds of medicines and the total amount of medicine in the normal medicine cabinet that needs discarding. Provide for the students copies of a chart on 11- x 14-inch paper with the headings "Medicine or Product," "Cost," "Purpose," and "Expiration Date."

Materials Needed: chart listing the headings just described
Processing Questions:

1. What type of medicine or product is found most often in your medicine cabinet?

2. What do these products do?

Scrambled-Up Health

Valued Outcome: The students will learn discretion when using health products or services.
Description of Strategy: Through various media, people are constantly being bombarded with ads about goods and services that supposedly improve health or appearance. The following items have some scrambled words that name some items that should be considered with caution and discretion. Unscramble the words and write them in the blanks (see following example).

Beware of . . .

1. Religious faith _____. (rsleahe)

2. Advertisements where the only "evidence" is _____ of other people. (nistmstoeie)

3. So-called doctors whose only degrees are from unaccredited or nonexistent _____. (tnisotsituin)

4. Products that miraculously cause weight _____ such as "body wrapping." (odcruetin)

5. High-potency _____ that make extravagant claims about their effect. (ansivitm)

6. Very expensive cures or remedies that may not be harmful by themselves, but are totally _____. (viftecefine)

7. Overuse of medicines that may be _____ forming. (bahti)

8. Medicines that may alleviate symptoms temporarily, but prevent a possibly sick person from seeking the _____ help that is needed. (oinspfolresa)

9. Using medicine that has been _____ for someone else whose symptoms are similar. This is especially dangerous because the problems causing the sickness and how two people react may be entirely different. (rsiepcbdre)

Answers: (1) healers, (2) ineffective, (3) institutions, (4) reduction, (5) vitamins, (6) ineffective, (7) habit, (8) professional, (9) prescribed.

Materials Needed: copy of "Beware Of" handout
Processing Questions

1. Have you heard or read health claims that might not be truthful?

2. How can you determine if a health claim is accurate and truthful?

Know Thy Medicine

Valued Outcome: The students will be able to describe the information found on over-the-counter and prescription drugs labels.

Description of Strategy: To give students an opportunity to become familiar with information provided on over-the-counter and prescription drugs, have them bring to class the label from an OTC product and a prescription drug. Mount the labels on index cards. These cards can then be used for a variety of activities. Students can classify the cards into two groups, OTC and prescription drugs, or classify them by kinds of medicine (for what purpose they are taken), or by the instructions on how often they should be taken—once, twice, three times a day.

Materials Needed: index cards, glue, signs listing (OTC, prescription, use)

Processing Questions:

1. What type of information is found on OTC product labels? on prescription products?

2. Are the directions clear on how to use the OTC products? the prescription products?

Slogans—Do They Sell?

Valued Outcome: The students will discuss the impact of slogans on the health products they purchase.

Description of Strategy: Provide each student with a copy of the following slogans. The students can also be asked to develop their own list.

Materials Needed: magazines or video with slogans for various health products

Slogans and Selling Worksheet

Directions: Listed are several slogans used to sell products. Can you identify them?

1.	Can't beat the feeling	a.	Burger King
2.	This is the new generation of . . .	b.	Pontiac
3.	Good time, great taste	c.	Chevrolet
4.	We build excitement	d.	Diet Coke
5.	Just for the fun of it	e.	Kodak
6.	The heartbeat of America	f.	Dr. Pepper
7.	You'll love this place	g.	Oldsmobile
8.	Really satisfies you	h.	Kellogg's Corn Flakes
9.	For the times of your life	i.	McDonald's
10.	Just what the doctor ordered	j.	Snickers
11.	You got the real thing, Baby	k.	Pepsi
12.	Taste it for the first time again	l.	Coca-Cola Classic

Answers: (1) Coca-Cola Classic, (2) Oldsmobile, (3) McDonald's, (4) Pontiac, (5) Diet Coke, (6) Chevrolet, (7) Burger King, (8) Snickers, (9) Kodak, (10) Dr. Pepper, (11) Pepsi, (12) Kellogg's Corn Flakes.

Materials Needed: handout listing slogans
Processing Questions:

1. How do slogans influence our purchasing?

2. What are some other slogans you can think of?

3. Why do slogans influence what we buy?

How Are Your Health Habits?

Valued Outcome: The students will be able to evaluate their health to determine what lifestyle changes they might make.
Description of Strategy: Students can develop and conduct a survey of health habits at their school. Answers can be either yes or no and can include questions dealing with superstitions and personal health habits; for example, Have you ever bought a product just because you saw it advertised on TV or in a magazine? Have you ever ordered anything through the mail and been disappointed with the merchandise? Do you take vitamins? Results can be tallied and reproduced in the form of a bulletin board for the classroom or published for the school to read the results. Medically correct answers can also be published at that time so people can get a feel for their own knowledge, or lack of knowledge, concerning health issues.
Materials Needed: A list of possible questions to be asked in survey. Enough questions should be provided to help students start the project.
Processing Questions:

1. What did you discover from the survey?

2. How should you change any negative lifestyle habits you identified?

3. What positive health habits did you identify?

4. What additional information would you like?

Health and Big Business

Valued Outcome: The students will work in groups to design a health-related business and present their plans to the class.
Description of Strategy: Guest speakers in the health field can be invited to describe their business operations and the service they provide to the community. Included in such a group could be local health officials, nurses and/or doctors, aerobics instructors, university health professors, fitness and wellness personnel, and health club personnel. Working in large groups, have the students study and design their own health-related businesses. Each group can then present its program to the class via lecture, bulletin board, poster board, and so forth for class review and discussion.
Materials Needed: provide list of health-related businesses
Processing Questions:

1. What health areas do you think would be most profitable from a business perspective?

2. What kinds of problems did you find when trying to set up a business (expenses, finding qualified personnel, obtaining equipment, and so on)?

3. Why did you choose your specific area to set up a business?

Deciphering What We Eat

Valued Outcome: The students will use nutrition labels to plan a healthy meal.

Description of Strategy: Have the students bring package labels to class that list the ingredients and the amounts of fat, carbohydrates, sugars, protein, and so on. In groups, have the students decide which of the foods they eat are really good for them and explain why or why not. Have students make note of added ingredients, such as salts, sugars, and hidden fats they may not be aware of eating. Using the labels in each group, students can plan a meal that will provide 33 percent of their daily needs without acquiring too much fat, cholesterol, or simple sugars.

Materials Needed: labels for various food products

Processing Questions:

1. Were there any foods that especially surprised you in the amount of fat, sugar, or other added ingredients?

2. Do you have any suggestions for getting the nutrients you need without adding ingredients that might not be as healthy?

3. Can you eat in a manner that is healthy and still eat appetizing food?

Old Wives and Health

Valued Outcome: The students will make a collection of health "myths" and state why they are accurate or inaccurate.

Description of Strategy: Students can research and collect "old wives' tales" such as "Feed a cold and starve a fever" "Toads cause warts" and "An apple a day keeps the doctor away." These can be used to develop a bulletin board or scrapbook listing and illustrating the adages as well as the truth or fiction of them. Discussion can include scientific accuracy for the sayings that may have relevance and why people continue to believe and follow such beliefs today.

Materials Needed: paper to list "myths" and "sayings"

Processing Questions:

1. Are all "old wives' tales" completely false?

2. Why do you think people first developed these myths?

3. Why do people continue to believe these myths today?

Health News

Valued Outcome: The students will gather current health information and present in newspaper form.

Description of Strategy: Have students research, develop, and publish a copy of an "underground" newspaper dealing with health issues. Included in the paper should be articles, cartoons, editorials, advertisements, and human interest stories. These should be based on information but rewritten by students in original form.

Materials Needed: magazines, newspapers, and other sources of health information

Processing Question: What did you learn about health that you did not know before?

Health Promotion Agencies

Valued Outcome: The students will learn what health agencies are responsible for specific activities.

Description of Strategy: The following is a list of agencies involved in health promotion programs. Each has a letter beside it. Have students write the letter of the agency next to the description of its functions. Not all letters will be used.

_____   **1.**   enforces laws for labeling and safety of cosmetics, medicines, and food

_____   **2.**   responsible for inspecting and grading meat and poultry

_____   **3.**   prevents false advertising from being sent through the mail

_____   **4.**   has offices all over the country to handle consumer complaints and keep track of businesses engaged in fraudulent practices

_____   **5.**   involved in examining and testing of electrical devices to ensure safety in operation

_____   **6.**   in charge of coordinating federal efforts in the field of health care

_____   **7.**   functions in the promotion of cancer research and educational programs dealing with all aspects of cancer

_____   **8.**   under the guidance of the United Nations, oversees programs dealing with disease, nutrition, and sanitation in all member countries

_____   **9.**   establishes regulations on the manufacture and sale of biological products, researches health problems and provides information to the public, and assists local and state health departments

_____   **10.**   within a specific political division, maintains clinics, laboratories, and staffs of nurses and other personnel to aid in the prevention and control of disease

a. Better Business Bureau

b. Department of Health, Education, and Welfare

c. U.S. Postal Service

d. National Association for the Prevention of Blindness

e. Underwriters Laboratory

f. American Heart Association

g. American Cancer Society

h. Public Health Service

i. Food and Drug Administration

j. World Health Organization

k. U.S. Department of Agriculture

l. state and local health departments

Answers: (1) i, (2) k, (3) c, (4) a, (5) e, (6) h, (7) g, (8) j, (9) h, (10) l.
Materials Needed: copy of agencies

Processing Questions:

1. What other agencies can you name?

2. What agencies do you think are most important to our personal protection?

Advertising: Don't Buy It Hook, Line, and Sinker

Valued Outcome: The students will be able understand the role of advertising in product purchases.

Description of Strategy: Distribute the following questionnaire (you may wish to expand the number of questions). Ask students to bring to class various advertisements. List on the board the various types of appeals used in advertising. Help students determine the appeal used in each advertisement. Then have students circle the appropriate letter to best complete the statement or question.

1. When a product's package says, "Free coupon inside," the advertising appeal being used is
- **a.** cost and rewards
- **b.** scientific appeal
- **c.** snob appeal
- **d.** testimonial or authority figure

2. People who purchase and use goods and services are called
- **a.** advertisers
- **b.** consumers
- **c.** researchers
- **d.** shopkeepers

3. Advertising is designed to do all of the following except
- **a.** entertain
- **b.** inform
- **c.** persuade
- **d.** promote

4. The most serious health-related effect of not understanding advertising techniques is
- **a.** dependence on a stimulant drug
- **b.** failure to seek out proper treatment
- **c.** feelings of total frustration
- **d.** loss of one's self-respect

5. In evaluating an advertisement that features an endorsement by a famous person, the most important question should be
- **a.** How is this person qualified to judge the product?
- **b.** How much money is this person being paid?
- **c.** Does this person really like the product?
- **d.** Does this person use the product regularly?

Answers: (1) a, (2) b, (3) b, (4) b, (5) a.

Materials Needed: copy of "Don't Buy It Hook, Line, and Sinker" questionnaire; teacher may add questions
Processing Questions:

1. What is the most important role advertising serves?
2. Why do famous people serve as spokespersons for various products?
3. Do any health products have potentially dangerous consequence?

Now for This Commercial Message

Valued Outcome: The students will be able to analyze commercials to determine misleading or overstated claims concerning health products.
Description of Strategy: Ask the students to work together in pairs or small groups to re-enact commercials they have seen on television for health care products or services. Let each group decide on the commercial they wish to re-enact. Draw up a master list so there will not be too much duplication. Then have the students who are working together study the commercial of their choice closely at home. Let them get together and rehearse their re-enactment. Each student should play a different role. For example, one student can be the person recommending the product, and another student can be the person trying out the product, as in many aspirin commercials. When the students are ready, have each commercial re-enacted in front of the class. After the re-enactment, the students who played the roles should explain what might have been misleading or overpromising about what they said or did. Videotaping will allow reuse of some of the commercial at a later time.
Materials Needed: none
Processing Questions:

1. What types of commercials seem to be the most misleading?
2. How do these commercials seem to overstate the effectiveness of the product?
3. What is misleading about the commercials you have just seen?

Dr. I. M. A. Quack

Valued Outcome: The students will learn to recognize phony health and medical treatment claims.
Description of Strategy: Let each student come up with a quack product or service and try to convince the class that this product or service is actually of value. Encourage imagination. For example, one student might try to convince the class that magnetic energy can cure arthritis. Another might claim to have invented a product that will cure the common cold. The class should listen to each presentation without interruption but then point out the fallacies of each presentation.
Materials Needed: a box containing props for role-playing
Processing Questions:

1. What were some of the statements made that might want us to buy the product or service?
2. What made some of the presentations believable?
3. Can you identify some points we should keep in mind when selecting health products or services?

Finding a Doctor

Valued Outcome: The students will be able to identify criteria for selection of a physician or a dentist.

Description of Strategy: After discussing the procedures that can be used for locating a qualified physician, have students role-play the techniques. For instance, let one student play the part of a representative from the county medical society who can recommend physicians who are accepting new patients. Another student can call on the telephone to ask for the names of such physicians, or one student can play the part of a doctor while the other plays the part of a prospective client. The latter should ask questions about availability of services, fees, qualifications of the doctor, and so forth.

Materials Needed: none

Processing Questions:

1. Where would you look to help identify the location of a physician or dentist?

2. How would you contact a physician or dentist?

3. What questions would you ask before using the services of a health professional?

Complaints

Valued Outcome: Students will practice appropriate ways to complain about defective or ineffective health products.

Description of Strategy: Have small groups of students role-play how they would act when complaining about a defective or ineffective product or service. One student should act the part of the disgruntled consumer, another the part of the seller, and a third the part of a consumer advocate or representative of a local Better Business Bureau or other consumer-oriented group.

Materials Needed: none

Processing Questions:

1. What are some agencies where consumers can seek help?

2. Where do you begin when filing a consumer complaint?

3. Who is ultimately responsible for protecting us in consumer issues?

Medicine Safety Rules

Valued Outcome: The students will be able to list the rules for safely taking medicine.

Description of Strategy: After discussing the medicine safety rules, divide the class into seven groups, and let each group develop a brief (two to five minutes) skit dramatizing each rule. The rest of the class can try to determine which rule is being acted out by each group. The medicine safety rules are listed here:

1. Don't take any medicine without asking an adult about it first.

2. Only take medicines that you really need.

3. Take only the medicine prescribed by your doctor especially for you.

4. Never take more than one medicine at a time, unless your doctor tells you to do so. Different medicines may interact in a way that can be dangerous or even fatal.

5. Don't take any medicine unless you are sure you know what it is.

6. Throw away medicine that doesn't have a label or that has passed the expiration date.

7. Keep all medicines out of the reach of younger children.

Materials Needed: Place rules on poster board.
Processing Questions:

1. Why are medicine safety rules so important?

2. Are there other medicine safety rules you could think of to help protect us?

Information or Puffery?

Valued Outcome: The students will be able to analyze health-related commercials.
Description of Strategy: Have the students closely watch and analyze a health-related commercial on television. Ask students to determine how much actual useful information is conveyed in the commercial and how much of what is said is mere puffery. Let each student present his or her findings and explain how the commercial attempts to appeal to consumers and manipulate their behavior and attitudes.
Materials Needed: index cards for student responses
Processing Questions:

1. Did the commercial you viewed contain misinformation?

2. How could the commercial be changed to reflect more accurate information?

3. What should we keep in mind as we view health-related commercials?

The Laws of Advertising

Valued Outcome: The students will be able to list at least three laws that protect consumers.
Description of Strategy: Students can learn about the laws that protect consumers against fraud or useless products and services. They can begin to learn about advertising laws by looking under "consumer protection" in the card catalog or the *Reader's Guide to Periodical Literature.* Write the laws on the poster board and discuss.
Materials Needed: poster board
Processing Questions:

1. Why was it necessary to pass laws to protect us against fraud?

2. Do you think most consumers know about these laws?

3. What is the key to consumers being protected against fraud?

Do Only Ducks Quack?

Valued Outcomes: The students will be able to describe quacks and quackery.
Description of Strategy: Develop a class discussion around the topic of quacks and quackery. Questions that can be used include

What is quackery?

Why does quackery continue to flourish?

Who are the people most likely to believe what quacks say?

How can consumers be protected from quackery?

What can be done if you think a legitimate physician is in error?

Why would people give testimonials about products that have no proven value?

What are some areas of health concern where it would be easiest to get people to buy products?

After the discussion, have students divide into groups. Each group is to develop and build a pretend fraudulent medical device and/or medicine to present to the class. Have the students formulate advertisements to stimulate interest in their phony product. After completion, projects can be displayed in the classroom. Presentations can be videotaped.
Materials Needed: poster board, videotaping equipment
Processing Questions:

1. Do you think fraudulent medicines and cures are very prevalent?

2. Should there be strong laws against people advertising phony remedies? Why or why not?

Health Options?

Valued Outcome: The students will identify different forms of treatment other than traditional medicine.
Description of Strategy: After dividing the class up into small groups, have the students investigate alternative forms of health choices. The following forms could be included: acupuncture, chiropractic, faith healing, holistic health, homeopathy, and visualization, laughter therapy, or positive self-talk. Reports could then be given to the class. Students can discuss the scientific basis of each, the feasibility of trying alternative kinds of medical care, under what circumstances they might try an alternative form, and the intrinsic value of each method. A master list of alternative treatments may be given to the class to help the students choose their topics. Presentations can be videotaped.
Materials Needed: video equipment
Processing Questions:

1. Would you try any of these alternative forms of treatment?

2. Do you think some or all of these alternative forms of treatment are useful?

3. What are some guidelines we should keep in mind when deciding if we might try an alternative treatment?

Is That So?

Valued Outcome: The students will analyze health-related commercials for truthfulness.
Description of Strategy: Ask each student to find a commercial or advertisement that appears to be quite truthful and informative. Have the students discuss the commercials or advertisements and explain their reasons for believing the claims made. Then ask the rest of the class to offer their own opinions. You may need to point out subtle approaches used in the commercial or advertisement to suggest greater informational content than is actually the case.
Materials Needed: magazines

Processing Questions:

1. What advertising techniques were you able to identify?
2. Why were the commercials effective?

Labels Are Important

Valued Outcome: The students will learn how to read and interpret health and drug labels correctly.
Description of Strategy: With the cooperation of parents, have each student analyze the information given on the package of a health product or OTC drug. Students should prepare individual reports about what they find.
Materials Needed: labels from over-the-counter drugs and health products
Processing Questions:

1. What did you learn from reading the label that you did not know before?
2. Are any drugs safe for everyone to take?
3. Why do you think the warnings were placed on the products that you brought in?
4. What do you think could happen if you had one of the conditions listed as dangerous to take the drug or product and you took it anyway?

Is There Any Difference?

Valued Outcome: The students will try different unlabeled cola drinks and try to determine what each one is.
Description of Strategy: Many products are indistinguishable once removed from their packaging. To demonstrate this, bring in some different brands of cola soft drinks. Pour small amounts of three or four different brands into paper cups, and have the students do taste comparisons. Let them try to guess which cup contains a particular brand.
Materials Needed: several different liters of cola, small cups
Processing Questions:

1. Do you have a favorite cola drink? Could you tell which one it was?
2. How much do you think advertising affects what you buy?

Which Is Better?

Valued Outcome: The students will exchange consumer products such as shampoo or soap to determine if there are actual differences between them.
Description of Strategy: Ask students to bring a particular health-related product such as a shampoo or soap to school, making sure that the brands are not the same. Then have volunteer students trade the products they now use with someone using another brand of shampoo or soap. Let each volunteer use the alternate product for a week or two and then report on the results.
Materials Needed: index cards or paper for recording comments
Processing Questions:

1. Did the alternate shampoo or soap do just as effective a job, or were differences noted?
2. Were any differences a matter of individual preference?

3. Are different products perhaps more or less effective for different individuals?

(Be sure to note that differences or a lack of difference in OTC products may not hold true for prescription medications.)

Slogans

Valued Outcome: The students will listen to a list of slogans used by various products that are used to manipulate buying of that product and attempt to recognize them.
Description of Strategy: Prepare a list of advertising slogans (such as "You got the right one, Baby—un-hunh!"), and have the class try to guess which product each slogan promotes. Students should be able to add to the list that you compile.
Materials Needed: index cards to list slogans
Processing Questions:

1. Do any of the slogans provide you with actual information about the product?

2. What is the main purpose of a slogan?

3. Do you find that you purchase products more if you like and remember the slogan it uses?

Consumer Riddles

Valued Outcome: The students will solve these riddles about consumerism.
Description of Strategy: Use the following riddles on consumerism to assess student knowledge of consumerism.

1. I am a fraud, but I sound like a duck. What am I? (a quack)

2. An inflated advertising claim is a huff and a _____. (puff)

3. My initials are BBB. I can help you if you have a consumer problem. What am I? (Better Business Bureau)

Processing Questions:

1. What other riddles can you identify that illustrate an aspect of consumerism?

2. Can you think of an example for each of the riddles?

Scrambled Words

Valued Outcome: The students will unscramble words that relate to consumerism.
Description of Strategy: Have students unscramble each of following words:

1. mocmlaceri (commercial)

2. qyuracek (quackery)

3. singiadevrt (advertising)

4. elagi githrs (legal rights)

5. aeetngura (guarantee)

Materials Needed: copy of the scrambled words; teachers may add to the list

Processing Questions:

1. Can you define all the scrambled words?

2. How does each word relate to consumerism?

Consumer Health Tic-Tac-Toe

Valued Outcome: The students will develop health-related questions and use them to beat an opposing team at tic-tac-toe.

Description of Strategy: This game can be played either by two players or by the whole class divided into two halves. Have each team come up with a health-related question for one of the tic-tac-toe squares. The opposing side or player tries to answer, to mark a particular square without knowing what the question is. If an incorrect answer is given, no mark on the tic-tac-toe board is to be made. Each side plays in turn until there is a winner.

Materials Needed: health-related questions, poster board with tic-tac-toe symbol

Processing Questions:

1. Can you correct all the answers that were missed?

2. What are some additional questions?

Consumer Reports

Valued Outcome: The students will learn about comparison shopping and where to obtain product information that is free from advertising.

Description of Strategy: Older elementary school children can learn about how products and services are evaluated objectively by reading copies of *Consumer Reports* magazine. Get some back issues from the public library, and discuss the products tested in the articles. Note that this magazine does not carry any advertising.

Materials Needed: Consumer Reports magazines

Processing Questions:

1. Why do you think this magazine has no advertising in it?

2. Pick a product that you find particularly attractive, such as a car. After reading the comparison of it with similar products, are you as convinced you like the product as before?

3. What is the advantage of reading a magazine such as *Consumer Reports*?

Comparison Shopping

Valued Outcome: Students will learn to compare similar products from a cost perspective.

Description of Strategy: Have the students develop a list of five or six health care products, such as toothpaste, deodorant, soap, eye drops, dental floss, and antiseptic cream. Let each student comparison-shop for these items and report on which stores in the community sell each brand of product for the best price. This can be done either by visiting stores or by checking prices in newspaper advertisements. You may wish to have the students comparison-shop for specific brands that they normally use, or you may suggest that the students look for the cheapest and most expensive brand of each type of product. Compare the results in a class discussion.

Materials Needed: sheet for listing products, price, comments

Processing Questions:

1. Do the same products cost the same at various stores?

2. What is the difference in cost between the most expensive of a certain item and the least expensive?

3. Is the most expensive product always the best? Is the least expensive product always the worst?

4. On what criteria should you base your purchases?

Food Labeling

Valued Outcome: The students will read and record data contained on a food label.

Description of Strategy: Labeling of foods transported interstate is controlled by the Federal Food and Drug Administration (FDA). According to FDA guidelines, food labels must be accurate, in English, and include information for each of the areas listed in Figure 21.1. Have students select a food product (or you can assign one), and then have them fill in information for each area.

Materials Needed: nutritional fact sheet (Figure 21.1)

Processing Questions:

1. How many times did you find salt and sugar listed in the product that you chose?

2. How many servings were contained in the package you selected?

3. How many additives and artificial ingredients were contained in your food product?

4. How does the product compare with a 2000- or 2500-calorie diet?

Packaging

Valued Outcome: The students will recognize the importance of attractive packaging in influencing the purchase of a product and will design a package for a product of their own.

Description of Strategy: Some of the appeal of a product results from the way it is packaged. Have the students bring in empty packages from various health care products. Discuss the visual appeal of each one, then have the students design packages of their own for the products. First, they should try to design a package they think would be very appealing to consumers. Then they should try to design a package that would not appeal to consumers. These can be shown to other students for feedback.

Materials Needed: students need to bring empty packages

Processing Questions:

1. Did you think it was difficult to design a package that would help sell your product?

2. What did you find the most attractive—certain colors or designs or wording?

3. How much do you think packaging influences what you and your family buys?

The Pharmacist and You

Valued Outcome: The students will learn what a pharmacist does.

Description of Strategy: Students can either visit a pharmacy or invite a pharmacist to class to discuss both his training and educational level and exactly what he or she does as a pharmacist. Students can work together to make a list of questions to ask the pharmacist about the job, how

Figure 21.1
*Food Label
Informational Form*

Name of product _____

Nutrition facts

Serving size: _____

Servings per container: _____

Amount per serving

Calories: _____   Calories from fat: _____

Percent daily value

Total fat: _____   _____ %

   Saturated fat: _____   _____

Cholesterol: _____   _____

Sodium: _____   _____

Total carbohydrates: _____   _____

   Dietary fiber: _____   _____

   Sugar: _____   _____

Vitamin A: _____   _____

Vitamin C: _____   _____

Calcium: _____   _____

Iron: _____   _____

*Percent daily values are based on a 2000-calorie diet. Your diet values may be higher or lower depending on your calorie needs.

	Calories	2000	2500
Total fat	Less than	65 g	80 g
Saturated fat	Less than	20 g	25 g
Cholesterol	Less than	300 g	300 g
Sodium	Less than	2400 g	2400 g
Total carbohydrates		300 g	275 g
Fiber		25 g	30 g

Calories per gram

Fat:_____   Carbohydrates:_____   Protein:_____

he or she likes it, his or her income level, and the decisions he or she makes in collaboration with both doctors and pharmaceutical salespeople. Questions can also be asked, or research done, into the history of pharmacy and how modern technology has enabled it to evolve into an exacting science today.

Materials Needed: list of questions to be asked at interview

Processing Questions:

1. Would you be interested in a career in pharmacy?

2. What kinds of questions could a pharmacist help you answer about drugs and medications?

3. What is the most important thing a pharmacist does?

Where Can I Go for Help?

Valued Outcome: The students will learn about services offered in their community.

Description of Strategy: Have students research legitimate health care services available in the community and write reports on their findings. Community health resources include private physicians, dentists, therapists, hospitals, clinics, health maintenance organizations (HMOs), telephone referral services, and so on. Keep a list of what type of services each student chooses, so that not too many will have the same topic. Students can discuss their resource in class.

Materials Needed: list of services offered in community with heading or phone numbers and services, to be filled in by the student

Processing Questions:

1. Are there many health organizations in your community?

2. What services does your organization provide?

3. How do the various health services differ?

Listen Carefully

Valued Outcome: Students will increase their awareness of meaningless phrases used in advertising.

Description of Strategy: Tape some radio or TV commercials using either audio or video tape and play them back for the class. First play the commercial in its entirety, asking students to listen or watch for any misleading statements. Play the commercial again, this time stopping the tape to discuss statements such as "Now more improved than ever" or "America's number one choice!" These types of statements are really meaningless since the comparison is not specifically stated. Singing commercials are among the least informative.

Materials Needed: tape or video of commercials, poster board to list misleading statements

Processing Questions:

1. What types of statements do you find used most often?

2. How are certain statements misleading?

3. Give examples of other commercials on TV or radio that are also uninformative or misleading.

I'm a Wise Consumer Because . . .

Valued Outcome: Students will list ways that they can be wiser consumers.

Description of Strategy: Ask each student to complete the statement "I'm a wise consumer because . . ." in twenty-five words or less. Each written answer should be based on actual behavior or attitudes. Talk about each student's response in a general class discussion.
Materials Needed: paper for writing response
Processing Questions:

1. On what values did you base your statements?

2. What consumer tips did you learn from others in your class?

3. How can these tips help you in the future?

Shopping Game

Valued Outcome: The students will participate in a game to increase their knowledge of consumer spending.
Description of Strategy: Prepare a game board as shown in Figure 21.2. The game can be played by from two to six players. Each player is given $200 in play money at the start. Participants roll dice in turn to determine the number of moves. The winner is the player with the most money at the end of the game. Play can continue until only one player has any money left. Let each player decide to what extent he or she "won" or "lost" by the consumer decisions the game dictated. Follow with a discussion of options in buying products and services.
Materials Needed: copy of shopping game board (Figure 21.2)

Resources

Books

Consumer health and safety. 1993. Contains ninety reproducible activities in a variety of formats. Available from Health Edco. Paperback. (FW50540)

Over-the-counter drugs: Harmless of hazardous? 1997. Resource on drugs and consumer use. Available from Chelsea House Publishers. Broomall, PA.

Schaller, W. E., C. R. Carroll, 1976. *Health quackery and the consumer.* Philadelphia: W. B. Saunders.

Your rights as a consumer. 1997. A clear, concise explanation of your rights when it comes to making purchases. Available from Chelsea House Publishers. Broomall, PA.

Videos

Supermarket persuasion.
How food is merchandised. A video tour through the world of consumer manipulation at the grocery store. Available from The Learning Seed. (23 minutes)

Invisible persuaders.
How persuasion pros control your decisions. Available from The Learning Seed. (22 minutes)

Web Sites

Healthlinks. Based at the University of Washington Health Sciences Center. Healthlinks has articles, guides, and links to other health sites on the Net.
http://www.hslib.washington.edu

Health Resources. This site offers a set of Netwide links and lists links to forty health care publications.
http://www.1hr.com

Figure 21.2
Shopping Game Board

Start			
Buy mouthwash. Spend $2.	Consult a quack. Spend $100.	Spend allowance on video games. Spend $10.	Go to HMO. Save $ and get $35 back.
Buy unneeded vitamin pills. Spend $8.	Buy defective product. Waste $50.	Have everything you need. No buying.	Buy most expensive shampoo. Spend $7.
Waste money on junk food. Spend $4.	Buy a new shirt that shrinks. Waste $15.	Find cheaper and better brand of toothpaste. Save $2. (Get $2 back.)	Buy a worthless acne cure. Waste $6.
Do comparison shopping. Save $12.	Resist silly commercial for cold remedy. No money spent.	Buy a new coat that you like on sale. Spend $25.	Buy a present for a family member. Spend $15.
Go fishing. No cost.	Buy a toy that breaks. Waste $11.	Visit the dentist for a checkup. Spend $30. Save $100 if dental problem avoided.	Buy a book that you want. Spend $7.
Develop dental problem that you could have prevented. Spend $100.	Buy a new brand of soap. Save $1. (Get $1 back.)	Buy a new bicycle. Spend $120 but get $20 back because of sale.	End *(continue until end.)*

Chapter Twenty-Two
Aging, Dying, and Death

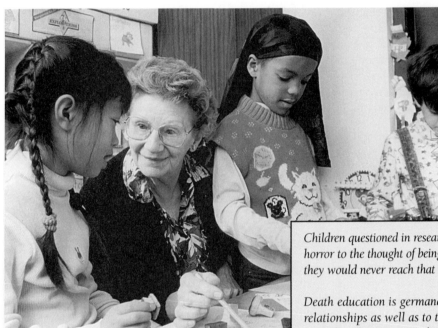

Children questioned in research studies react with horror to the thought of being old. Most are convinced they would never reach that undesired state.
—Belsky (1990, 4)

Death education is germane to the sphere of social relationships as well as to the confrontation with mortality that comes in the most private, personal moments of solitude and introspection."
—DeSpelder and Strickland (1992, 567)

Valued Outcomes

After reading this chapter, you should be able to

- ○ discuss aging as a normal part of the life cycle
- ○ describe how ageism affects the elderly in our society
- ○ describe the current demographic aspects of the American elderly
- ○ explain the factors that can help delay or retard the physiological changes that occur in aging
- ○ list the reasons why elderly people have problems with nutrition
- ○ describe Alzheimer's disease
- ○ suggest intergenerational contact programs for school-age students and the elderly
- ○ discuss the factors that will lead to better quality lives for the elderly in the future
- ○ discuss the fears of a dying person

○ describe the relationship of personal beliefs in facing dying and death

○ list ways in which family members cope with and help in times of a relative's death

○ describe healthy ways to grieve

○ discuss the purposes of funerals, hospice care, and living wills

○ describe effective methods of teaching death education

The Normalcy of Aging

Aging is a normal developmental process, not a pathological phenomenon, as it is often viewed. When we speak of aging, we must avoid the misconception that the process affects only those over sixty-five; each of us is aging every day. We generally consider the changes taking place in the body as "development" until postadolescence, and "aging" after that. Most people in our society view growth as positive and aging as negative. But in fact both are part of one process. The process of aging is a continuous experience that begins at birth and ends at death.

Exactly how we age is not clearly understood. Many theories have been advanced, but some aspects of the aging process are still mysteries. In any case, the number of elderly in the United States has risen sharply in the past two decades, and this trend will continue. Because of advances in medical technology, improved health care delivery, reduced infant mortality, and control of diseases, more people are living longer. In the first part of this chapter, we examine the ramifications of this fact and consider the ways in which aging is viewed in our society.

The Significance of Aging Education

Aging education is relatively new compared to other health topics. Because the number and proportion of elders are expanding rapidly in the United States, education about aging and the aged is becoming increasingly important. The presentation of correct facts and figures about the elderly and the aging process can counteract many misconceptions (Ferrini and Ferrini 1993, 11). Elders are having a tremendous impact on our society through their talents, wisdom, and psychological support for younger age groups.

People face many changes and challenges in life as they age. The problems of the elderly are problems that affect all of us. Major challenges facing the elderly include income, fitness, acute illness, nutrition, housing, sexuality, mandatory retirement, and the changing character of American society.

Our society places a great deal of emphasis on youth and productivity; the elderly person's role is considered less significant. Also, because of financial reasons (sharing housing costs) and social factors (desiring to live with or near peers and living nearer service-oriented agencies), some elderly people have opted to move into housing and communities for the aged. This further segregates them from the remainder of society and makes them less visible.

Students today are more likely to lose significant contact with the older generations than in the past. Some students see older persons daily (such as grandparents), but the interaction is often not as meaningful as in the past (Blieszner and Bedford 1995, 224). This lack of meaningful contact with the elderly, coupled with misleading stories they read and hear, often leads to fears and misconceptions. Students need to be taught about the elderly and aging early in their lives. They need to see that they themselves will one day be old. They also need to understand that the elderly were once students like themselves.

If the schools fail to include aging education, myths and stereotypes about aging will continue to abound. The goal of health education is to teach all aspects of growth and development through the life cycle, including the latter stages. Through the study of aging, secondary school students will become more aware of issues facing their parents and grandparents today. It will also prepare them for their own aging. Effective aging education can lead to more satisfactory living for today's elderly by promoting understanding and empathy among those who will one day also be old. A major objective of aging education is to promote and enhance the quality of life in all the years that a person lives.

Demographic Aspects of the Elderly

Life expectancy for both men and women has been increasing in our country. Those born today can expect to live more than twenty-five years longer than those born in 1900. The life expectancy for white women born in 1990 was 79.3 years; for white men, 72.6; for black women, 74.5 years; and for black men, 66.0 years. Females reaching age sixty-five can expect to live another nineteen years; and men fifteen years (Ferrini and Ferrini 1993, 19).

Elderly people over sixty-five make up 12.5 percent of the U.S. population. Of these elderly, 14.4 percent are females and 10.4 percent are males; 6.5 percent of females and 3.7 percent of males are over seventy-five years of age. Percentages of ethnic elderly show that blacks are 12.1 percent; Asians and Pacific Islanders, 2.9 percent; Native Americans, 0.8 percent; Hispanics, 9 percent (Ebersole and Hess 1994, 14–15).

The number and proportion of those over sixty-five have grown faster during most of this century than any other segment of the population. In 1985, there were 28.5 million people age sixty-five and older in the United States. At the beginning of the century, less than one in twenty-five people was sixty-five or over. Now, one person in nine (or 12 percent) fell into this category. The number of those aged fifty-five and over in our population is expected to double by the year 2050.

A popular myth is that most elderly are in nursing homes or other homes for the aged. In fact, only 5 percent of older people in this country live in such institutions. The majority, 67 percent, live in a family setting. Because more women outlive their spouses, older women are less likely to live with a spouse than older men. Florida has the highest percentage of elderly in a state population over 20 percent. Many social statistics regarding the elderly are dismal. For example, 12 percent of older people live below the poverty level. This is due to a variety of reasons, the chief among them being mandatory retirement; low income levels during the working years, leading to lower retirement incomes; poor planning for retirement income; and lack of opportunity to work, either for social or physical reasons. Just over 10 percent of elderly males and about 8 percent of elderly females participate in the labor force. Again, some have been forced to retire, many are women who have never been in the labor force, and some are physically incapable of working. Less than one-half of today's elderly have completed a high school education, and only 9 percent have graduated from college (Ferrini and Ferrini 1993, 20–21; Ebersole and Hess, 1994, 14–15).

Factors Related to Aging

Aging is a complex function, influenced by physiological, psychological, and sociological factors. Some of these factors are as follows.

Sex

Women have a longer life expectancy than men. This is primarily due to the fact that men are more susceptible to disease at every stage of life, especially chronic diseases. Also, men are more prone to stress than women.

Race

Whites have a higher life expectancy than nonwhites. This difference can be partly attributed to the fact that some nonwhites, especially black males, are more prone to hypertension than whites. Also, the general differences in education, economic levels, living conditions, nutrition, and health care between whites and nonwhites are factors.

Personality

People who are very nervous will probably not live as long as those who are more relaxed. Also, some personality types may be more prone to taking risks or may pursue a more physically taxing lifestyle.

Genetics

The genetic code in our bodies provides a blueprint that may dictate how long we will live. Also, genetic diseases affect the number and quality of our years.

Employment and Income

The more money an individual has, the better diet and lifestyle the person usually enjoys. Also, people with higher incomes generally have less financial stress.

Education

The more education an individual has, the better job the person might get. Better educated individuals are also more likely to be aware of the importance of a good diet, proper exercise, and the dangers of tobacco and alcohol misuse. College graduates have a greater life expectancy than nongraduates.

Social Attitudes

Many of the elderly in our country today feel "old" because they are behaving in the way they are expected to by the younger generation. Our society often treats the aged as sickly and unproductive. If people accept these social expectations of behavior, their lifestyles will certainly be affected as they age.

The Aging Process

Before the specific changes associated with the aging process are discussed, it should be emphasized that the changes occur to different people at different times. Most of these changes are gradual, and adjustments can often be made to offset them. Further, many of the changes can be retarded through proper exercise and other preventive health maintenance.

Biological Aspects of Aging

The following physical changes occur to the body with the passage of time (Spirduso 1995, 58–85):

1. slight loss of height
2. gradual reduction of muscle mass
3. loss of elasticity in the lungs, which causes more effort in breathing
4. loss of calcium from the bone (possible osteoporosis)
5. cellular dehydration
6. thinning of epidermis
7. gradual reduction in strength and endurance

Another biological phenomenon associated with aging is organic brain syndrome (OBS), also known as *senility* or *senile dementia*. OBS is a general term to describe a progressive disease that results in abnormal intellectual function. The personality and the behavior of the victim of OBS may be affected along with intellect. OBS may be caused by a series of small strokes, nutritional deficiencies, or atherosclerosis.

The most common and the most perplexing form of OBS is Alzheimer's disease (or presenile dementia), which is characterized by a progressive and irreversible decline in mental functioning that interferes with daily living. Alzheimer's is a cerebral degenerative disorder of unknown origin. It should be emphasized that Alzheimer's disease is not a normal process of aging, but is typically associated with older persons. It can occur as early as forty-five years of age, in which case it is called *presenile dementia*. The victim of Alzheimer's becomes confused, suffers memory loss, suffers physical and mental decline, and is unable to recognize even close family members. Little is yet known about the cause, prevention, and treatment of Alzheimer's. There seems to be a genetic link, because relatives of a person who developed symptoms before age sixty-five are more likely to contract Alzheimer's; however, many Alzheimer's victims have had no family history of the disease. Also, viral residue from remote disorders, such as herpes simplex and viral encephalitis, is providing researchers with questions about a possible relationship to later development of Alzheimer's and some other dementias (Ebersole and Hess 1994, 628–629).

Psychological Aspects of Aging

The psychological changes that accompany the aging process affect some elderly more than others. Many of these are the result of negative attitudes and behavior toward the elderly by the younger generation. Better treatment of and more positive attitudes toward the elderly would do much to limit many of these detrimental attitudes and behaviors. In helping individuals cope with changes that do occur, it must be recognized that the elderly face many losses, including peers, jobs, spouse, and physical senses. These problems of adjustment overwhelm some elderly people, whereas others are able to face the challenges and find satisfaction.

Sociological Aspects of Aging

Sociological aspects of aging in America include

1. a loss of the child-rearing function (the empty nest syndrome)
2. loss of one's spouse
3. mandatory retirement (or if voluntary, still a change in role)
4. problems with transportation
5. lack of community involvement
6. lack of knowledge of community resources
7. inadequate medical services
8. financial problems
9. a need for leisure activities and use of time
10. loneliness
11. loss of role identification
12. victimization through crime or abuse

Again, it should be noted that many of these sociological aspects of aging are the result of the discrimination and inappropriate treatment from younger people. With proper education and attitudinal changes in the general population, many of these detrimental changes could be alleviated among some of the elderly in America. The validity of this premise can be demonstrated by contrasting the role of the elderly in America with that of the elderly in some other cultures, such as that of Japan. In Japan, individuals enjoy higher social status and prestige as they grow older—almost the opposite of what happens in our country.

One factor that will determine the quality of life in the elderly is access to medical services

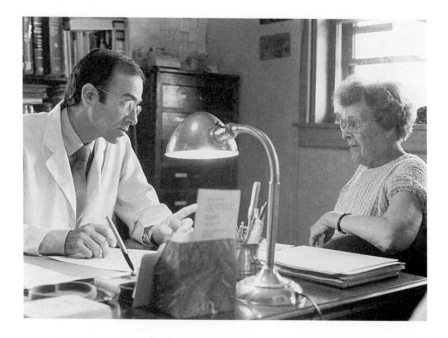

Major Challenges Facing the Elderly

Chief among the challenges facing the American elderly is the lack of financial resources. As mentioned earlier, many elderly live below poverty level. Lack of sufficient income is the result of inflation that has eroded the savings many elderly acquired during their working years. Retirement benefits from Social Security are not sufficient to meet all their needs. As of 1992 an elderly person over the age of sixty-five who earns more than $10,200 above their Social Security benefits is taxed on the additional income (this does not apply to individuals over the age of seventy).

Housing continues to be a major issue for the elderly. Nearly two-thirds of the elderly in our country own their own homes. But even if the house is paid for, the owners are still responsible for taxes and insurance costs. Also, if the home is older, it has higher maintenance costs. Some elderly have to make a decision between drastic improvements in their current home and moving. They are sometimes limited financially as to where they can move. Some government housing is available based on current income—the less the income, the less the monthly payment. Some elderly share housing to reduce the monthly costs. For many elderly, however, there are few housing options. Other housing alternatives are apartments for the aged, sponsored by private, public, and nonprofit church-related groups. Also, for the aged dependent, boarding homes and nursing homes that provide both intermediate and skilled care are available.

Maintaining good health is a major challenge of growing old. An individual's health affects every aspect of life—relationships to spouse, family, and community; income-producing ability; and leisure pursuits. The health problems that beset the elderly are usually associated with the aging process, in addition to those related to environmental causes, trauma, and heredity. Chronic ailments, such as heart disease, are the most common affliction of the elderly.

Escalating medical and health-related expenditures are a major concern for the older population. Of economic necessity, the health care of many elderly people is crisis oriented. Because they cannot afford to visit a physician every time they are ill, many do not seek help until they feel it is absolutely necessary. In addition, there are many areas in which the elderly needlessly spend money on health remedies or could spend their money more wisely for greater health benefits. Federal programs such as Medicare and Medicaid have helped in some ways, but even these programs do not pay enough of the health care bills of some elderly, because of the ever-increasing costs of health care delivery.

Medicare is a health insurance program for those age sixty-five and over that is designed to help pay for hospital insurance and medical insurance. Currently about 95 percent of the elderly population in our country are beneficiaries. The hospital insurance helps pay for hospital care and certain follow-up care after the person leaves the hospital. The medical insurance primarily pays for a doctor's services and outpatient hospital services. Medicare pays for about half of the medical expenses incurred, but the remaining amount must come from the elderly person (Ferrini and Ferrini 1993, 375).

Some of the health problems faced by the elderly are due to improper nutrition. Nutrition is as important for the elderly as it is for other age groups. Because of limited finances, loneliness, various disease states, and a reduction in the senses of smell and taste, many elderly skip meals or do not otherwise eat well. Sometimes emotional problems, such as depression, keep elderly people from eating. Because an elderly person's basal metabolism is reduced, the person's caloric need is also reduced. For this reason, better planning is required to ensure proper nutrition. Less food is required, but the quality must remain high. Programs such as Meals on Wheels, which delivers meals to homebound elderly, and the federal government's Food Stamp Program and Nutrition Program for the Elderly (Title VII of the Older Americans Act of 1965, which is updated every three years) help defray the cost and improve the nutrition of the poor elderly.

Drug use in older adults may cause greater problems than in younger people because of slower metabolic rates and more illnesses. It is very common for older people to be taking many different drugs. Some recommendations to help prevent drug problems among the elderly are for the patient to make sure when the medication is to be taken, to keep an up-to-date record of the drugs taken, to keep the physician informed of all medications taken, and to discard old medicines (Ebersole and Hess 1994, 307–319).

Medical quackery also affects the elderly. Arthritis sufferers, mostly older individuals, spend $300 million yearly on quack remedies. Other types of crime against the elderly range from muggings and theft to financial exploitation and physical abuse by members of their own family. Transportation is a major challenge for some elderly Americans; many of them do not drive. Others drive but have not adjusted to today's complicated traffic patterns. Also, those who drive with failing eyesight and hearing are more likely to be involved in accidents. The cost of automobile maintenance and gasoline prohibits some older people from operating a car. Nondrivers must seek other means of transportation. Taxis can be expensive, and public transportation, although cheaper, is much less convenient; it requires more walking and takes more time. Often it is not designed with the elderly in mind. For these reasons, many elderly are restricted to their homes and apartments except for going out to get health care, groceries, and other necessities.

Ageism

Ageism is a term used to describe the discrimination that often accompanies old age. The elderly are described as being the least capable, least healthy, and least alert. Our society promotes ageism by exalting youth and vigor and emphasizing efficiency, speed, and mobility. We are critical of those considered unproductive. This attitude causes much discrimination and fosters many false beliefs about the elderly (Spirduso 1995, 374).

Intergenerational misunderstandings are reduced when the old and young work, play, study, and socialize together. When the young and old see each other frequently and interact in meaningful ways, they generally express a high regard for each other (Blieszner and Bedford 1995, 224). Younger people are quick to emphasize the problems that occur with aging and the aged. Although people do face special problems and challenges as they grow older, the problems are not so widespread as many younger people believe. For example, it is a myth that most elderly are incapacitated. In fact, most older people are able to work and live independently. Only 5 percent of the elderly are institutionalized, and elderly individuals average less than fifteen days a year in bed because of ill health. Here are some other misconceptions about the elderly (Ferrini and Ferrini 1993, 12–17):

1. "After age sixty-five, life goes steadily downhill."
2. "Old people are all alike."
3. "Old people are lonely and ignored by their families."
4. "Old people are senile."
5. "Old people have the good life."
6. "Most old people are sickly."
7. "Old people no longer have any sexual interest or ability."
8. "Old age used to be better."
9. "Most old people end up in nursing homes."

Health Highlight

Stereotypes of Elder Sexuality

There is much misinformation and bias regarding elder sexuality, most of which is borne of ageism. These myths add to younger people's fears of losing sexual function with age. Some of the more common myths are as follows:

○ *Sexuality is reserved for the young.* Americans generally associate sexuality with the physical characteristics of youth: beautiful young people with shapely or muscular bodies. This myth is perpetuated by the media, which offer us ways to stay young and remain sexy. Sometimes the elderly become victims of their own negative attitudes in this area.

○ *Elders' sexual needs are amusing or insignificant.* Elders expressing affection in public is often described as "cute" or is commented on as if they were children.

○ *Older people don't enjoy sex. If they do, it's abnormal.* Many younger people find it difficult to accept that older people engage in sexual intercourse—perhaps because they envision the old as an extension of their parents.

○ *Sexual ability is lost with age.* This myth is also promoted on television and in print. Impotence is not a result of the aging process, but is due to factors that can happen at any age. Studies consistently show sexual activity is possible into the eighties and nineties

Source: A. F. Ferrini and R. L. Ferrini. 1993. *Health in the later years.* 2nd ed. Madison, WI: Brown & Benchmark, 341–343.

Intergenerational Contact

Intergenerational contact programs can be one of the most effective ways for secondary teachers to implement an aging education program. Such an experiential approach to intergenerational contact has been implemented in programs throughout the country. Notable examples are the Foster Grandparent Program and the Retired Seniors Volunteer Program. Volunteers and paid aide programs, tutoring projects, free lunches, and guest speaker days have all served as ways to involve the elderly with the schools. Only as students are given the opportunity to understand aging and the aged will many false beliefs be dissolved. The positive attitudes gained from aging education can help students realize their full potential throughout their lives as they themselves age. By studying aging, students will be better able to understand and interact with their parents and grandparents.

There are several things for young adults to consider when planning for later life. For example, those elderly with a better education will be better able to cope with the challenges of later life; therefore, younger adults should place an emphasis on continuing their education. A related factor that will help a young adult prepare for later life is the development of hobbies; therefore, one's education does not have to include a program that would result in a formal degree. Some courses can be taken to investigate various interests and hobbies. Young adults should become active in organizations and/or movements in which they have concerns or interests—such as environmental issues, women's rights, and charitable organizations. This activity contributes to one's self-concept by providing a purpose in life, and can add to the quality of life in later years. Finally, young adults should carefully consider financial planning for later years. It is difficult for a young adult to contemplate financial needs that are thirty to forty years away—especially in a society that promulgates "instant gratification." Financial concerns usually top the list of problems for elderly people in our society, and this trend is likely to continue; therefore, it is vital for young adults to develop a sound financial plan in order to ensure quality health care, housing, and living standards for themselves in later life.

Considering Death

Death is a vital part of the life cycle for every creature on earth. Death is included in the natural order of birth, growth, aging, and dying. Death is very democratic—a respecter of no person. Death is a certainty—it will come to every person. These seem like elementary statements, but many people in contemporary society believe that life and death are mutually exclusive phenomena.

The contemplation of death can be trying. The various aspects of dying and death are extremely complex and confusing because there is so much about death we do not comprehend. Many questions regarding death, such as "If we are born to die, then why do we live?" "If death is natural, why do so many people regard it as bad?" have still not been answered satisfactorily. None of the numerous attempts to come up with answers to these and similar questions have been able to satisfy everyone. The "unknowns" have caused much confusion and put an aura of mystery around death, but they have also been the source of many interesting attitudes and philosophies on the subject.

Recognizing that death is a natural end to our lives can have a profound influence on our lives.

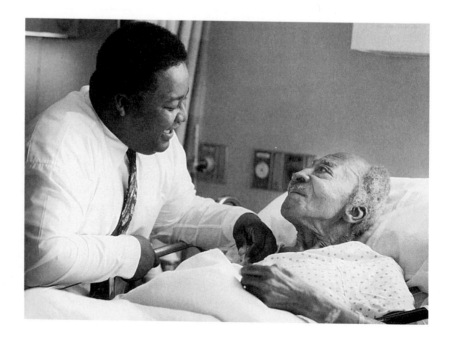

Death is as much a part of human existence, of human growth and development, as birth. Death sets a limit on our time in this world, and life culminates in death. Recognizing that death is a natural end to life can have a profound influence on our lives. Our lifestyles can depend on our attitudes toward death. Much information on death and dying is now available. Many misconceptions and problems concerning issues of death and dying still exist. For example, many physicians and clergy have had little training in caring for the emotional needs of dying people and their families. Physicians are trained to cure, but some are lacking in ability to be caring and comforting. Often they avoid the crucial issues, thereby complicating the dying process. Even today, such courses are conspicuously absent at many of the seminaries and medical schools in our country (Oaks and Ezell 1993, 51).

Another problem with death and dying concerns students of secondary school age. Parents often "protect" their children from the trauma of death-related events, thinking they are doing the best thing for the student. However, this treatment tends to propagate fears and misconceptions. For example, students tend to regard death as happening only to the old. This is a result of parents telling them not to worry about death until they are older.

In the remainder of this chapter, we examine these and other death-related issues. We also look at attitudes toward death, the needs of dying people and their families, the grief experience, funerals and related rituals, and death education for students.

Common Attitudes Toward Death and Dying

The current attitude of Americans toward death is contradictory. We are both intimidated and fascinated by death. We enjoy living, but we take risks by driving dangerously and taking part in high-adventure sports. We want safety and happiness, but we behave in self-destructive ways, for instance by abusing drugs. We consider the subject of death to be a social taboo, but insist on reading and talking more about it. We say we need nuclear weapons, but at the same time we are concerned about spiritual rebirth.

Our typical response to death is denial of death. This results from our resistance to imagining death, and is predicated on our fears of death, such as fears of abandonment, loss of self-control, suffering and pain, physical disfigurement, loss of dignity, and fear of the unknown (Marrone 1997, 79–81). We deny death by not planning for it (for example, not making out a will), and by participating in high-risk activities as if we were impervious to dying.

Furthermore, many people display an outright hatred of death. They hate death because they think people die too young or because they are afraid of what comes after death. The hate and fear might not result so much from the "unknown" factor as from the hopelessness regarding what is beyond death.

Others believe that death should be considered a taboo topic for discussion. Being taboo means that death is considered forbidden, profane, or unclean. We are therefore denied open, honest discussions of dying and death. Death is also a taboo topic because of the mystery and danger associated with it. This latter attitude is influenced by society's emphasis on youth and secularism.

Attitudes toward death are influenced by past experiences with death, by early parental messages, cultural influences, life experiences, religious beliefs, level of education, and maturity. Attitudes are formed largely by childhood experiences and carried into adulthood. Findings from research indicate that negative attitudes toward death tend to be higher among females, blacks, youth, and those who do not characterize themselves as "religious" (DeSpelder and Strickland 1992, 109–118, 576).

It is interesting that many people today who would rather not discuss death in an open and frank manner actually talk about death every day. For example, we hear "You'll be the death of me yet" or "My shoes are killing me" or "That loud noise scared me to death!" In other cases, death is the subject of jokes and humor, like the jokes about Saint Peter at the "Pearly Gates." People who talk about death in these ways show both an aversion to death as a topic of conversation, and a fascination with death. They may be subconsciously trying to show themselves and others that death really doesn't bother them, even though serious contemplation of the subject makes them extremely uncomfortable.

We also treat death in a very special way. We set aside special places for death—the funeral home, cemeteries, hospices, and hospitals. We set aside special times for remembering deaths—Memorial Day, the Day of the Dead in Mexico, and Good Friday, a day for remembering the death of Jesus. In addition, the deaths of other celebrated and martyred persons have been remembered with special days. We have special symbols for death, such as black armbands worn by athletes when a teammate has died, or a flag flown at half-mast in memory of someone who has died.

Several factors have contributed to our very narrow and stereotyped attitudes toward death and dying. We are so far removed from death that we fail to accurately contemplate its nature. We blindly believe in modern medicine to the point that we subconsciously feel we may never die. Many never come to realize that death is a fact of life with which all people must cope and reason out for themselves. Most Americans say they want to die quickly or in their sleep. This response reflects a negative attitude and lack of preparation for accepting a painful or slow death, where one is conscious of what is going on.

Our attitudes toward death and dying are confusing and contradictory. We normally detest the taking of another person's life, as in homicide, yet we train soldiers to do just that in war. In fact, we make heroes of soldiers who tempt death and kill the enemy. In every state in the nation there is serious debate regarding capital punishment. Is it right to kill people because they have committed heinous crimes, such as murder? Is the use of capital punishment a statement that we condone the killing of a criminal and that killing under these circumstances is the way to solve the problem? Another controversial issue involving death is abortion. Such groups as the "Right to Life" organization say that abortion is murder, akin to genocide. Yet abortion is legal if certain guidelines are followed, for example, if it is performed in the first trimester of pregnancy.

Most Americans have very negative attitudes toward death, primarily because they are uncomfortable with their own mortality. Many people associate death only with loss, pain, suffering, frustrated desires, and uncompleted goals. They see death as a separation from people we love, from places or objects we treasure, and from a part of our own self-identity, and they fail to see anything positive in death.

Otherwise mature individuals often find themselves unable to cope with the thought of death. These people generally choose to try to ignore death, to pretend on a subconscious level that they are immortal. This attitude is assumed primarily out of a fear of death. Furthermore, other people's deaths remind us of our own vulnerability, causing us to feel totally helpless, as if nothing we can say or do can change a thing.

Many people try to avoid even mentioning death. When it is brought up in conversation, it is usually in the form of a joke. When the subject of personal death, or the death of someone close comes up, there are often looks of dismay and discomfort until someone changes the subject, much to everyone's relief. When people refer to death, they often use euphemisms that do not imply the finality, totality, and complete separation from life that death is. These euphemisms include "expired," "passed away," "departed," "gone to his rest," and "gone to her great reward." Such phrases make it easier to talk about and think about death, because they soothe the harshness of its reality. The use of euphemisms is an extension of the denial attitude that many

Americans take toward death. This denial is carried over to other aspects of death as well. For example, many families request embalming of a body so the body in the casket will "look alive" and "seem real."

These attitudes toward death can have a profound influence on people's lives. If death is nothing but fear, and if fear prevents people from thinking and acting, they then become less than human. Also, if the fear of death does limit an individual's view of the future, this negative attitude can hinder the person's ability to plan ahead, to anticipate both hazards and opportunities in life.

Positive Approaches to Death

Death should not be considered taboo. It should be seen as a natural part of our existence. The more absolute death becomes, the more meaningful our life can become. Death is as much a part of human existence and the life cycle as birth. It is not an enemy to be conquered, but an integral part of life that gives meaning to human existence. Death sets a limit on our time in this life, urging us to do something meaningful with that time as long as it is ours to use. Dying is the final chance to grow, to become more truly who you are. Those who truly are reconciled to their own mortal existence are the ones who get the most out of life. Such a positive approach to death frees one to focus on the daily tasks of living life more fully.

A normal and healthy fear of death is considered essential to the preservation of life, because this fear leads us to take certain precautions. But we should not allow this fear to affect our emotional health in a negative way. We must find ways to cope effectively with death and dying, and it is not enough to intellectualize. The quality of our life depends on our ability to acknowledge reality and to deal appropriately with death and dying. The first step in overcoming a fear of death is to face it openly and resolve any unrealistic fears by looking into the causes of those fears. Frank and open discussion about death can help a person to diminish fear, anxiety, aggression, and other conflicts associated with death and to develop a positive attitude.

Other media that have been used to help people confront death are religion, art, music, poetry, and love. For example, those who characterize themselves as "religious" tend to report less death anxiety than those who do not characterize themselves in this way (DeSpelder and Strickland 1992, 576). Most religions believe that death comes only to the physical self and that one's spirit (or soul) will survive.

Furthermore, people who have shared in the death of someone who understood death's meaning tend to develop a more positive attitude toward dying and death. Those who have a healthy attitude toward death and who consider it truly one phase of existence have profited from this frame of mind. Positive attitudes toward dying can enhance the meaningfulness and richness of life for many, even for the terminally ill. The awareness of one's finiteness can bring on a feeling of ecstasy at being freed from social constraints, for example (Oaks and Ezell 1993, 11).

Personal Beliefs about Death

Personal beliefs are helpful in coping with the reality of death and dying, whether these beliefs are called ethics, thoughts, meditations, or religion. People rely on personal beliefs to find comfort in the face of death. Some use religious beliefs as an escape, as if to gain personal exemption from the reality of death. However, belonging to any religious group does not guarantee that death will be faced any more positively. Research does appear to show that maintaining a strong religious belief system does diminish the fear of death (Backer, Hannon, and Russell 1994, 27).

Needs of a Dying Person

Most Americans, when asked how they would want to die, will say they wish to die in a sudden, unexpected way, or in their sleep. In other words, they want to die without knowing what is happening; however, the majority of Americans will die of chronic illnesses. Those in this situation tend to feel powerless over their own destiny. They begin to realize their own mortality and sense a loss of independence.

Fear is the most typical psychological response that a dying person experiences. Dying people often fear humiliation, a sense of failure, a loss of self-worth, and anxiety about the future. Other common fears of the dying are the fear of the unknown (that is, not knowing what will happen after death), fear of being disfigured, fear of pain, fear of indignity, and a fear of abandonment by friends and relatives (Marrone 1997, 79–81).

In a sense, dying people have no model to follow. They feel like strangers to the healthy living because no one understands what they are going through. Most dying people want to talk about death and their own illness, but unfortunately, sometimes they cannot find anyone willing to discuss these matters.

Adjusting to Dying

Adjusting to dying during the grief process consists of a number of phases, such as shock and numbness, intense grief (which consists of yearning, anger, guilt and disorganization) and finally reorganization or resolution. This adjustment period occurs differently in each individual, and does not necessarily happen in sequential process. Understanding these stages of adjustment to impending death is critical in understanding the needs of the dying person. These phases occur to the person who learns that he or she is going to die as well as to the bereaved person grieving the loss of the deceased.

Shock and numbness is the most immediate reaction to death—the dying person cannot accept the fact that he or she is going to die, and the bereaved cannot consciously believe that the death just occurred. This is the body's normal reaction to protect the person from something he or she may not be able to handle emotionally at that time.

Intense grief includes a collection of fears (as discussed earlier in this chapter) on the part of the dying person, and a subconscious searching for the deceased because the thoughts and behavior of the bereaved are focused on the deceased. Hallucinations are not uncommon because of the intense desire for the return of the deceased. Anger is manifested by irritability directed at anyone who comes in contact with the dying person or the bereaved, sometimes even directed at God. The anger may be directed at oneself because of thoughts such as "If I had only done this with my life" or "If I had only done this while he/she was alive." During this intense grief, the dying person and the bereaved often experience despair. Apathy, aimlessness, futility, emptiness, and disorganization are all manifested during this time.

Reintegration is a time of recovery or resolution. This phase occurs when the dying person "comes to grips" or resolves his or her own mortality, and when the bereaved begins to function normally once again. This indicates that the bereaved has resolved the meaning and the purpose of the death, and has decided that he or she is going to be healthy and can function even in light of the loss that has occurred. Even when reintegration occurs, there can still be pain during special times, such as anniversaries, birthdays and holidays (Backer, Hannon, and Russell 1994, 263–265).

It should be noted that each person is unique in death as in life, and everyone responds differently. Some may progress naturally through these phases, whereas others might reach one of the latter phases of adjustment, then regress. Further, not all dying people will reach the phase of resolution before they die.

The Family of a Dying Person

Impending death affects family members of the dying person in various ways. Sometimes there is a strong prohibition in the family against talk of death, because they feel this may bring about death more quickly. Some family members think that a discussion of death would make the others more uncomfortable, and any discussion may seem to be related to an undue interest in the estate of the dying person. The loss of an important family member, such as the head of a household, can threaten certain social and psychological arrangements. This can lead to enormous stresses and cause tension among all remaining members.

Besides grief, emotional reactions to the death of a family member may range from guilt and anger to fear, anxiety, and money worries. Sometimes the anger is directed toward the person that died: "He died and left me with all these debts" or "She deserted us during a crucial time of our lives." Further, death is a reminder of the survivors' own vulnerability, which evokes fear in itself. If the dying person lives in the home before death, tension and resentment can develop. When family members have to sacrifice their own friends and activities to provide care, feelings of hostility and anger toward the dying person can develop. Then the anger turns to guilt, which has been described as anger turned inward. Some family members tend to feel inadequate when confronted with this overwhelming situation. They tend to want to protect themselves and the dying relative by not speaking to the person. This is wrong, because it leads to emotional abandonment, making the situation all the more difficult for the dying person. Compassion, not isolation, should be given.

The family can help the most by, when circumstances permit, maintaining an emotional and social environment consistent with the person's past life. This means keeping the person at home or hospice rather than in a hospital or nursing home. The family should include the dying relative as a participant in every discussion, especially those that involve decisions about that person's care and welfare. The family should do all they can to show their love and concern without doing it in ways that make the person feel guilty for being a burden to them. Family members should not allow their inability to face death to hinder the dying person's adjustment. When the person is ready to accept the reality of dying, the family should share that acceptance. An absence of support at this crucial time will mean that the person will die without dignity.

The Grief Experience

Grief is usually described as sorrow, mental distress, emotional agitation, sadness, suffering, and related feelings caused by a death. *Bereavement* refers to a state of experiencing grief. Mourning is comprised of culturally defined acts that are usually performed when death occurs.

The closer the relationship of the bereaved to the deceased, the stronger the emotional response. Among these emotions and patterns of behavior are sadness, anger, fear, anxiety, guilt, loneliness, tension, loss of appetite, weight loss, loss of interest in things once interesting, a decrease in socialization, and disrupted sleep. These responses are usually greater when the death is unexpected.

Funerals meet many emotional needs of the survivors.

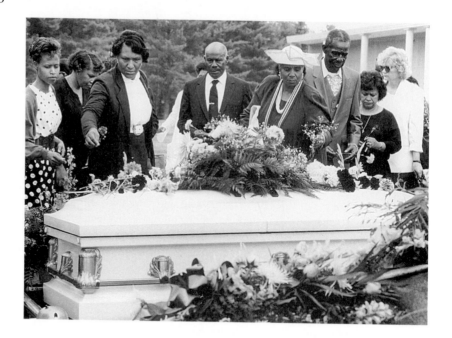

Grief and mourning are generally much less formal in the United States than in some other cultures, or than it was in early America. Today people generally have greater freedom to determine for themselves what kind of grieving, bereaving and mourning is appropriate (DeSpelder and Strickland 1992, 235).

Studies of mourning show that it is therapeutic for survivors to talk about the deceased and work through their death-related problems in counseling sessions (Corless, Germino, and Pittman 1994, 269). Another form of therapy involves going to work, going to school, or participating in organizational activities. Americans seem in need of much more elaboration of death ceremonies than many other cultures. This helps explain why many in our society place a strong emphasis on the rituals of funerals and burials.

Funerals and Related Rituals

The funeral is an organized, group-centered response to death. It involves rituals and ceremonies during which the body of the deceased is present. The traditional funeral includes speaking to the needs of the mourners. Some religions include a eulogy of the deceased, and some include an open casket that survivors view as part of the ceremony.

An alternative to the traditional funeral is a memorial service. Memorial services are sometimes held in conjunction with a cremation (with the urn present or absent) or when the body is not present for some reason (such as being donated to a medical school immediately on death or the family preferring not to have the body present). This service is held in a church, chapel, home, or whatever place is considered appropriate by the family. The service is not a eulogy but a chance to show thankfulness for having known the person. It also gives an opportunity for the expression of grief and sharing with family members. Generally, individuals who hold a memorial service are using this time to celebrate the life of the deceased while on earth, as opposed to a mourning. Memorial services are most common among families who have strong religious convictions and the belief in life after death. Memorial services are becoming more common even among the nonreligious.

A primary purpose of the funeral is to dispose of the body. It also meets many emotional needs, like grief and mourning, of the survivors. The visitation part of the funeral ceremony is important for friends to show their respect for the deceased and support for the survivors. Also, viewing the casket, which is part of some funeral home visits, is important to some for realization (seeing and thus believing that the person is dead) and recall (providing an acceptable image for recalling the deceased). For these reasons, the funeral home visitation can be therapeutic for friends as well as family.

Cemeteries, with markers for each grave, formerly were thought of as very sacred places where relatives could go in quiet and peace to show their respect to the dead. Now, however, many cemeteries are crowded, congested, and impersonal. The relatives of the deceased might also live many miles from the burial site. For these reasons, cemetery visits are less common than they once were. This ritual is not used as often in working out grief and mourning among the survivors.

Issues Surrounding Death

Some topics related to death have become the focal point of controversy in recent years. These issues include the definition of death, the right to die, organ transplants and donations, wills, and suicide.

Definitions of Death

For thousands of years, the time of death was clearly defined as the time of cessation of the life functions. Now, however, with advanced medical technology, life can be sustained beyond when death formerly would have occurred. The problem of defining it is much more complex—for example, not just knowing when a person is dead, but being able to determine the exact moment of death. This is important in the case of potential organ transplants, when every second is critical.

Some say that a person is brain dead when the entire brain is dead, even if respiration and circulation could be maintained artificially. Others argue that a person is dead when the outer surface of the cerebrum of the brain has ceased to function. (This individual may still breathe spontaneously via control of the brain stem, but thinking and reasoning ability would have ceased.)

Definitions of death center around "brain," "heart," or "physiological" death when various organs cease to function and "clinical" death when there is a total lack of response to any external or internal stimuli, lack of spontaneous respiration, fixed and dilated pupils, lack of brainstem reflexes, and a flat EKG (no heartbeat). The significance of the definition of death is not just for the purpose of organ transplants. It also indicates which human lives can be saved, possibly with life support systems such as heart–lung machines.

Organ Donation and Transplants

Some people wish to donate their organs or entire body for scientific and medical uses. This sometimes involves an urgent decision at the time of the donor's death. Biological, medical, and legal ethics are all involved in this issue. For those who wish to donate an organ, the Uniform Anatomical Gift Act of 1978 sets guidelines underlying the donor laws of each state. Some individuals donate their entire bodies to medical schools for dissection. Other parts of the body that can be donated include eyes, for corneal transplants; ear bones, to temporal bone banks for use in research into ear diseases; kidneys, for kidney transplants; pituitary glands, for use in producing growth hormone for those who lack this vital substance; and hearts, for heart transplants.

Virtually no religion in our country places any restrictions on organ donations to help another patient regain health. Further, the donation of an organ does not have to interrupt or modify the planned funeral service for the donor in any way. A donor needs to have a signed and witnessed donor card, usually carried at all times. These donor cards are available from many agencies in the community, such as the local kidney dialysis clinic or the Department of Motor Vehicles.

Currently only organ donations of kidneys, liver, heart, and the pancreas are accepted for donation. This acceptance is based on the definition of death discussed early in this chapter. The donor must die in a hospital, since surgery must be performed within hours if the organ(s) is to be used. For example, the heart is suitable for transplantation for only four to five hours. For this reason, surgeries are usually begun simultaneously for the donor and the recipient. The liver must also be transplanted within four to five hours, but the kidneys are suitable for transplantation for thirty-six to forty-eight hours.

It is not always known for sure who will receive the transplant, nor is such information as the donor's name or home town usually given. General information is provided, though. An example of this would be the information that the kidney of a thirteen-year-old who died in an auto accident was used. Anyone eighteen years or older and of sound mind may donate by signing a donor card. Anyone under eighteen years may become a donor if either parent or the legal guardian gives permission. Body parts from a person who is over fifty-five are not accepted for donation.

Although much of transplant surgery is still classified as experimental, the future is encouraging. Medical knowledge and technology is improving every day. Today two-thirds of the liver transplants live beyond the first year. Even when a transplant patient lives only a few months, most families consider the operation worthwhile, because the patient's quality of life was probably vastly improved.

The Right to Die and Euthanasia

Euthanasia, or "death with dignity," is not just a medical problem because it also involves legal, ethical, social, personal, and financial considerations. For this reason, the debate over euthanasia involves many professionals and paraprofessionals, as well as the patients and their families. The arguments now have to do with the dignity of the patients, the quality of their lives, their mental state, and sometimes their usefulness to society. For example, the patient who is in a vegetative state is considered dead by some but not by others, and this case presents substantial ethical and logistical problems. Some say that to intervene in any way is to "play God," while others maintain that the rights of the patient are violated if the medical staff does not allow the patient to die. Such procedures as using a life support machine to sustain life are sometimes seen as heroic acts, but others think this only prolongs the suffering of the patient. Therefore, the line between heroic procedures (or unnecessary care) and "giving up" (or neglecting the patient) is difficult to draw. This distinction would be simple if we could just ask patients which treatment they wanted, but this is not possible in a majority of such cases.

Today we are being forced to rethink our ideas and choices about life, dying, and death. The issue of euthanasia is an excellent example of this. Currently, there is a change in emphasis in the euthanasia debate. The focus is less on allowing people to die a natural and painless death and more on allowing death to occur by withholding "heroic" medical treatment. Typically, patients involved in a case of euthanasia are the terminally ill or severely deformed, or severely diseased infants. Often the decision to practice euthanasia is more of a decision between letting the person die now or later, rather than a choice between life and death. Some argue that the movement in favor of euthanasia may be rooted in our fear of facing death, and that euthanasia is used to hasten death so that we will not have to cope with the consequences associated with the actual process of dying. A related issue that intensifies the problem is that many times the life, living, dying, or death decision is made by medical staffs or families about someone else's life or death.

The term *euthanasia* has come to imply a contract for the termination of life in order to avoid unnecessary suffering at the end of a fatal illness. Direct (or active) euthanasia is defined as a deliberate action to shorten life. It involves a procedure such as injecting air or a chemical substance into the bloodstream. This is termed *mercy killing* and is still considered murder in our country, although some feel it should be permissible. A related phenomenon is physician-assisted suicide, in which the physician supplies the equipment and medicine needed, and the patient performs the act necessary to cause death (Williamson and Shneidman 1995, 280). Physician-assisted suicide is currently being discussed by the U.S. Supreme Court.

In indirect, or passive, euthanasia, death is not induced; it is permitted death accomplished through the omission of an act or acts rather than commission of a life-taking act. For example, doctors might halt treatments that would prolong the life of a patient, or they might withhold treatment altogether. According to several national polls and surveys, the majority of Americans support passive euthanasia (Williamson and Shneidman 1995, 280).

Rapid advances in medical technology have given the medical profession the ability to sustain or prolong life through extraordinary methods, so that those who might have died quickly now have a chance of survival with life-sustaining artificial support mechanisms. An adult in this country is considered to have the right to determine whether this type of medical technology should be employed. The person has the right to expressly prohibit life-saving surgery or other medical treatments. In other words, the right to die with dignity is inherent for every individual, as much so as the right to live. Some individuals fear the indignity and humiliation of existing merely as a vegetable, with others making decisions for them and caring for their every need. These people would rather die a "good death" than exist in this manner. The proponents of euthanasia, or the right to die, state that saving a life is not always the same as saving people, as some do not wish to go on living or be revived. They argue that further extension of life should not be forced on the person just so life itself is preserved. This places an emphasis on the quality of life rather than just the literal existence of life.

Some states have passed laws to ensure their citizens of the right to die. This type of legislation provides death with dignity to those who sign a legal document known as a *living will*. Signers of a living will anticipate a time when they cannot make or communicate decisions about their condition and treatment, but wish to reject artificial means of prolonging life and ask, in most cases, for such treatment to be withheld. The majority of states have passed similar legislation or are currently considering such a bill.

Wills

The last will and testament is a legal instrument declaring a person's intentions concerning the disposition of property, the guardianship of students, or the administration of the estate after a person's death. A will is a legal document in which a person states how he or she wants property and possessions to be distributed after his or her death. By making such a document, people can ensure how their property will be distributed, the cost and time of settling the estate can be reduced, an executor can be named, family quarrels can be avoided, a guardian can be appointed, and a testamentary trust can be created. For most people, ensuring the desired distribution of their property and possessions is sufficient reason for writing a will. Further, a person can enact a living trust that entrusts an estate to another person while the owner of the estate is still alive. A living trust keeps the estate private instead of public, even when the owner of the estate dies. A living trust can avoid probate, attorney fees, and some taxation when the owner of the estate dies.

Perhaps because ours is a society that denies death, most people delay writing a will. It is not surprising that most Americans, even many with sizable estates, do not have a will, because writing a will reminds people of their own mortality.

What Happens When No Will Is Left

A will is needed to ensure that personal property gets distributed as the testator desires, to avoid the consequences of estate and inheritance taxes, and to have some control over one's estate after death. For individuals who die without wills, property passes according to state law. In other words, the state will decide which relatives get which part of the estate, even if the deceased person may have wished otherwise.

Near-Death Experiences

The near-death experiences that have been recorded have remarkable similarities, leading many to believe that they are not merely dreams, as previously thought. Some physicians report not only that their resuscitated patients have similar experiences but also that the events occur in much the same sequence. Generally, people who have such experiences tell about a sensation of being out of their bodies, traveling through some tunnel or tubular conveyance and entering into another world before they return to their bodies. Some of these people experience an "enlightenment," as if their knowledge had been broadened considerably. Others see cities of light, like heaven, or other light imagery. Many report a feeling of being "exposed" in other words, they were not able to hide behind an emotional "mask" and their every thought and deed were portrayed openly (DeSpelder and Strickland 1992, 551–552).

Many people who experience near-death experiences as hospital patients undergoing surgery can recall procedures used on them and remembering what each person in the room said. One patient, a nurse in a coma, recalled the exact procedures used, with total recall. These patients also reported an instant replay of their own lives. Some patients have multiple experiences during a prolonged illness—some of these experiences are bad (usually the first ones), while others are very good. The patients themselves interpret whether the experience is good or bad. Sometimes the unpleasant experiences are so frightening that the conscious mind cannot cope with them, and the patient suppresses them into the subconscious.

Hospices

A hospice is a program, type of care, or facility that cares for the terminally ill and their families. Sometimes hospice care is given in the patient's home, and at other times in a separate wing of a hospital. Generally the goal of hospice care is to enhance the quality of a dying person's life during the last days and to allow the person to live as comfortably and inexpensively as possible.

Suicide

During the last half of this century, suicide among school-age students has increased dramatically. Suicide is now one of the leading causes of death for young Americans (Marrone 1997, 187).

Health Highlight

Warning Signs of Suicide

Suicidal people often give warning signs, consciously or unconsciously, indicating that they need help. Several warning signs often will be apparent. Some of the typical warning signs are as follows:

○ withdrawing from friends and family

○ loss of interest in usual activities

○ showing signs of sadness, hopelessness, irritability

○ changes in appetite, weight, level of activity, or sleep pattern

○ making negative comments about self

○ previous attempts

○ giving away possessions

Source: R. Marrone. 1997. *Death, mourning, and caring*. Pacific Grove, CA: Brooks/Cole.

There is more guilt associated with suicide than with any other type of death. The parents or relatives feel they are somehow to blame for needless death. Some feel that a suicide reflects badly on the parents and family, but this is not always the case. Some hold a religious view that suicide is morally wrong or that one who commits suicide cannot enter heaven.

Any suicidal threat, however subtle, must be taken seriously. Most individuals who commit suicide provide significant clues to their contemplated action. These include obvious changes in mood or behavior, excessive use of drugs, changes in any set of habits, preoccupation with personal health, decreased academic performance, and insomnia.

There are four commonly recommended steps for helping someone who seems in danger of suicide. First, one should talk to the person who threatens suicide and determine how deeply troubled the individual really is. Second, one should not challenge the individual to act on the threat. Such a challenge may force the person to act to prove the validity of the threat. Third, someone can help the person postpone the decision and offer other options to consider. Fourth, one can be knowledgeable about resources that can provide aid. The person might have exhausted all personally known avenues of assistance and might need professional help.

Suicide prevention is a community responsibility, and everyone can play an important part in its resolution. However, many people hold various misconceptions regarding suicide.

Students and Death

Students in our society no longer experience many aspects of the life cycle. Most do not live with grandparents or on farms, so they do not observe aging and death in their immediate environment. Death education is necessary for the proper development of students. Death education should be viewed as a natural topic for inclusion in education because students are not immune to experiencing the death of a loved one, a pet, or a classmate.

Death is inseparable from the whole of human experience. Education about death can bring insights concerning the true nature of the student and help them discover more about themselves. The study of death and dying leads naturally to choices of an emphatically personal nature. Death education is germane to the sphere of social relationships as well as to the confrontation with mortality that comes in the most private, personal moments of solitude and introspection (DeSpelder and Strickland 1992, 567).

Death Education

Positive attitudes toward death can help prepare succeeding generations to face death more realistically. We can help students accept the reality of death by preparing them properly for funerals and by allowing them to mourn, cry, recover from the loss of a pet or a relative, and express grief as part of a healing process. We should talk to students about death in whatever terms they can understand. This discussion can be either from a religious or a factual point of view, depending on the preference of the parents and on the student.

We should explain the cause of death, in order to eliminate any fear or guilt the student might develop as a result of experiencing a death. Do not deceive the student by using euphemisms or half-truths. Parents can even allow the student to go through a funeral and burial ceremony to teach the student cultural customs and rituals related to death.

Another way to teach students about death is to allow—not force—a student to attend a funeral. A recommended method is to take the student first to the funeral of a neighbor or distant relative. Because the parents would not be as physically or emotionally involved in such a situation, they could devote time and energy to the student. Make the funeral a learning experience. Prepare the student before the funeral, ask him or her to watch for certain things during the funeral, and encourage questions afterward. Educating the student through attendance at a funeral will help the student gain a more complete understanding of death and make it more likely that the student will develop a healthy attitude about death.

Finally, students should be encouraged to talk openly about their fears and feelings. This will help eliminate any misgivings the students have and help the parents to respond more appropriately to the emotions expressed. Of course, this assumes that the parents know how to respond and that they will share their own emotions with the student.

Fortunately, people today are more willing to discuss death and dying. The many books available on the subject, the courses being taught in schools and universities, the increased number of bereavement societies and hospice groups, and the increasing number of documentaries, specials, and films in the media are evidence of this. The new openness about death is refreshing—a challenge to the previous treatment of death as a taboo topic for conversation, research, and writing. Communication about death can improve the quality of our lives and help us grow as individuals. Even if we fumble through a discussion on death, as a friend or parent, our effort is very helpful.

Death is a universal part of living, even though it is a taboo topic in our society. Students are interested in knowing more about the subject of death, but they are generally shielded from such exposure. Many parents are reluctant to talk with their students about death because they wish to protect their children (and themselves) from the pain of loss. Students are often prohibited from some hospital wards, health care institutions, and other places where people are dying. As a result, they tend to learn about death through the media, which can be confusing and misleading.

Sooner or later, students must confront death to understand the needs of the dying, to have some preparation for the experience, and to deal with their own feelings. Education about death is a legitimate subject for students. It is an important topic worthy of open, informed, and sensitive discussion. Death education can guide students toward greater understanding about death and dying, and, even though it might be painful for them and for the teacher, gaining such understanding can be essential for sound mental health.

In death education, the teacher should come to terms with her own feelings about death and not just learn the material. She needs to be aware of her students' willingness to express their feelings on this sensitive topic and be ready to let them discuss the subject openly and frankly. One should never tell students they need to wait until they are older to talk about death. Many times adults use this ploy as an excuse to avoid their own insecurities about death. Teachers need to answer any question at the students' level of understanding. Feelings and emotions related to death (the teacher's and the students') should also be allowed to be expressed in the classroom, even encouraged. Teachers can use experiences in the classroom, such as the death of a flower, a pet, or a classmate to teach students about death feelings and rituals.

▤ Summary

- ○ Aging is a normal part of the life cycle, not a pathological condition. We are all aging every day.
- ○ The number of elderly has risen sharply in the past two decades, and this trend is likely to continue.
- ○ The life expectancy for all Americans is increasing.
- ○ The majority of older Americans still own their own homes, and only 5 percent are institutionalized.
- ○ For the most part, the aging process remains poorly understood.
- ○ Many factors, both intrinsic and extrinsic, also affect the aging process for each individual.
- ○ Many biological, psychological, and sociological changes occur as a person ages. Some of these changes present unavoidable problems for the elderly, but other changes can be successfully adjusted to.
- ○ Elderly Americans face many challenges in life, but these issues affect all members of society, not just the aged. Among these challenges are income, retirement, housing, health problems, nutrition, crime, and transportation.
- ○ Some of the problems facing the elderly are the result of discrimination and misconceptions.
- ○ Stereotypes about the elderly largely result from lack of knowledge and insufficient contact with the elderly.
- ○ Intergenerational contact programs in schools can be one of the most effective ways to help students understand aging and the elderly, helping dissolve some of the many myths about aging.
- ○ The elderly of the future will generally enjoy a better standard of living.
- ○ Death is the natural end to life, yet many in our society try to deny its existence.
- ○ Death is mysterious because we do not know what is beyond death.
- ○ Many people fear death and refuse to discuss the topic openly and frankly.
- ○ Everyone has personal beliefs about death. Some of these beliefs are helpful in facing death because they help demystify it.
- ○ Facing death is a traumatic experience for the dying person and survivors alike.

○ The dying person has many emotional needs that often go unmet by relatives and the medical profession. This may leave the dying person very lonely and feeling abandoned.

○ The individual goes through various stages of adjustment to impending death. If we understand these stages, we can better help the dying person.

○ Many controversies and issues surround death, including the definition of death, the person's right to die, organ donation and transplants, wills, and suicide.

○ Most students in our society do not experience death close to home anymore.

○ These students go through definite stages in their understanding of death.

○ Students are interested in knowing more about the subject of death. Thus death education is a legitimate, worthy topic in schools.

Discussion Questions

1. Discuss the significance of aging education and death education in the school curriculum.
2. Describe the benefits of intergenerational contact.
3. Discuss the current demographics of the American elderly.
4. Predict the lifestyle of the American elderly in the year 2000.
5. Why do most people fear death?
6. How can the family help in the adjustment of a dying person?
7. Differentiate among grief, bereavement, and mourning.
8. Why is there more guilt associated with a suicidal death than with other types of deaths?

References

Backer, B. A., N. Hannon, and N. A. Russell. 1994. *Death and dying: Understanding and care,* 2nd ed. Albany, NY: Delmar.

Belsky, J. K. 1990. *The psychology of aging,* 2nd ed. Pacific Grove, CA: Brooks/Cole.

Blieszner, R., and V. H. Bedford, eds. 1995. *Handbook of aging and the family.* Westport, CT: Greenwood Press.

Corless, I. B.,B. B. Germino, and M. Pittman, eds. 1994. *Dying, death, and bereavement: Theoretical perspectives and other ways of knowing.* Boston: Jones & Bartlett.

DeSpelder, L. A., and A. L. Strickland. 1992. *The last dance,* 3rd ed. Mountain View, CA: Mayfield.

Ebersole, P., and P. Hess. 1994. *Toward healthy aging: Human needs and nursing response,* 4th ed. St. Louis: Mosby.

Ferrini, A. F., and R. L. Ferrini. 1993. *Health in the later years,* 2nd ed. Madison, WI: Brown & Benchmark.

Hockey, J., and A. James. 1993. *Growing up and growing old.* London: Sage.

Marrone, R. 1997. *Death, mourning, and caring.* Pacific Grove, CA: Brooks/Cole.

Oaks, J., and G. Ezell. 1993. *Dying and death,* 2nd ed. Scottsdale, AZ: Gorsuch Scarisbrick.

Spirduso, W. W. 1995. *Physical dimensions of aging.* Champaign, IL: Human Kinetics.

Williamson, J. B., and E. S. Shneidman. 1995. *Death: Current perspectives,* 4th ed. Mountain View, CA: Mayfield.

Chapter Twenty-Three
Strategies for Teaching about Aging, Dying, and Death

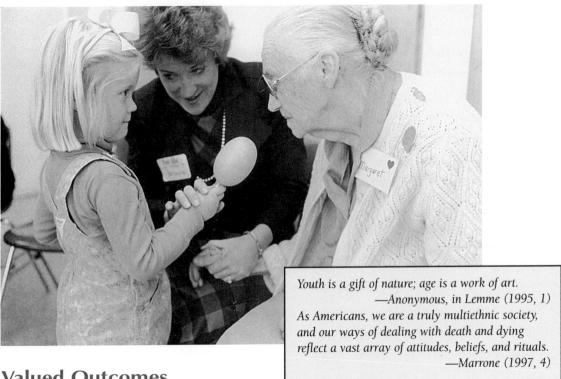

> Youth is a gift of nature; age is a work of art.
> —Anonymous, in Lemme (1995, 1)
> As Americans, we are a truly multiethnic society,
> and our ways of dealing with death and dying
> reflect a vast array of attitudes, beliefs, and rituals.
> —Marrone (1997, 4)

Valued Outcomes

Aging

After doing the exercises in this chapter, the students should be able to explain and illustrate the following statements.

○ Aging is a natural part of the total life cycle.

○ The body changes as a person ages.

○ Exercise and proper diet can retard the aging process to some degree.

○ Most elderly people are healthy and alert.

○ Responsibilities change as a person ages.

○ People use their retirement years for different activities.

○ Elderly people make positive contributions to society.

○ Grandparents and grandchildren can share activities.

○ Older people face many changes and challenges.

○ Medications affect older people differently from younger ones.

○ Nutritional needs differ as one ages.

○ Everyone needs to continue to exercise throughout one's lifetime.

○ The elderly in America are often discriminated against.

○ Many social agencies provide services for the elderly.

Dying and Death

○ Death is a natural end to the life cycle.

○ There are many different ways to determine the exact moment a person dies.

○ Our society generally avoids the topics of death and dying in discussion and conscious thought.

○ Personal beliefs about death and dying can affect mental health and lifestyle.

○ There are vastly contrasting views on what happens to us after we die.

○ There are many misconceptions about how to treat a dying person.

○ Dying people have special needs.

○ The family of a dying person also has special needs.

○ Grief and bereavement naturally follow the death of a close friend or relative.

○ Funeral and burial rituals have significant meaning in our society.

○ People are choosing alternative methods of burials and funerals in order to save money.

○ Wills and testaments are beneficial legal documents.

○ The right to die is a basic human right.

○ Suicide attempts among young people are increasing.

○ There are ways each of us can help a friend who is contemplating suicide to reconsider the action.

○ Organ donation can be considered an "ultimate gift of life."

Introduction

Aging

The percentage of our elderly population is growing extremely fast; therefore, the study of aging is becoming important to everyone. Our culture typically propagates ageism through inaccurate portrayals of elderly people in television, movies, and literature. These stereotypes are shared by young people in this country, primarily because of a lack of opportunity to learn about aging and the aged, and through a lack of contact with older people. Young people often fear older people and the aging process.

We need to present realistic and accurate information to students about aging and the aged. This type of education will allow students to decide for themselves what aging and the elderly are

*Most elderly people are
healthy and alert.*

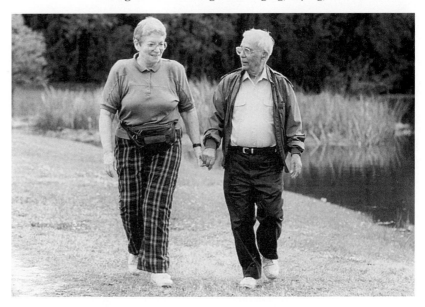

really like. When students are able to understand and develop healthy attitudes toward aging (including their own aging), they will be able to live a higher-quality life as they grow older.

Dying and Death

The death of a relative, or even a pet, can be traumatic to people of all ages, including children. For this reason, some parents approach the problem by trying to shield their children from experiences related to dying and death. Rather than solving the problem, this avoidance leaves the child unprepared to face a natural part of the life cycle. Many children, though they may not have an accurate concept of death, want to know about the many aspects of life related to dying and death, such as funerals and cemeteries. Death education in the elementary schools can help meet this need. Its objectives are to allow children to clarify their values about death and dying, to provide factual information about the subject, and to encourage children to discuss openly the vital issues concerning the natural end of the life cycle.

Value-Based Activities

Aging

Relationships with Elders

Valued Outcome: Students will evaluate relations between younger and older adults.
Description of Strategy: Working in small groups, have students relate how they can interact with older adults in ways that are beneficial to everyone. Each group should share their suggestions with the class.

Materials Needed: paper and pencil
Processing Questions:

1. How would I feel if I were an older adult and wanted to converse with a young person?

2. What might my fears be? my joys, if given this opportunity?

Source: Health: Choosing wellness, Teacher's edition. 1989. Needham, MA: Prentice Hall.

The Aging Process

Valued Outcome: Students will participate in an activity to become aware of issues related to the aging process.
Description of Strategy: Ask the students to answer the following questions, that you will read verbally, on their own sheet of paper. Give them several minutes to write a thoughtful answer to each question.

1. The most important things in life to me right now are . . .

2. When I am seventy years old, the most important things to me will probably be . . .

3. The things that I look forward to about aging are . . .

4. The things that I dread the most about aging are . . .

5. If my parents are no longer able to care for themselves, I will . . .

6. If I am no longer able to care for myself, I will . . .

7. The terms that come to mind when I think of "old" people are . . .

8. To ensure that I will live a full and healthy life, I am doing the following things right now . . .

When the students have finished answering these questions, ask volunteers to report on their answers. Incorporate answers into a group discussion on feelings associated with aging.
Materials Needed: paper and pencil
Processing Questions:

1. Do your responses seem appropriate to you? Why/why not?

2. How do you think other people your age would respond?

3. How would an elderly person respond?

Source: Adapted from R. Donatelle, L. Davis, and C. Hoover. 1988. *Access to health,* Annotated Instructor's Edition. Englewood. Cliffs, NJ: Prentice Hall, p. 434.

Rank Ordering

Valued Outcome: The students will be able to decide which qualities associated with aging s/he most desires.
Description of Strategy: Prepare a list of positive qualities often associated with aging. After discussing these qualities, have students individually rank order each, using the format shown here. Follow with a discussion of why some students feel certain qualities are more desirable than others. Note the importance of individual preferences. Number each of the following from 1 to 5. Use 1 to show that quality or condition about becoming older that appeals to you most, 2 for the second most appealing quality or condition, and so on.

__ Retirement

__ Wisdom

__ Grandchildren

__ Leisure time

__ Satisfaction

Materials Needed: overhead or sheet with these conditions on it
Processing Question: Why are some qualities more desired than others?

Aging Time Line

Valued Outcome: The students will be able to state the most important events in their lives.
Description of Strategy: The teacher will draw a long line on the board. Have different students come to the board, and mark on the line the most important dates in their lives, such as date of birth, birthdates of other siblings, date entering school. Stress that many events happen during our lives, but some are most important. Have them notice on the line how much more time they have for important events.
Materials Needed: none
Processing Question: Do you think events in the future will be as significant to you as events that have already happened?

Aging Voting

Valued Outcome: The students will be able to determine for themselves if they agree with aging-related statements.
Description of Strategy: Have students vote by raising their hands if they agree or disagree with the following statements about aging:

1. Good health habits may affect the length of your life.
2. Good health habits always mean that you are going to live longer than people with bad health habits.
3. Bad health habits can cause a shorter life span.
4. It is important to develop good health habits to enjoy more years of life.
5. Retirement is the worst part about growing old.
6. Grandparents are fun to be around.
7. Growing old makes a person wiser.
8. Growing old is a normal part of life.
9. Old people are not very bright.

Materials Needed: none
Processing Question: What factors determine your attitudes about growing old?

Sentence Completion

Valued Outcome: The students will be able to complete statements related to aging.
Description of Strategy: Instruct students to complete each sentence by writing down their

immediate reaction to the statement. Point out that statements should be honest, even if some are negative. After the exercise, discuss the responses on a volunteer basis. Note varying points of view and discuss possible reasons for these opinions.

1. Aging is . . .

2. Growing old is . . .

3. My grandparents . . .

4. Retirement from full-time work is . . .

5. I think that old people are . . .

Materials Needed: handouts with the preceding statements, pencils for all students
Processing Question: Are your immediate responses the same as they would be if you thought about the statement for awhile?

Decision Stories

Aging

Valued Outcome: The students will be able to answer the focus question in each of the following decision stories.
Description of Strategy: The teacher and students will follow the procedures outlined in chapter 4 for discision stories.

Going for a Visit

Martha's grandparents live in a retirement village in another state. Her family is going to fly there for a visit next month. But Martha doesn't want to go. She visited her grandparents a few years before, when she was younger. She remembers that there was nothing for her to do at her grandparents' home. There were no other kids around. And her grandparents made such a fuss over her. They were nice, but they treated her like a baby. Martha didn't like that, and she wished her grandparents would realize that she was growing up now.
Focus Question: What should Martha do?

Death

Death of a Loved One

Valued Outcome: Students will identify how it feels to lose someone they care about.
Description of Strategy: Propose the question "How did you feel when you once lost something of great value?" to the students. Ask them to write down detailed descriptions. Have students share their responses on a voluntary basis. Explain to students that these common reactions are akin to what people feel when someone dies. Allow class discussion following this activity. (This would be a good activity to use as an introduction to the stages of dying.)
Materials Needed: paper and pencil
Processing Question: Why did I feel the way I did when I lost this item?

Source: M. B. Merki. 1990. *Teen health: Decisions for healthy living*, Teacher's manual. Mission Hills. CA: Glencoe/McGraw-Hill, p. 172–173.

How It Felt

Valued Outcome: Students will demonstrate, through artistic expression, what they think a funeral is.

Description of Strategy: Allow students to tell stories about a funeral they have attended or what they think a funeral involves, using felt boards with felt cutout figures and objects that represent things associated with funerals (such as flowers, angels, crosses, cemeteries, coffins, guns, blood, crashed cars, and so on). Offer each child an opportunity to create a story about being at the funeral home, the funeral or memorial service, the cemetery, or the family gathering after the funeral.

Materials Needed: felt board and cutouts

Processing Questions:

1. What do you associate with funeral experiences?
2. Are they positive or negative things? Why?

Anagrams

Valued Outcome: Students will create an anagram to increase awareness of feelings.

Description of Strategy: Have children choose a phrase, word or name (such as "I remember . . ." family, Sarah, Mom, and so on). Then have them write it down vertically on a piece of paper. Next have the children write down sentences or phrases using the first letter of the chosen word. This activity will help students identify feelings about people, places, things that are special to them.

Materials Needed: paper, markers

Processing Questions:

1. What are some things that are important to me, and what is it about these things (or people) that make them special to me?
2. Why do I like them?
3. What will I always remember about them?

Source: Waving goodbye: An activities manual for children in grief. 1993. Activity submitted by The Dougy Center, Portland, OR, p. 36.

Memorial Quilt

Valued Outcome: Students will have the opportunity to memorialize the death of a pet or loved one.

Description of Strategy: Each child is given a blank square of fabric to decorate with the name of their deceased. The squares don't have to be washable—so there is a lot of leeway for how they are decorated. A 1/2-inch seam allowance should be allowed all around the square so it can be seamed or sashed together. The group can vote on a favorite fabric to sash it together. A sleeve can be sewn on the back so the piece can be hung.

(*Variation:* Using squares or circles of colored paper, design a block to represent a deceased family member. Hole punch corners or circle quadrants and tie them together with colored yarn.)

Materials Needed: white cotton fabric 9-x 9-feet square, fabric paints, markers, appliqué items, and decorative glitter.

Processing Question: What things help me remember my deceased pet or person?

Source: *Sharing our best, A collection of activities and ideas to use in bereavement groups for children and teens, compiled Spring of 1995* by: The Kids Grief Network of Western Washington, Puyallup, WA, p. 3. Activity submitted by BRIDGES: A Center for Grieving Children.

Clarifying Values on Suicide

Valued Outcome: Students will clarify their values on the subject of suicide.
Description of Strategy: Read the following Associated Press article, and have the students discuss their opinions about the issue at hand.

Golden Gate Bridge authorities have beefed up security to delay as long as possible the inevitable 500th fatal leap from the western hemisphere's most famous suicide spot.

Authorities don't doubt someone will jump from the 6,451-foot span that stands at the gateway to San Francisco Bay. Number 499 took the 240 foot plunge Monday—and Dr. Richard H. Seiden, who is conducting an intensive three-year study of bridge suicides, said he half expected someone obsessed with a bizarre kind of fame of being number 500 to take the leap right afterward.

Bridge directors are currently considering an eight-foot-high fence of pencil-thick steel rods to replace the present low barrier. Its estimated cost is $800,000.

Dale W. Luehring, the bridge general manager, said, "my mail is running three to one against a suicide barrier." Reasons for opposing the barrier, he said range from those who say bridge officials don't have any authority to tell people whether they should live or die to those saying the $800,000 should be put into new mass transit facilities for people who want to live.

Source: AP, September 1973.
Processing Questions:

1. Do you feel that persons with authority have the right to tell people whether they can or cannot commit suicide?

2. How do you think the $800,000 should be spent?

Source: D. Read. 1980. *Creative teaching in health*, 3rd ed. Prospect Heights, IL: Waveland Press, p. 135.

Body Map

Valued Outcome: Students will participate in an activity and will validate that emotional pain is felt physically.
Description of Strategy: Talk about how we hold our feelings—store them somewhere inside our bodies. Give the students a copy of a handout of an outline of a body, and inform them that this is a "picture of you." Ask them to think of a particular situation when they lost something or someone. Have them put their names on it, and color their "feelings" in different parts of their bodies, using different colors. Give the feelings a name. Discuss the final products of the students; ask them to comment on their work.
Materials Needed: body outline handouts, pens or crayons
Processing Questions:

1. What are the feelings you felt when you lost something or someone?

2. Did you have physical feelings in your body? Where are/were they?

3. Do you still feel them?

Source: *Sharing our best, A collection of activities and ideas to use in bereavement groups for children and teens, compiled Spring of 1995* by: The Kids Grief Network of Western Washington, Puyallup, WA, p. 27. Activity submitted by Journey Program.

Values Statements

Valued Outcome: The students will be able to clarify their values regarding death.
Description of Strategy: Have the students complete each of the following statements with their first reactions. Afterwards, discuss how different individuals react and feel about each issue raised in the statements.

1. When I think about death, I . . .
2. To me, death means . . .
3. If I could choose how I will die, I would . . .
4. My greatest fear about dying is . . .
5. When I think about relatives who have died, I . . .

Materials Needed: handouts with the preceding statements, pencils for all students
Processing Question: What events in your life have determined your attitudes about death?

Personal Views on Suicide

Valued Outcome: The students will be able to clarify their values regarding suicide.
Description of Strategy: Have students answer and discuss these questions:

1. Do you feel that an individual has the right to make the ultimate decision as to whether he or she should live or die?
2. What would you do if a friend said to you, "I think I might commit suicide—would you help me?" Would you:

    a. call the police
    b. do nothing
    c. ask why
    d. call a doctor
    e. send your friend away with the statement "Sorry, but I am unable to help you!"
    f. try to help by talking

3. What do you feel might be one possible answer to suicide prevention?

Materials Needed: none
Processing Question: Why do some people feel differently about suicide deaths as opposed to other types of deaths?

Me Boxes

Valued Outcome: Students will reflect on self-image, and the changes in one's self following a loss.

Description of Strategy: Each person decorates the outside of a box showing how others see him or her. Then decorate the inside of the box with how you see yourself or how you would like to be. Share boxes with group as comfortable. Group gives positive feedback on each. *Hint:* Try to ask everyone to help collect boxes a few weeks in advance.

Materials Needed: small cardboard boxes (shoe boxes work well), stickers, construction paper, glue/tape, markers, colorful contact paper, magazine cutouts, and so on

Processing Questions:

1. What do I really like about myself?

2. What do others see in me?

3. How might I change the things about myself that are not so good?

Source: Burrell, R., B. Coe, G. Hamm. 1994, November. *Fernside idea book: A guidebook for group facilitators at Fernside: A center for grieving children.* Cincinnati, OH, p. 107.

On Living and Dying

Valued Outcome: The students will be able to decide if death-related ideas are acceptable to them.

Description of Strategy: Have students look over the various statements. They relate to death, dying and living. Have the students ask themselves, "Would this idea be acceptable or unacceptable to me?" They can use a rating scale as follows:

1 = very acceptable

2 = acceptable

3 = unsure

4 = unacceptable

5 = not acceptable at all

1. being killed in an auto accident

2. living forever

3. dying slowly

4. dying of cancer

5. being saved through medical help but unable to walk again

6. being able to choose when you will die

7. dying before your spouse

8. living to age 110

9. dying after your spouse

10. choosing how you will die

Materials Needed: handouts with the preceding statements, pencils for all students

Processing Question: Why should we consider our own death?

Value Voting

Valued Outcome: The students will be able to verbalize his or her bio-ethical values regarding death-related issues.

Description of Strategy: Present a series of statements such as the following to your class. First, explain that each statement represents the way some people feel about death-related issues. Then ask students to raise their hands if they basically agree with the stance or to keep hands down if they disagree. After each show of hands, allow students who wish to comment on the statement to do so. Follow the activity with a general discussion of issues that came up.

1. Euthanasia is murder.

2. Euthanasia is a peaceful way to die.

3. Euthanasia is murder only if the patient is conscious.

Materials Needed: none
Processing Question: Why is euthanasia such a controversial issue?

First Encounters

Valued Outcome: The students will be able to describe their first encounter with death.
Description of Strategy: On a sheet of paper, ask the students to write down a description of their very first encounter with death. Let volunteers relate their experience to the class. Divide the class into small groups, and have group members compare answers and discuss their feelings.
Materials Needed: paper and pencils for all students
Processing Question: How did your first encounter with death shape your current views about dying and death?

Source: J. Oaks and G. Ezell. 1993. *Dying and death*, 2nd ed. Scottsdale, AZ: Gorsuch-Scarisbrick.

Decision Stories—Dying and Death

Valued Outcome: The students will be able to answer the focus question in each of the following decision stories.
Description of Strategy: The teacher and students will follow the procedures outlined in chapter 4 for decision stories.

Sally's Grief

The mother of Karen's best friend, Sally, died in an automobile accident. Sally had not called Karen yet, but Karen knew that she needed to talk to Sally. She had heard that Sally was not coping with her mother's death well at all. Karen also wanted to see Sally, but she was unsure of what to say or do once she saw Sally.
Focus Question: What could Karen say or do?

A Gift of Life

Loretta is dying of kidney disease. She knows it and has accepted the fact of her coming death. Now her doctors would like to use her heart in a transplant operation. They tell her that her heart could be used to help another person to live. Loretta isn't sure about the matter.
Focus Question: What should Loretta do?

Good relationships with grandparents can enhance a child's life.

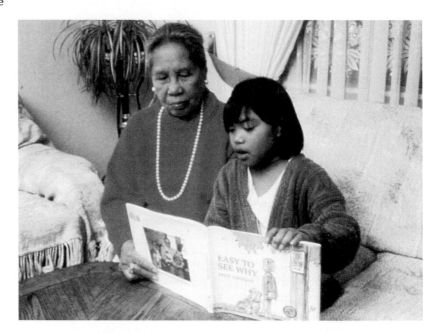

Dramatization

Aging

Role-Playing Life Stages

Valued Outcome: Each student should have a better understanding of the aging process.
Description of Strategy: Assign different roles to students—any role from the family baby to a teenager to a grandparent. Students should be encouraged to use costumes and other props to support their role-playing. The role-playing may be performed in mime or otherwise, but it should clearly demonstrate the characteristics of the people they represent. The role-playing exercise in this case would be best performed when showing the response of family members and the individuals to aging.
Materials Needed: costumes and props
Processing Questions:

1. What is your response to getting older?
2. What is your favorite stage of life? Why?

Grandparents/Grandchildren

Valued Outcome: The students will be able to discuss relationships with grandparents.
Description of Strategy: Assign several students to role-play a situation involving grandchildren and grandparents. The roles will be: grandfather, grandmother, mother, father, sister, and broth-

er. The scene is a visit from the grandparents. The dad will ask the children to remain at home for the day to spend visiting with the grandparents. One child will be instructed to play the role with a lot of enthusiasm, while the other child will resent being made to stay home because of missing the afternoon playing with friends.

Materials Needed: none

Processing Questions:

1. How should a child relate to grandparents?

2. Do you have any meaningful relationships with an elderly person?

Elderly Puppet Show

Valued Outcome: The students will be able to describe physical attributes of the elderly.

Description of Strategy: Have three students enact the following: A young boy and girl set out on a hike in the morning and come to a bridge. An old troll there is angered by their presence and casts a spell on them to make them "old for a day." They examine themselves and find the following traits, which they discuss with each other: wrinkled skin with aging spots, gray hair (boy becomes bald), cannot move as quickly and not as strong, quickly out of breath on their hike.

Materials Needed: none

Processing Question: What physical effects occur during the aging process?

Now I Am Old

Valued Outcome: The students will be able to differentiate between an active and inactive retirement lifestyle.

Description of Strategy: Have two volunteers role-play situations where two elderly retirees are planning the day's activities. One situation could include two retirees who are very active, and another where the two retirees are inactive. Follow up the activity by asking the students with which of the characters they most identified.

Materials Needed: none

Processing Questions: Can a retiree be healthy if he or she chooses an inactive lifestyle during retirement?

Dying and Death

Grandpa is Dying

Valued Outcome: Students will simulate what it is like to experience the death of a loved one.

Description of Strategy: Working in pairs, have students role-play a conversation between two young people (cousins or siblings) whose grandparent is dying. Discuss ways to support your grandparent, the rest of your family, and each other.

Materials Needed: none

Processing Questions:

1. How would I feel if my grandparent were dying or how did I feel when my grandparent died?

2. How do you think you would feel if you were your grandparent who is dying?

Source: Health: Choosing wellness, Teacher's edition. 1989. Needham, MA: Prentice Hall, p. 361.

Bereavement Role-Play

Valued Outcome: Students will feel the feelings of bereavement by acting out situations and life experiences.

Description of Strategy: Suggest various scenarios that are common to bereaved teens. Let the group act them out. Brainstorm for scenarios that teens want to act out or have someone else act them out for them. Write the scenarios on index cards for future activities.

Materials Needed: index cards, pencil

Processing Question: What are some behaviors I have noticed in friends, family, or in myself, who were dealing with the death of a loved one?

Source: N. Flynn and M. Erickson. 1996. *Teen talk: Grief support group for teenagers.* Puyallup, WA: Good Samaritan Hospice, p. 16.

Coping with a Death

Valued Outcomes:

1. The students will be able to describe some ways to help himself or herself cope with a death of a pet, friend or relative close to him or her.

2. The students will be able to role-play characters affected by death or offering sympathy.

Description of Strategy: The teacher will start the lesson by asking the students to divide into groups of two. Give each group of two a role-play situation card.

Examples:
You are the one who must tell your five-year-old sister that the family pet has been run over by a car.

Your teacher's mother died unexpectedly of a heart attack. Today is her first day back to school. Also, give each child a puppet to role-play with. Get puppets by making them with the students a day in advance with some paper bags.)

Have the groups practice the situations out with the puppets. After each group is through, have the groups go back to the big discussion group circle. Have each group perform the card situation out in front of the rest of the class. After each situation, discuss with the students how it felt to be the person affected by the death or the person offering sympathy. Also, after the discussions are over, hand each student a piece of paper. Tell each student to write down several things that a best friend could say that would make him or her feel better if someone special they were close to had died.

Materials Needed: enough situation cards for all pairs of two students, puppets, white construction paper

Processing Questions:

1. What things should be said to a friend whose relative has died?

2. What should a person do to help him or her cope with a close relative's death?

Source: L. Landy. 1992. *Child support: Through small group counseling.* Charlotte, NC: Kids Right.

Suicide

Valued Outcome: The students will be able to discuss ways to help a suicidal friend.

Description of Strategy: Have two students role-play that one friend is calling the other to tell him or her that their best friend just attempted suicide by taking an overdose of pills. Let the students bring the role-play to closure by discussing ways they can help their mutual friend.

Materials Needed: a sample prescription bottle with "fake" pills

Processing Question: How can an untrained person help a suicidal friend?

Talk Can Help

Valued Outcome: The students will be able to describe how to visit a friend who is dying in the hospital.

Description of Strategy: Have one student play the part of a dying patient in a hospital. Have another play the role of a close friend who comes to visit. Role-play the situation for five minutes per pair of students. Ask each student to play the part in the way that seems most comfortable and natural. Have the students switch roles so all will have the opportunity to play the "dying patient." Discuss the different approaches used in acting out this situation.

Materials Needed: bed for "dying" patient

Processing Question: What should one say when visiting a dying friend in the hospital?

Only One Week To Live

Valued Outcome: The students will be able to discuss what they would consider most important in their lives if facing death.

Description of Strategy: Have volunteers role-play an interviewee who has just been asked what he or she would do if he or she only had one week to live. This activity could be spontaneous, or you could allow the volunteers some time to think about the activities and list them.

Materials Needed: none

Processing Question: How does facing death affect our values and desires?

Discussion and Report Techniques

Aging

A Long Time Ago

Valued Outcome: Students will be able to think about and discuss changes and what causes them.

Description of Strategy: This is a peer support group activity. Talk about changes in people. Do you know anyone who seems to have changed? Have students complete the following statements:

A long time ago I was . . .	But now I am . . .
A long time ago I thought . . .	But now I am . . .
A long time ago I felt . .	But now I feel . . .
A long time ago I wanted . . .	But now I wish . . .
A long time ago I couldn't imagine . . .	But now I realize . . .
A long time ago I . . .	But now I . . .

After students complete the statements divide the class into small groups for sharing and discussion of their responses. Ask a representative from each group to report on the similarities and differences that arose from their discussion.

Materials Needed: paper and pencil

Source: Burrell, R., B. Coe, G. Hamm. 1994, November. *Fernside idea book: A guidebook for group facilitators at Fernside: A center for grieving children.* Cincinnati, OH, p. 105.

Life Collage

Valued Outcome: The students will create and present a visual representation of their lives from birth to present.

Description of Strategy: Have students bring in articles from home that are special to them and that they feel helps explain who they are. Encourage them to bring things from their early childhood as well as newer things. Stress that items should be small enough to be glued or taped to poster board (which they should also bring from home). Distribute magazines, and have students cut out anything that relates to their life up to the present (toys they have or had, baby for sibling). Remind them only to cut out things that already apply to them, not that they hope will in the future. Have students glue or tape items to their poster board. When they have finished, have students tell the class about their collage and explain how the things they chose are significant to their life.

Materials Needed: magazines, personal items, poster board, glue, tape, scissors

Processing Questions:

1. Why is it important to include items from your early childhood?

2. What part of your collage do you think best represents who you are? Why?

Me—When I Am Old

Valued Outcome: The students will understand the aging process, along with the effects of aging.

Description of Strategy: Have students draw pictures showing how they might look when they are old. What losses do they depict in the drawings? a loss of hair? eyesight (eyeglasses)? hearing (hearing aids)? What things are new in their lives? canes? walkers? medications? Have students stand and present their drawings. At this time ask the children to explain their pictures and talk about how they think they might feel being old.

Materials Needed: 8 1/2- x 11-inch paper, markers, coloring crayons

Processing Questions:

1. Do you think it will matter what you look like when you are old?

2. Will you care what you look like?

Source: R. Loya, ed. 1983. *Health-education teaching ideas,* Secondary Level. Reston, VA: American Alliance for Health, Physical Education, Recreation and Dance, pp. 75–76.

Panel Discussion

Valued Outcome: The students will be able to discuss the social and emotional problems faced by elderly people.

Description of Strategy: Divide the class into small groups, and have each group research a problem area for elderly Americans. These areas should include health problems, financial problems, problems due to stereotypes and misconceptions, forced retirement, crime, and loneliness. After research is complete, have each group present a panel discussion of their findings. Group members should be prepared to answer questions from the class about the problem area that they have researched.

Materials Needed: research books, such as *World Book* or *Encyclopedia Britannica*

Processing Questions:

1. What health problems do elderly people face?

2. What social problems do elderly people face?

3. What financial problems do elderly people face?

Services for the Elderly

Valued Outcome: The students will be able to explain how the Social Security program benefits the elderly.

Description of Strategy: Ask a member of a local Social Security office to come to class and explain the Social Security system provided to elderly people. Or have students research the Social Security program and present a lecture to the class.

Materials Needed: none

Processing Questions:

1. How does the Social Security program benefit elderly people?

2. How does an elderly person become involved in this program?

Quality Time with Grandparents

Valued Outcome: The students will be able to relate a positive experience with an elderly person.

Description of Strategy: Have students write a paragraph on the best time they have spent with a grandparent or elderly friend. Have volunteers share the essay with the class.

Materials Needed: paper and pen/pencil

Processing Questions: What type of positive experiences can a young person have with an elderly person?

Fountain of Youth

Valued Outcome: The students will be able to discuss the implications of a population which never grew old and died.

Description of Strategy: Have students debate whether a fountain of youth would be good or bad for humans.

Materials Needed: none

Processing Questions:

1. What if everyone stayed young and did not die?

2. What implications for overpopulation would there be?

Time Line

Valued Outcome: The students will see all the important events in his or her life.
Description of Strategy: Have children draw a horizontal line on a piece of paper and fill in the last birthday they had. Have them choose the next event in his or her life that feels important (they can draw pictures, too). Fill that in with corresponding age. Continue to have them fill in the important events in their life. Provide time for each child to share his or her work. Suggest that the students may wish to do this again with their family and that we all may see very different things as important.

   Note: For older children, an additional concept of a graph can be added to this activity. High, medium, and low graph lines allow the event to reflect the feelings of the time.
Materials Needed: paper, pencils and crayons
Processing Questions:

1. What are some major events that have occurred in my life thus far?

2. What gave them meaning?

Source: Waving goodbye: An activities manual for children in grief. 1993. Activity submitted by The Dougy Center, Portland, OR, p. 34.

Dying and Death

Good Grief!

Valued Outcome: Students will be able to understand normal process and validate normality.
Description of Strategy: Prepare a handout of ten to twenty experiences that are common to grief. Through discussion, compare the class experiences with those on the handout.
Materials Needed: copies of handout
Processing Questions:

1. How do my experiences compare to those on the handout?

2. Are they normal responses and feelings related to grief and loss?

Source: N. Flynn and M. Erickson. 1996. *Teen talk: Grief support group for teenagers.* Puyallup, WA: Good Samaritan Hospice, p. 12.

Stages of Grief

Valued Outcome: Students will be acquainted with the stages of grief in relation to death.
Description of Strategy: Have students think about movies or TV programs they have seen. Ask them to describe the different ways people show their grief. Emphasize that expressing grief is positive because it serves as an outlet for emotions. Also emphasize that, like the stages of dying, there are stages of grief. Again, a person may go through some of the stages or all the stages. Some of the stages may occur simultaneously.
Materials Needed: none
Processing Questions:

1. What are the stages of dying? Of grief?

2. In what ways do we express emotions in each of these stages?

Source: L. Meeks and P. Heit. 1991. *Health: A wellness approach,* Teacher's edition. Blacklick, OH: Meeks Heit, p. 220.

The Truth about Bereavement

Valued Outcome: Students will learn how to communicate with those experiencing the grieving process.

Description of Strategy: Explain that the peak time of grief for most people begins in the week after a loved one's funeral. Realizing that there is no one guaranteed formula for helping the bereaved, friends and caregivers can help by performing some or all of the following points. Give this True or False quiz to the students (have them circle the correct letter) and then discuss each point. The students should realize that all their answers are "true," thus giving them the "Truth about Bereavement."

T/F   1.   Make few demands on the bereaved; allow him or her to grieve.

T/F   2.   Help with the household tasks.

T/F   3.   It is okay if the bereaved person vents anguish and anger, even if some of it is directed at you.

T/F   4.   The bereaved person has painful and difficult tasks to complete; mourning cannot be rushed or avoided.

T/F   5.   You should not be afraid to talk about the deceased person; this lets the bereaved know that you care for the deceased.

T/F   6.   Express your own genuine feelings of sadness, but avoid pity. Speak from the heart.

T/F   7.   Reassure bereaved persons that the intensity of their emotions is very natural.

T/F   8.   Advise the bereaved to get additional help if you suspect continuing major emotional or physical distress.

T/F   9.   Keep in regular contact with the bereaved; let him or her know you continue to care about them.

Materials Needed: a copy of the preceding True/False activity for each student.

Processing Question: How would I want to be treated or cared for by my family and friends in the event that I should lose a loved one?

Source: Information adapted from W. Payne and D. Hahn. 1992. *Understanding your health,* 3rd ed. St. Louis: Mosby-Year Book, p. 606.

Dear Aunt Blabby . . .

Valued Outcome: Students will participate in an activity that encourages sharing and problem solving.

Description of Strategy: Prepare a fictitious letter that asks "Aunt Blabby" for advice concerning a common situation that teens may face after a death in their family. Read this letter to the group, and ask the teens to respond with their own advice. The teens take on the role of Aunt Blabby (like "Dear Abby"). Read some of the anonymous responses. Remind the students that if we expect others to treat us respectfully and with caring when we are in pain, then we want to also be gentle and compassionate toward others.

Materials Needed: pencil and paper
Processing Question: How would I want to be helped if I were on the receiving end of advice concerning a death in my family?

Source: N. Flynn and M. Erickson. 1996. *Teen talk: Grief support group for teenagers.* Puyallup, WA: Good Samaritan Hospice, p. 22.

Keys to Communication

Valued Outcome: Students will be able to communicate thoughts, feelings, and opinions appropriately.
Description of Strategy: Make a construction paper key for each student. On one key, write the word *communication*, but do not call attention to it. Prepare a box with a keyhole cut to fit the "communication" key. Tell students that each of them is to try to unlock the box with their keys. None of the keys will work, except the "communication" key. When that key is tried, the box will open. Tell students that "communication" is the key to understanding each other. Let the student who opened the box distribute the worksheets (each with one of the following topics) previously placed inside the box. After the students discuss the topics, lead a class discussion on communication. Ask students to name other topics that might be difficult to talk about with another person. Examples of topics to place in the box are

attraction to a special boy or girl

depression

financial problems

anger toward someone

death in the family

divorce in the family

one's weight or complexion

Ask students to suggest why these topics are difficult to discuss. Point out that listeners can make it easier for a person to express his or her feelings by being attentive, responsible, and sensitive to the person's feelings. Discuss the following ways that students can improve their listening skills: Give full attention to the person talking, show the person talking that you understand his or her feelings, restate the person's thoughts and feelings to show that you are really listening. If time permits, allow students to create role-play situations in which they can practice their communication skills. Use the preceding list of difficult situations listed above as topics.
Materials Needed: "topic sheets," construction paper, box
Processing Question: What are some things I can do to improve my listening skills?

Source: American School Health Association. 1994. The key to healthy communication. *Journal of school health* 64(3): 123–125.

Preventing Premature Death

Valued Outcome: Students will recognize that many causes of premature death can be prevented by positive health practices and appropriate health care.
Description of Strategy: Obtain two pictures of automobiles—one of a new car and the other of a classic older car that is in mint condition. The second car should be at least twenty years old but

in outstanding condition. You can get these pictures from a magazine, or you can visit your local new car dealer who should have many promotional brochures containing pictures of cars from which you can choose. Bring the car pictures to class. Begin this strategy by showing the pictures of the cars to students. Ask the students to share what they see as the differences between the cars. Ask the students to make comments about the conditions of the cars. They most likely will say, "Although the two cars are different, they both look like they are in excellent condition." Tell students that although both cars appear to be in excellent condition, one is new and the other is old. Explain that in many respects, people of all ages, whether young or old, can be in great condition if they have taken the time to care for their bodies and their minds. Discuss aging, heredity, and other factors that are present in the aging process. Tell the students that one way to stay healthy during older age is to practice healthful behaviors at a young age. Explain that the two leading causes of death among all people are heart disease and cancer. Explain that, to a large degree, the premature development of these two diseases is influenced by one's lifestyle.

Materials Needed: two pictures of automobiles; one of a new car and one of a classic older car that is in mint condition.

Processing Questions:

1. What are some of the lifestyle habits of your parents and/or grandparents and how have they affected their health through the years?

2. What lifestyle habits do I want to incorporate into my life to keep me healthy?

Source: Adapted from L. Meeks and P. Heit. Awsome aging. 1996. *Totally awesome health*, Sixth grade manual. Blacklick, OH: Meeks Heit, pp. 73–74.

Obituary

Valued Outcome: The students will write their own obituaries as they would appear in the newspaper.

Description of Strategy: Read several obituaries from the newspaper aloud to the class. Have students write their own obituaries, modeling the ones that they heard. Require students to include the date and cause of death and a list of survivors. Any other information provided is the student's choice (such as occupation, achievements, residence, and so on). Have students type and print out their obituaries on the computer. Display the obituaries on the class bulletin board.

Materials Needed: newspapers, paper, pencils, computer

Processing Question: Why did you choose the lifestyle that you did for yourself?

Dealing with Death

Valued Outcomes:

1. Students will recognize that all human beings will eventually die.

2. Students will recognize that in the face of death sadness is a fitting emotion.

Description of Strategy: Use the subject of the death of pets to lead into a general discussion of death. Tell students about a pet you or one of your family members had that died, and read one of the many excellent books on the death of a pet. Although these books focus on the death of pets, many of them obliquely refer to death of people. Some available book titles are:

Father's Laika, by Mats Wahl

Jim's Dog Muffins, by Miriam Cohen

Goodbye, Max, by Holly Keller

The Dead Bird, by Margaret Wise Brown

Better With Two, by Catherine Stock

It Must Hurt A Lot: A Child's Book About Death, by Doris Sanford

Materials Needed: books of choice

Processing Questions: After reading the story, have students identify some of the feelings that the main character or characters had. Allow time for students to ask questions or to talk about family pets that have died. For those who have had a family member or pet die, ask what kind of feelings they felt at the time? How did they start to feel better? (Maybe a new pet, counseling, and so on.) Stress that sadness is an appropriate feeling when a loved pet dies.

Source: G. Ezell. 1992. *Healthy living 2: Healthy and growing*. Grand Rapids, MI: Christian Schools International, p. 68.

Elderly I.Q.

Valued Outcome: Students will test their knowledge about the elderly and will be able to discriminate between truths and misconceptions with regard to the aging process.

Description of Strategy: Have the student write "yes" or "no" to the following questions as you read them out. Explain that this will be a personal assessment of what they know about aging. Quiz them before and after you cover aging as a topic of discussion. This will stimulate thought about aging and will demonstrate their success in understanding aging after this section is taught.

What Do You Know about Aging?

1. A person's height tends to decline in old age.
2. Older people have more acute (short-term) illnesses than do people under age sixty-five.
3. The aged are more fearful of crime than are people under sixty-five.
4. More of the aged vote than any other group.
5. There are proportionately more older people in public office than in the total population.
6. Most old people live alone.
7. All five senses tend to decline in old age.
8. When the last child leaves home, the majority of parents have serious problems adjusting to their "empty nest."
9. Aged people have fewer accidents per driver than drivers under sixty-five.
10. One-tenth of the aged live in long-stay institutions like nursing homes.
11. Most old people report they are seldom angry or irritated.
12. Most old people are socially isolated and lonely.
13. Most old people work or would like to have some kind of work (including housework or volunteer work).
14. Medicare pays more than half of the medical expenses for the aged.
15. Social Security benefits automatically increase with inflation.

Answers: Odd-numbered questions are "yes"; even-numbered questions are "no."
Materials Needed: pencil and paper
Processing Questions:

1. What were the sources of the information on which you based your responses?

2. How would you describe the quality of the relationships you have had thus far with older adults?

3. What aspects of middle age do you find the most and least attractive?

4. Have you identified any misconceptions about older adults that you may have had?

Source: W. Payne and D. Hahn. 1992. *Understanding your health,* 3rd ed. St. Louis: Mosby-Yearbook, p. 574.

Elderly True-False

Valued Outcome: The students will better understand dying.
Description of Strategy: The teacher will write on the chalkboard the following facts and have students determine whether or not they are true or false.

1. Mature individuals often find themselves unable to cope with the thought of death.

2. Individuals generally choose to ignore death.

3. When death is brought up in conversation, it is usually in the form of a joke.

Then engage the class in a round robin to discuss the responses.
Materials Needed: none
Processing Question: Why is our society considered a "death denying" society?

Why Should I Have a Will?

Valued Outcome: The students will be able to explain why each adult should have a will.
Description of Strategy: Discuss with the class the reasons for having a will. Describe the format of the will, and have the students prepare wills for themselves, with two classmates acting as "witnesses." Have students list their important possessions and the people to whom they would like to bequeath these things.
Materials Needed: paper and pencils for all students
Processing Question: Should adults without a lot of possessions have a will?

Dying

Valued Outcome: Students will see that adjusting to dying and understanding these stages is critical to understanding the needs of a dying person.
Description of Strategy: The teacher will give the following directions to the students: "There are five stages of dying and they are listed here out of order. Please put the stages back in order by placing the number of the stage beside the sentence where it belongs."

Depression: The patient is saddened by the fact that death is approaching and then starts the grief process for the losses death will entail.

Denial and isolation: Learning of the diagnosis of a terminal condition, the patient reacts with disbelief.

Bargaining: The patient is accepting the inevitability of death and begins to bargain (with God or others) for more time.

Anger: The reality of impending death begins to seep into the patient's consciousness, and anger is the reaction.

Acceptance or Resolution: The patient resolves the issue of death.

Materials Needed: handouts with the preceding descriptions of stages, pencils for all students
Processing Question: Why is it important for each of us to understand the stages of grief?

Dying and Death Individual Rights

Valued Outcome: Students will establish what they think their rights are as human beings facing death.

Description of Strategy: Divide class into groups of four or five. Have the students brainstorm what they perceive as their rights as human beings who will be faced with death at some point in their lives. Ask them to list the things that are important to them regarding their feelings about personal issues in their lives and what they would have done to preserve these things in the event that they knew they were dying. Have the students report on their findings. Assign yourself the role of recorder, and on the board, write "The Dying Person's Bill of Rights." As the students report their findings, add them to the list of the Bill of Rights. Discuss the importance of coming to terms with one's rights as a human being facing death.

Materials Needed: chalk/chalkboard
Processing Questions:

1. How do I want to be treated as an individual?

2. Should this treatment change if I may be dying? Why or why not?

Describing the Stages of Grief

Valued Outcome: The students will be able to identify feelings that he or she might feel when a grandparent dies.

Description of Strategy: The teacher will start the lesson by showing a chart with the five stages of grief on it. Talk about the chart with the students. Divide students into four or five equal groups. Give each group a poster, a marker and a ruler. Have each group make a new chart of the five stages of grief like the one that you show them. Have each group make up their own sentence for each stage. After the groups are finished, bring all groups together and look at the charts that they made. Talk about each chart and go over the sentences they made for each stage of grief.

Give each student a piece of white paper. On the paper, have the students write about one special gift that they could give to a grandparent that is still living. (*Example:* poem, flowers, colored picture)

Materials Needed: five or six poster boards, five or six markers, sheets of white paper for every student

Processing Question: Have you ever experienced any of these stages of grief?

Source: L. Landy. 1992. *Child support: Through small group counseling.* Charleston, NC: Kids Right.

Holiday Memories

Valued Outcome: The students will be able to identify some holidays or memories in a group setting to remember his or her parent who has died.

Description of Strategy: The teacher will start the lesson by handing out two magazines and a piece of white construction paper to each student. The students will look through the magazines and find pictures that describes a parent's physical features or what the parent likes to do. The students will cut out pictures and then, make a collage of the pictures. After students make their collages, have every student display his or her picture on a bulletin board.

Give each group a sheet of paper. Have the group come up with ideas of what they could do in memory of a parent who dies. For example, draw a picture of a vase or write a poem. When everyone is finished, have all groups share their ideas with class .

Materials Needed: two magazines per student, white construction paper, scissors and glue, markers, student journals

Processing Question: Why is it important to recall memories of loved ones who have died?

Source: L. Landy. 1992. *Child support: Through small group counseling.* Charleston, NC: Kids Right.

My Pet Died

Valued Outcome: The students will be able to describe the experience of having a pet die.

Description of Strategy: Most students have had pets that died—either dogs, cats, hamsters, or other small animals. Ask students who have had the experience of having a pet die to write a short report about the event. The reports should emphasize the things about the pet that the child liked most. Explain that we can remember those qualities and talk about the pleasure or companionship of a past pet even though the pet will never return to us. Note the comfort that such fond memories can bring.

Materials Needed: paper, pen/pencil

Processing Question: Why should we recall qualities of pets who have died?

Experiments and Demonstrations

Aging

Last Year's Clothing

Valued Outcome: The students will be able to discuss how they are aging, and the implications of the aging process for them.

Description of Strategy: Have students bring in articles of clothing that they wore a year before and try them on. Use this activity as a springboard for a discussion of growth and aging. Note that the process is a continuum and a normal part of the life cycle.

Materials Needed: clothing (brought in by students)

Processing Questions:

1. Why do we grow in childhood as we age?

2. Is aging a positive part of the life cycle?

Aging in Plants

Valued Outcome: The students will be able to explain the aging process in a plant.
Description of Strategy: As a year-long project or seasonal project, have the children observe the changes that take place in plants. Observation of annuals, such as many flowers, will permit a view of an entire life cycle, from budding stage, through flowering, to withering. Long-term growth can be observed and compared in different trees.
Materials Needed: pots, soil, and plant seeds
Processing Question: How does the life cycle of a plant help us understand aging in ourselves?

Aging in Humans

Valued Outcome: The students will be able to describe how the aging process affects a person's facial features.
Description of Strategy: Bring in photographs of some well-known person taken over a period of many years. Have the students note the aging process in the person's features from year to year.
Materials Needed: photographs of a person taken at several stages of his or her life
Processing Question: How does a person's features change as he or she ages?

Life Cycle

Valued Outcome: The students will observe and record the stages in the life cycle of a frog.
Description of Strategy: Order tadpoles for classroom, and place them in a shallow, clear container. Explain the different stages of a frog's life (growing back legs, growing front legs, losing tail). When the tadpoles start to go through the first noticeable change, have students observe and record these changes in their journals. They may either write the information or draw a picture. Have students repeat this procedure for each stage in the life cycle until the tadpoles have all lost their tails.
Materials Needed: tadpoles, container, journals, pencils
Processing Questions:

1. How long did it take for the tadpoles to start growing their back legs?
2. What is the very first stage in a frog's life?

Puzzles and Games————————————————————

Aging

Games People Should Play

Valued Outcome: The students will be able to describe the implications of the physical aspects of aging on everyday activities.
Description of Strategy: Do you really understand what it feels like to be old or chronically ill? Try these simulations and see how your attitudes change.

1. *Arthritis/Stiff Joints.* In order to simulate stiff knees, get two elastic bandages (3 or 4 inches wide), wrap one firmly, but not too tightly, around each knee, and try walking. First move around the room; then climb some steps. Place these same elastic bandages around your

elbows, and try to put on a coat, or eat or drink something. To feel what it's like to have arthritis of the hands and wrists, put on a pair of bulky gloves and try to button your shirt or blouse.

2. *Stroke or Paralysis.* If you are right handed, take a pencil in your left hand (vice versa for you southpaws) and try to write your name. Would the teacher give you an *A* in penmanship? Simulate the speech problems that follow a stroke by placing a ping-pong ball or a small rubber ball (please wash it first) in your mouth. Now recite the Pledge of Allegiance. Call a friend on the telephone and chat for a few minutes. Did he recognize your voice? Hold a yardstick against the outside of one leg, and secure it with pieces of heavy rope at six-inch distances. Walk around the room, then try going up and down stairs. Feel awkward?

3. *Hearing Loss.* Place a cotton ball in each exterior ear canal, then don a pair of earmuffs. (If you have stereo headphones, use them, because they're more soundproof.) Then call someone in from the next room and strike up a conversation with her. How many times did you have to ask her to repeat something? Did you find yourself lipreading? Turn the TV set down to its lowest level, sit at the opposite end of the room, and listen to the evening news or the local talk show. Hard work, isn't it?

4. *Visual Problems.* Take a pair of swim goggles or old glasses and cover them with wrinkled cellophane or clear food wrap. Read the newspaper for a few minutes or watch TV. It won't be long before your eyes feel strained. Again, watch TV. But this time turn it slightly out of focus. See how long you can watch before you become irritated.

5. *Loss of Smell.* Take a sheet of tissue paper, tear it in half, and gently push one piece into each nostril. Or simply clamp your nose between your thumb and index finger of your left hand. Then grab an apple or your favorite snack and eat it while still holding your nose. Not very tasty, is it?

6. *Loss of Touch.* Cover your fingers with rubber cement. Let it dry and then try to thread a needle. Not so easy, is it? This time cover your hand with a sandwich bag or sandwich wrap. Again try threading that needle and see how long it takes.

Materials Needed: elastic bandages, bulky gloves, shirts that button, pencils, ping-pong balls, yardsticks, cotton balls, earmuffs (or stereo headphones), television set, swim goggles, old eyeglasses, cellophane or clear food wrap, newspaper, tissue paper, apples, rubber cement, needle, thread
Processing Questions:

1. What is it like to be old?

2. What changes in your lifestyle would you need to make if you were old?

Source: K. W. Sehnert. 1976, April. Put yourself in their place. *Family health*, p. 28–40, 53.

Aging Word Search

Valued Outcome: The students will be able to find specific aging-related words in a word search.
Description of Strategy: The teacher will provide a sheet with the following word search on it. Instruct the students to find the following aging-related words in the puzzle:

life expectancy, sex, personality, race, education, ageism, Medicare, Medicaid, retirement, income, employment, calcium, strength, fear, smell, financial, medical, touch, visual

```
R  L  F  I  N  A  N  C  I  A  L
V  I  N  C  O  M  E  S  B  L  S
I  F  M  E  D  I  C  A  L  M  M
S  E  D  U  C  A  T  I  O  N  E
U  E  C  A  R  A  C  K  U  V  L
A  X  X  R  A  O  A  E  T  U  L
L  P  E  A  S  I  M  E  O  W  H
P  E  R  S  O  N  A  L  I  T  Y
S  C  A  L  C  I  U  M  A  N  T
T  T  D  M  D  Y  O  E  S  E  T
R  A  G  E  I  S  M  D  O  M  O
E  N  E  D  I  C  A  I  D  Y  U
N  C  T  I  H  I  N  C  A  O  C
G  Y  T  C  A  L  L  A  U  L  H
T  D  S  A  H  U  T  I  P  P  W
H  H  A  R  T  D  I  D  Y  M  O
S  R  A  E  F  A  S  R  A  E  Y
T  N  E  M  E  R  I  T  E  R  F
```

Dying and Death

Scavenger Hunt

Valued Outcome: Children will be encouraged to verbalize their feelings of grief.

Description of Strategy: Prior to the class meeting, hide six to twelve "symbols" throughout the classroom. The symbols will have questions written on them that ask children to share feelings about someone they know who died (or a pet). *Example:* "Share with the group a special memory you have of your pet (who died)." Once the class meets, children search for symbols with clues from the teacher. After they have all been found, children gather in a circle. The children who find the symbols take turns reading and answering the questions. If a student does not wish to answer, let them know it is okay to use the "I Pass Rule." Then the question may be passed to another student who would like to share their response.

Materials Needed: paper or index cards

Processing Question: How did (or would) it feel to lose someone (or a pet) that I loved?

Source: Waving goodbye: An activities manual for children in grief. 1993. Activity submitted by Evergreen, Portland, OR, p. 6.

Dying and Death Puzzle

Valued Outcome: Students will identify terms related to coping with death and dying by completing a fill-in-the-blank puzzle.

Description of Strategy: Have students fill in the blanks to complete the following puzzle. Choose from the following list of words:

death	anger	attitudes	funeral	communicate
deny	hospices	life	memorial	brain waves
diary	burial	support	negative	death certificate
comforting	reality	drugs	decisions	life-sustaining
funeral	property	grief	numbness	bereavement
cremation	living will	depression	euthanasia	

Death is an inevitability of life. _____ toward death vary greatly. They may be based on our attitudes toward _____. And they may depend on whether _____ is anticipated. The five stages identified by Elisabeth Kübler-Ross that dying people go through are denial, _____, bargaining, _____, and acceptance or resolution. Places where the dying are cared for include hospitals, nursing homes, _____ and home. Most people prefer to die at home, where they are comfortable and the surroundings are familiar. Three things that are measured to determine if death has occurred are breathing, heartbeat, and _____ _____.

In American society, we tend to _____ death. In other cultures, however, death is not seen as _____. Rituals that are associated with death in American society include the completion of a _____ _____, funeral or _____ services, and disposal of the body by _____, _____, placement in crypts or mausoleums, or donation to science. Services help the living to acknowledge death's _____. _____ the survivors is another goal of these services.

Methods of coping with death and dying include keeping a _____. Groups that offer _____ can be of great help, also. _____ should only be used when prescribed by a physician and only if absolutely necessary. _____ involves taking direct action to enable a person to die. It is a very controversial issue. Expressing feelings is a healthy way to show that a person is dealing with his or her _____. _____ is the initial period of profound grief and is characterized by _____ and bewilderment.

Preparations for one's own death involve _____. Whether one wants to be kept alive by extraordinary _____ measures can be addressed through a _____ ____. Distribution of _____ can be handled by a last will and testament. _____ services entail many details and expenses; it is best to _____ one's wishes to others.

Materials Needed: pencil and paper

Source: Information adapted from J. Luckmann. 1990. *Your health!* Englewood Cliffs, NJ: Prentice Hall, p. A60-A61.

Other Ideas

Aging

Adopt a Grandparent

Valued Outcome: The students will be able to develop a meaningful, positive relationship with an elderly friend.

Description of Strategy: Have the class choose (possibly with the cooperation of the local senior citizens' group) an elderly person(s) as an adoptive grandparent. The class could invite the elderly person to class for special occasions, such as birthdays, art projects, storytime, and so forth.

Materials Needed: none

Processing Questions: How can a positive relationship with an elderly person enhance the quality of life as a child?

Elderly Health Fair

Valued Outcome: The student will be able to discuss the positive aspects of the talents of elderly people.

Description of Strategy: Have the students plan a health fair designed for the elderly. Provide health screening services, information about health services in the community. Present arts, crafts, and hobbies made by the elderly. This is a great opportunity for the students to interact with the elderly and acquire an appreciation for the talents of another generation.

Materials Needed: arts, crafts, and hobbies made by elderly people

Processing Question: Do elderly people have talents that can be appreciated by younger people?

What Was It Like Then?

Valued Outcome: The students will be able to explain how society during an elderly person's childhood was different from now.

Description of Strategy: Present a living American heritage lesson to your students. Have an older person in the community report on past lifestyles, historic moments for your community and country. Another suggestion is to find a veteran of World War I and/or the Depression, and have that person report on his or her activities during the war or Depression, and explain how society was different then.

Materials Needed: none

Processing Question: How was the world different during the time of present-day elderly people?

Dying and Death

Poetry

Valued Outcome: The student will be able to compose a poem about dying and death.
Description of Strategy: Some of the greatest works of poetry in literature concern death and dying. Find short poems about death, appropriate to the level of your class, and read them aloud. Discuss the meaning of each poem. Then ask the children to write poems of their own on aspects of death and dying. Post the completed poems around the room for all to see and appreciate.
Materials Needed: poems about death and dying
Processing Question: Why do so many poems have dying and death as a central message?

Take A Walk!

Valued Outcome: Students will gain an understanding of living and nonliving things in their environment.
Description of Strategy: Take your students on a walk outside and touch different things such as grass, rocks, leaves, sticks, bugs. Is it alive or dead? Was it ever alive? How can you tell? Have you ever touched a dead animal? How did it feel? The next time you find one—touch it! Death is not dirty. There may be bacteria on the animal, but you can wash your hands well later with soap and hot water. Your eyes and fingers can help you understand what is hard to understand only in words. Discuss how the students felt during this activity.
Materials Needed: none
Processing Questions: Why do I feel the way I do about death? Is it a negative perspective? Why or why not?

Source: V. Fry. 1995. *Part of me died, too.* New York Dutton Children's Books, p. 21.

What Does a Funeral Director Do?

Valued Outcome: The students will be able to discuss the funeral arrangements that need to be made when a family member dies.
Description of Strategy: Invite a funeral director to speak to the class about how funeral arrangements are made. Ask your guest to explain what is done, how costs are determined, and how family members are involved. The funeral director should explain any special considerations that must be taken into account for religious, cultural, or family reasons. Allow time for a question-and-answer session after the presentation.
Materials Needed: none
Processing Questions:

1. What funeral arrangements have to be made when a family member or relative dies?

2. What is the significance of funeral rituals?

References

American School Health Association. 1994, March. The key to healthy communication, *Journal of school health* 64(3), pp. 123–124.

Donatelle, R., L. Davis, and C. Hoover. 1988. *Access to health*, Annotated Instructor's Edition. Englewood Cliffs, NJ: Prentice Hall.

Ezell, G. 1992. *Healthy living, Level 2: Healthy and growing*. Grand Rapids, MI: Christian Schools International.

Fernside idea book: A guidebook for group facilitators at Fernside: A center for grieving children. 1994. Cincinnati, OH: Fernside Center.

Flynn, N., and M. Erickson 1996. *Teen talk: Grief support group for teenagers.* Puyallup, WA: Good Samaritan Hospice.

Fry, V. 1995. *Part of me died, too.* New York: Dutton Children's Books.

Health: Choosing wellness, Teacher's edition. 1989. Englewood Cliffs, NJ: Prentice Hall.

Landy, L. 1992. *Child support: Through small group counseling.* Charleston, NC: Kids Right.

Lemme, B. H. 1995. *Development in adulthood.* Boston: Allyn and Bacon.

Loya, R., ed. 1983. *Health-education teaching ideas*, Secondary Level. Reston, VA: American Alliance for Health, Physical Education, Recreation and Dance.

Luckmann, J. 1990. *Your health!* Englewood Cliffs, NJ: Prentice Hall.

Marrone, R. 1997. *Death, mourning, and caring.* Pacific Grove: Brooks/Cole.

Meeks, L., and P. Heit. 1996. *Totally awesome health*, Sixth grade manual. Blacklick, OH: Meeks Heit.

Meeks, L., and P. Heit. 1991. *Health: A wellness approach*, Teacher's edition. Columbus, OH: Merrill.

Merki, M. B. 1990. *Teen health: Decisions for healthy living*, Teacher's manual. Mission Hills, CA: Glencoe/McGraw-Hill.

Oaks, J. and G. Ezell. 1993. *Dying and death*, 2nd ed. Scottsdale, AZ: Gorsuch-Scarisbrick.

Payne, W., and D. Hahn. 1992. *Understanding your health*, 3rd ed. St. Louis: Mosby-Yearbook.

Sharing our best: A collection of activities and ideas to use in bereavement groups for children and teens. 1995. The Kids Grief Network of Western Washington.

Read, D. 1980. *Creative teaching in health*, 3rd ed. Prospect Heights, IL: Waveland Press.

Sehnert, K. W. 1976, April. Put yourself in their place. *Family health*, pp. 28–40, 53.

Suggested Readings

Backer, B. A., N. Hanoi, and N. A. Russell. 1994. *Death and dying: Understanding and care*, 2nd ed. Albany, NY: Delmar.

Belsky, J. K. 1990. *The psychology of aging*, 2nd ed. Pacific Grove, CA: Brooks/Cole.

Blieszner, R., and V. H. Bedford, eds. 1995. *Handbook of aging and the family*. Westport, CT: Greenwood Press.

Corless, I. B., B. B. Germino, and M. Pittman, eds. 1994. *Dying, death, and bereavement: Theoretical perspectives and other ways of knowing.* Boston: Jones & Bartlett.

DeSpelder, L. A. and A. L. Strickland. 1992. *The last dance*, 3rd ed. Mountain View, CA: Mayfield.

Ebersole, P., and P. Hess. 1994. *Toward healthy aging: Human needs and nursing response*, 4th ed. St. Louis: Mosby.

Ferrini, A. F., and R. L. Ferrini 1993. *Health in the later years*, 2nd ed. Madison, WI: Brown & Benchmark.

Hockey, J., and A. James. 1993. *Growing up and growing old.* London: Sage.

Marrone, R. 1997. *Death, mourning, and caring.* Pacific Grove, CA: Brooks/Cole.

Spirduso, W. W. 1995. *Physical dimensions of aging.* Champaign, IL: Human Kinetics.

Williamson, J. B., and E. S. Shneidman. 1995. *Death: Current perspectives*, 4th ed. Mountain View, CA: Mayfield.

Resources

Videos

The following videos are available from Films for the Humanities and Sciences, P.O. Box 2053, Princeton, NJ 08543

Teen suicide: A Phil Donahue show
This show brings together parents of teen suicide victims, teens who have attempted suicide, and a psychotherapist. This program seeks ways to stem the tide of increasing suicide rates among young people, and to help youngsters and adults recognize the signals and warning cries of potential suicides.

The right to die
In this program, the medical, ethical, and legal dilemmas of cases are discussed by a physician-attorney and a nurse.

Children die, too
A couple whose three-year-old daughter died suddenly, a teenage girl whose sister died from leukemia, a mother whose six-month-old died from multiple birth defects, and a young woman who has undergone two miscarriages and two stillborns talk about their experiences.

Video focus on health
This video discusses several topics related to aging, dying and death, such as successful aging and medically assisted suicide.

The biology of death
This video discusses the importance of knowing when a patient dies for the purpose of organ transplantation. Also, discusses the various definitions of death.

The following videos are available from Schoolhouse Videos & CDs, 4205 Grove Ridge Drive, Durham, NC 27703

Health aging
Healthy aging shows the connection between your daily lifestyle habits and your potential for both a longer life and health span. (60 minutes, Item 6066)

Someone I love has Alzheimer's disease
The message of this video is you are not alone. You will meet kids aged 7 through 15. All are caring for and coping with a loved one with this confusing disorder. (17 minutes, Item 7917)

Web Sites

Alzheimer Disease Web Site
http://med.www.by.edu/Alzheimer/home.html

Batesville Casket Company
http://www.batesville.com

Bereavement Resources Director
http://asa.ugl.lib.umich.edu/chdocs/support/bereave.html

Children and Grief Resources
http//www.psych.med.umich.edu/web/aacap/factsFam/grief.html

Cremation
http://www.twoscan.com/2s...erals/cremation.htm

Eldercare Web
http://www.ice.net/~kstevens/ELDERWEB.HTM

Heart Mind Body Institute
http://www.power.net/hbm/hbm1.html

Internet Resources on Aging and Loss
gopher://gopher.rivendell.org/11/resources/aging

OncoLink
http://www.oncolink.upenn.edu/

Suicide save.org
http://www.save.org

United States Public Health Services
http://phs.os.dhhs.gov/phs/

General Sites

American Medical Association
http://www.ama-assn.org

MedicineNet
http://www.medicinenet.com

Medscape
http://www.medscape.com

Oncolink
http://www.oncolink.upenn.edu

ParentsPlace.com
http://www.parentsplace.com

Thrive@ pathfinder
http://pathfinder.com/thrive

Links Only

Hardin Meta Directory of Internet Health *Sources*
http://www.arcade.uiowa.edu/hardin-www/md.html

Medical Matrix
http://www.5lackinc.com/matrix

Surveillance and Data Systems

Agency for Health Care Policy and Research Data and Methods
www.ahcpr.gov:80/data

CDC National Center for Health Statistics
www.cdc.gov/nchswww/nchshome.htm

Educational and Community-Based Programs

CDC National Center for Chronic Disease Prevention and Health Promotion
www.cdc.gov/nccdphp/nccdhome.htm

Health Resources and Services Administration
www.hrsa.dhhs.gov

Healthy Cities Online
www.healthycities.org

Office of Minority Health Resource Center
Washington State Department of Health
www.doh.wa.gov

Death/Dying

Donor Network of Arizona
http://www.donor-network.org/organ/organ.html

Emotional Support Guide
http://asa.ugl.lib.umich.edu/chdocs/support/emotional.html

Euthanasia Research and Guidance Organization
http://www.efn.org/~ergo/

GriefNet
http://rivendell.org/

Hospice Hands
http://gator.net/~jnash/hospice.html

Chapter Twenty-Four
Environmental Health

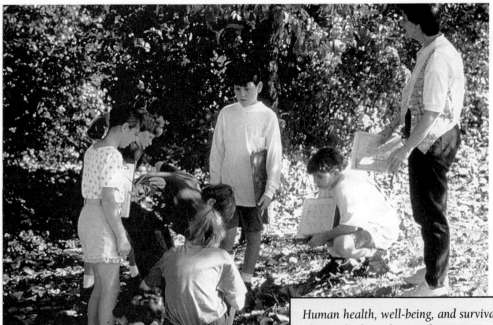

> Human health, well-being, and survival are ultimately dependent on the integrity of the planet on which we live.
>
> —Donatelle and Davis (1996, 590)

Valued Outcomes

After reading this chapter, you should be able to

○ discuss the responsibility of every human being in caring for the environment

○ describe the impact of pollution on all members of the ecosystem

○ describe an ecosystem

○ relate the connection between overpopulation and environmental pollution

○ explain the impact of acid rain on the environment

○ detail the conditions that lead to water pollution

○ suggest what individuals can do to remedy the different types of environmental pollution

○ discuss the Environmental Protection Agency's "Superfund" attempt at solid waste cleanup and control

○ give examples of legislation designed to control environmental pollution
○ describe the Clean Air Act that is enforced by the Environmental Protection Agency

Human Impact on the Environment

Maintaining personal health is largely an individual responsibility. Yet none of us lives in a vacuum. We are all subject to the influences of our environment. Thus a person may attempt to exercise the most positive of personal health behavior and still be subjected to health hazards in the form of contaminated drinking water, polluted air, and urban-caused stress factors, such as noise and overcrowded living conditions. Clearly, our environment has an impact on health.

Human beings are the dominant species on earth because of our power to control, manipulate, and alter our surroundings. To a large extent, we have learned to use the natural resources of the planet for our own benefit. But in doing so, we have also created a host of environmental problems. For a long time, many of these problems went unrecognized. However, with the growth of technology and industry the problems became more and more obvious. Even then, many preferred to ignore what was happening to our environment, putting it down to "the price of progress." In any case, there seemed to be no way of correcting many of the problems.

Today, more and more people are becoming aware of the negative impact human activity has had on the environment. Many of the negative changes that have occurred did not have to happen. Certainly, most do not have to keep getting worse. We can no longer plead ignorance about how our activities affect the world in which we live. We also are increasingly recognizing our responsibility toward protecting the environment and preserving our natural resources for future generations.

Ecology is the study of interactions in the environment. From this study, three basic natural laws have been determined:

1. Every system within nature is connected to every other system.

2. Once created, matter is never destroyed but is recycled in one way or another.

3. Natural resources are finite, and nature's capacity to absorb the by-products of human technology is limited.

The implications of these three laws, separately and together, have great bearing on the health of all people and the state of the environment. At first, it may seem that these principles are beyond control of the individual, but this is not so. Each of us has a responsibility both to understand the laws of ecology and to realize that as individuals what we do affects the operation of these laws. This is the most important single concept in the teaching of environmental health education.

Children must become aware that they are part of the overall ecosystem of our planet and as intelligent members of that ecosystem have both rights and responsibilities concerning the environment. This is a vital concept that must be stressed.

The basic teaching plan for environmental health involves three main areas: ecosystems and ecology, pollution of the ecosphere, and preservation of the ecosphere. Each of these areas will be discussed in this chapter.

Ecosystems and Ecology

Each living thing, whether plant or animal, is part of an immediate ecosystem, or habitat in which the living and nonliving components interact and interrelate. For example, all the organisms in a particular field or pond form an ecosystem. By interacting in a balanced fashion with all other parts of the ecosystem, a given species within that ecosystem can generally continue to thrive while perpetuating its population. This interrelationship and interdependence with other animals and plants in the environment produces a web of common sharing of most natural resources, including air, water, territorial space, sunlight, and soil minerals. Nonliving natural resources are usually referred to as the *physical environment* of the given ecosystem, while living organisms are referred to as the *biotic environment* of the ecosystem.

Both environmental components of an ecosystem influence the other. When the physical environment is altered significantly, the biotic environment will be altered significantly, and vice versa. As a result, ecosystems are governed and operate through an interwoven natural organization of cycles between groups within the system so that balance and stabilization of the community are sustained. Yet balance and stability are dynamic processes, always changing to adapt to the alterations in these cycles as they themselves are changed by the varying interactions between the residents of the neighborhood and their use of natural resources. Thus, since ecosystems are inherently unstable, an input of energy is required in order to maintain equilibrium or homeostasis. This input of energy produces a closed and self-sustaining cycle wherein chains of interconnections arise. For example, life is nurtured from decomposition within the system, one species feeds off another, and so forth. All resources, by nature's rules, are recycled and continually reused in one form or another, because energy is always constant.

In addition, ecosystems are in continuous interaction with one another and are joined by the actions of the various physical and biotic environments to form a total worldwide ecosystem called the *ecosphere* or *biosphere*.

The human species, unlike any other species, can extensively manipulate both the physical and biotic environments of ecosystems, indirectly affecting the ecosphere as a whole. Although many of these alterations in and of themselves are not inherently damaging, the cumulative impact on the ecosphere has taken its toll and the natural recycling mechanisms have sometimes been overwhelmed. Ecologists have pleaded for all of us to develop a greater understanding of the scientific principles that govern ecosystems so that an increased awareness about our impact on the ecosphere will result. Then more of our decisions regarding the ways in which we choose to interact with the environment will be based on knowledge and logic rather than ignorance or greed. Ecologists have also warned of the grave danger facing our entire planet from depletion or pollution of its rich natural resources, which are finite and must be preserved for future generations.

Pollution of the Ecosphere

Pollution is the contamination of the environment that results from an overabundance of substances that render the physical surroundings unfit, unsafe, or unsanitary for use or habitation by the residents of the ecosystem. Although pollutants may initially appear to directly affect only a limited or select population within the ecosystem, such as birds and marine life, these substances

Environmental problems arise from overpopulation.

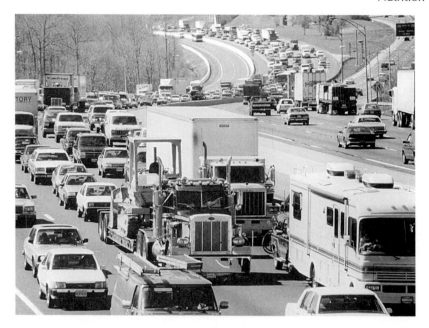

eventually have an impact on all members of the ecosystem because of the interdependence and interaction between organisms. Human activity is the major cause of environmental pollution, but humans often experience the results of contamination much less quickly than other members of the ecosphere. As a result, although pollution of the environment has been occurring for centuries, only relatively recently has an awareness developed that polluting constitutes self-destructive behavior. The most crucial areas of concern include problems caused by overpopulation, air pollution, water pollution, hazardous chemical pollution, solid waste pollution, radiation pollution, and noise pollution.

Overpopulation

Many environmental health problems arise not so much from misuse of technology but from the sheer numbers of people who exist. There are simply not enough natural resources to support an unlimited human population.

A rapidly growing population often exceeds the food resources. World shortages of food have already been occurring, because the population appears to be increasing twice as fast as the food supply. Nutrient deficiencies result in a high infant mortality rate and shortened life expectancy. When food stores are low, the risk of famine is great (Smolin and Grosvenor 1994, 552).

The consequences of uncontrolled world population growth go beyond the issue of food. In addition to hunger, joblessness, environmental devastation, and uncontrolled urban growth would result. In many countries in the last decade or two, attempts have been made to deal with the problem of overpopulation by means of governmental incentives to limit births. However, ethical and moral controversy surrounds the issue, which is understandably a very delicate and highly personal one to most individuals. Regardless of the ethical or moral considerations, however, overpopulation is a serious environmental problem that must be addressed—not only by governmental and private agencies but by the schools as well. Information about family planning and parenthood should be provided to junior high and high school students after a foundation about families and population has been provided at the elementary school level. Children need to understand that our planet will soon be unable to house the growing human population if reproduction continues at the present rate. Although the solutions are not easy and decisions must ultimately be made by each individual, a world perspective should be provided.

Population Control

In the year 1800, about 1 billion people lived on earth; in 1900, about 2 billion. By the year 2020, there may be more than 7.7 billion people on our planet. With the increase in the number of people comes an increase in the demand for resources (Hales 1994, 567–568).

The problems resulting from overpopulation are well recognized in such countries as China and India, where governmental incentives have been established to limit childbearing. Before condoms and diaphragms became available in the nineteenth century, birth control methods were generally unsafe and did not enjoy widespread use. However, particularly with the introduction to the general public of the birth control pill and the intrauterine device (IUD) in the 1960s as well as improved female sterilization and male vasectomy techniques introduced in the 1970s, birth control has become more accepted throughout the world. In addition, dissemination of information about contraceptive methods has been increased to include preteens, teenagers, young adults, and older adults alike. Although some individuals and groups believe instruction about birth control is ill advised in a school setting, many school systems nevertheless have incorporated such instruction into the curriculum. The establishment of various kinds of family planning services throughout the United States and in many other nations has also aided in increasing contraceptive education.

In the United States, population growth has stabilized. The average age for marriage has increased, and many young couples delay parenthood in order to advance educationally or professionally. In Third World countries, where population control is more of a problem, efforts must be made to provide the same kind of education and services that are offered in the more technologically advanced nations. It must be recognized, however, that decisions about pregnancy are deeply personal, cultural, religious, and social in nature and should be based on free choice.

Air Pollution

Human beings—all 5.3 billion of us—need air more desperately than any other material for survival. People can endure drought, famine, and drastic temperature changes, but oxygen deprivation will result in death after only a few minutes. Yet most of us think very little about the air we breathe, what it is composed of, or how as a finite supply it is replenished and kept clean. Almost no oxygen was present in the atmosphere at the earth's creation, but an abundance of carbon dioxide was available for sustaining plant life. Green plants, over an evolutionary period, were responsible for producing oxygen as a waste product of photosynthesis so that today the atmosphere is composed of approximately 80 percent nitrogen and 20 percent oxygen. Whereas plants have been responsible for producing the oxygen humans and other animals need for life, humans have been largely responsible for polluting the atmosphere with a variety of harmful gases and other substances. The result is air pollution, an increasing environmental health problem in the United States and many other nations.

Exposure to high-enough concentrations of air pollutants can cause a variety of health problems ranging from sneezing and coughing to labored breathing and death. Those individuals who are most sensitive to air pollution are usually older adults and people who have chronic

Health Highlight

Health Effects of Global Warming and Ozone Layer Depletion

○ Fertile areas will turn into deserts, thereby decreasing food supplies.

○ Polar ice caps will melt, which will, in turn, raise the sea level by three to twenty feet and displace millions of people living near the coasts.

○ Increased precipitation, resulting in increased flooding.

○ Increased respiratory irritants and thereby increase lung diseases.

○ Increased ultraviolet C radiation and raise the incidence of skin cancers, cataracts, and infectious diseases.

Source: C. Bruess and G. Richardson. 1994. *Healthy decisions.* Madison, WI: Brown & Benchmark, pp. 343–344.

respiratory or cardiovascular conditions. The chief air pollutants include carbon monoxide and nitrogen oxides, sulfur oxides, hydrocarbons, and particulate matter.

Carbon Monoxide and Nitrogen Oxides. Carbon monoxide, which is by far the most plentiful air pollutant, is a colorless, odorless poisonous gas produced by the incomplete burning of carbon in fuels. The chief source of carbon monoxide is internal combustion engines, most of which are gas-powered motor vehicles. Because hemoglobin has a greater affinity for carbon monoxide than for oxygen, carbon monoxide replaces oxygen in the blood. An environment in which heavy traffic is present provides significant levels of carbon monoxide, and diminished physical and mental functioning can result from long-term exposure. Adverse effects include affected breathing, heart failure, impaired perception, and thinking (Pruitt and Stein 1994, 505).

Nitrogen oxides, which account for about 6 percent of air pollutants, are chemically very similar to carbon monoxide, and poisonous nitrogen oxides, such as nitrogen dioxide and nitric acid, produce comparable physiological disturbances in the circulatory system. Nitrogen oxide combines with water vapor in the air to form nitric acid, a brown gas capable of corroding metal and destroying vegetation. As with carbon dioxide, the major emitter of nitric acid is the automobile.

Pollution from automobiles and other internal combustion engines is a major source of air pollution. This source produces most man-made carbon monoxide. Most experts agree that shifting away from automobiles as the primary source of transportation is the only way to reduce air pollution significantly. Many cities have encouraged this shift by setting high parking fees, imposing bans on city driving, and establishing high road use tolls. Also, community governments should be encouraged to provide convenient, inexpensive, and easily accessible public transportation for citizens. Furthermore, auto makers must be encouraged to manufacture automobiles that provide good fuel economy and low rates of toxic emissions (Donatelle and Davis 1996, 599).

Sulfur Oxides. Next to carbon monoxide, sulfur oxides are the most abundant air pollutant. These are poisonous gases that come from combustion of sulfur-containing coal and fuel oil. Sulfur dioxide, a poison that irritates the eyes, nose, and throat, damages the lungs, is highly injurious to human health, to property, and to vegetation (Green and Ottoson 1994, 511).

Hydrocarbons. Although no specific ailments or irritations can be directly attributed to the release of hydrocarbons—compounds comprised of hydrogen and carbon—these substances constitute an important component of smog. They account for 10 percent to 15 percent of all air pollution emissions.

Particulate Matter. Particulate matter is any nongaseous pollutant found in the air, whether liquid or solid. These pollutants include such substances as ash, soot, asbestos, and lead. It is estimated that particulate matter comprises approximately 8 percent of air emissions. Prolonged exposure to these pollutants can cause deterioration of the respiratory tract surfaces, particularly the cilia.

Lead. Sources of airborne lead are primarily smelters and automobile exhausts. (Unleaded gasoline has eased the problem of automobile exhaust pollution somewhat.) Health hazards from high concentrations of lead include irritability, anemia, convulsions, severe intestinal cramps, loss of consciousness, and kidney and brain damage. Lead enters the body primarily through the respiratory tract and sometimes through the stomach walls. Signs of lead poisoning are behavior problems, anemia, decreased mental functioning, vomiting, and cramps.

Asbestos. In the past, asbestos was widely used in construction and manufacturing, and most exposures occur in occupational settings. Asbestos can cause serious respiratory problems, such as emphysema, and has been implicated in lung cancer.

Toxic substances, the final major source of air pollution, are generally the products of technology and have not been studied extensively. These substances include natural elements such as arsenic and mercury and man-made products such as polyvinyl chlorides, asbestos, and pesticides. Some are highly toxic, causing cancer and death.

Damage Resulting from Air Pollution

Air pollution causes serious damage in terms of human well-being, property, and plant and animal life. In addition, two air pollution conditions can lead to serious environmental problems. They are acid rain and temperature inversions.

In terms of human welfare, air pollution negatively affects such respiratory illnesses as coughs, colds, asthma, pneumonia, and bronchitis, as well as cancer and even heart disease. Animals and plant life can also be severely harmed by air pollution. When pesticides are sprayed by crop dusters, only one-fourth lands on the crop, less than 1 percent may hit the target insects, and the rest drifts miles away. The insecticides kill birds, frogs, and predatory insects. Falcons and eagles have become extinct in some local areas, as a result of pesticide spraying. Herbicides sprayed on forest lands have caused miscarriages, cancer, and birth defects and often wipe out local wildlife as well as pets and livestock. Vegetation may change color or fail to pollinate. Animals grazing on affected land can be contaminated. Finally, our houses, apartments, and public buildings are damaged by air pollution. Buildings become darkened and discolored as a result of air pollution. Public works of art and monuments are damaged by contaminants. Unfortunately, today's high technology produces pollutants faster than the scientific community is able to study their results. These by-products may pose serious health problems that are currently unknown.

Acid Rain. The primary cause of acid rain is the burning of fossil fuels in electricity-generating plants. The sulfur in fuel is converted to sulfur oxides. If rain, snow, dew, or mist is present, sulfuric and nitric acids are formed. Most sulfur pollution in the United States originates east of the Mississippi River. Much of the pollution that originates in the United States is deposited in Canada. Throughout the eastern parts of Canada and the United States, acid rain changes soil acidic levels, ruins the eggs of amphibians and fish, and causes lakes and streams to become more acidic. As the water becomes more acidic, life begins to disappear from the water, thus disrupting the ecosystem and eventually affecting all of our lives.

Temperature Inversions. When a warm air mass moves over cooler air near the ground, a temperature inversion results. The cooler air cannot be dissipated. Temperature inversions decrease visibility and allow a buildup of pollutants, making the air unsafe for breathing. The pollutants are trapped and subjected to the acting of sunlight and produce other pollutants, such as ozone. The temperature inversion eventually disperses, but illness and even death have resulted from this condition.

Air Pollution Control

The Environmental Protection Agency (EPA) was established in 1970 by Congress to become the federal environmental watchdog agency. Under the provision of the Clean Air Act of 1970, the EPA set national ambient air quality standards for "criteria" pollutants, the most common air pollutants. Examples of criteria pollutants are ozone, particulate matter, carbon monoxide, sulfur dioxide, lead, and nitrous oxides. For example, acid rain is produced when sulfur dioxide and nitrous oxides are released into the atmosphere through the smokestacks of power plants and industry, and the exhaust of automobiles. According to the EPA, at least 74 million people have lived in areas that still exceeded at least one air quality standard, and as many as 140 million people may have lived in areas that had ozone levels, or smog, in excess of national standards during that year. Progress in controlling air pollution has been made in the area of reducing lead levels by switching from leaded to lead-free gasoline in automobiles, but the United States has not been able to meet the 90 percent improvements mandated by the Clean Air Act for any of the other criteria air pollutants (Mullen et al. 1996, 614).

The EPA also lists "hazardous" air pollutants and establishes safety standards for them. For example, new regulations will ban most uses of asbestos by the mid-1990s (Green and Ottoson 1994, 518). Other examples of hazardous pollutants are asbestos, beryllium, mercury, vinyl chloride, arsenic, benzene, and coke oven emissions.

Water Pollution

Like air, water is essential to life. The demand for clean water has increased correspondingly with the growth in population, in irrigation demands and in manufacturing. These areas of growth, plus the conversion of land that formerly held water has caused a significant and dangerous reduction in water tables in many areas of the country. Current contamination of drinking water supplies in the United States ranges from 1 percent to 2 percent, and this may expose as much as 10 percent of the population. As a result, health problems abound due to infectious agents and toxins in the water (Green and Ottoson 1994, 419).

Despite water's importance, we dump everything from animal fertilizer and detergents to industrial wastes and sewage into our precious water supply. In addition, when pollutants are channeled into nonflowing bodies of water, such as lakes, eutrophication, or accelerated growth

Health Highlight

Objectives for Regulation of Contaminants by the Year 2000

○ Reduce human exposure to toxic agents by confining total pounds of toxic agents released into the air, water and soil to no more than 0.24 billion pounds of those toxic agents included on the Department of Health and Human Services list of carcinogens. Baseline: 0.32 billion pounds in 1988.

○ Reduce human exposure to solid waste-related water, air, and soil contamination, as measured by a reduction in average pounds of municipal solid waste produced per person each day to no more than 3.6 pounds. Baseline: 4 pound per person each day in 1988.

○ Increase to at least 85 percent the proportion of people who receive a supply of drinking water that meets the safe drinking water standards established by the EPA. Baseline: 75 percent of 58,099 community water systems serving approximately 80 percent of the U.S. population in 1988.

Source: L. Green and J. Ottoson. 1994. *Community health.* 7th ed. St. Louis: Mosby, p. 422.

of algae, occurs. As algae growth skyrockets on a diet of inorganic pollutants, especially nitrogen and phosphorous, a blanket of slime covers the water. Eventual death of the algae results in bacterial decomposition that consumes the oxygen present. This oxygen deficit kills off fish and other lake inhabitants, many of which are valuable as food resources. Eventually, the body of water becomes contaminated beyond use. Even flowing bodies of water, such as streams and rivers, that undergo natural purification can be badly polluted if sufficient amounts of wastes are dumped.

There are numerous sources of water pollution. The main ones are industrial wastes, animal fertilizers, human sewage, and thermal pollution.

Industrial Wastes. Chemical by-products from the manufacture of paper, steel, oil, pesticides, and the like account for more than half of the water pollution in this country. Despite water pollution laws, an abundance of diverse industrial wastes continues to be disposed of in lakes, streams, and rivers throughout the country. Many, like lead and mercury, are known to be toxic to humans. Of great concern regarding the danger of any industrial waste product is the length of time it takes to be broken down by the environment and the amount of concentration that is tolerable by given organisms, particularly humans.

Animal Fertilizers. Agriculture is one of the major sources of water pollution. Many animal fertilizers are particularly rich in nitrogen, thus adding to the problem of eutrophication and oxygen depletion of bodies of water. Also, the use of fertilizer often results in diminishing returns: The more fertilizer that is used, the less it helps (Levy, Dignan, and Shirreffs 1992, 522).

Human Sewage. Although contamination of water from human waste is much less serious than it once was, it nevertheless can occur in varying degrees if a community's sewage treatment system is antiquated or not inspected regularly. It is recommended that sewage treatment consist of two stages: primary and secondary. The primary stage rids the water, which has been allowed to settle in a holding tank, of large objects through a filtration process of passing the liquid over a series of screens. During the secondary stage of treatment, smaller particles of organic material and microbes are removed through additional filtration techniques, dispersement over beds of stone, and chemical purification. The final step usually involves the addition of chlorine in order to disinfect the water of any remaining bacteria in order for it to be safe for recycling.

Thermal Pollution. Numerous industries, including those involved in generating nuclear power, use water as a coolant for their equipment. Water absorbs heat from the equipment and is channeled back to its source, where it produces a rise in temperature of the source water itself. Although this process seems harmless enough, the warmer water is, the less oxygen it will absorb, and the less oxygen absorbed, the less quickly the lake or river decomposes its organic material. Since power-generating plants in particular heat large volumes of water, the parent waterway is certainly at risk. In addition, much of the aquatic life is drastically affected by extreme temperature variation from the norm.

The Effects of Water Pollution. Polluted water can be responsible for transmitting many pathogens. For example, typhoid fever, dysentery, cholera, and parasitic worms are just a few of the diseases that can be transmitted through polluted water. Viruses from human wastes carried in contaminated water can cause hepatitis. Bacteria found in polluted water can cause intestinal disorders. Other materials found in polluted water, such as asbestos fibers, can cause cancer.

Polluted water can be particularly harmful to fish, birds, and animals. For example, herbicides, phosphates, fertilizers, sewage, and industrial wastes kill numerous fish and birds. These products also promote the growth of algae, which changes the ecological balance. These same products produce odors and foul-tasting drinking water. In addition, fish may be affected by rising water temperature, which retards their reproduction, destroys their food supplies, or kills them.

The oil slicks of recent years have been widely publicized. The devastation to birds and fish has been apparent. The oil coats the gills of fish, thus killing them. Feathers of birds are coated so that they cannot fly. Oil-covered beaches are also expensive to clean, and the public loses recreational areas.

Water Quality Control. Although federal controls regarding water pollution have not been as extensive as those for air pollution, the enactment of the Federal Water Pollution Control Act in 1973 was conceived as a means of developing a national system that would require any institution, industry, or company that discharges substances into waterways to meet EPA standards. In addition, Congress passed the Safe Drinking Water Act in 1974, which covers 40,000 community water supply systems and another 200,000 private systems. This act provided for the periodic updating of water standards (Green and Ottoson 1994, 431).

Hazardous Chemical Pollution

The hazardous chemicals that pollute our environment are numerous and varied. They include not only the toxins deposited in our air and waterways but also the pesticides sprayed on crops, the chemicals transported along our railways and highways for use in industry, and those contained in commonly used household products.

Pesticides. With the 1962 publication of Rachel Carson's *Silent Spring*, people began to become more conscious of the hazards of pesticides, toxic chemicals used to kill insects, and other pests that destroy crops. In past decades, the harm caused by the widespread use of chlorinated hydrocarbons such as aldrin, dieldrin, and DDT (dichlorodiphenyltrichloroethane) as pesticides was not fully recognized. DDT is a synthetic chlorinated insecticide that kills insects by attacking biochemical processes in their nervous systems. It is a persistent pesticide, sometimes remaining in the environment for as long as fifteen years before degrading. These chemicals are particularly dangerous not only because they are toxic, but also because they accumulate in human fat tissue (they are fat soluble). Traces of DDT, probably the most widely disseminated pesticide in the world, are said to exist in all Americans. DDT appears to be a potent cancer promoter. DDT was banned from use in the United States, but is still used in underdeveloped nations around the world (Mullen et al. 1996, 611).

Chlorinated hydrocarbons decompose very slowly and remain toxic to a wide variety of animal life for long periods. Organophosphorous pesticides such as diazinon, parathion, and malathion exhibit similar properties and are even more poisonous than the chlorinated hydrocarbons.

Although worldwide food production needs to be increased to meet the demands of a growing population, extensive use of pesticides can cause great harm to environmental health in the process. Questions still need to be answered concerning the implication of long-term exposure to moderate or even minimal levels of pesticides. There is evidence that these chemicals can damage the human reproductive and nervous systems, for example. It is obvious, therefore, that the use of pesticides must be limited and controlled in order to protect all inhabitants of our ecosphere.

Industrial Chemicals. One of the newer and most dangerous environmental threats is the transportation of industrial chemicals from state to state and from country to country. Although transportation itself is not inherently deleterious, leakage or spills of chemical substances most certainly is. In fact, hardly a week goes by without news of such an accident that causes disability or death. In addition, accidents involving the transportation of oil and other petroleum products have resulted in several major oil spills that have damaged some of our nation's most beautiful beaches and killed or endangered countless birds and marine life.

In response to this increasingly dangerous threat, many state governments as well as the federal government have formed special subcommittees to study the problem of transportation of industrial chemicals. Particularly in regard to the movement of radioactive material across states for industrial and burial purposes, many states have indicated an unwillingness to continue to allow such toxins to be brought in. More controls and safeguards need to be implemented in transporting hazardous chemicals of any kind, whether by trucks, ships, or trains.

Household Products. Before the recent ban on spray cans containing propellant fluorocarbons and detergents containing phosphates, numerous household products served as contaminators of the environment by releasing these agents into the air and water, respectively. Fluorocarbons destroy the protective ozone layer of the atmosphere that shields us from damaging ultraviolet rays of the sun, while phosphates serve as excellent nutrients for bacteria, protozoa, and algae, promoting eutrophication of lakes, streams, and rivers. These examples serve as an excellent illustration of the dangers involved in releasing seemingly harmless compounds into our surroundings from heavily used household products like cleansers, polishes, waxes, and sprays of all kinds without first studying their environmental impact before marketing them.

Hazardous Chemical Control. With governmental regulation of DDT in 1973, national attention was focused on the dangers of pesticides in general. As a result, more sensible approaches to crop spraying have evolved. Nonetheless, the widespread use of pesticides still poses a danger to environmental health.

Solid Waste Pollution

Until recently, the public virtually ignored the problems related to the disposal of solid wastes. By the year 2000, solid waste generation is projected to reach 216 million tons daily, or 4.2 pounds per person. Approximately 73 percent of this waste is buried in landfills. To date, 32,500 potentially hazardous waste sites have been identified across the nation. The U.S. Public Health Service has declared over 90 percent of the thousands of authorized hazardous waste disposal sites as posing "unacceptable" health risks. Hazardous wastes consist of materials that are flammable, corrosive, toxic, or chemically reactive (Donatelle and Davis 1996, 604–606).

Today, we use more and more "convenience" products that are easily disposed of and replaced. Everything from disposable diapers, dishes, and food containers to plastic wraps, sanitary products, and paper napkins are available. The price of this convenience has been the growing problem of solid waste disposal. The unsightly junkyards, dumps, and scattered litter that dot our land are more than just eyesores. They are a public health hazard as well.

Many solid waste materials are not biodegradable and remain in the environment for long periods of time because they do not decay or cannot be burned easily. The piles of refuse serve as excellent breeding grounds for micro-organisms, rats, insects, and other disease carriers. In addition, agricultural waste products from orchards, feedlots, and farms add significantly to the total solid waste that must be disposed of each year. How then do we rid ourselves of all our refuse? Current methods primarily used include dumps, sanitary landfills, recycling, and incineration.

Dumps. Most solid waste in this country is deposited in open, minimally managed dumps. Some burning of garbage does take place in order to condense the material. Besides being extremely unsightly, open dumping grounds can pose a serious threat to a community's health if the insect or rodent population gets out of control. The widespread use of dumps results from the short-term cheapness of this method of solid waste disposal.

Sanitary Landfills. Unlike the procedures of open disposal in a dump, those in a sanitary landfill require that the solid waste be covered by dirt each day after it has been compacted. Once covered with dirt, the landfill is bulldozed in order to smooth out and compress the area. A properly operated sanitary landfill requires predetermined designing and engineering of the site as well as continued daily maintenance from a crew of workers within a city sanitation department. However, the benefits of a well-functioning landfill can be numerous. Because refuse is covered daily, risk of a contaminated water supply or of disease due to the breeding of flies, mosquitoes, rats, and the like is diminished considerably. Because burning is not necessary, the technique does not contribute to air pollution. In addition, after the location has been completely filled in, it can serve some other valuable purpose, such as a site for housing, recreation, or industry.

There are problems, nevertheless, associated with the use of sanitary landfills. Land itself is becoming more scarce and more expensive, not all types of terrain are suitable to serve as landfills, and the surrounding water table must be low enough. In addition, residents are often opposed to the establishment of a sanitary landfill nearby for fear that it will lower property values.

Recycling. Many products can be recycled, or reused in another mode. For example, paper, glass, and metal products can all be recycled. This method of solid waste control gained some popularity during the environmentally conscious era of the late 1960s and early 1970s. Today many communities require households to recycle some materials. Other communities provide recycling centers to which residents can bring recyclable materials. Some communities merely ask

The benefits of a well-functioning landfill can be numerous.

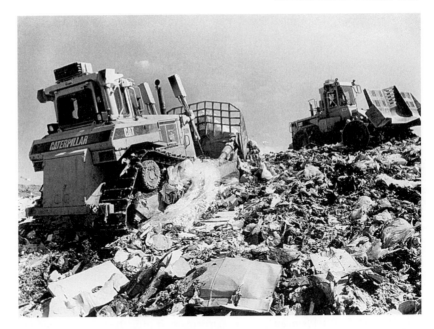

residents to place recyclable materials out for pickup in front of their homes. These projects have significantly decreased the amount of unrecycled solid waste.

Incineration. Like dumping, incineration is a very old method of waste disposal that adds to environmental pollution because of the release of particular matter into the atmosphere during burning. Of particular danger is the release of hydrogen chloride from burning plastic materials, which are mainly composed of polyvinyl chloride. On contact with moisture in the air, hydrogen chloride forms hydrochloric acid, an especially corrosive agent that causes respiratory irritation.

However, the energy and heat produced as a by-product of incineration can be used in homes and industry. Incineration of solid wastes has been employed successfully for this purpose in many locations throughout Europe and is now being used in the United States. To accomplish this in the United States, many incinerators would have to be redesigned and rebuilt. As it stands, incineration is already one of the more costly waste disposal methods. Nevertheless, incineration as a generator of energy deserves more investigation. It is important to emphasize to students that all plants and animals have interdependent functions in our environment.

Solid Waste Control. In 1980, the United States created the Superfund, a $1.6-billion trust fund designated to clean up abandoned hazardous waste sites. Under this law, the EPA can clean up a dump site, and then recover the costs, through lawsuits, from those responsible. In 1986, realizing the problem was greater than originally thought, another $8.5 billion was added to the Superfund. Progress has been slow in this area. In 1990, the EPA reported that cleanup had been completed in only 52 of the 1,207 waste dump sites on the National Priorities List (Mullen et al. 1996, 623). Also, the EPA set forth a plan in 1988 that called for Americans to recycle 25 percent of their household trash by 1992. Voluntary recycling efforts aid these mandatory efforts (Levy, Dignan, and Shirreffs 1992, 518–519).

The United States, like many other nations, is still struggling with the problem. Until citizens recognize that many solid waste disposal programs are ineffective or unacceptable the situation is unlikely to change. More public awareness and action are needed to draw attention to the problem of solid waste disposal. In addition, individual efforts toward decreasing the daily use of disposal products that are not easily biodegradable as well as efforts aimed at recycling can assist greatly.

Radiation Pollution

Individuals are exposed to radiation daily both from natural sources, such as sunlight, and manmade sources. The manmade sources of radiation are of most concern. Radioactive materials release energy in the form of a stream of particles generally referred to as *radiation*. Alpha and beta radioactive particles do not easily penetrate the human body, but gamma radiation does. Gamma rays are much like X rays. If an individual is exposed to a high-enough dosage of gamma radiation, several adverse effects occur, ranging from nausea, hair loss, and diarrhea to cell mutation, anemia, and death.

In the United States, individuals come into contact with radiation mainly through medical testing and X rays. Although X rays are generally "safe," many instances of unnecessary exposure have been reported. Several month intervals should elapse before undergoing continued exposure to X rays. Pregnant women, particularly during the first trimester, should avoid being X-rayed if at all possible because radiation can cause cell damage and mutation to the developing fetus.

Exposure to low-level radiation for a prolonged period is also of great concern for individuals whose work surroundings or home environment may be near a radioactive source. The health effects of radiation exposure depend on many factors, including the duration, type, dose of exposure, and individual sensitivity. Lesser exposure can affect egg and sperm production, embryonic development and irreversible changes to the eyes and skin. Heavy exposure can produce radiation sickness or immediate death (Hahn and Payne 1997, 436). As a result, opponents to the use of nuclear power as an energy source are becoming more vocal. They fear both the potential for a nuclear accident like that which occurred at Three Mile Island in Pennsylvania in March 1979 and at the Chernobyl plant in the Soviet Union in April 1986, and the dangers of mishandling the disposal of nuclear wastes. On the other hand, supporters of nuclear power believe that through the implementation of the Nuclear Regulatory Commission's guidelines, nuclear power can be a safe, viable, and much needed energy source for the future.

Radiation Exposure Control

Guidelines exist that indicate allowable ranges of radiation exposure from medical testing, X rays, and consumer products emitting small amounts of radiation, such as television sets. However, the long-term effects on health of even low or "safe" levels of radiation are still poorly understood. Any radiation at all may in fact be deleterious to health. Certainly as individuals we must become more educated and aware of both the benefits and dangers of using radiation and nuclear power.

Noise Pollution

With more and more of the American people living in metropolitan areas, the problem of noise as a pollutant is also growing. Noise pollution is a problem for almost every urban dweller, and a particular cause of concern among people living near airports, employees working in manufacturing or industry, and commuters who must endure hours of noise each week traveling in cars, trains, buses, and subways. Also, listening to loud music, especially through earphones, is a noise pollutant that is a potential cause of hearing loss.

Noise levels are calculated in decibels (dB), a measurement for which 1 dB represents the minimum level of hearing for humans. A sound that is 10 times as loud would be 10 dB, another 100 times as loud would be 20 dB, one 1000 times as loud would be 30 dB, and so forth. Some typical noise levels include whispering (30 dB), air conditioner at 20 feet (60 dB), busy traffic (70 dB), truck noise (90 dB), airplane overhead or chainsaw (100 dB), rock band concert in front of speakers (120 dB), shotgun blast (140 dB), rocket pad during launch (180 dB). Intensity of sound exceeding 80 to 85 decibels can cause hearing damage. The damage is initially reversible; however, with continued exposure, the changes become permanent (Hahn and Payne 1997, 438–439).

Many detrimental effects apart from hearing impairment can occur due to noise because of its stressful nature. Headaches, difficulty in sleeping, increase in anxiety, and elevated blood pressure are just a few. As a result, increased efforts must be made toward minimizing noise pollution.

Noise Pollution Control

No uniform standards regarding acceptable noise levels for school, home, or work environments have been formulated. Therefore each individual must exercise personal judgment in deciding how much noise exposure is not only tolerable but safe. Employees in industry are, of course, issued protective ear devices, but the general public is not guaranteed the same protection on

Health Highlight

What You Can Do to Protect Our Planet

○ Buy green—e.g., switch from plastic wrap to wax paper and buy products packaged in recycled materials.

○ Recycle—collect, reprocess, market, and use materials once considered trash. Promote recycling of bottles, cans, newspapers, and mixed paper.

○ Composting—Mix organic products, such as leftover food and vegetable peels with straw and keep damp.

○ Don't smoke cigarettes—which pollutes the air.

○ Switch to light bulbs of lower wattage for those not used for reading.

○ Learn to enjoy music at lower volumes.

○ Reduce use of aerosol spray cans.

○ Turn your automobile off when you would be idling for a long time.

○ Reduce your time in taking a shower.

○ Switch from paper products to cloth handkerchiefs, napkins, and towels.

Source: D. Hales. 1994. *An invitation to health.* 6th ed. Redwood City, CA: Benjamin/Cummings, pp. 570–573.

noisy highways or in neighborhoods near loud noise sources. Greater awareness of the harmful effects of noise, both physical and psychological, may lead to public action and legislation in the years ahead.

Preservation of the Ecosphere

Conservation and protection of our natural resources must stem from both individual and public action. Both are needed to stabilize and eventually reverse the harmful cycle of contamination that currently plagues the ecosphere. Legislation and implementation of healthier environmental practices have been instituted. The enactment of additional measures could serve to improve the quality of living for us and for future generations.

☰ Summary

- Individuals should act responsibly and diligently with regard to their environment to ensure high-level wellness.
- The environment in which one lives must be free of dangerous levels of pollutants and therefore conducive to quality living—not just mere survival.
- In order to maintain the natural resources on which all living things depend, it is essential that we understand how we interact with and influence our ecosystem, our immediate habitat.
- Many man-made changes have caused havoc in the natural ecological chains or webs within ecosystems.
- Because ecosystems, like the residents within them, are interdependent and thus form one worldwide ecosphere, the harmful impact of human growth and technology is felt through the entire planet.
- In sheer numbers alone, our species is stretching the capacity of land, water, and food supplies to accommodate us.
- Particularly in the highly industrial nations, human lifestyles have resulted in an abundance of pollution problems that cannot be dealt with by the natural cycles within the ecosphere.
- With our automobiles, we release dangerous pollutants into the air.
- Industry adds still other toxins, and runoff from agriculture and industrial dumping contaminates our water.
- Hardly a week goes by without some incident involving the accidental leakage or spilling of highly lethal substances being transported.
- These environmental health problems, coupled with those of solid waste disposal, radiation exposure, and noise pollution, have resulted in ecological crises never before witnessed.
- Through continued research and education, which will spark responsible action on the part of both governments and individuals, preservation of the ecosphere is possible.
- It is our job as educators to provide instructional and consciousness-raising experiences to the children we teach so that their children and grandchildren will enjoy continued health and well-being in a sound environment.

Discussion Questions

1. Define and differentiate between the terms *environment* and *ecology*.

2. What is the ecosphere, and how do human beings interact with elements of the ecosphere?

3. What impact does overpopulation have on the state of the environment, and what problems directly or indirectly stem from overpopulation?

4. Discuss the health effects of global warming and ozone layer depletion.

5. What are the major sources of air pollution? Describe the harmful effects of specific air pollutants on human health.

6. What are the objectives that the U.S. government has set for regulation of contaminants by the year 2000?

7. What individual steps can be taken to more effectively manage and control air pollution?

8. What threats to environmental health does the transportation of hazardous substances pose?

9. What is noise pollution? How does it affect environmental health?

10. How can each individual help to preserve the ecosphere? Give specific suggestions.

References

Bruess, C., and G. Richardson. 1994. *Healthy decisions.* Madison, WI: Brown & Benchmark.

Donatelle, R., and L. Davis. 1996. *Access to health*, 4th ed. Boston: Allyn and Bacon.

Green, L., and J. Ottoson. 1994. *Community health*, 7th ed. St. Louis: Mosby.

Hahn, D., and W. Payne. 1997. *Focus on health*, 3rd ed. St. Louis: Mosby-Yearbook.

Hales, D. 1994. *An invitation to health*, 6th ed. Redwood City, CA: Benjamin/Cummings.

Levy, M., M. Dignan, and J. Shirreffs. 1992. *Life & health: targeting wellness.* New York: McGraw-Hill.

Mullen, K., R. McDermott, R. Gold, and P. Belcastro. 1996. *Connections for health*, 4th ed. Madison, WI: Brown & Benchmark.

Pruitt, B., and J. Stein. 1994. *Healthstyles: Decisions for living well.* Fort Worth, TX: Saunders College.

Smolin, L., and M. Grosvenor. 1994. *Nutrition: Science and applications.* Fort Worth, TX: Saunders College.

U.S. Department of Health and Human Services. 1990. *Healthy people 2000.* Washington, DC: U.S. Government Printing Office.

Chapter Twenty-Five
Strategies for Teaching Environmental Health

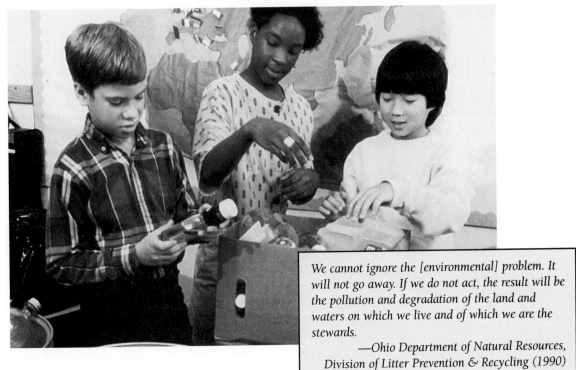

> *We cannot ignore the [environmental] problem. It will not go away. If we do not act, the result will be the pollution and degradation of the land and waters on which we live and of which we are the stewards.*
>
> —Ohio Department of Natural Resources, Division of Litter Prevention & Recycling (1990)

Valued Outcomes

After doing the activities in this chapter, the students should be able to explain and illustrate the following statements:

○ High levels of personal wellness can only be sustained if the environment is conducive to well-being.

○ All the animals, plants, and natural resources in any particular habitat form a self-sustaining ecosystem.

○ All parts of an ecosystem are interdependent.

○ Each ecosystem is linked to all other ecosystems to form a global network called an *ecosphere*. Thus change in one ecosystem has the potential to affect any other ecosystem and the ecosphere as a whole.

○ Because human beings have the ability to alter and manipulate the environment, human activities have the greatest impact on ecosystems.

○ Human activities have caused extensive harm to the environment, which has affected environmental health.

○ The major sources of pollution are air impurities, water contaminants, hazardous chemicals, solid waste, radiation, and noise.

○ Overpopulation has also resulted in environmental problems.

○ Conservation of natural resources, preservation of ecosystems, and protection of the environment from pollution are essential for preserving the ecosphere.

○ Preservation of the ecosphere must stem both from individual and public action.

Fostering Environmental Appreciation

Every species of plant and animal has had to adapt to its environment or face extinction. This adaptation has resulted in an amazing variety of lifeforms on the planet. Thick-skinned cacti have adapted to the harsh environment of our deserts. Luminescent fish live successfully in the perpetual darkness of the ocean depths. Polar bears carry on their life cycles in the frozen landscape beyond the Arctic Circle.

Human beings have also had to adapt to the physical environment. But unlike any other form of life on the planet, human beings can also extensively adapt the environment to suit their needs. We build cities, dam rivers, mine the earth, and farm the land. To a large extent, we can manipulate and control our environment. This unique ability has sometimes resulted in the misconception that we are the masters of our environment. This has led to abuse of natural resources and consequent pollution, waste, and lowering of environmental quality.

In the last few decades, we have become more aware that human beings are not free to alter the environment—we pay a price. We have recognized that we are part of a worldwide ecosystem, interacting and interrelating with every other part. This increased environmental awareness has not come too soon. We now know all too well that nature's resources are finite and must be conserved and used wisely. We have begun to see that change to any part of the environment can have a wide-ranging impact on many other parts. Failure to understand the consequences could mean disaster not only for ourselves but for the entire planet.

Children need to learn about the importance of healthy environment. They must recognize that it is up to each of us to maintain the environment. Doing so will more easily foster high-level wellness. Instruction about environmental health should build a sense of appreciation for all life and natural resources and encourage personal practices that will help to ensure the continued preservation of the ecosphere. The activities suggested in this chapter will help you attain this goal for your students.

Value-Based Activities

Value-based activities are designed to assist children in developing their critical thinking skills, personalize information, and establish concepts that are conducive to high-quality wellness. Teachers can design a variety of value-based activities depending on the content being discussed. Some suggestions follow:

Health Highlight

Things Kids Can Do to Protect the Environment

Our natural resources are important, and there are many things we can do to protect and preserve them. Some things kids can do include the following:

○ Recycle all aluminum.

○ Purchase recycled products.

○ Ask parents to reuse grocery shopping bags.

○ Recycle metals.

○ Recycle newspapers.

○ Use as few paper products as possible.

○ Recycle cardboard.

○ Recycle plastics.

○ Recycle tin cans.

○ Recycle glass containers.

Major Environmental Problems

Valued Outcome: Students will identify the biggest problem affecting our environment.
Description of Strategy: This activity is designed to help children discuss the problems affecting our environment. Topics may include overpopulation, pesticides, land pollution, air pollution, water pollution, and noise pollution.
Processing Questions:

1. Why do you believe this is the biggest problem?

2. How is this affecting the environment?

3. How does this problem affect you and your family?

4. What can your family do to help relieve this problem?

Ecological Food Chain

Valued Outcome: Students will be able to describe the ecological food chain.
Description of Strategy: The following items are the major parts of the ecological food chain. Have the students place them in order to make an ecological food chain model. The students may add links to make a more elaborate food chain: water, birds, fish, humans.
Processing Questions:

1. What happens when pesticides affect one link in the ecological model?

2. What is an example of an endangered animal or bird that has been affected by pesticides or pollution?

3. What are some ways you can help eliminate environmental pollution?

*We are the stewards of
our land and water.*

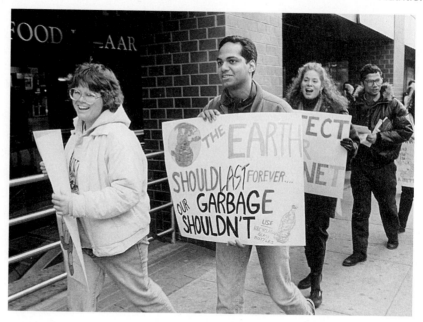

Let's Rank Our Environmental Problems

Valued Outcome: The students will be able to identify the most hazardous environmental problems.

Description of Strategy: Have the students rank the environmental problems from most hazardous to least hazardous, 1 being the most and 3 being the least. Once the class is finished, write the problems on the board and rank them as a group. Have an open class discussion about the answers.

Air Pollution

____ carbon monoxide and nitrogen

____ sulfur oxides

____ lead

Water Pollution

____ animal fertilizers

____ human sewage

____ industrial wastes

Solid Waste Pollution

____ dump

____ sanitary landfills

____ recycling

Hazardous Chemical Pollution

____ pesticides

____ industrial chemicals

____ household products

Materials Needed: copy of the various environmental hazardous. May wish to develop own list.
Processing Questions:

1. Why are some hazards more dangerous than others?

2. What are some ways we can prevent pollution of our environment?

Decision Stories

Present decision stories such as these, using the procedures outlined in Chapter 4.

The Fishing Trip

Johnny is going fishing with his grandfather. He is very excited. They have fixed a picnic lunch because they plan to stay all day. Johnny and his grandfather drive to the river. As they walk along the riverside, Johnny notices some dead fish floating in the water. "Grandfather, what killed those fish?" Johnny asks. "They were killed because people put garbage into the river," Grandfather replies. Then they sit down and start to fish. Johnny and his grandfather catch several fish apiece.
Focus Questions: Should they take the fish home and cook them? Why or why not? What can Johnny and his grandfather do to make the river cleaner?

A Bird's Nest

Jim and Richard are good friends who live next door to one another. They are now old enough to walk home from school, and today is their first time to do so. On the way home they cut through a small park. Richard discovers a bird's nest with three eggs in it. He wants to take it home. Jim has been taught to respect living things. He knows it is important not to disturb the natural surroundings, but Richard is such a good friend.
Focus Question: What should Jim do?

Is Recycling Worth the Work?

Kathy has heard about a recycling center in her town. People can bring bottles and aluminum cans there. The material is crushed and then sold to industry to be used again. Kathy tells her mother about the recycling center and asks if the family can bring in their bottles and cans. "It sounds like a good idea," Kathy's mother says. "But it's too much work. We would have to clean and sort all our old bottles and cans. Anyway, the recycling center has enough bottles and cans without us."
Focus Questions: Should Kathy try to convince her mother that recycling is worth the effort? How could she do this?

Bad Air

One day, Sarah's mother comes home from work coughing and wheezing. "What's wrong, Mom?" Sarah asks. "It's all that dirty air I have to breathe riding the bus to and from work," her mother replies. "Maybe you could find a job closer to home," Sarah says. "It's not that easy to find jobs these days," her mother says. "I guess I'll just have to put up with the bad air on the bus."
Focus Questions:

1. Is there anything Sarah can do to help her mother?

2. Whom can Sarah contact to find out about lowering air pollution?

Dramatizations ———————————————————

Role-Playing

Valued Outcome: The students will be able to discuss several environmental hazards.
Description of Strategy: Divide the students in groups of four to five students. Have the groups pick an environmental hazard. Then have one group at a time come up and act out the problem. If a group is having trouble picking an environmental hazard, then the instructor can help the group. Examples of hazards that can be used are water pollution, air pollution—pretend to be using hair spray, littering, and so on. The group that can guess what environmental hazard is taking place receives a point. If no one can guess the environmental hazard, then that group receives a point. Keep playing until everyone has gone several times. At the end of the lesson, have the students brainstorm all the hazards and write them down on the board.
Materials Needed: none
Processing Question: Where can environmental hazards be found?

Water Pollution

Valued Outcome: The students will be able to describe how oil spills hurt the environment.
Description of Strategy: Have five and ten students pretend that they are living plants, fish, animals, and other living things in a body of water. Have three or four other students act as if they were the sun shining on the water and helping the plants and other living things to live. Then have five to ten students come marching in and pretend they are an oil spill in the water. Once the oil blocks the sun, have all the living organisms pretend to die.
Materials Needed: none
Processing Questions:

1. What exactly happens during an oil spill?

2. What other environmentally dangerous events can oil spill cause?

Population Problems

Valued Outcome: The students will be able to discuss how to conserve resources.
Description of Strategy: Have three of the students act as if they were wild horses in the wild. Provide several bottles around the room for water and little snacks for food. Tell the horses they

must eat and drink to survive. The snack can represent the grass they must have, and the water will represent a stream of water. Add three more horses, then three more, and keep going until everyone is a horse. Have them "go to sleep," and tell them that when they wake up there will only be a small amount of water and food left. Ask them to explain to you what they will do. Have several of the horses die. Then ask a variety of questions about what actually happened. Relate the story to us as human beings and our resources. Explain what happens when this happens to other animals and the whole ecology system.

Materials Needed: three water bottles, bags of corn flakes or another cereal

Processing Questions:

1. What was the problem?

2. What would happen once there was no more food or water?

Plants and Animals Need Protection, Too

Valued Outcome: The students will role-play a community of plants and animals in environmental danger.

Description of Strategy: Divide students into groups and use a story such as "Smokey the Bear," "Bambi," or any other suitable example for the specific grade level to inspire students to role-play a community of plants and animals who are in danger from an environmental threat. Tell students not only to voice their concerns as the animals and plants, but to also try to decide whether they as plants and animals can do anything to either prevent or diminish the environmental threat.

Materials Needed: none

Processing Question: How do environmental health dangers affect animals?

Home Hunting

Valued Outcome: The students will role-play selling a house and identify several examples of a safe neighborhood.

Description of Strategy: Divide the class into small groups. Each group is responsible for describing a home in a neighborhood that is for sale. One or two people in the group act as the sellers, while one or two people act as the buyers. The buyers come to look at the house and ask all sorts of questions, many of which focus on environmental concerns, such as: What is the average monthly heating bill? cooling bill? How many miles from downtown is the neighborhood? How far away are the schools and shopping centers? Where is the nearest industrial site? Is there much noise in the neighborhood? Give only minimal guidance, such as a few examples of environmentally related questions. Allow each group five minutes for the presentation, and keep track of the commonly asked questions. Then summarize by emphasizing the importance of living in a safe, wholesome environment.

Materials Needed: none

Processsing Question: What environmental concerns are involved with owning and maintaining a house?

Future Lifestyles

Valued Outcome: The students will be able to portray what life will be like in the future.

Description of Strategy: Divide students into small groups. Assign each group a different social role. For example, one group could be factory workers; another group, business professionals;

and a third group, small farmers. Ask groups to portray what they think life will be like for their members fifty years in the future, paying particular attention to possible environmental changes and their influences on the surroundings.

Materials Needed: none

Processing Question: What environmental changes will affect people's lives fifty years from now?

City Crisis

Valued Outcome: The students will enact a hypothetical dilemma concerning an environmental issue.

Description of Strategy: Provide the class with a hypothetical dilemma involving a voting question about a proposed city ordinance concerning an environmental issue. Give enough detailed information about the city and its problems so that the viewpoints of various special interest groups can be developed. This may best be accomplished with a descriptive handout outlining pertinent information about the city. Then divide the class into three groups. Assign two groups the task of presenting a scenario and possible solution to the problem at a town meeting. Let students within each group volunteer to role-play identical characters, such as meeting moderator, mayor, union representatives, conservation spokespeople, and so forth. Allow both groups a few days to prepare a fifteen-mininute dramatization. Dramatizations are presented as the third group acts as observers. Following the presentations, the third group then objectively critiques the ideas by highlighting strong points of each presentation and suggesting additional alternatives.

Materials Needed: none

Processing Questions:

1. What environmental concerns are being debated, discussed, and voted on by your city politicians?

2. How will their discussions affect you and your family?

Disaster Preparation Practice

Valued Outcome: The students will identify an environmental disaster and its effects on communities.

Description of Strategy: Divide the class into moderate-size groups, and assign each group to research an environmental disaster that could affect communities, such as an air pollution crisis, train derailment of hazardous chemicals, or a highly toxic pollutant entering municipal water system. Ask each group to dramatize a preparation plan that demonstrates the actions that should be taken or contributions that could be made by various community organizations in dealing with the environmental danger, should it ever occur.

Materials Needed: none

Processing Questions:

1. What are examples of environmental danger plans?

2. Does your school and/or city have such a plan for a radiation disaster or other danger?

Alien Impressions

Valued Outcome: The students will be able to discuss how foreigners to our country would react to our environmental conditions.

Description of Strategy: Divide the class into groups of about five students. Tell each group that they are aliens from outer space who have suddenly landed in the heart of the city. Ask the groups to act out their reactions to our earthly surroundings, placing special emphasis on impressions about noise levels, traffic, air pollution, crowding, and use of natural resources.
Materials Needed: none
Processing Question: How would our environmental conditions appear to someone not familiar to our country?

Discussion and Report Strategies

Nature Watch

Valued Outcome: The students will observe behaviors in the environment with regard to plants and animals.
Description of Strategy: Group students into threes and place each group in a spot on or near the school premises in as "natural" an environment as possible. Have each group silently observe the happenings in the environment for ten to fifteen minutes, particularly those associated with plants and animals. Then have each group discuss their observations. Later, ask the members of the class as a whole to focus on their feelings and attitudes about nature, based on this observation experience.
Materials Needed: pen and paper
Processing Questions:

1. What aspects of nature did you observe?
2. How did you feel about the environment you observed?

Activities and Their Environmental Effects

Valued Outcome: The students will list ten activities and describe how these activities affect the environment.
Description of Strategy: Ask each student to list ten hobbies or activities he or she enjoys doing. After listing the activities, students should examine each activity in terms of its effects, if any, on the environment. As a result of this exercise, students will observe the relationship between their behavior and the environment in which they live.
Materials Needed: pen and paper
Processing Question: What effects, if any, does your hobby have on the environment? Is it positive or negative?

Me and My Surroundings

Valued Outcome: The students will recognize his or her perceptions of the environment.
Description of Strategy: Ask each student to keep a daily log for a week about his or her perceptions of environmental influences by writing a short paragraph that describes each day in terms of environmental awareness. Students should emphasize not only facts but also feelings about these influences. For example, "Heavy rain against my window last night sounded nice. The noisy and crowded school bus made me feel irritable." At the end of the week, divide the class

into small discussion groups, each one representing one day of the week. Have groups compare their logs for that day and summarize major perceptions about surroundings. One group member should then present a five-minute report to the class outlining summary findings.
Materials Needed: pen and paper
Processing Questions:

1. What environmental influences did you observe?

2. Are there any influences that need to be changed in order to protect the environment?

Environmental Stories

Valued Outcome: The student will create a story regarding a picture of the environment.
Description of Strategy: Select a colorful, eye-catching, and appropriate picture depicting an aspect of the environment. Have each student write a story about the picture. Allow about twenty minutes, and encourage both creativity and the exploration of values. Several volunteers may want to read their stories to the class.
Materials Needed: picture of environment, pen, paper
Processing Questions:

1. What did you notice about the environment from the picture?

2. Was the environment in the picture a pleasant scene?

Resource Reduction

Valued Outcome: The students will identify common products and compare the usage of different products.
Description of Strategy: Divide the class into small groups, and assign each group a common environmental product or resource, such as paper, plastic, water, electricity, or natural gas. For a few days, ask each group member to keep a daily list of his or her specific uses of the resource. Then have group members compare lists and prepare a master list on wall-size sheets of paper outlining the most typically used products, frequency or most common uses, amount students think has been used by the total group, and ways to reduce the use. Tack the master lists to the wall. Lists might look something like this:

Product	Frequency	Amount	Ways to Reduce
Paper napkins	_____	_____	_____
Facial tissues	_____	_____	_____
Toilet paper	_____	_____	_____
Notebook paper	_____	_____	_____

Materials Needed: poster board, markers
Processing Questions:

1. What did you observe about the products you use?

2. Do you think you can conserve products in order to help the environment?

Environmental Newswatch and Commentary

Valued Outcome: The students will identify various environmental articles as to the articles' lesson or moral value.

Description of Strategy: Divide students into small groups. Provide each student with three sheets of colored construction paper, and ask students to paste a newspaper or magazine article on each sheet that deals with an environmental topic. Use of newsletters, supplementary magazines, and books that are written for the students' grade level should be encouraged. Underneath each article, have the students write a caption that describes the "moral" or "lesson" of the article. Have each group then compile their articles into a booklet. Similar articles should be grouped within the booklets.

Materials Needed: construction paper, markers, newspapers, magazines, glue

Processing Questions:

1. What was your environmental article about?

2. Did the story portray a lesson about conservation?

Environmental Worksheet

Valued Outcome: The students will illustrate ideas concerning various environmental resources.

Description of Strategy: Ask each student to draw or illustrate his or her ideas in the appropriate section about the following:

1. Most important environmental resource
2. Most abundant environmental resource
3. Most depleted environmental resource
4. Most dangerous environmental threat to the world
5. Most environmentally helpful family measure practiced
6. Least environmentally helpful family measure practiced
7. Most environmentally helpful personal measure practiced
8. Least environmentally helpful personal measure practiced

Let students share their global pictures with each other to compare ideas.

Materials Needed: pencil and paper

Processing Questions:

1. Did you learn anything from this activity that will help protect our environment?

2. What can you personally do to protect the environment?

Let's Be Creative

Valued Outcome: The students will be able to present solutions for various environmental hazards.

Description of Strategy: Have the students draw a cartoon series, write a story, or make up a poem about an environmental problem. Then have volunteers share what they did with the class. Discuss what was said, problems, and solutions for the environmental hazard. After completing the activity, have them tape their work around the room. Let the students walk around and observe each other's displays.

Materials Needed: paper, markers, and so on
Processing Questions:

1. What environmental hazards did you identify?

2. What solutions did you present for each hazard?

Recycling Centers

Valued Outcome: The students will be able to discuss the recycling plan in their community.
Description of Strategy: Have the students tell you where they can go to recycle in their community and what they can recycle. Then have a guest speaker come in from one of the recycling centers to talk with the students. Ask them to explain the plant, what they do, and what the students should do.
Materials Needed: none
Processing Question: What is the purpose of a recycling plant or center?

What Do You Think?

Valued Outcome: The students will be able to discuss alternatives to activities that are environmental hazards.
Description of Strategy: Divide the students in groups of four to six students. Give each group an environmental hazard. Have the group think of all the pros and cons for the item. Ask them to think of what hazards it can cause and of different alternatives that can be used. If it is a problem, have them think of a solution. Depending on what the environmental factor is, suggest a variety of things for them to think about. Then have each group discuss what their item is and their conclusions from it. Have the whole class discuss the problem, and ask the group different questions concerning the item.
Materials Needed: cans, paper, hair spray, oil, and so on
Processing Questions:

1. What are some environmentally dangerous activities you participate in every day?

2. Are there alternatives to these activities that are less dangerous to our environment?

Banner

Valued Outcome: The students will be able to describe the positive and negative environmental aspects of their surroundings.
Description of Strategy: Place a long blank banner on one side of the room and another long banner on the other side of the room. Write positive on one and negative on the other. Have the student draw and write positive and negative environmental factors on the correct banner. Then have the students volunteer to show what they drew or wrote to the class and discuss it.
Materials Needed: two long banners, markers or crayons
Processing Questions:

1. What environmental factors in your surroundings should be considered?

2. What are the positive and negative aspects of each of those factors?

Ecosystem Explanation

Valued Outcome: The students will be able to explain an ecosystem.
Description of Strategy: Using the dairy cow as an example of the relationships that exist in an ecosystem, explain with pictures, posters, and diagrams how cows eating grass produce milk we drink. Then ask each student to think of another animal that is part of a food chain, and have the students describe the workings of that food chain.
Materials Needed: none
Processing Questions:

1. What is an ecosystem?
2. How does an ecosystem affect your environment?

Population Problems

Valued Outcome: The students will be able to discuss overpopulation as an environmental hazard.
Description of Strategy: To stimulate discussion about the concerns of overpopulation for very young students, have them recite the nursery rhyme, "There was an old woman who lived in a shoe./She had so many children she knew not what to do." Have students tell you what this rhyme means to them. Older students can be asked to make a graph of the world's population increases since the beginning of recorded years. Note especially the curve for the last twenty years. Then provide further information about the problem of overpopulation, and have students discuss suggestions to curb overpopulation.
Materials Needed: pen and paper
Processing Questions:

1. Does your community have an overpopulation problem?
2. What measures can be taken to reduce the overpopulation problem?

Hunger Hurts

Valued Outcome: The students will be able to discuss world hunger.
Description of Strategy: As a class, have students research information about the impact of hunger on children throughout the world. This may be done by asking the librarian to suggest a few sources that each class member can read. Also have students determine the three leading causes of death among infants and children in America as compared to those of several other countries you select. Be sure to include both European and Third World countries. Allow students to discuss their ideas concerning the reason for these differences.
Materials Needed: library books
Processing Questions:

1. What is the nature of hunger in Europe and other countries?
2. Is hunger a problem in our country? in your community?

General Pollution Problems

Valued Outcome: The students will be able to describe the impact of major environmental problems.

Description of Strategy: Divide the class into several small groups, and assign each group a different major pollution problem. After researching the general aspects of the problem, each group should give a short oral panel presentation. Within the groups, each member is then assigned a specific aspect of the given pollution problem, such as oil spills, effects of sulfides in the air, or the banning of DDT. Have the students prepare individual written reports.
Materials Needed: pen and paper
Processing Question: What are the major environmental problems that affect you?

Energy Savings

Valued Outcome: The students will be able to explain how citizens can save energy.
Description of Strategy: Have a general class discussion concerning ways Americans can save energy. Discuss how rising costs of fuel have made Americans more energy conscious in recent years. Individual students may wish to volunteer how their families are doing more to save energy.
Materials Needed: none
Processing Questions:

1. What are the types of energy used in your homes?

2. What are ways you and your family can save energy?

Experiments and Demonstrations

Recyclable Containers

Valued Outcome: The students will be able to explain the positive aspects of recycling.
Description of Strategy: Have the students bring a flat box or paper bag to class. Ask the students to draw, color, write, or whatever they want on their containers. The student will either make a box or bag that can recycle paper or cans. Place the boxes and bags around the school and in different classes. At the end of the week, collect the recyclable cans and paper. Discuss with the class how they feel about the project and the results from it.
Materials Needed: box or bag, marker, crayons, and so on
Processing Questions:

1. What is the purpose of recycling?

2. How does recycling help our environment?

Signs

Valued Outcome: The students will be able to produce some helpful environmental hints.
Description of Strategy: Have the students make a variety of signs to display around the school; for example, "Turn off the water when you're finished," "Throw away your trash," "Recycle your cans." After a week, discuss the results. Note the changes. If there are no changes, ask why. Think of another alternative, and go with it. If it works, congratulate them for a job well done.
Materials Needed: paper, markers, pens, and so on
Processing Question: What can we do to help advance the cause of environmental conservation?

Water Conservation

Valued Outcome: The students will be able to describe ways to conserve resources in order to help the environment.

Description of Strategy: Bring two toothbrushes to class, with some toothpaste. Have two students volunteer to brush their teeth. One student will leave the water running, while brushing his or her teeth, and the other student will turn the water off. Ask students to notice how much water was wasted. Have them explain what will happen to our water supply if everyone did this. Have them also tell you some other ways we waste water. Ask them to explain how we can prevent this from happening.

Materials Needed: two toothbrushes, toothpaste

Processing Question: What are some habits that you can change in your daily life that will conserve resources and help the environment?

Water Pollution

Valued Outcome: The students will be able to describe the negative effects of used engine oil on the environment.

Description of Strategy: Take a little jar, and place some engine oil within the jar. Show the students what happens to the water. Then use the bigger container and place the same amount of oil in it. Show the students the results. Have them explain what they observed. Explain to them how it doesn't matter how much oil is spilled because it spreads. Ask the students how many of their parents change the oil in their own cars. Ask what they do with the oil once they are through. Tell them that the average car uses 4 quarts of oil. Have them guess how much water would be polluted with 4 quarts of oil (30–40 square feet). Have them tell you how their parents can recycle the engine oil.

Materials Needed: one jar, bucket, pail, or container, bottle of engine oil

Processing Question: What are some ways you and your family can recycle oil in order to protect the environment?

Waste Production

Valued Outcome: The students will be able to discuss the impact of solid waste (such as trash, garbage) on the environment.

Description of Strategy: Have the students observe in their homes how many bags of trash they fill a day. Have them do this for three days. Every day before class starts, tally up the bags of trash used the day before. After three days, have the students place a recyclable bag or box by the trash. Calculate the bags of trash for the next three days. Make sure you do the same thing in the classroom. Have the students explain what has happened and what they have observed. This will show how much they waste and how much our country wastes. Discuss what will happen if we keep doing this. Discuss what might happen if we start recycling.

Materials Needed: none

Processing Questions:

1. What is the impact of solid waste products on our environment?

2. What are some ways you and your family can dispose or recycle some solid wastes to help protect the environment?

Seasonal Adjustments

Valued Outcome: The students will be able to explain the environmental influences of trees and plants.

Description of Strategy: Divide students into small groups, and ask each group to select a favorite tree or shrub in the school yard to observe once a month for the school year. Let groups record their observations in relation to environmental influences on the changes of the tree or shrub.

Materials Needed: none

Processing Questions:

1. What changes take place in trees from season to season?

2. What effects do these changes have on our environment?

Terrariums and Aquariums as Ecosystems

Valued Outcome: The students will be able to describe the interrelationships involved in ecosystems.

Description of Strategy: As a class project, help students make a terrarium and an aquarium. Refer to science texts as resources to help you do this. Use the terrarium and aquarium to demonstrate the interrelationships among residents in each particular ecosystem.

Materials Needed: terrarium and/or aquarium

Processing Question: How do residents in a terrarium and/or aquarium depend on each other for their existence?

Trees can have a positive influence upon our environment.

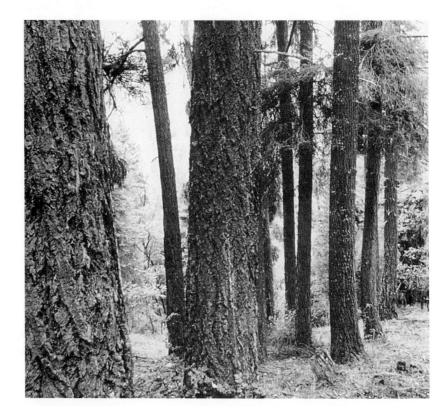

Water Impurities

Valued Outcome: The students will be able to discuss the environmental implications of impurities in drinking water.
Description of Strategy: Have each student bring in a small jar of water from a tap at home. Even though the water may all come from the same municipal supply, there will be differences in the samples because of rust or chemical residues in the water pipes in each home. Examine under a microscope.
Materials Needed: jars, water from tap
Processing Questions:

1. What are the implications of impurities in drinking water?

2. How can we ensure that we have safe water to drink?

Crowding Problems

Valued Outcome: The students will be able to discuss the effects of overcrowding (overpopulation) on the environment.
Description of Strategy: Divide students in groups, and give each group two milk cartons with a few holes punched in the bottom for drainage. Ask students to fill each carton about two-thirds full of potting soil and in one carton plant two or three bean seeds about one inch apart and just under the surface of the soil. In the other carton, students should plant fifteen seeds about one-half inch apart. Let them water the cartons every four days and record their observations. As an extension of this activity, crowd students into a confined space for a few minutes and then ask them to describe how it felt.
Materials Needed: two milk cartons, potting soil, bean seed, water
Processing Question: What are the problems of overcrowding as it relates to the use of natural resources?

Noise Levels

Valued Outcome: The students will be able to discuss unwanted noise as an environmental hazard.
Description of Strategy: Use a decibel meter to check noise levels in varous locations throughout the school. Noise levels will vary during different times of day. Which locations are noisiest? Are there any sources of particularly loud sounds, such as school bus engines?
Materials Needed: decibel meter
Processing Questions:

1. How can some sounds become environmental hazards?

2. What are some ways to diminish noise pollution in the school environment?

Puzzles and Games

Health Hazard

Valued Outcome: The students will be able to name and suggest solutions to environmental hazards.

Description of Strategy: Ask the students various questions about their environmental health. Examples: How many of you like to drink soda? (Raise your hand.) How many of you recycle your cans when you're done? Why? Why not? How many of you have an electric can opener in your house? Do you think you're wasting electricity by using it instead of a manual one? What are some other hazards we do that can threaten our environmental health? Examples: not conserving water or electricity; polluting the air, water, environment; not recycling; and so on.

Have a student put on a jersey and make him or her one of the health hazards in our environment. The student will be "it." He or she will try to tag the other students. Once the students are tagged, they must sit down because they are now health hazards. After two minutes, have all the students who have not been tagged come to you. Ask the students to tell you something that we can do to correct the problem. For instance, if the health hazard was "waste" the students may suggest that we recycle. The game starts again with another health hazard. At the end of the lesson, have three or four health hazards be "it." This will suggest that the more health hazards we have, the more of a chance of having a really unhealthy environment.

Materials Needed: open areas, optional—jerseys or bandannas

Processing Question: What are some specific ways that each of us can correct some environmental hazards?

Treasure Hunt

Valued Outcome: The students will be able to describe the recycling process and how recycling helps protect the environment.

Description of Strategy: Divide the students in groups of five to eight students. On each table there should be a variety of items (recyclable, nonrecyclable, hazards, and helpful things for our environment). Examples: notebook paper, a coin, a leaf, plastic wrap, clean water, rubber stopper, cleansers, oil bottle, and so on. Ask the students various questions about environmental health. Some questions might relate to the items on the table, and some questions may not. Students must write the answer down. An example of a question that might be asked is "Who can show me a recyclable item?" Whichever group raises a hand first and can give the right answer will get a point. Another example: "Name three types of pollution" (water, air, noise, radiation, chemical). The game continues until the instructor has asked all the questions he or she wants about environmental health. The group that answers the most questions correctly is considered the winner.

Materials Needed: different objects that are, variously, recyclable, nonrecyclable, harmful, or helpful to the environment

Processing Questions:

1. What is the purpose of recycling?
2. How does recycling help protect the environment?
3. How can recycling help your health?

Brainstorm

Valued Outcome: The students will be able to discuss the meaning of several environmental terms.

Description of Strategy: Divide the class in groups of four to six students. Write a word on the board, such as *recycle*. The students brainstorm everything that comes to their minds when they hear the word *recycle*. The groups work together as a team to make a list of words; for example, glass, paper, plastic, newspapers, water, and so on. After one minute, start with group 1 and have them tell one item on their list. Group 2 will then go, telling another item different from group 1. Ask each group. Write all the words on the board for the class. After each group has been asked, go around the room again. The group who has the most responses gets a point. Then the game starts again with another word. Specific questions can also be asked. For example, what are the effects of water pollution? Answers: "destroys animals," "depletes food supplies," "harms reproduction," "produces odors," "makes foul tasting drinking water," "causes diseases," "pollutes beaches," and so on.

Materials Needed: paper, pencils

Processing Question: What are the effects of various types of pollution on the environment?

Other Ideas

Poster Contest

Valued Outcome: The students will be able to create a poster with an environmental message.

Description of Strategy: Ask each student to make a poster entitled "Energy." Give minimal details about what might be included. Let the students use their creativity. Number each poster anonymously and tack them around the room. Have another class view the posters and select the five best.

Materials Needed: poster board

Processing Question: What are some environmental messages we can portray through posters?

Survival Lists

Valued Outcome: The students will be able to compile a list of supplies needed in the time of an environmental disaster.

Description of Strategy: Divide students into small groups. Ask each group to prepare two lists. One list should include necessary supplies for a family of four to survive on the earth for the next year in the event of a disaster. The other list should include the twenty most important items to take on a trip to outer space. Let groups compare lists and discuss ideas. If enough agreement can be reached, make a class master list.

Materials Needed: paper, pen or pencil

Processing Questions:

1. What are some environmental disasters that might necessitate the prior accumulation of supplies?

2. What supplies would be the most important to gather prior to such a disaster?

Reference

Ohio Department of Natural Resources, Division of Litter Prevention & Recycling. *Super saver investigators.* Columbus, OH: Author, 1990.

Resources

Books

Environmental action groups. 1996. Broomall, PA: Chelsea House.

Toxic materials. 1996. Broomall, PA: Chelsea House.

Videos

Can buildings make you sick?
Discussing "bad" air in buildings, homes, schools, and hospitals. Library Video Company.

Environmental S.W.A.T. team.
Scientists fight against time, disease, and adversity. Library Video Company.

The greenhouse effect.
Computer animation and live action video combine to develop a fundamental understanding of the greenhouse effect. Library Video Company.

Web Sites

The Enviro Link. This site has several links to sources of environmental information. For instance, there is a list of environmentally sound consumer information. *http://envirolink.org/start_web.html*

Environmental Education Network. This site offers links to environmental resources for researchers and students. *http://www.environlink.org/enviroed*

Environmental Protection Agency. This site offers a searchable database and comprehensive directory. *http://www.epa.gov*

The Use Less Stuff Report Page. Waste reduction, EPA materials. Simple and fun page. *http://garnet.msen.com:70/1/vendor/cygnus/uls*

If our values are straight and we value human health above all else, then health education becomes one of the master areas in all of American education, along with language. It deals, or should deal, with all those phenomena indigenous to being human, that develop or retard, create or kill. Nothing is more important. Time must be found for it.

—Delbert Oberteuffer, April 24, 1982

It is the intention of the authors that this textbook portray the necessity for providing a sound cognitive base for health education complemented by opportunities for weighing and formulating a value system. This process enables students to begin to make more intelligent decisions pertaining to their health. The message is that all teaching efforts are aimed at the development of a value system resulting in a positive and healthy lifestyle. Ultimately, the decisions about lifestyle rest with each individual. Although the ability of children to fully control their health patterns may be limited, the seeds of critical thinking, wise decision making, and positive health choices must be planted and nourished. It is the teacher's professional, societal, and personal responsibility to facilitate the understanding of a wellness lifestyle that will result in the highest quality of life possible for every student.

We believe that health education should be viewed as a planned series of experiences that promote disease prevention behaviors and reinforce positive health experiences in each student. The ultimate goal of health education is the development of individuals who take charge of their lives and promote their own well-being, as well as that of their family and their community. To accomplish this goal, our nation must strive for the development of a comprehensive health education program. This necessitates effort beginning in grade K and continuing through grade 12. Each step in the educational ladder should be predicated on what has previously occurred in the learning situation. Health is the most fundamental of the basics. Health education must be allotted time in the same manner as mathematics, reading, and science.

The content areas of health education are many and varied. Health is not just physical education, although this is an important component. Truly healthy individuals are more able to accept themselves and others, are more physically fit, and are more capable of making informed decisions concerning the many components of living a more healthy wellness type of lifestyle. Without the best possible health, people become less productive, less satisfied in their personal lives, and less capable of contributing to other people's lives and the society of which they are a part.

As health educators, we should seek to enhance the life of each person we touch. It is our desire to help people feel better about themselves, to enhance their personal esteem, to help them select positive health habits, and to become better critical thinkers. There is no one blueprint to accomplish these goals. Each state, many school systems, and individual teachers have plans and strategies that can serve as springboards to facilitate in providing responsible health education.

Each year new crises evolve requiring health educators' efforts. The issues are constantly changing. New need and new knowledge are continually evolving. New challenges in the areas of HIV education, nutrition education, substance abuse, family life education, and environmental education are ongoing. The one constant in all this is the classroom teacher. His or her professional dedication and love for the student must remain, if health education is to be successful. Other than parents, no one person has a greater impact on a child than a teacher. What children learn about themselves, others, and their society begins with the classroom teacher.

We hope this book helps point out the necessity for health education and provides part of the blueprint for becoming successful in the teaching of health education. After all, each teacher deals with our most precious of resources—our children.

Checking Someone Who Appears Unconscious

Check the scene and the victim.

Check for consciousness:

- ○ Tap and gently shake person.

- ○ Shout "Are you okay?"

If person responds . . .

- ○ Do check for conscious person.

If person does not respond . . .

- ○ Send someone to CALL 9-1-1 or local emergency number then . . .

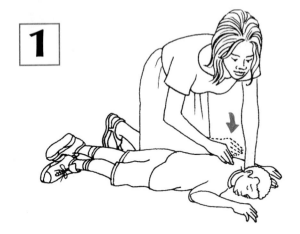

Check for breathing

- ○ Look, listen, and feel for breathing for about 5 seconds.

If person is not breathing or you cannot tell . . .

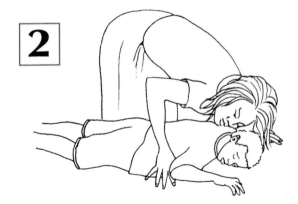

Roll the person onto the back

- ○ Roll person toward you while supporting head and neck.

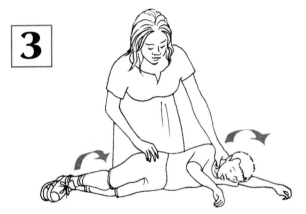

Checking Someone Who Appears Unconscious (cont'd)

Open the airway:
○   Tilt head back and lift chin.

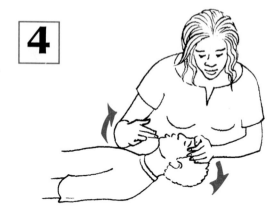

Recheck for breathing:
○   Look, listen, and feel for breathing for about 5 seconds.

If person is not breathing . . .

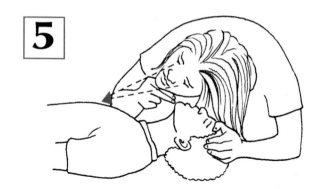

Give 2 slow breaths:
○   Keep head tilted back.

○   Pinch nose shut.

○   Seal your lips tightly around person's mouth.

○   Give 2 slow breaths, each lasting about $1\frac{1}{2}$ seconds.

○   Watch to see that your breaths go in and out.

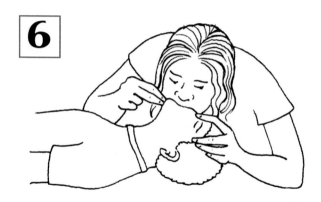

Checking Someone Who Appears Unconscious (cont'd)

Check for pulse:

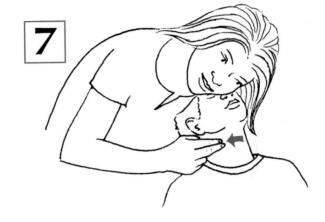

○ Locate Adam's apple.

○ Slide your fingers down into groove of neck on side closer to you.

○ Feel for pulse for about 5–10 seconds.

Check for severe bleeding:

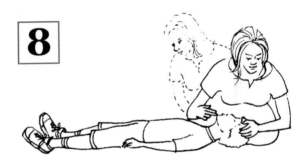

○ Look from head to toe for severe bleeding.

CARE for the conditions you find.

If person has pulse and is not breathing . . .

○ Do rescue breathing.

If person does not have pulse . . .

○ Do CPR.

If person is bleeding severely . . .

○ Attempt to quickly control bleeding.

Checking Someone Who Is Conscious

CHECK the scene and the victim.

Interview the person

○ Introduce yourself and get permission to give care.

○ Ask—

   ○ His or her name?
   ○ What happened?
   ○ Do you feel pain anywhere?
   ○ Do you have any allergies?
   ○ Do you have any medical conditions or are you taking any medication?

Note: Send someone to CALL 9-1-1 or the local emergency number any time a life-threatening emergency becomes apparent.

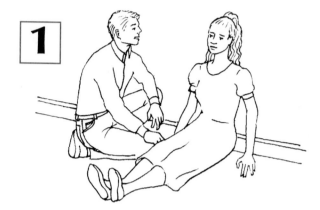

Check head to toe:

○ Visually inspect body.

○ Before you begin, tell person what you are going to do.

○ Look carefully for bleeding, cuts, bruises, and obvious deformities.

○ Look for medical alert tag.

Note: Do not ask the person to move any areas in which he or she has discomfort or pain or if you suspect injury to the head or spine.

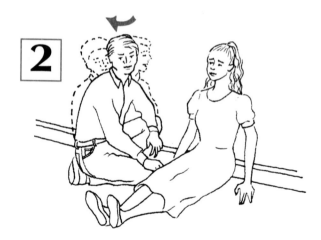

Check the head:

○ Look at scalp, face, ears, eyes, nose, and mouth for cuts, bumps, bruises, and depressions.

○ Notice if victim is drowsy, not alert, or confused.

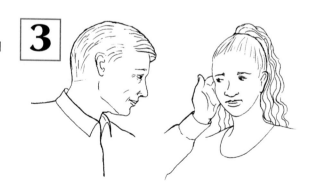

Checking Someone Who Is Conscious (cont'd)

Check skin appearance and temperature:

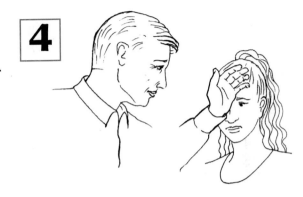

○ Feel person's forehead with back of your hand.

○ Look at person's face and lips.

○ Ask yourself, is the skin—
  ○ Cold or hot?
  ○ Unusually wet or dry?
  ○ Pale, bluish, or flushed?

Check the neck:

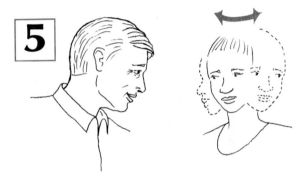

○ If there is no discomfort and no suspected injury to neck, ask person to move head slowly from side to side.

○ Note pain, discomfort, or inability to move.

Check the shoulders:

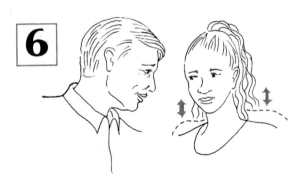

○ Ask person to shrug shoulders.

Check the chest and abdomen:

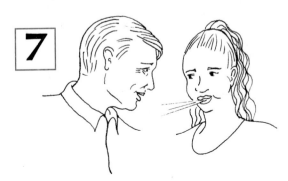

○ Ask person to take a deep breath and blow air out.

○ Ask if he or she is experiencing pain during breathing.

Checking Someone Who Is Conscious (cont'd)

Check the arms:

○ Check one arm at a time.

○ Ask person to—
  ○ Move hands and fingers.
  ○ Bend arm.

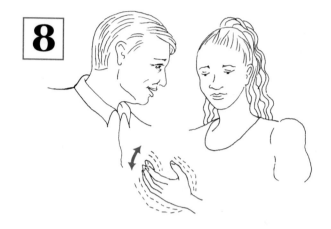

Check the hips and legs:

○ Check one leg at a time.

○ Ask person to—
  ○ Move toes, foot, and ankle.
  ○ Bend leg.

CARE for any conditions you find.

If person can move all body parts without pain or discomfort and has no other apparent signs of injury or illness—

○ Have him or her rest for a few minutes in sitting position.

○ Help person slowly stand when he or she is ready, if no further difficulty develops.

If person is unable to move a body part or is experiencing pain on movement or dizziness—

○ Help him or her rest in most comfortable position.

○ Keep person from getting chilled or overheated.

○ Reassure him or her.

○ Determine whether to call EMS personnel.

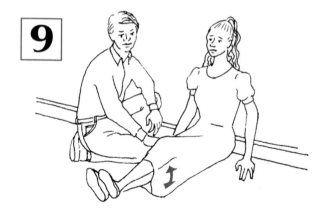

Rescue Breathing for an Adult or Child

CHECK-CALL-CARE

If person is not breathing . . .

Give rescue breathing

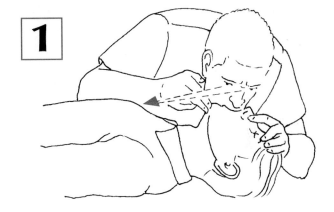

- Keep head tilted back.
- Pinch nose shut.
- Seal lips tightly around person's mouth.
- Give 1 slow breath every 5 seconds (1 slow breath about every 3 seconds for child).
- Watch to see that breaths go in and out.
- Continue for 1 minute—about 12 breaths (adult); about 20 breaths (child).

Recheck pulse and breathing about every minute:

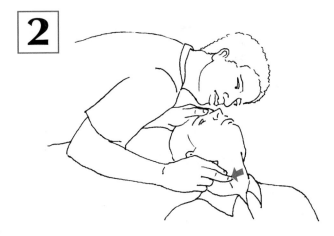

- Feel for pulse for about 5 seconds.
- Look, listen, and feel for breathing.

If person has pulse and is breathing . . .

- Keep airway open.
- Monitor breathing.
- Wait for EMS personnel to arrive.

If person has pulse but is still not breathing . . .

- Continue rescue breathing until EMS personnel arrive.

If person does not have pulse and is not breathing . . .

- Begin CPR.
- Wait for EMS personnel to arrive.

Rescue Breathing for an Infant

CHECK-CALL-CARE

If infant is not breathing . . .

Give rescue breathing,

○   Keep head tilted back.

○   Pinch nose shut.

○   Seal lips tightly around infant's mouth and nose.

○   Give 1 slow breath about every 3 seconds.

○   Watch to see that breaths go in and out.

○   Continue for 1 minute—about 20 breaths.

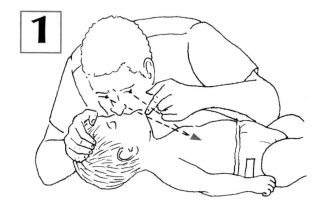

Recheck the pulse and breathing every minute:

○   Feel for pulse for about 5 seconds.

○   Look, listen, and feel for breathing.

If infant has pulse and is breathing . . .

○   Keep airway open.

○   Monitor breathing.

○   Wait for EMS personnel to arrive.

If infant has pulse but is still not breathing . . .

○   Continue rescue breathing until EMS personnel arrive.

If infant does not have pulse and is not breathing . . .

○   Begin CPR.

○   Wait for EMS personnel to arrive.

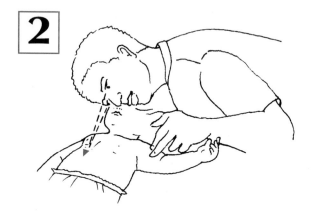

Care for a Conscious Choking Adult or Child with an Obstructed Airway

CHECK-CALL-CARE

If, when you check, the person is unable to speak, cough, cry, or breathe . . .

Position hands:

- ○ Wrap your arms around person's waist.
- ○ With one hand find navel. With other hand make fist.
- ○ Place thumb side of fist against middle of person's abdomen just above navel and well below lower tip of breastbone.

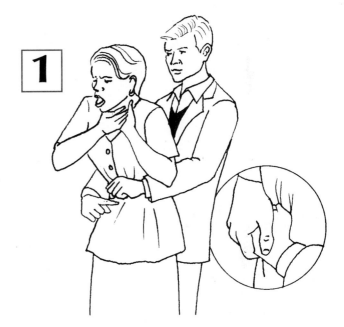

Give abdominal thrusts:

- ○ Press fist into person's abdomen with quick upward thrust.
- ○ Each thrust should be separate and distinct attempt to dislodge object.

Repeat abdominal thrusts until . . .

- ○ Object is coughed up.
- ○ Person starts to breathe or cough forcefully.
- ○ Person becomes unconscious.
- ○ EMS personnel arrive.

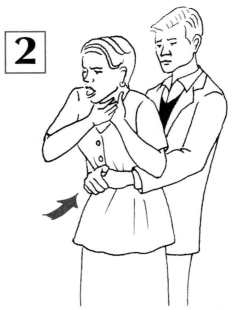

Care for an Unconscious Choking Adult or Child with an Airway Obstruction

CHECK-CALL-CARE

If, when you check, person is not breathing and your breaths do not go in . . .

Reposition the person's head:

○   Tilt person's head further back.

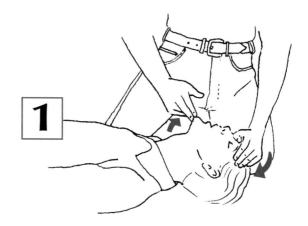

Reattempt 2 slow breaths:

○   Give 2 slow breaths, each lasting about 1¹/₂ seconds.

If breaths still do not go in . . .

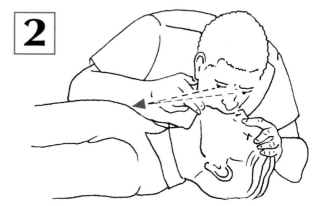

Position hands:

○   Place heel of 1 hand against middle of person's abdomen, just above navel.

○   Place other hand directly on top of first hand.

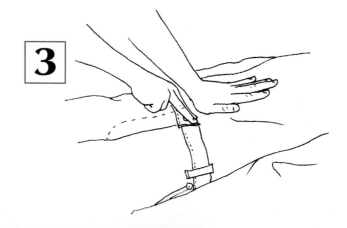

Care for an Unconscious Choking Adult or Child with an Airway Obstruction (cont'd)

Give up to 5 abdominal thrusts:

○ Press into abdomen with quick upward thrusts.

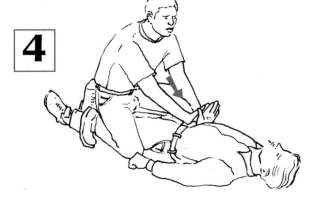

Do finger sweep (simulate):

○ Grasp tongue and lower jaw and lift.

○ Slide finger down inside of cheek and attempt to sweep object out. (For child, sweep only if you see object.)

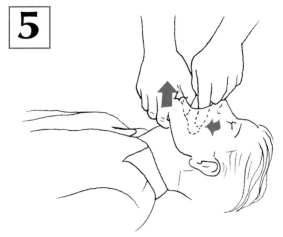

Open the airway and repeat breaths:

○ Tilt head back.

○ Pinch nose shut.

○ Seal lips tightly around person's mouth and give breaths.

If breaths go in . . .

○ Check pulse and breathing.
○ If person has pulse but is not breathing, do rescue breathing.
○ If person does not have pulse and is not breathing, do CPR.
○ Check for and control severe bleeding.
○ Wait for EMS personnel to arrive.

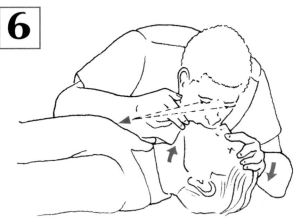

If breaths do not go in . . .

○ Reposition head, reattempt breaths, finger sweep, and breathing steps until . . .
○ Obstruction is removed.
○ Person starts to breathe.
○ EMS personnel arrive.

Care for a Conscious Choking Infant with an Obstructed Airway

CHECK-CALL-CARE

If, when you check, the infant is unable to cough, cry, or breathe . . .

Position the infant face down on your forearm:

○ Carefully support infant's head and neck.

○ Lower forearm onto thigh.

○ Infant's head should be lower than feet.

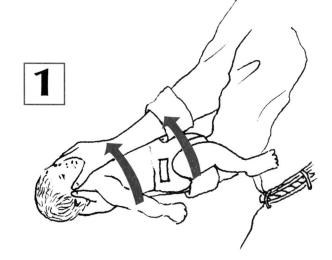

Give 5 back blows:

○ Using heel of your hand, give forceful back blows between infant's shoulder blades, 5 times.

○ Each blow should be separate and distinct attempt to dislodge object.

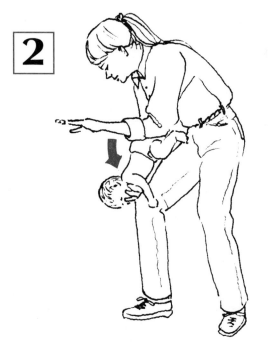

Care for a Conscious Choking Infant with an Obstructed Airway (cont'd)

Position the infant face up on your forearm:

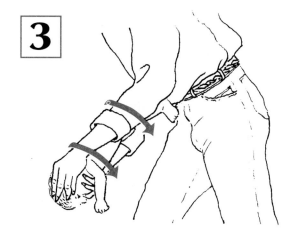

○ Carefully support the infant's head and neck.

○ Lower forearm onto thigh.

○ Infant's head should be lower than feet.

Give 5 chest thrusts:

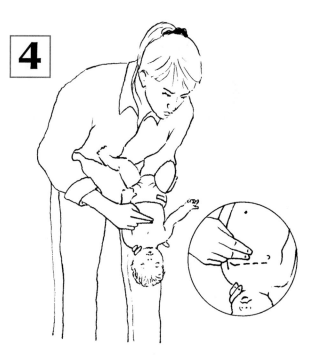

○ Locate finger position for chest thrusts.

○ Using pads of two fingers, smoothly compress breastbone $1/2$ to 1 inch, 5 times.

○ Each thrust should be separate and distinct attempt to dislodge object.

Repeat back blows and chest thrusts until . . .

○ Object is coughed up.

○ Infant starts to breathe or cough forcefully.

○ Infant becomes unconscious.

○ EMS personnel arrive.

Care for an Unconscious Infant with an Airway Obstruction

CHECK-CALL-CARE

If, when you check, the infant is not breathing and your breaths do not go in . . .

Reposition the infant's head:

○ Tilt infant's head further back.

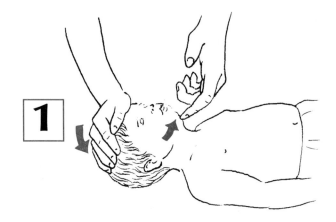

Reattempt 2 slow breaths:

○ Give 2 slow breaths, each lasting about 1¹⁄₂ seconds.

If breaths still do not go in . . .

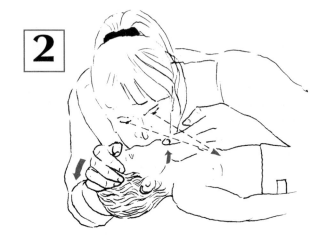

Position the infant face down on your forearm:

○ Carefully support infant's head and neck.

○ Lower forearm onto thigh.

○ Infant's head should be lower than feet.

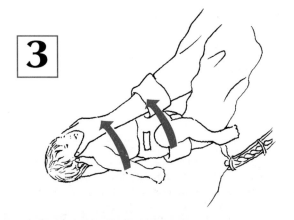

Care for an Unconscious Infant with an Airway Obstruction (cont'd)

Give 5 back blows:

○ Using heel of your hand, give forceful back blows between infant's shoulder blades, 5 times.

○ Each blow should be separate and distinct attempt to dislodge object.

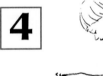
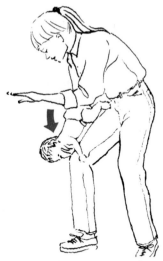

Position the infant face up on your forearm:

○ Carefully support infant's head and neck.

○ Lower forearm onto thigh.

○ Infant's head should be lower than feet.

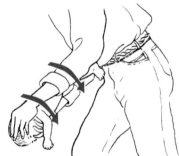

Give 5 chest thrusts:

○ Locate finger position for chest thrusts.

○ Using pads of two fingers, smoothly compress breastbone $1/2$ to 1 inch, 5 times.

○ Each thrust should be separate and distinct attempt to dislodge object.

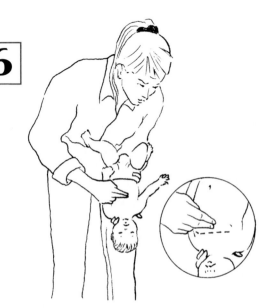

Care for an Unconscious Infant with an Airway Obstruction (cont'd)

Do a foreign body check:

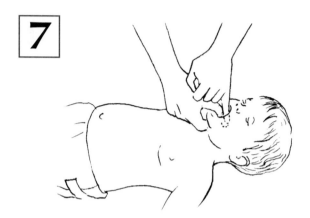

○ Grasp tongue and lower jaw and lift.

○ If object can be seen, slide little finger down inside of cheek and attempt to sweep object out.

Open the airway and repeat breaths:

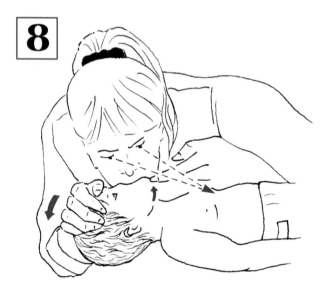

○ Tilt head back.

○ Seal lips tightly around infant's mouth and nose and give breaths.

If breaths go in . . .

○ Check pulse and breathing.

○ If infant has pulse but is not breathing, do rescue breathing.

○ If infant does not have pulse and is not breathing, do CPR.

○ Check for and control severe bleeding.

○ Wait for EMS personnel to arrive.

If breaths do not go in . . .

○ Reposition head, reattempt breaths, back blows, thrusts, foreign-body check, and breathing steps until . . .

    ○ Obstruction is removed.
    ○ Infant starts to breathe or cry.
    ○ EMS personnel arrive.

CPR for an Adult

CHECK-CALL-CARE

If, when you check, the person is not breathing and has no pulse . . .

Find hand position:

○ Locate notch at lower end of sternum.

○ Place heel of other hand on sternum next to fingers.

○ Remove hand from notch and put it on top of other hand.

○ Keep fingers off chest.

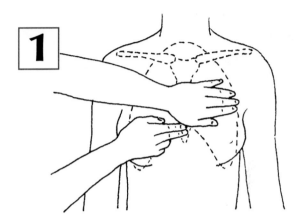

Give 15 compressions:

○ Position shoulders over hands.

○ Compress chest 1 $^1/_2$ to 2 inches.

○ Do 15 compressions in about 10 seconds.

○ Compress down and up smoothly, keeping hand contact with chest at all times.

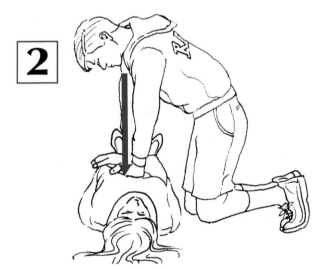

Give 2 slow breaths:

○ Open airway with head-tilt/chin-lift.

○ Pinch nose shut and seal your lips tightly around person's mouth.

○ Give 2 slow breaths, each lasting about 1$^1/_2$ seconds.

○ Watch chest to see that your breaths go in.

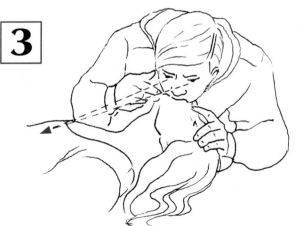

CPR for an Adult (cont'd)

Repeat compression/breathing cycles:

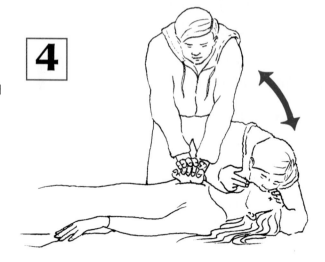

○ Do 3 more sets of 15 compressions and 2 breaths.

Recheck pulse and breathing:

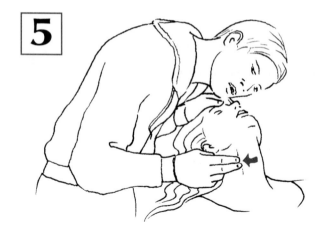

○ After 1 minute, feel for pulse for about 5 seconds.
○ Look, listen, and feel for breathing.

If person has pulse and is breathing . . .

○ Keep airway open.
○ Monitor breathing.
○ Wait for EMS personnel to arrive.

If person has pulse but is still not breathing . . .

○ Do rescue breathing.
○ Recheck pulse about every minute.
○ Wait for EMS personnel to arrive.

If person does not have pulse and is not breathing . . .

Continue compression/breathing cycles:

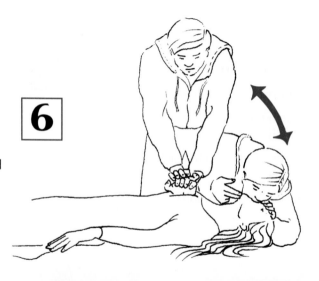

○ Locate correct hand position.
○ Continue cycles of 15 compressions and 2 slow breaths.
○ Recheck pulse every few minutes.
○ Wait for EMS personnel to arrive.

CPR for a Child

CHECK-CALL-CARE

If, when you check, the person is not breathing and has no pulse . . .

Find hand position:

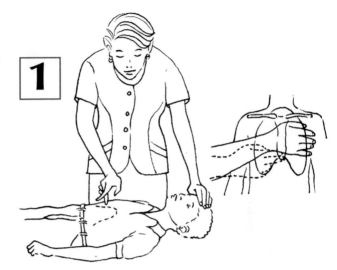

- ⭕ Maintain head tilt with hand on forehead.
- ⭕ Locate notch at lower end of sternum with other hand.
- ⭕ Place heel of same hand on sternum immediately above where fingers were placed.

Give 5 compressions:

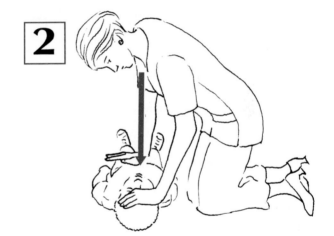

- ⭕ Position shoulders over hands.
- ⭕ Compress sternum 1 to 1 $1/2$ inches.
- ⭕ Do 5 compressions in about 3 seconds.
- ⭕ Compress down and up smoothly, keeping hand contact with chest at all times.
- ⭕ Maintain head tilt with your hand on forehead.

Give 1 slow breath:

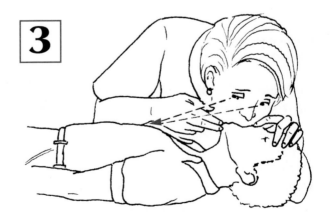

- ⭕ Open airway with head tilt/chin lift.
- ⭕ Pinch nose shut and seal lips tightly around child's mouth.
- ⭕ Give 1 slow breath lasting about $1 1/2$ seconds.
- ⭕ Watch chest to see that breath goes in.

CPR for a Child (cont'd)

Repeat compression/breathing cycles:

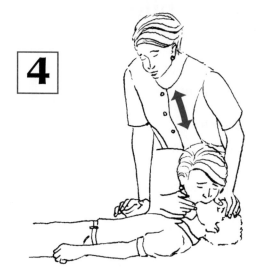

○ Repeat cycles of 5 compressions and 1 breath (about 20 cycles).

Recheck pulse and breathing:

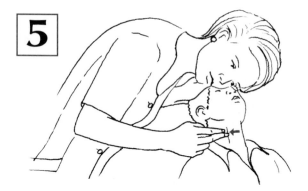

○ After about 1 minute, feel for pulse for about 5 seconds.
○ Look, listen, and feel for breathing.

If child has pulse and is breathing . . .
○ Keep airway open.
○ Monitor breathing.
○ Wait for EMS personnel to arrive.

If child has pulse but is still not breathing . . .
○ Do rescue breathing.
○ Recheck pulse about every minute.
○ Wait for EMS personnel to arrive.

If child does not have pulse and is not breathing . . .

Continue cycles of 5 compressions and 1 slow breath:

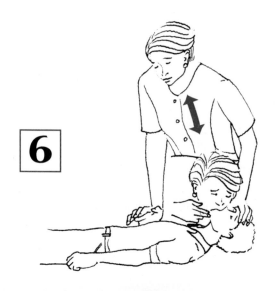

○ Locate correct hand position.
○ Continue cycles of 5 compressions and 1 slow breath.
○ Recheck pulse every few minutes.
○ Wait for EMS personnel to arrive.

CPR for an Infant

CHECK-CALL-CARE

If, when you check, the infant is not breathing and has no pulse . . .

Find finger position:

- ○ Maintain head tilt with hand on forehead.
- ○ Place pads of fingers below imaginary line running across chest connecting nipples.
- ○ Relax your index finger.
- ○ Adjust finger position if necessary.

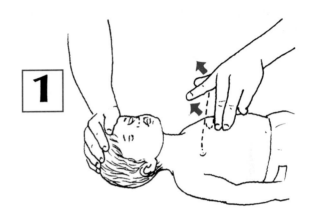

Give 5 compressions:

- ○ Position hand over fingers.
- ○ Compress sternum $1/2$ to 1 inch.
- ○ Do 5 compressions in about 3 seconds.
- ○ Compress down and up smoothly, keeping finger in contact with chest at all times.
- ○ Maintain head tilt with hand on forehead.

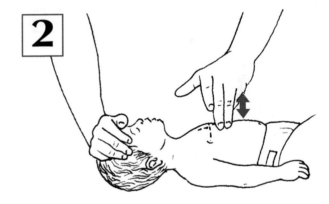

Give 1 slow breath:

- ○ Maintain finger contact with chest.
- ○ Seal lips tightly around infant's mouth and nose.
- ○ Give 1 slow breath lasting about $1 1/2$ seconds.
- ○ Watch chest to see that breath goes in.

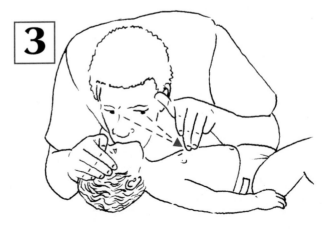

CPR for a Infant (cont'd)

Repeat compression/breathing cycles:

O   Repeat cycles of 5 compressions and 1 breath (about 20 cycles).

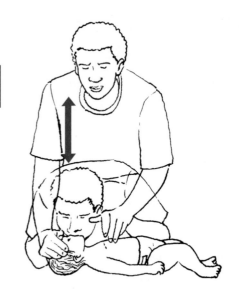

Recheck pulse and breathing . . .

O   After about 1 minute, feel for pulse for about 5 seconds.

O   Look, listen, and feel for breathing.

If infant has pulse and is breathing . . .

O   Keep airway open.
O   Monitor breathing.
O   Wait for EMS personnel to arrive.

If infant has pulse but is still not breathing . . .

O   Do rescue breathing.
O   Recheck pulse about every minute.
O   Wait for EMS personnel to arrive.

If infant does not have pulse and is not breathing . . .

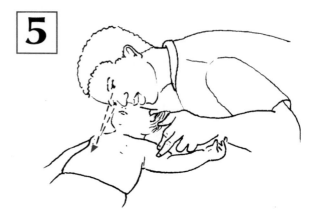

Continue compression/breathing cycles:

O   Locate correct hand position.
O   Continue cycles of 5 compressions and 1 slow breath.
O   Recheck pulse every few minutes.
O   Wait for EMS personnel to arrive.

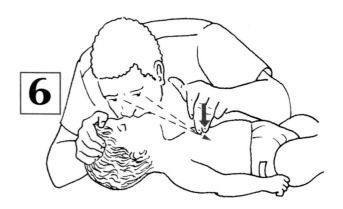

Controlling Bleeding

CHECK-CALL-CARE

If, when you check, the person is bleeding . . .

Apply direct pressure:

○ Place sterile dressing or clean cloth over wound.

○ Press firmly against wound with your gloved hand.

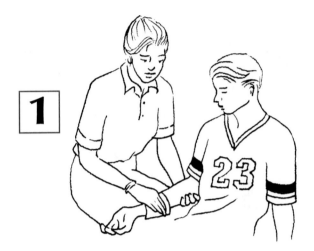

Elevate the body part:

○ Raise wound above level of heart.

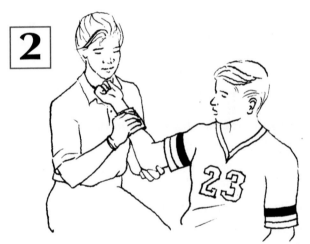

Apply a pressure bandage:

○ Using a roller bandage, cover dressing completely, using overlapping turns.

○ Secure bandage.

○ If blood soaks through bandage, place additional dressings and bandages over wound.

If bleeding stops . . .
• Determine if further care is needed.

If bleeding does not stop . . .
• Send someone to call EMS personnel.

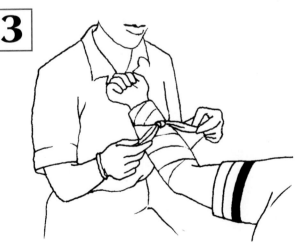

Controlling Bleeding (cont'd)

Then . . .

Use a pressure point:

- ○ Maintain direct pressure and elevation.
- ○ Locate brachial artery.
- ○ Press brachial artery against underlying bone.

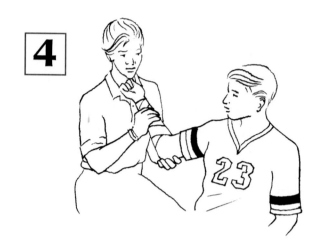

If bleeding is from leg, press with the heel of your hand where leg bends at hip.

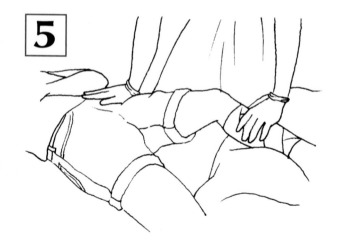

Continue to take steps to minimize shock:

- ○ Maintain direct pressure, elevation, and pressure point.
- ○ Position person on back.
- ○ Monitor breathing and pulse.
- ○ Keep person from getting chilled or overheated.
- ○ Apply additional dressings and/or bandages as necessary.

Index